Neuroinflammation: Latest Findings

Neuroinflammation: Latest Findings

Edited by Alfred Galswells

hayle
medical

New York

Hayle Medical,
750 Third Avenue, 9ᵗʰ Floor,
New York, NY 10017, USA

Visit us on the World Wide Web at:
www.haylemedical.com

ISBN: 978-1-63241-681-0

Cataloging-in-Publication Data

   Neuroinflammation : latest findings / edited by Alfred Galswells.
      p. cm.
   Includes bibliographical references and index.
   ISBN 978-1-63241-681-0
   1. Nervous System--Diseases. 2. Inflammation. 3. Inflammation--Immunological aspects.
   4. Neuroimmunology. I. Galswells, Alfred.
RC346.5 .N48 2019
616.804 6--dc23

Table of Contents

Preface

This book has been a concerted effort by a group of academicians, researchers and scientists, who have contributed their research works for the realization of the book. This book has materialized in the wake of emerging advancements and innovations in this field. Therefore, the need of the hour was to compile all the required researches and disseminate the knowledge to a broad spectrum of people comprising of students, researchers and specialists of the field.

Neuroinflammation refers to the inflammation of the nervous tissue, triggered due to traumatic brain injury, infection, autoimmunity or toxic metabolites. The central nervous system exhibits inflammation due to the activation of microglia. The immune response of the peripheral nervous system is through the expression of major histocompatibility complex molecules. Such an immune response though defensive in nature can present itself as a risk of toxicity and widespread inflammation. There is an association of neuroinflammation and neurodegenerative diseases such as Alzheimer's disease, Parkinson's disease and multiple sclerosis. There is thus clinical interest in the strategy of inflammation reduction to reverse neurodegeneration. This book discusses the fundamentals as well as modern approaches in the study of neuroinflammation. The topics included in this book on neuroinflammation are of utmost significance and bound to provide incredible insights to readers. It is an essential guide for both academicians and those who wish to pursue this discipline further.

At the end of the preface, I would like to thank the authors for their brilliant chapters and the publisher for guiding us all-through the making of the book till its final stage. Also, I would like to thank my family for providing the support and encouragement throughout my academic career and research projects.

Editor

ZIKV infection activates the IRE1-XBP1 and ATF6 pathways of unfolded protein response in neural cells

Zhongyuan Tan[1,2], Wanpo Zhang[3], Jianhong Sun[1], Zuquan Fu[3], Xianliang Ke[1], Caishang Zheng[1], Yuan Zhang[1], Penghui Li[1,2], Yan Liu[1], Qinxue Hu[4], Hanzhong Wang[1*] and Zhenhua Zheng[1*]

Abstract

Background: Many viruses depend on the extensive membranous network of the endoplasmic reticulum (ER) for their translation, replication, and packaging. Certain membrane modifications of the ER can be a trigger for ER stress, as well as the accumulation of viral protein in the ER by viral infection. Then, unfolded protein response (UPR) is activated to alleviate the stress. Zika virus (ZIKV) is a mosquito-borne flavivirus and its infection causes microcephaly in newborns and serious neurological complications in adults. Here, we investigated ER stress and the regulating model of UPR in ZIKV-infected neural cells in vitro and in vivo.

Methods: Mice deficient in type I and II IFN receptors were infected with ZIKV via intraperitoneal injection and the nervous tissues of the mice were assayed at 5 days post-infection. The expression of phospho-IRE1, XBP1, and ATF6 which were the key markers of ER stress were analyzed by immunohistochemistry assay in vivo. Additionally, the nuclear localization of XBP1s and ATF6n were analyzed by immunohistofluorescence. Furthermore, two representative neural cells, neuroblastoma cell line (SK-N-SH) and astrocytoma cell line (CCF-STTG1), were selected to verify the ER stress in vitro. The expression of BIP, phospho-eIF2α, phospho-IRE1, and ATF6 were analyzed through western blot and the nuclear localization of XBP1s was performed by confocal immunofluorescence microscopy. RT-qPCR was also used to quantify the mRNA level of the UPR downstream genes in vitro and in vivo.

Results: ZIKV infection significantly upregulated the expression of ER stress markers in vitro and in vivo. Phospho-IRE1 and XBP1 expression significantly increased in the cerebellum and mesocephalon, while ATF6 expression significantly increased in the mesocephalon. ATF6n and XBP1s were translocated into the cell nucleus. The levels of BIP, ATF6, phospho-elf2α, and spliced xbp1 also significantly increased in vitro. Furthermore, the downstream genes of UPR were detected to investigate the regulating model of the UPR during ZIKV infection in vitro and in vivo. The transcriptional levels of atf4, gadd34, chop, and edem-1 in vivo and that of gadd34 and chop in vitro significantly increased.

Conclusion: Findings in this study demonstrated that ZIKV infection activates ER stress in neural cells. The results offer clues to further study the mechanism of neuropathogenesis caused by ZIKV infection.

Keywords: Zika virus, Neural cell, Neuropathogenesis, ER stress, Unfolded protein response

* Correspondence: wanghz@wh.iov.cn; zhengzh@wh.iov.cn
[1]CAS Key Laboratory of Special Pathogens and Biosafety, Center for Emerging Infectious Diseases, Wuhan Institute of Virology, Chinese Academy of Sciences, Wuhan 430071, China
Full list of author information is available at the end of the article

Background

The mosquito-borne flavivirus, Zika virus (ZIKV), was first isolated in 1947 from a rhesus monkey in the East African country of Uganda [1]. ZIKV infection in humans was first reported in 1952 and only 14 cases of sporadic infection have been previously documented until an outbreak was reported by physicians on Yap Island in 2007 [2–4]. The unprecedented epidemics of ZIKV among the Americas in 2015 have raised alarm due to its rapid transmission and association with microcephaly in newborns and serious neurological complications in adults, such as Guillain–Barre syndrome [4–7]. The World Health Organization declared a public health emergency to maintain international concern regarding the virus [8]. The relationship between ZIKV infection and neurodevelopment abnormalities has attracted more and more attention [5, 7, 9, 10]. ZIKV, like other members of the *Flavivirus* genus, is a positive (+) single-strand RNA virus. An approximately 10.7 kb genome of ZIKV encodes a single polyprotein precursor that is posttranslationally cleaved into three structural proteins (C, prM/M, and E) and seven nonstructural proteins (NS1, NS2A, NS2B, NS3, NS4A, NS4B, and NS5) by viral and host proteases [11–13]. Nonstructural proteins induce the formation of a membranous network with ER where viral replication occurs [14]. Immature virions assemble within the ER, where viral RNA is complexed with the C protein and packaged into an ER-derived lipid bilayer containing heterodimers of prM and E proteins [15]. Immature virions then bud into the ER lumen and are transported through the *trans*-Golgi network. In the Golgi apparatus, glycan modification and structural cleavage (furin-mediated cleavage of the prM to M) are accomplished, and mature infectious virions are secreted into extracellular space via exocytosis [14, 15].

The ER is an important location for posttranslational modification, folding, and oligomerization of secretory and cell surface proteins. It is also a main intercellular signal-transducing organelle for responding to environmental changes. Many viruses depend on the extensive membranous network of the ER for their translation, replication, and packaging [16]. The *Flaviviridae* family, including the dengue virus (DENV) [16, 17], West Nile virus (WNV) [18, 19], yellow fever virus (YFV), hepatitis C virus (HCV) [20], and Japanese encephalitis virus (JEV) [17], depend on the ER for their life cycles and are called endoplasmic reticulum tropic (ER-tropic) viruses [16]. Infection by an ER-tropic virus disrupts the normal ER function, and then ER stress is induced. To alleviate ER stress, the UPR is activated and mainly functions in translational attenuation, protein folding, protein degradation, and cellular apoptosis [21, 22]. PKR-like ER kinase (PERK), transcription factor 6 (ATF6) and inositol-requiring enzyme 1 (IRE1) are the sensors of the UPR pathway. In unstressed cells, the ER chaperone immunoglobulin heavy-chain-binding protein (BIP) binds to the ER luminal domain of the three sensors. Under the condition of ER stress, however, BIP is dissociated from the three sensors and preferentially binds to misfolded and unfolded proteins. Then, the three response pathways are activated to deal with different ER stress states in a time-dependent manner [16]. Phosphorylated PERK phosphorylates the α-subunit of eukaryotic translation initiation factor 2 (eIF2α). Phosphorylated eIF2α (phospho-eIF2α) forms a complex with guanine nucleotide exchange factor (eIF2B) and inhibits catalysis of GDP-GTP exchange, thereby leading to the translation attenuation and contradictory expression by activating transcription factor 4 (ATF4). Activated ATF4 upregulates a series of genes related to encoding metabolism and redox regulation and helps cells recover from ER stress. Growth arrest and DNA damage-inducible protein (GADD34), which is regulated by ATF4, interacts with protein phosphatase 1 (PP1) to dephosphorylate eIF2α, thereby acting as a negative feedback loop to restore protein translation [23]. PERK-mediated eIF2α phosphorylation is triggered in early DENV-2 infection and suppressed in mid and late DENV-2 infection because the inhibition of eIF2α phosphorylation is necessary for viral protein synthesis [16]. The RNase activity of phosphorylated IRE1 (phospho-IRE1) has only one substrate, X-box binding protein 1 (XBP1), and removes a 26-nucleotide intron from unspliced *xbp1*mRNA (*xbp1u*) [24, 25]. The spliced *xbp1*mRNA (*xbp1s*) results in a frameshift mutation and encodes spliced XBP1 (XBP1s), a transcription factor that binds to the sequences of ER stress response elements (ERSEs) and UPR elements (UPREs), and upregulates the transcription of ER-association degradation (ERAD) proteins, proapoptotic proteins, and some ER chaperones [26]. JEV infection activates the IRE1-XBP1 pathway and has a beneficial effect on the activation of the regulated IRE1-dependent decay (RIDD) pathway during the viral life cycle [17, 27]. Cleaved ATF6 (ATF6n) also can bind to the ERSE and UPRE sequences and upregulate transcription chaperones, foldases, and lipid synthesis genes [26]. ATF6 is required for efficient WNV replication by maintaining cell viability and modulating the innate immune responses [28]. In brief, ER is an important location in viral life cycle, and UPR is closely associated with the regulation of viral replication. ZIKV is a flavivirus that its life cycle also closely depends on the extensive membranous network of the ER [29]. However, whether ZIKV activates and benefits from ER stress to regulate viral replication needs to be investigated.

Many neurological diseases are linked to abnormal protein accumulation in the ER and activation of UPR to deal with ER stress [30]. Khajavi and Lupski reported that the UPR is responsible for the demyelination in peripheral neuropathy [31]. Yang and Paschen proposed that the UPR dysfunction after brain ischemia contributes to neuronal death [32]. Several studies found a clear activation of the UPR in toxicological models of Parkinson's disease. ATF6, XBP1, and pro-apoptotic transcription factor CCAT/enhancer-binding protein (CHOP) play functional roles in controlling dopaminergic neuron survival [33]. In addition, whether the UPR plays an important role in the neuropathogenesis caused by ZIKV infection has yet to be studied in animal models or cellular level. In the present study, we found that ZIKV infection activated ER stress both in vitro and in vivo, showing that the expression of ER stress markers, namely, BIP, cleaved ATF6, phospho-IRE1, and phospho-eIF2α, significantly increased. The regulating model of UPR was developed, with ZIKV infection activating the IRE1-XBP1 pathway to regulate cellular apoptosis mediated by CHOP. This study could serve as a reference for elucidating ZIKV neuropathogenesis.

Methods
Cells, viruses, and infection
Aedes albopictus clone C6/36 cells (ATCC-CRL-1660) were cultured in Dulbecco's Modified Eagle's medium. SK-N-SH cells (ATCC-HTB-11) and African green monkey kidney epithelial Vero cells (CCL-81, American Type Culture Collection) were cultured in MEM. CCF-STTG1 cells (ATCC-CRL-1718) were cultured in RPMI 1640. All cells were maintained in a medium containing 10% fetal bovine serum (Life Technology, Australia) in 5% CO_2 at 37 °C. ZIKV strain (Zika virus/SZ01/2016/China, GenBank: KU866423.2) was obtained from the Wuhan Institute of Virology, Chinese Academy of Science [34]. It was propagated using C6/36 cells. Virus titers were measured using 50% tissue culture infectious dose (TCID50) in Vero cells and analyzed using Reed–Muench formula [35]. The cells were infected with ZIKV at a multiplicity of infection (MOI) of 5. Positive controls were treated with tunicamycin at a final concentration of 2 μM.

Animals and treatments
C57BL/6 mice deficient in type I and II IFN receptors (AG6 mouse, *ifnagr*$^{-/-}$) were acquired from Prof. Qibin Leng in the Institute Pasteur of Shanghai, Chinese Academy of Sciences. Three-week-old AG6 mice were infected with 1×10^5 PFU/mouse (each dose, $N = 3$) via intraperitoneal injection. Mock-infected controls were administered with PBS through the same route. At 5 days post infection (dpi), the mice were perfused with 4%

paraformaldehyde, and the brain tissues were obtained and treated according to further assay.

Western blot analysis
Cells were washed once with PBS and then lysed on ice in RIPA buffer (Beyotime) supplemented with phenylmethanesulfonyl fluoride (PMSF) (Beyotime) and protease inhibitor cocktail tablets (Roche) in accordance with the manufacturer's instructions. Total protein was separated via SDS polyacrylamide gel electrophoresis containing 10% polyacrylamide gels and then transferred onto Immobilon-P polyvinylidene fluoride membranes (Millipore) in transfer buffer [30 mM Tris, 200 mM glycine, 20%(V/V) methanol] for 150 min at 4 °C. Immunoblots were blocked using 5% bovine serum albumin (BSA) dissolved in TBS-T for 1 h at 37 °C and then incubated with primary antibodies diluted using primary antibody dilution buffer (Beyotime) overnight. After washing with TBS-T three times for 7 min each, immunoblots were incubated with horseradish peroxidase (HRP)-conjugated secondary antibodies diluted using TBS-T with 0.5% BSA for 1 h at 37 °C. After washing with TBS-T five times for 7 min each, immunoblots were visualized and analyzed by using a Bio-Rad imaging system with an Immobilon Eastern Chemiluminescent HRP substrate (Millipore). The band was analyzed by using Image Lab 4.0.1.

The primary antibodies used in this study were as follows: ATF6 (Beyotime, 24,169–1-AP), phospho-IRE1 (Abcam, ab48187), BIP (Beyotime, AB310), phospho-eIF2α (Cell Signaling Technology, #9721), total elf2α (Cell Signaling Technology, #9722), XBP1 (Abcam, ab37152), β-actin (Beyotime, AF0003), and ZIKV envelope protein (BioFront Technologies, BF-1176-56). All antibodies were diluted in accordance with the manufacturer's protocol.

RT-qPCR analysis
Total RNA was extracted from cells and mouse brains by using TRIZOL Reagent (Invitrogen) in accordance with the manufacturer's protocol. The first strand cDNA was reverse transcribed from 1 μg of total RNA by using PrimeScript RT reagent Kit with gDNA Eraser (Takara) in accordance with the manufacturer's protocol. Each 20 μL of quantitative PCR reaction mix contains cDNA, forward primer, reverse primer, and iTap™ Universal SYBR Green® Supermix (Bio-Rad). Amplification in a Bio-Rad CFX real-time quantitative PCR system involved activation at 95 °C for 3 min followed by 40 amplification cycles of 95 °C for 5 s and 60 °C for 45 s. All primers for PCR are shown in Table 1. Virus RNA copies were quantified by the

Table 1 Primers used for RT-qPCR assay

Gene	Forward primer (5'→3')	Reverse primer (5'→3')
ZIKV	AARTACACATACCARAACAAAGTG	TCCRCTCCCYCTYTGGTCTTG
gadd34-human	GATGGCATGTATGGTGAGCG	GAGACAAGGCAGAAGTAGAG
atf4-human	CACCGCAACATGACCGAAAT	GACTGACCAACCCATCCACA
chop-human	GAACCAGGAAACGGAAACAG	ATTCACCATTCGGTCAATCA
xbp1s-human	AAGAACACGCTTGGGAATGG	CTGCACCTGCTGCGGAC
T-xbp1-human	GACAGAGAGTCAAACTAACGTGG	GTCCAGCAGGCAAGAAGGT
edem-1-human	CTGGTGGAATTTGGGATTCT	GTATCATTGCTCCGGAGG
gapdh-human	GTCTCCTCTGACTTCAACAGCG	ACCACCCTGTTGCTGTAGCCAA
bip-mouse	CCATCCCGTGGCATAAAC	GACTCCTCCCACAGTTTCA
ire1	GGACAGGCTCAATCAAATGG	CGGTCAGGAGGTCAATAACA
atf6	TCGGTCAGTGGACTCTTATT	CCAGTGACAGGCTTATCTTC
gadd34-mouse	CCGCTTATCCCACATCAC	GGTTTGTATCCCGGAGCT
atf4-mouse	TTAGAGCTAGGCAGTGAAGTT	CTGTCATTGTCAGAGGGAGT
chop-mouse	CACATCCCAAAGCCCTCG	CGTTCTCCTGCTCCTTCTC
xbp1s-mouse	CTGAGTCCGCAGCAGGTG	GACCTCTGGGAGTTCCTCCA
T-xbp1-mouse	GGGACTACAGGACCAATAA	ACCATAGCCAGGAAACGT
edem-1-mouse	GGAGTCCCATTCTACAACC	GCAATCCGAAAGCCACCA
gapdh-mouse	AACGACCCCTTCATTGAC	TCCACGACATACTCAGCAC

standard curve method and relative expression level of genes were analyzed by using the $2^{-\Delta\Delta Ct}$ method.

Confocal immunofluorescence microscopy

For localization assay, SK-N-SH and CCF-STTG1 cells were grown on glass slides with 5×10^4 cell per dish. Mock, tunicamycin-treated, and ZIKV-infected cells were designed and manipulated as described above. At 24 h post infection, the slides were washed with PBS, fixed with 4% paraformaldehyde, and then permeabilized with 0.2% Triton X-100 for 15 min. The cells were blocked by using 5% BSA and 3% normal goat serum (NGS) dissolved in PBS for 1 h at 37 °C. The cells were then washed with 3% NGS dissolved in PBS two times and then incubated in primary antibodies (1:200) diluted with 3% NGS dissolved in PBS overnight at 4 °C. After washing five times, cells were incubated with Goat anti-Rabbit IgG secondary antibody, FITC (Thermo Fisher Scientific, #F-2765), and Goat anti-Mouse IgG secondary antibody, Texas Red®-X (Thermo Fisher Scientific, #T-6390) (1:200) diluted with 3% NGS dissolved in PBS for 1 h at 37 °C. After washing two times, cell nucleus was dyed with Hoechst 33258 for 10 min at 37 °C. Microscopic analysis was performed as previously described [36]. The primary antibody used in this study was as follows: XBP1 (Abcam, ab37152), ZIKV envelope protein (Bio-Front Technologies, BF-1176-56).

Immunohistochemistry and immunohistofluorescence

For immunohistochemistry assay, the paraffin blocks of tissues were divided into 5-μm sections. After deparaffinization and rehydration, the sections were treated with 3% hydrogen dioxide solution for 30 min at room temperature and then washed two times with PBS for 5 min each. The sections were incubated in citrate buffer solution for 30 min at 95–100 °C, cooled, and then washed three times with PBS for 5 min. The sections were then blocked with 5% BSA for 1 h at room temperature and then incubated in primary antibodies (1:300) overnight at 4 °C. After washing three times, the sections were incubated in HRP-conjugated second antibodies for 1 h at 37 °C. Subsequently, the sections were covered with 0.02% DAB solution and counterstained with hematoxylin for 3 min. The sections were then washed for 10 min, dehydrated, transparentize, and then sealed with neutral resin sheets. Images were captured by using a NIS-Elements system under a Nikon 80iMicroscope. Aperio ImageScope viewing software was used to analyze the percentage of positivity (algorithm, positive pixel count). For immunohistofluorescence assay, the whole brain sections of AG6 mice were stained with DAPI, anti-ZIKV-ENV antibody, and anti-XBP1 or anti-ATF6 antibody. The experimental procedure accorded to the normal protocol. Images were captured by using a digital slice scanning analysis system (Pannoramic MIDI). The primary antibodies used in this study were as follows: XBP1 (Abcam, ab37152), ATF6 (Abcam, ab37149), phospho-IRE1 (Abcam, ab48187), ZIKV envelope protein (BioFront Technologies, BF-1176-56).

Statistical analysis

All experiments were reproducible and carried out in triplicate. Data are represented as mean ± SD when indicated and Student's t test was used for all statistical analyses with the GraphPad Prism 6.0 software. Differences were considered significant when P value was less than 0.05.

Results

ZIKV infection activates the IRE1-XBP1 and ATF6 pathways of UPR in the nervous tissues of the mouse brain

AG6 mice succumb to ZIKV infection and sustain high viral loads in many tissues, including the spleen, liver, kidney, serum, testes, brain, and spinal cord [37, 38]. To study whether ZIKV infection causes ER stress in the nervous tissues of the mouse brain, AG6 mice were infected with 1×10^5 PFU of ZIKV (SZ01/2016/China). The total mRNA of the mouse brain was extracted for the detection of ZIKV mRNA by RT-qPCR, revealing 6.2×10^4 copies/µg RNA at 2 dpi and 8.6×10^5 copies/µg RNA at 5 dpi (Fig. 1a), respectively. Total lysates of mouse brain were analyzed via western blot and ZIKV envelope protein (ZIKV-ENV) could only be detected at 5 dpi (Fig. 1b). The cerebrum, cerebellum, and mesocephalon were extracted for immunohistochemistry assay, showing that these tissues were all infected by ZIKV (see Additional file 1: a, b). These results together indicate that ZIKV infects and replicates in the nervous tissues of the mouse brain, and this infection model can be used in future studies.

The ER chaperone BIP, which is dissociated from three UPR sensors under stress and acts as the primary indicator or regulatory factor [16], was analyzed by using total lysates and mRNA from the nervous tissues of the mouse brain. Following ZIKV infection, BIP expression significantly increased at the levels of protein and mRNA (Fig. 1c, d, e). These results suggest that BIP was likely activated to regulate the homeostasis of ER in the nervous tissues of the mouse brain infected with ZIKV.

IRE1-XBP1 is an important arm of the UPR. Phospho-IRE1 splices a 26-nt intron from full-length $xbp1u$, resulting in the formation of $xbp1s$. $Xbp1s$ encodes the transcription factor XBP1s which activates the expression of genes involved in chaperone and protein degradation [39, 40]. Phospho-IRE1 and XBP1 were analyzed by western blot. Compared with mock-infected samples, the ZIKV-infected nervous tissues of the mouse brain exhibited an upregulation of phospho-IRE1 and XBP1

(Fig. 1c, d). The genes encoding IRE1 and XBP1 were also analyzed via RT-qPCR. As there are two forms of $xbp1$, primers that specifically amplified $xbp1s$ and total $xbp1$ (t-$xbp1$, including both $xbp1u$ and $xbp1s$) were used [41]. We found that the expression of $ire1$ increased. The ratio of $xbp1s$/t-$xbp1$ between mock-infected and ZIKV-infected was 2.08-fold (Fig. 1e). Collectively, the findings demonstrated that ZIKV infection in the nervous tissues of the mouse brain activated phospho-IRE1 and induced the post-transcriptional cleavage of $xbp1$.

The targets of ATF6 are prominent ER-resident proteins involved in protein folding, such as BIP. Upon accumulation of the unfolded proteins, ATF6 is transported to the Golgi apparatus and cleaved by two proteases. The 50-kDa N-terminal cytosolic fragment, ATF6n, moves into the nucleus to activate the UPR genes [25]. The expression of ATF6 was analyzed by using total lysates and mRNAs from the nervous tissues of the mouse brain. We found that, following ZIKV infection, ATF6n expression was moderately upregulated at the protein level, and $atf6$ at the mRNA level (Fig. 1c, d, e). The results indicated that ATF6 pathway was activated in the ZIKV-infected nervous tissues of the mouse brain.

Sections from the cerebrum, cerebellum, and mesocephalon of AG6 mice were stained using anti-phospho-IRE1 antibody, anti-ATF6 antibody (recognizing both cleaved and full forms of ATF6), and anti-XBP1 antibody (recognizing both non-spliced and spliced isoforms of XBP1). Immunohistochemistry assay was used to detect the expression changes of phospho-IRE1 (Fig. 2a), XBP1 (Fig. 2b), and ATF6 (Fig. 2c) in the cerebrum, cerebellum, and mesocephalon. Through positive pixel count and statistical analysis, we found that the protein level of phospho-IRE1 was higher in the cerebellum and mesocephalon of ZIKV-infected compared with the mock-infected (Fig. 2d). The protein level of XBP1 was higher in the cerebellum and mesocephalon of ZIKV-infected compared with the mock-infected (Fig. 2e). The protein level of ATF6 was higher in the mesocephalon of ZIKV-infected compared with the mock-infected (Fig. 2f). The results indicated that the expression of phospho-IRE1 and XBP1 significantly increased in the cerebellum and mesocephalon during ZIKV infection. The expression of ATF6 significantly increased in the mesocephalon. Activated ATF6n and XBP1s are translocated into the cell nucleus and regulated the transcription of target genes [32, 42]. In order to verify the activation of ATF6n and XBP1s, immunohistofluorescence was used to analyze the nuclear localization of XBP1s (Fig. 3a) and ATF6n (Fig. 3b) during ZIKV infection. The whole brain sections of AG6 mice were stained with DAPI (blue), anti-ZIKV envelope protein

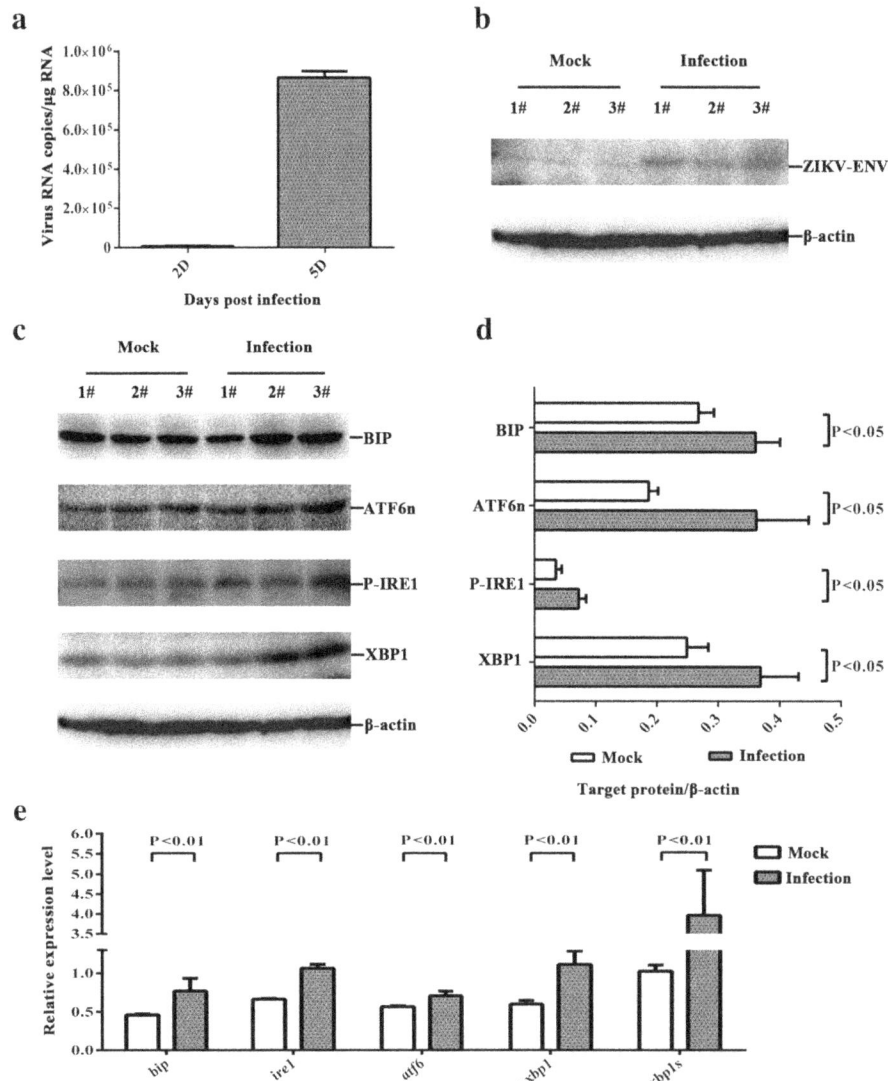

Fig. 1 ZIKV infects the nervous tissues of the mouse brain and activates the ER stress markers. Three-week-old AG6 mice were infected with 1×10^5 PFU/mouse (each dose, $N = 3$) via intraperitoneal injection. **a**. The total mRNA of the mouse brain was extracted, and ZIKV mRNA was detected at 2 dpi and 5 dpi via RT-qPCR. **b, c** The total lysates of mouse brain were analyzed at 5 dpi via western blot. An equal amount of lysates were analyzed with anti-ZIKV envelope protein antibody (**b**), anti-BIP antibody, anti-ATF6n antibody, anti-phoshpo-IRE1 antibody, and anti-XBP1 antibody (**c**). **d**. The band was analyzed by using Image Lab 4.0.1. The fold change of the *target protein/β-actin* was calculated. The protein expression of mock-infected and ZIKV-infected samples were normalized with the internal control β-actin. **e**. Primers that specifically amplified *bip*, *ire1*, *atf6*, *t-xbp1*, and *xbp1s* were used. The relative expression levels of the genes were calculated according to the $2^{-\Delta\Delta Ct}$ method. Data represented three independent experiments and *error bars* indicate mean ± SD. Statistical analyses were performed using multiple *t* tests ($N = 3$) ($P < 0.05$ or $P < 0.01$)

antibody (red), and anti-ATF6 or anti-XBP1 antibody (green). Images of the whole brain section were captured by using a digital slice scanning analysis system. We found that ZIKV infection stimulated ATF6n and XBP1s to translocate into the cell nucleus (Fig. 3c). These results further demonstrated that IRE1-XBP1 and ATF6 pathways were activated in the nervous tissues of the mouse brain during ZIKV infection, while ATF6n and XBP1s were translocated into the cell nucleus to target the downstream genes of UPR.

ZIKV infection activates ER stress sensors in human neural cells

In order to verify the ER stress at the cellular level which occurred on the nervous tissues of the mouse brain during ZIKV infection, we selected two representative neural cells, neuroblastoma cell line (SK-N-SH), and astrocytoma cell line (CCF-STTG1), to perform experiments. Neural cells were infected with ZIKV at an MOI of 5 PFU/cell. Viral growth was analyzed at different hours post infection (hpi) via RT-qPCR for the quantification of the viral

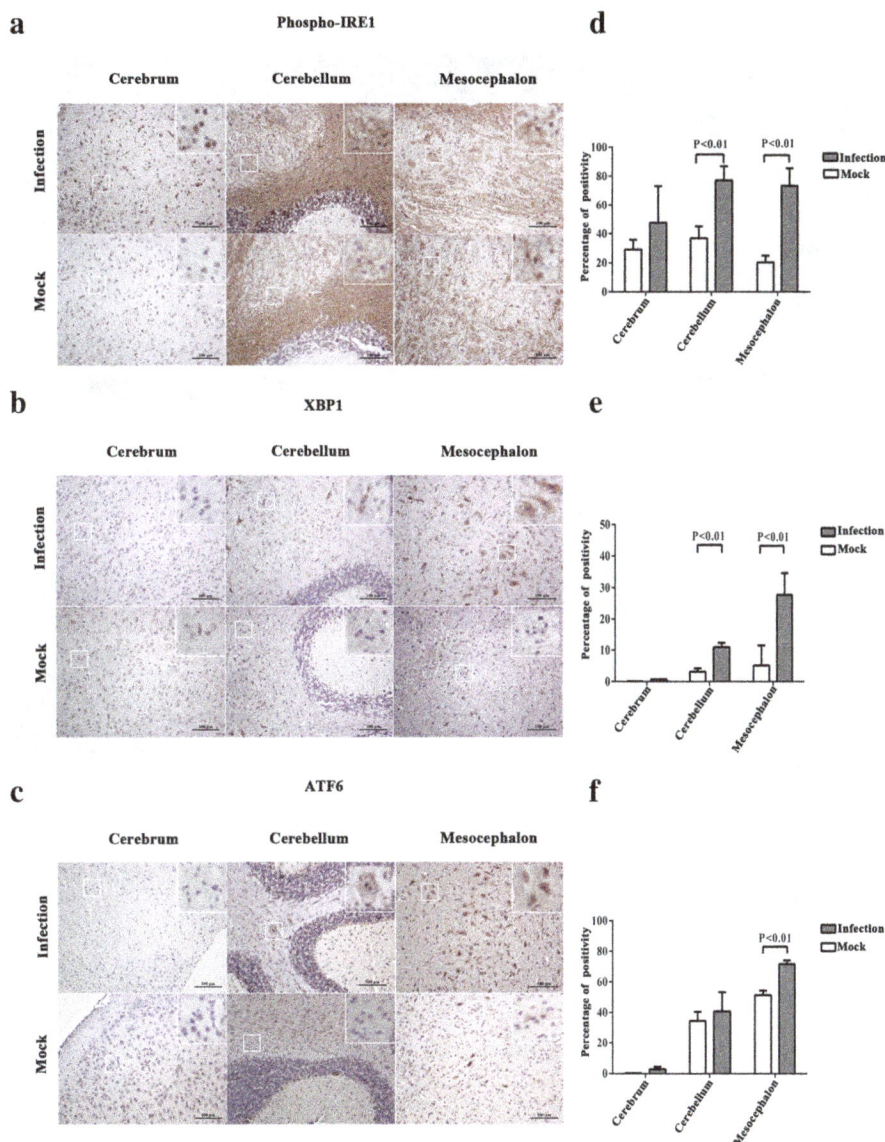

Fig. 2 ZIKV infection upregulates the expression of phospho-IRE1, XBP1, and ATF6 in the mouse brain. Three-week-old AG6 mice were infected with 1×10^5 PFU/mouse (each dose, $N = 3$) via intraperitoneal injection. **a**, **b**, **c** Sections of the cerebrum, cerebellum, and mesocephalon were obtained at 5 dpi, and anti-phospho-IRE1 antibody (**a**), anti-XBP1 antibody (recognizing both non-spliced and spliced isoforms of XBP1) (**b**), and anti-ATF6 antibody (recognizing both cleaved and full forms of ATF6) (**c**) were used for immunohistochemistry assay. Purple dots represent the cell nucleus. Brown spots represent the ZIKV envelope protein. A representative of three independent experiments is shown. Positive cells marked by white squares were magnified nine times and showed on the top-right corner. **d**, **e**, **f** Aperio ImageScope viewing software was used to analyze the percentage of positivity (algorithm, positive pixel count). Data represented three independent experiments and *error bars* indicate mean ± SD. Statistical analyses were performed using multiple *t* tests ($N = 3$) ($P < 0.05$ or $P < 0.01$)

nucleic acid (see Additional file 2: a, b). The maximum virus RNA copies of SK-N-SH and CCF-STTG1 were 1.103×10^8 copies/μg RNA at 48 hpi and 1.201×10^8 copies/μg RNA at 36 hpi respectively. Confocal immunofluorescence microscopy also revealed the presence of envelope protein at 24 hpi (see Additional file 2: c, d). The results indicated that ZIKV could infect and replicate in SK-N-SH and CCF-STTG1 cells. These results offered a model to study the ER stress of ZIKV at the cellular level.

To determine whether ZIKV infection in human neural cells also activates cellular ER stress, we detected the expression of ER stress sensors. Comparison of ZIKV infection with mock infection showed that the expression of BIP, phospho-elF2α, phospho-IRE1, and ATF6n significantly increased at 48 hpi in CCF-STTG1 (Fig. 4a). However, only phospho-elF2α significantly increased at 48 hpi in SK-N-SH (Fig 4b). The expression change of BIP, phospho-IRE1, and ATF6n was not

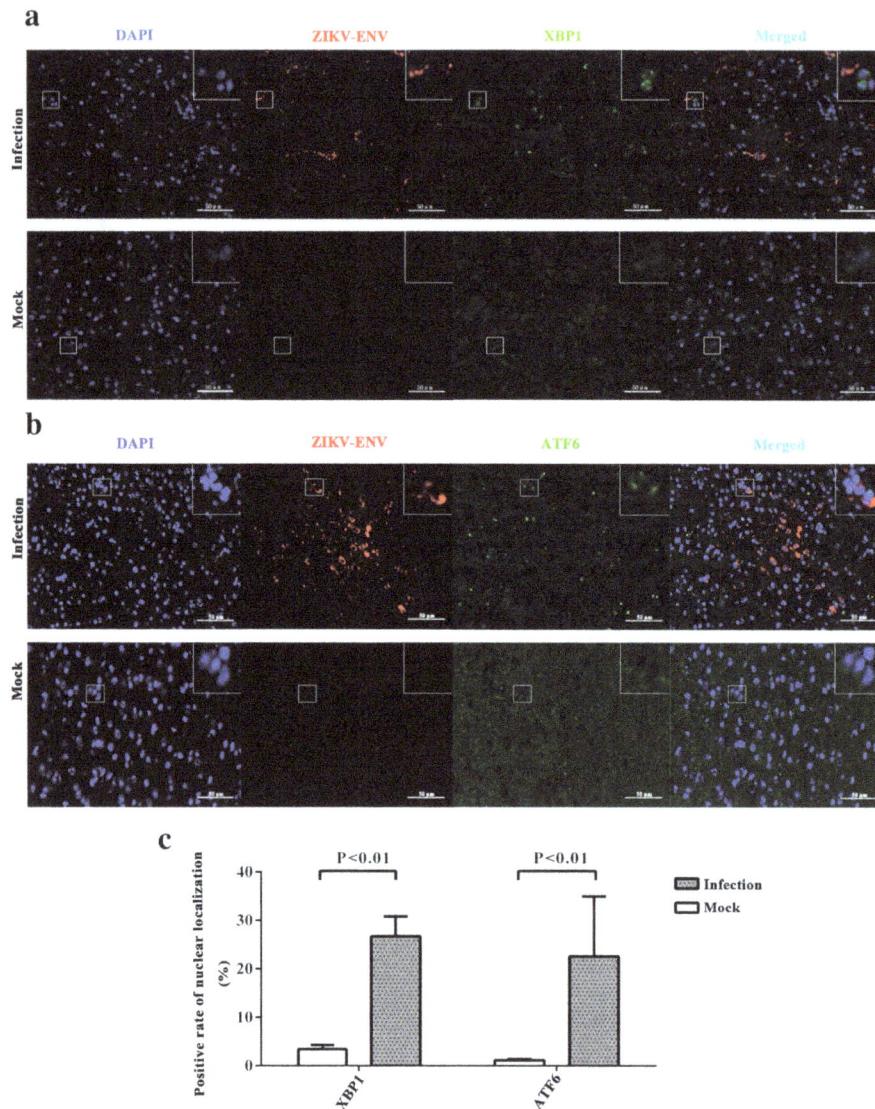

Fig. 3 ZIKV infection stimulates ATF6n and XBP1s to translocate into the cell nuclei of neural cells in the mouse brain. Three-week-old AG6 mice were infected with 1×10^5 PFU/mouse (each dose, $N = 3$) via intraperitoneal injection. **a**, **b** The whole brain sections of AG6 mice were stained with DAPI (blue), anti-ZIKV envelope protein antibody (red), and anti-XBP1 (**a**) or anti-ATF6 (**b**) antibody (green) and were used for immunohistofluorescence assay at 5 dpi. Images of the whole brain were captured by using a digital slice scanning analysis system (Pannoramic MIDI). A representative sub-area of mesocephalon is shown. Positive cells marked by white squares were magnified nine times and shown on the top-right corner. **c** Positive rates of nuclear localization were counted. Data represent three area of mesocephalon through random selection and *error bars* indicate mean ± SD. Statistical analyses were performed using multiple *t* tests ($N = 3$) ($P < 0.05$ or $P < 0.01$)

significant in SK-N-SH. The results indicated that ZIKV infection strongly activated the UPR in CCF-STTG1 and slightly activated in SK-N-SH.

ZIKV infection induces the splicing of *xbp1* and the translocation of XBP1s into the nuclei of human neural cells

To determine whether the IRE-XBP1 pathway is activated in response to ZIKV infection in human neural cells, *xbp1s* was detected via RT-PCR. Similar to that induced by tunicamycin, the spliced *xbp1s* was detected at 24 and 48 hpi. The ratios of *xbp1s*/t-*xbp1* between mock

and ZIKV infection were 15.8-fold (24 hpi) and 32.6-fold (48 hpi) in CCF-STTG1 cells, and 3.1-fold (24 hpi) and 10.9-fold (48 hpi) in SK-N-SH cells (Fig. 5a,b). RT-qPCR results indicated that *xbp1s* significantly increased during ZIKV infection. It implied that ZIKV infection induced the splicing of *xbp1*.

Confocal immunofluorescence microscopy was performed to further confirm the synthesis and nuclear localization of XBP1s. Guided by RT-qPCR data, SK-N-SH and CCF-STTG1 cells were grown on glass slides and infected with ZIKV at an MOI of 5 PFU/cell.

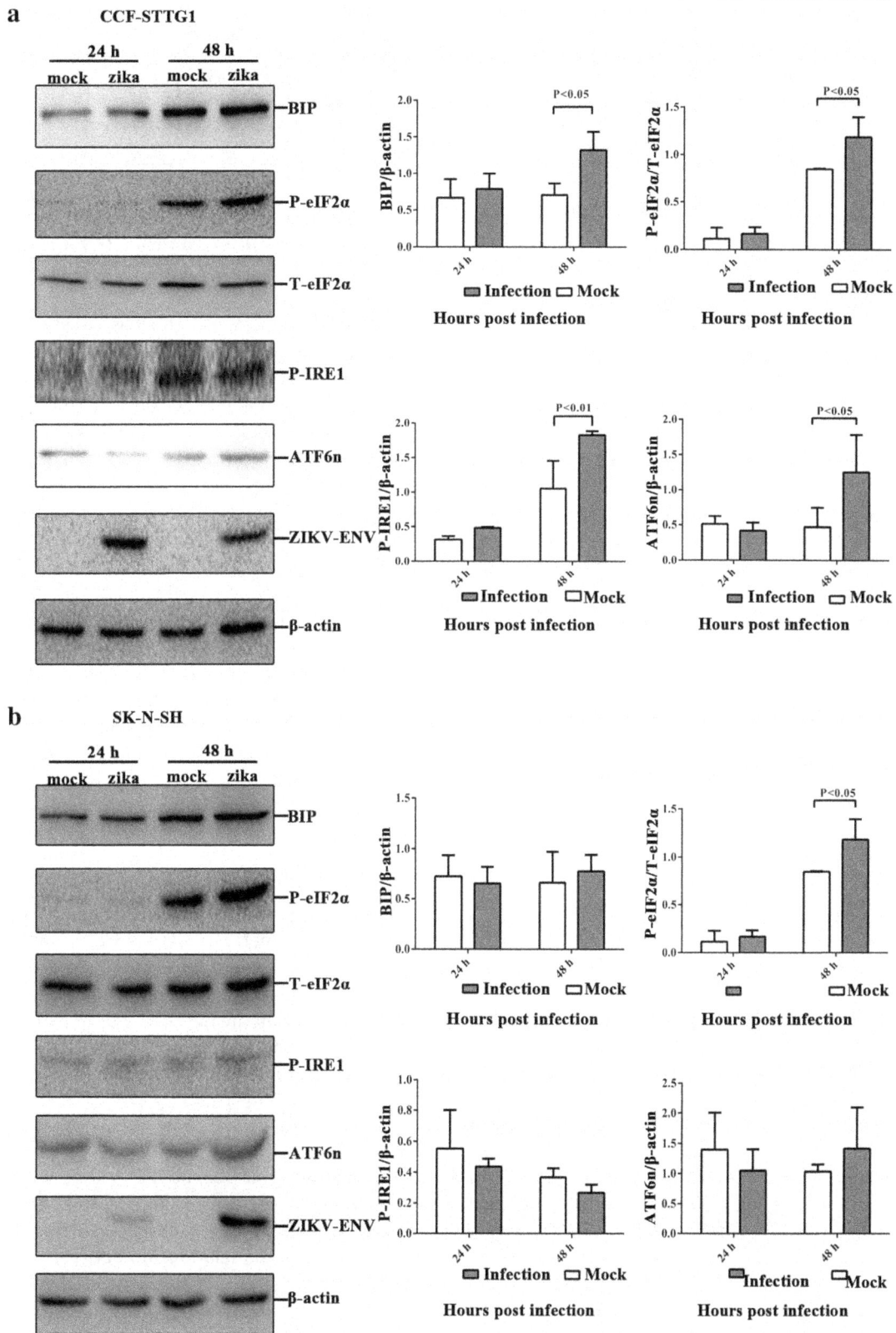

Fig. 4 (See legend on next page.)

(See figure on previous page.)

Fig. 4 ZIKV infection increases the expression of ER stress sensors in human neural cells. **a**, **b** CCF-STTG1and SK-N-SH were infected with ZIKV at an MOI of 5 PFU/cell, and cellular lysates were obtained at 24 and 48 hpi. An equal amount of cell lysates were analyzed with anti-BIP antibody, anti-phospho-eIF2α antibody, anti-total-eIF2α, anti-phoshpo-IRE1 antibody, anti-ATF6n antibody, anti-ZIKV envelope protein antibody, and anti-β-actin antibody. The bands were analyzed by using Image Lab 4.0.1. The fold change of *target protein/β-actin* was calculated. The protein level between mock-infected and ZIKV-infected compared with internal control β-actin. Data represented three independent experiments and *error bars* indicate mean ± SD. Statistical analyses were performed using multiple *t* tests (*N* = 3) (*P* < 0.05 or *P* < 0.01)

The cells were fixed at 24 hpi, at which time *xbp1* starts to be spliced and stained by using Hoechst 33258 (blue), anti-ZIKV envelope protein antibody (red), and anti-XBP1 antibody (green) (recognizing both non-spliced and spliced isoforms of XBP1). XBP1 was located in the cytoplasm in the mock-infected group. However, XBP1s translocated into the cell nucleus in both ZIKV-infected CCF-STTG1 and SK-N-SH cells and positive controls (tunicamycin treatment) (Fig. 5c,d). Confocal immunofluorescence results showed that ZIKV infection induced the translocation of XBP1s in the cell nucleus, consistent with the positive controls. In contrast to ZIKV infection, mock infection did not induce the translocation of XBP1s in the cell nucleus (Fig. 5e). The results indicated that ZIKV infection-induced ER stress triggers the synthesis and transport of XBP1s into the cell nucleus.

ZIKV infection activates the UPR downstream genes in the nervous tissues of the mouse brain and human neural cells

Phosphorylated PERK mediates eIF2α phosphorylation and regulates many ER stress-related genes through ATF4, such as amino acid metabolism, *gadd34*, and cell apoptosis [43]. Our results indicated that ZIKV infection induced eIF2α phosphorylation in human neural cells which is similar with the previous study [44]. ATF4 is regulated by phospho-eIF2α, and its activation results in the function of the PERK-eIF2α pathway [16, 43]. To determine whether the increasing amount of phospho-beIF2α in ZIKV infection is sufficient to induce ATF4 translation, the mRNA level of *atf4* was measured using RT-qPCR. The results indicated that *atf4* significantly increased in the nervous tissues of the mouse brain (1.60-fold) (Fig. 6) and at 48 hpi in CCF-STTG1 cells (1.40-fold) but not in SK-N-SH cells (Fig. 7a,b,). Although the mRNA level of *atf4* increased slightly, the fold change was negligible. This result suggests that phospho-eIF2α weakly activates ATF4. GADD34 is a negative feedback loop that restores protein translation by targeting PP1 to phosphor-eIF2α and making it dephosphorylate [45, 46]. RT-qPCR results demonstrated that the mRNA level of *gadd34* significantly increased in the nervous tissues of the mouse brain (1.86-fold) (Fig. 6) and at 48 hpi (2.6-fold) in CCF-STTG1 (Fig. 7c) cells and at 48 hpi (1.9-fold) in SK-N-SH cells (Fig. 7d). Those

results suggest that GADD34 expression is increased to restore protein translation during ZIKV replication, implying that ZIKV may take advantage of the protein synthesis of the host cell.

To deal with ER stress, the activated UPR causes translation attenuation, cellular apoptosis, and protein degradation. CHOP is one of the components of the ER stress-mediated apoptotic pathway. Activated CHOP further induces apoptotic markers, such as Bcl-2, Caspase-9, and Caspase-3 [16]. Its expression is mainly regulated at the transcriptional level. The transcriptional level of *chop* increased significantly in the nervous tissues of the mouse brain (1.65-fold) (Fig. 6) and at 24 hpi (1.6-fold) and 48 hpi (1.8-fold) in CCF-STTG1 cells (Fig. 7e), and at 24 hpi (1.5-fold) and 48 hpi (4.2-fold) in SK-N-SH cells (Fig. 7f). The transcription of *chop* was regulated by both ATF4 and XBP1s [16, 47]. However, ATF4 was weakly activated during ZIKV infection. The changing trends of *chop* were consistent with *xbp1s*. Thus, activated *chop* may be mainly regulated by XBP1s. ER degradation-enhancing α-mannosidase-like protein (EDEM) family proteins are the main members of ERAD activated during ER stress. XBP1 is involved in ERAD by the induction of EDEM [48]. Many studies demonstrated that EDEM-1 increases during virus infection or directly interacts with the viral proteins [49]. The transcriptional level of *edem-1* significantly increased in the nervous tissues of the mouse brain (1.76-fold) (Fig. 6), but no change was detected in neural cells (Fig. 7g,h). Therefore, the results implied that ZIKV infection mediates XBP1s to activate CHOP and may mediate cell apoptosis, but not EDEM-1 to activate protein degradation.

Discussion

ZIKV is a mosquito-borne flavivirus which causes microcephaly in newborns and serious neurological complications in adults, such as Guillain–Barre syndrome. Although the relationship between ZIKV infection and microcephaly is demonstrated in vivo [50], the neuropathogenesis caused by ZIKV infection is still unclear. Ivan Gladwyn-Ng et al. reported that ZIKV induced ER stress and UPR in human cortices in vivo and in hNSCs in vitro, and their findings were confirmed in the mouse embryonic brain in vivo. They

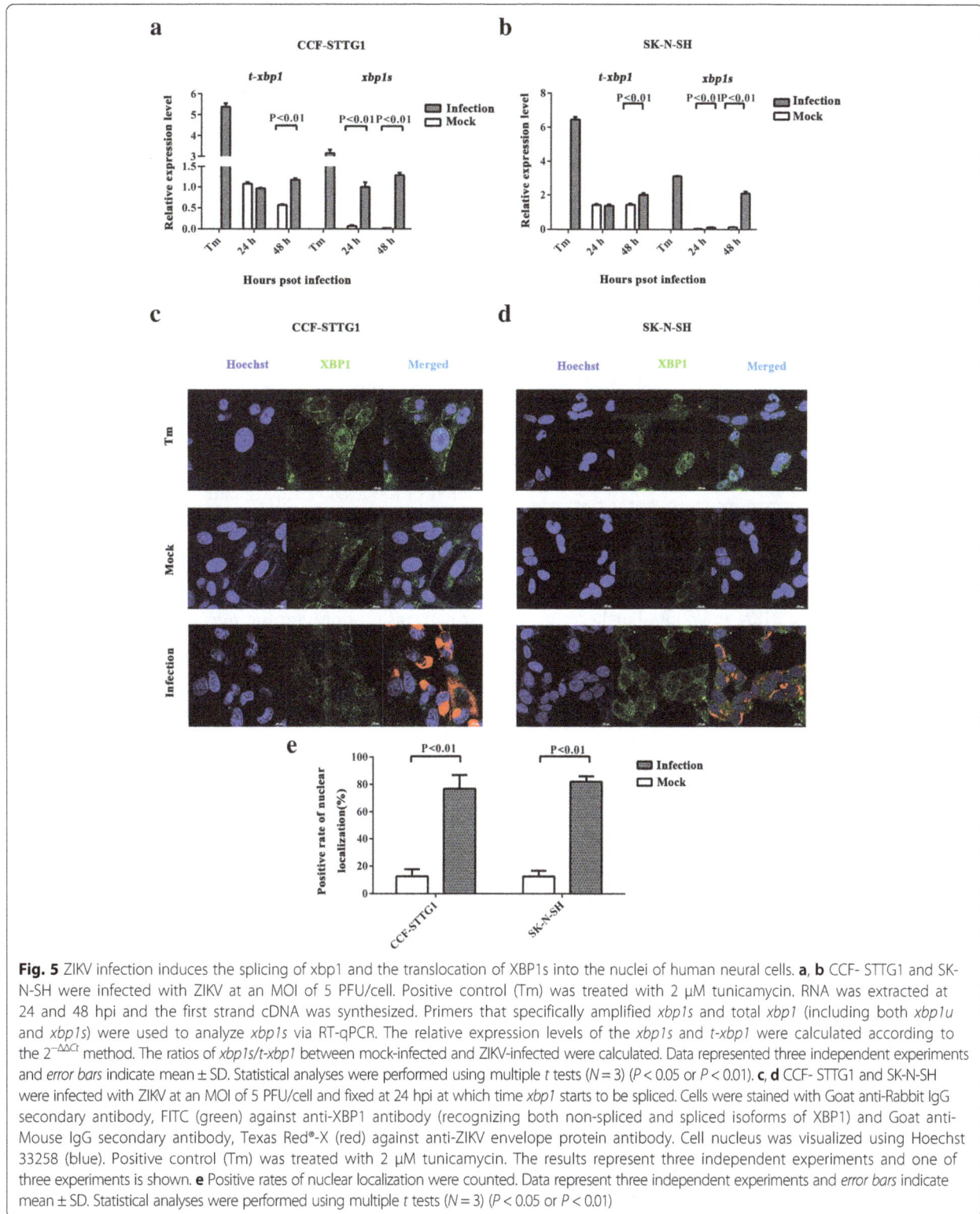

Fig. 5 ZIKV infection induces the splicing of xbp1 and the translocation of XBP1s into the nuclei of human neural cells. **a, b** CCF- STTG1 and SK-N-SH were infected with ZIKV at an MOI of 5 PFU/cell. Positive control (Tm) was treated with 2 μM tunicamycin. RNA was extracted at 24 and 48 hpi and the first strand cDNA was synthesized. Primers that specifically amplified xbp1s and total xbp1 (including both xbp1u and xbp1s) were used to analyze xbp1s via RT-qPCR. The relative expression levels of the xbp1s and t-xbp1 were calculated according to the $2^{-\Delta\Delta Ct}$ method. The ratios of xbp1s/t-xbp1 between mock-infected and ZIKV-infected were calculated. Data represented three independent experiments and error bars indicate mean ± SD. Statistical analyses were performed using multiple t tests (N = 3) (P < 0.05 or P < 0.01). **c, d** CCF- STTG1 and SK-N-SH were infected with ZIKV at an MOI of 5 PFU/cell and fixed at 24 hpi at which time xbp1 starts to be spliced. Cells were stained with Goat anti-Rabbit IgG secondary antibody, FITC (green) against anti-XBP1 antibody (recognizing both non-spliced and spliced isoforms of XBP1) and Goat anti-Mouse IgG secondary antibody, Texas Red®-X (red) against anti-ZIKV envelope protein antibody. Cell nucleus was visualized using Hoechst 33258 (blue). Positive control (Tm) was treated with 2 μM tunicamycin. The results represent three independent experiments and one of three experiments is shown. **e** Positive rates of nuclear localization were counted. Data represent three independent experiments and error bars indicate mean ± SD. Statistical analyses were performed using multiple t tests (N = 3) (P < 0.05 or P < 0.01)

also investigated the mechanism of ZIKV-associated microcephaly by administration of pharmacological inhibitors of the UPR and found that the PERK-eIF2α pathway is the principal dependence [51]. In the current study, however, we observed that ZIKV infection activated the IRE1-XBP1 and ATF6 pathways in the mouse nervous tissues in vivo and human neural cell line in vitro. Those two pathways are different

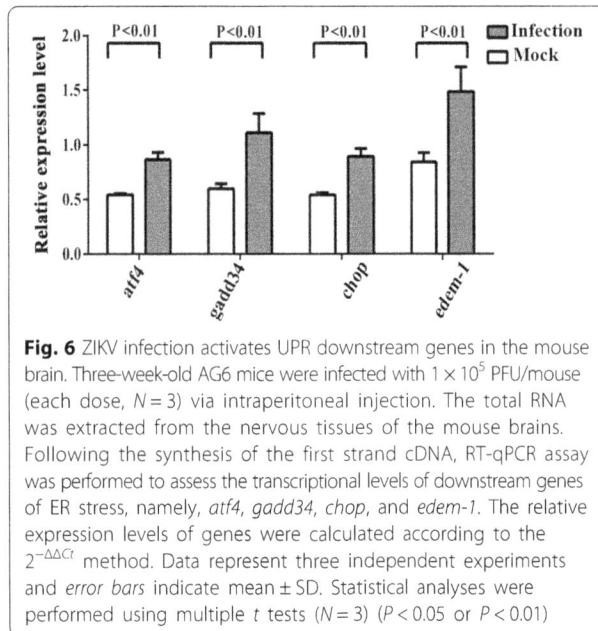

Fig. 6 ZIKV infection activates UPR downstream genes in the mouse brain. Three-week-old AG6 mice were infected with 1×10^5 PFU/mouse (each dose, $N = 3$) via intraperitoneal injection. The total RNA was extracted from the nervous tissues of the mouse brains. Following the synthesis of the first strand cDNA, RT-qPCR assay was performed to assess the transcriptional levels of downstream genes of ER stress, namely, atf4, gadd34, chop, and edem-1. The relative expression levels of genes were calculated according to the $2^{-\Delta\Delta Ct}$ method. Data represent three independent experiments and error bars indicate mean ± SD. Statistical analyses were performed using multiple t tests ($N = 3$) ($P < 0.05$ or $P < 0.01$)

from the PERK-eIF2α for regulating ER stress, so we speculated that the UPR also may deal with ER stress in another way during ZIKV infection. Furthermore, it is reported that ER stress can directly initiate inflammatory pathways. In turn, pro-inflammatory stimuli can trigger ER stress and the resulting UPR activation can further amplify inflammatory responses [52]. However, because of the limitation of IFNR-deficient mice, we cannot investigate the interplay between the UPR activation and inflammatory responses, especially innate immune response and its role in ZIKV pathogenesis. In order to build a cellular model for the verification of ER stress in vitro, we demonstrated that ZIKV replication was highly efficient in human neural cells, SK-N-SH, and CCF-STTG1 cells. It is easy to study the neuropathogenesis caused by ZIKV infection in vitro by using this cellular model which is firstly reported. Using this cellular model, we investigated the activation and regulation of three UPR pathways in neural cells. We found that ZIKV infection in neural cells activated the IRE1-XBP1, PERK-eIF2α, and ATF6 pathways respectively. Comparing the effects of each pathway, we found that phospho-eIF2α-mediated transcriptional attenuation was slightly activated. IRE1-XBP1 and ATF6 pathways are mainly activated during ZIKV infection in vitro and in vivo. Considering their effect on cell apoptosis, protein degradation, and ER homeostasis mediated by IRE1-XBP1 and ATF6, we found chop was upregulated in vitro and in vivo. Edem-1 was only upregulated in vivo. The chaperone, BIP, which participates in the regulation of ER homeostasis was upregulated in vitro and in vivo. Those

results demonstrated that ZIKV infection activated the ER stress and regulated the UPR in neural cells.

ZIKV infection activates the IRE1-XBP1 pathway to respond to ER stress

The IRE1-XBP1 signaling pathway plays an important role in viral infection. A number of viral infections activate IRE1-XBP1, triggering many cell responses. Firstly, ERAD activation accelerates protein degradation [53]. Secondly, CHOP expression induces apoptosis markers to guide cell death and plays a role in autophagy induction. Thirdly, IRE1 mediates the selective degradation of a subset of ER-located mRNAs. However, each virus causes different cell responses mediated by IRE1-XBP1. HCV glycoprotein E2 is an ERAD substrate that interacts with EDEM to accelerate glycoprotein degradation, which interferes with viral replication and particle production [53]. DENV infection induces CHOP but does not trigger apoptosis markers [16]. JEV induces the activation of the RIDD cleavage pathway, which is beneficial for viral infectivity [27, 49]. Findings in this study indicated that ZIKV infection induced the IRE1-XBP1 pathway to respond to cell stress. And the expression of ZIKV-ENV do not correlate with the XBP1 expression or its translocation into the nucleus, this suggested that ZIKV-ENV may not be responsible for induction of IRE1-XBP1 pathway or IRE1-XBP1 pathway activated in the infection state with the low expression level of ZIKV-ENV. The IRE1-XBP1 pathway triggered the cell responses of CHOP, which may activate cellular apoptosis. However, ZIKV infection did not trigger the EDEM-1 to increase the degradation of misfolded and unfolded proteins which alleviated the accumulation of abnormal proteins. We speculate that ZIKV infection facilitates neural cell apoptosis which may relate to the nerve injury and may also benefit from the virus release and contributes to viral replication [18].

ZIKV infection activates the ATF6 pathway to respond to cell stress

The activation of ATF6 is critical to the UPR. ATF6 increases the expression of many ER chaperone genes. BIP, as a major ER chaperone, facilitates protein folding, preventing intermediates from aggregating, and promoting misfolded protein for proteasome degradation. BIP acts as a central regulator of ER homeostasis. BIP is essential for the correct protein folding of nascent viral peptides in the ER, including viral core protein expression. BIP also plays a role in the replication of viral genetic material as well as the formation of new viral capsid complexes [54]. Our results reveal that ATF6 and BIP upregulated during ZIKV infection in vitro and in vivo. ATF6 may promote the expression of BIP. Activated BIP expression sustains the ER homeostasis and contributes

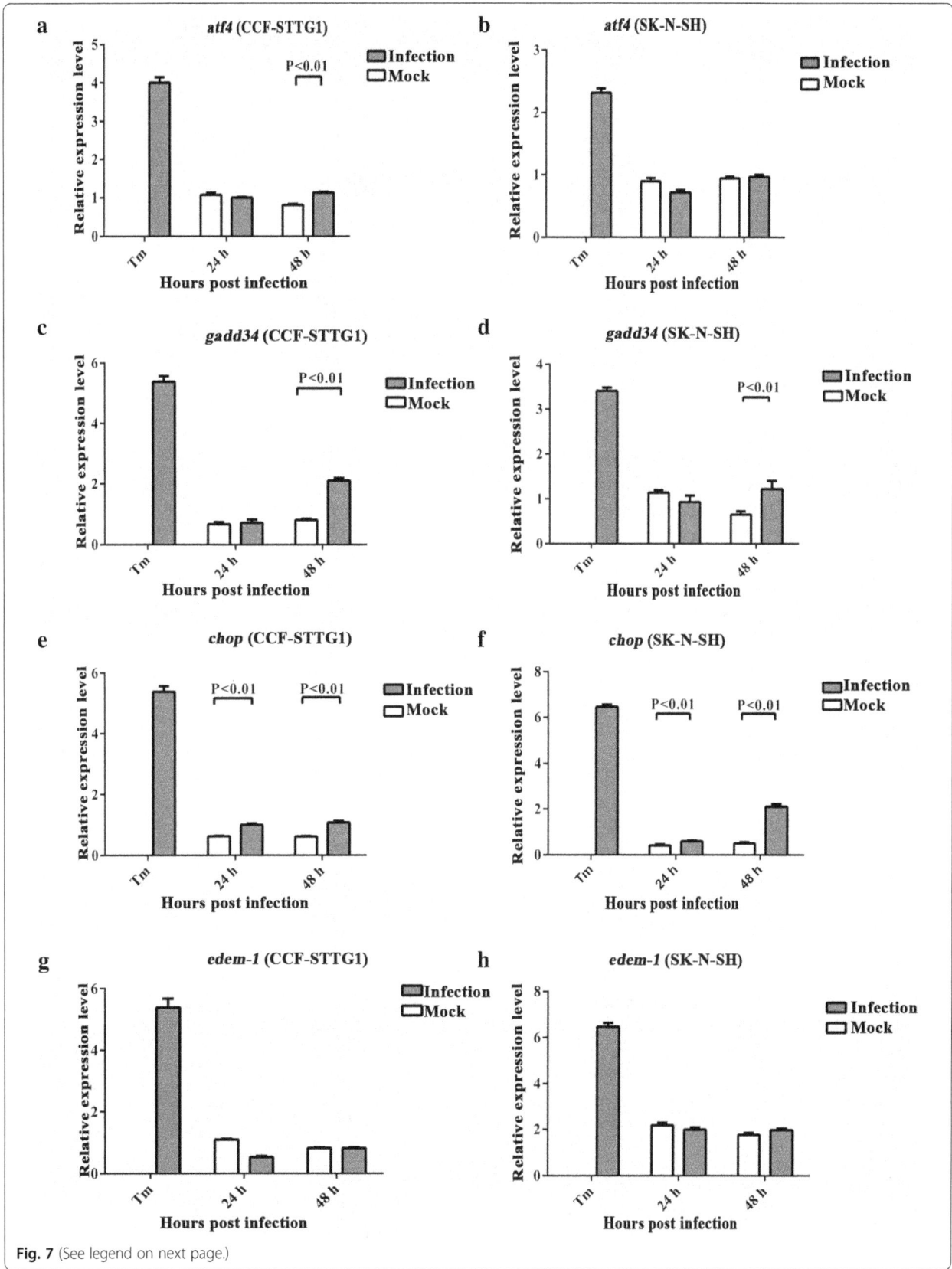

Fig. 7 (See legend on next page.)

(See figure on previous page.)
Fig. 7 ZIKV infection activates the UPR downstream genes in human neural cells. **a–h** CCF-STTG1 and SK-N-SH were infected with ZIKV at an MOI of 5 PFU/cell. RNA was extracted at 24 and 48 hpi and the first strand cDNA was synthesized. Primers that specifically amplified *atf4* (**a**, **b**), *gadd34* (**c**, **d**), *chop* (**e**, **f**), and *edem-1* (**g**, **h**) were used. The relative expression levels of the genes were calculated according to the $2^{-\Delta\Delta Ct}$ method. Data represented three independent experiments and *error bars* indicate mean ± SD. Statistical analyses were performed using multiple *t* tests ($N = 3$) ($P < 0.05$ or $P < 0.01$)

to the ZIKV replication. In addition, inducing the mRNA expression of *xbp1s* is one of the important functions of ATF6 [39, 49]. The mRNA level of *xbp1s* significantly increases, and XBP1s is translocated into the nucleus. ATF6n may participate in inducing *xbp1s* expression and mediate XBP1s activation.

ZIKV infection induces the phosphorylation of eIF2α but does not increase the expression of ATF4

Phospho-eIF2α transiently attenuates global mRNA translation, thereby helping cells reduce the accumulation of misfolded proteins and cope with temporary ER stress [49]. DENV-2 infection suppresses PERK-mediated eIF2α phosphorylation [16]. We detected the phosphorylation of eIF2α and found that the level of phospho-eIF2α significantly increased during ZIKV infection. The mRNA level of *gadd34*, which recruits PP1 to dephosphorylate phospho-eIF2α, increased significantly during ZIKV infection. However, ATF4 was hardly activated during ZIKV infection. Therefore, eIF2α-ATF4 did not mediate translation attenuation. Inversely, ZIKV may suppress the translation attenuation through increasing the expression of GADD34.

Many neurological diseases are linked to ER stress. For example, the accumulation of misfolded protein such as β-amyloid, α-synuclein, and huntingtin is apparently associated with selective nerve cell death in Alzheimer's, Parkinson's, and Huntington's diseases [47]. ATF6, XBP1, and CHOP play functional roles in controlling dopaminergic neuron survival [33]. In Parkinson's disease studies, the activation of UPR maintains the protein homeostasis in ATF6-deficient mice. ATF6 controls the level of BIP and ERAD components in dopaminergic neurons [33]. We found that ZIKV infection activated the UPR in the mouse nervous tissues and verified in the neural cells. The results offer some clues to further study the mechanism of neuropathogenesis caused by ZIKV infection.

Conclusions

Taken together, ZIKV infection significantly upregulated the expression of ER stress markers in the mouse nervous tissues and the neural cells. The results of this study provide evidence that ZIKV infection activated the UPR and offer some clues to further study the mechanism of neuropathogenesis caused by ZIKV infection.

Additional files

Additional file 1: Immunohistochemistry assay for ZIKV infection in the mouse brain. a Three-week-old AG6 mice were infected with 1×10^5 PFU/mouse (each dose, $N = 3$) via intraperitoneal injection. Sections of the cerebrum, cerebellum, and mesocephalon were obtained at 5 dpi, and anti-ZIKV envelope protein antibody was used for immunohistochemistry assay. Purple dots represent the cell nucleus. Brown spots represent the ZIKV envelope protein. Shown is representative one of three independent experiments. b Aperio ImageScope viewing software was used to analyze the percentage of positivity (algorithm, positive pixel count). Data represented three independent experiments and *error bars* indicate mean ± SD. Statistical analyses were performed using multiple *t* tests ($N = 3$) ($P < 0.05$ or $P < 0.01$). (EPS 474 kb)

Additional file 2: The model of ZIKV infection in human neural cells, CCF-STTG1, and SK-N-SH cell lines. a, b CCF-STTG1 and SK-N-SH were infected with ZIKV at an MOI of 5 PFU/cell. RNA was extracted and first strand cDNA was synthesized. A standard curve of RT-qPCR was built and the absolute quantification of the viral nucleic acid was calculated respectively. Data represented three independent experiments and *error bars* indicate mean ± SD. c, d Detection of viral envelope protein at 24 hpi by confocal immunofluorescence microscopy. The nucleus was visualized using Hoechst 33258 (blue), and the envelope protein was stained with the anti-ZIKV envelope protein antibody followed by Goat anti-Mouse IgG secondary antibody, Texas Red®-X (red). All the images were captured at × 10 magnification. One out of three independent experiments is shown, (c) CCF-STTG1 and (d) SK-N-SH. (EPS 1006 kb)

Abbreviations
ATF4: Activating transcription factor 4; ATF6: Transcription factor 6; ATF6n: Cleaved ATF6; BIP: ER chaperone immunoglobulin heavy -chain-binding protein; BSA: Bovine serum albumin; CCF-STTG1: Astrocytoma cell line; CHOP: Pro-apoptotic transcription factor CCAT/enhancer-binding protein; DENV: Dengue virus; dpi: Days post infection; EDEM: ER degradation-enhancing α-mannosidase-like protein; eIF2B: Guanine nucleotide exchange factor; eIF2α: α -subunit of eukaryotic translation initiation factor 2; ER: Endoplasmic reticulum; ERAD: ER-association degradation RIDD: regulated IRE1-dependent decay; ERSEs: ER stress response elements; GADD34: Growth arrest and DNA damage-inducible protein; HCV: Hepatitis C virus; hpi: Hours post infection; HRP: Horseradish peroxidase; IRE1: Inositol-requiring enzyme 1; JEV: Japanese encephalitis virus; MOI: Multiplicity of infection; NGS: Normal goat serum; PERK: PKR-like ER kinase; phospho-eIF2α: Phosphorylated eIF2α; phospho-IRE1: Phosphorylated IRE1; PMSF: Phenylmethanesulfonyl fluoride; PP1: Protein phosphatase 1; SK-N-SH: Neuroblastoma cell line; TCID50: 50% tissue culture infectious dose; t-xbp1: Total *xbp1*; UPR: Unfolded protein response; UPREs: UPR elements; WNV: West Nile virus; XBP1: X-box binding protein 1; XBP1s: Spliced XBP1; *xbp1s*: Spliced *xbp1*mRNA; *xbp1u*: Unspliced *xbp1*mRNA; YFV: Yellow fever virus; ZIKV: Zika virus; ZIKV-ENV: ZIKV envelope protein

Acknowledgements
The funders had no role in the study design, data collection and interpretation, or the decision to submit the work for publication. The authors thank the Core Facility and Technical Support, Wuhan Institute of Virology, for Ding Gao's help with confocal immunofluorescence microscopy and Xuefang An's help in animal experiments. The authors thank Prof. Qibin Leng in the Institute Pasteur of Shanghai, Chinese Academy of Sciences, for providing AG6 mice.

Funding
This work was supported by the National Key R&D Program of China (2016YFD0500406 to HanzhongWang), the National Natural Science Foundation of China (NSFC) (NO. 81471953 to ZhenhuaZheng), and Youth Innovation Promotion Association of CAS (2016302 to Zhenhua Zheng).

Authors' contributions
Z.T. and Z.Z. conceived and designed the experiments. Z.T., J.S., and Z.F. performed the experiments. Z.T., Z.Z., W.Z., J.S., Z.F., C.Z., P.L., X.K., Y.Z., and Y.L. analyzed the data. Z.T. wrote the manuscript. Z.Z., Q.H., and H.W revised the manuscript. All authors read and approved the final manuscript.

Competing interests
The authors declare that they have no competing interests.

Author details
[1]CAS Key Laboratory of Special Pathogens and Biosafety, Center for Emerging Infectious Diseases, Wuhan Institute of Virology, Chinese Academy of Sciences, Wuhan 430071, China. [2]University of Chinese Academy of Sciences, Beijing 100049, China. [3]College of Veterinary Medicine, Huazhong Agricultural University, Wuhan 430070, China. [4]State Key Laboratory of Virology, Wuhan Institute of Virology, Chinese Academy of Sciences, Wuhan 430071, China.

References
1. Simpson DI. Zika virus infection in man. Trans R Soc Trop Med Hyg. 1964;58: 339–44.
2. MacNamara FN. Zika virus: a report on three cases of human infection during an epidemic of jaundice in Nigeria. Trans R Soc Trop Med Hyg. 1954; 48:139–45.
3. Duffy MR, Chen T-H, Hancock WT, Powers AM, Kool JL, Lanciotti RS, Pretrick M, Marfel M, Holzbauer S, Dubray C, et al. Zika virus outbreak on Yap Island, Federated States of Micronesia. N Engl J Med. 2009;360:2536–43.
4. Petersen LR, Jamieson DJ, Powers AM, Honein MA. Zika virus. N Engl J Med. 2016;374:1552–63.
5. Johansson MA, Mier-y-Teran-Romero L, Reefhuis J, Gilboa SM, Hills SL. Zika and the risk of microcephaly. N Engl J Med. 2016;375:1–4.
6. Didier Musso DJG. Zika virus. Clin Microbiol Rev. 2016;29:487.
7. Brasil P, Jr JPP, Moreira ME, Nogueira RMR, Damasceno L, Wakimoto M, Rabello RS, Valderramos SG, Halai UA, Salles TS. Zika virus infection in pregnant women in Rio de Janeiro. N Engl J Med. 2016;375:2321.
8. Haug CJ, Kieny MP, Murgue B. The Zika challenge. N Engl J Med. 2016;374: 1801–3.
9. Schulerfaccini L. Possible association between Zika virus infection and microcephaly — Brazil, 2015. MMWR Morb Mortal Wkly Rep. 2016;65:59–62.
10. Calvet G, Aguiar RS, Aso M, Sampaio SA, De FI, Fabri A, Esm A, de Sequeira PC, Mcl DMA, De OL: Detection and sequencing of Zika virus from amniotic fluid of fetuses with microcephaly in Brazil: a case study. Lancet Infect Dis 2016, 16:653–660.
11. Kuno G, Chang GJ, Tsuchiya KR, Karabatsos N, Cropp CB. Phylogeny of the genus Flavivirus. J Virol. 1998;72:73–83.
12. Hamel R, Dejarnac O, Wichit S, Ekchariyawat P, Neyret A, Natthanej L, Perera-Lecoin M, Surasombatpattana P, Talignani L, Thomas F. Biology of Zika virus infection in human skin cells. J Virol. 2015;89:8880–96.
13. Kuno G, Chang GJJ. Full-length sequencing and genomic characterization of Bagaza, Kedougou, and Zika viruses. Arch Virol. 2007;152:687–96.
14. Valadão ALC, Aguiar RS, de Arruda LB. Interplay between inflammation and cellular stress triggered by Flaviviridae viruses. Front Microbiol. 2016;7:1–19.
15. Fernandez-Garcia MD, Mazzon M, Jacobs M, Amara A. Pathogenesis of flavivirus infections: using and abusing the host cell. Cell Host Microbe. 2009;5:318–28.
16. Pena J, Harris E. Dengue virus modulates the unfolded protein response in a time-dependent manner. J Biol Chem. 2011;286:14226–36.
17. Yu CY, Hsu YW, Liao CL, Lin YL. Flavivirus infection activates the XBP1 pathway of the unfolded protein response to cope with endoplasmic reticulum stress. J Virol. 2006;80:11868–80.
18. Medieshi GR, Lancaster AM, Hirsch AJ, Briese T, Lipkin WI, Defilippis V, Früs K, Mason PW, Nikolich-Zuqich J, Nelson JA. West Nile virus infection activates the unfolded protein response, leading to CHOP induction and apoptosis. J Virology. 2007;81:10849–60.
19. Ambrose RL, Mackenzie JM. West Nile virus differentially modulates the unfolded protein response to facilitate replication and immune evasion. J Virol. 2011;85:2723–32.
20. Tardif KD, Mori K, Kaufman RJ, Siddiqui A. Hepatitis C virus suppresses the IRE1-XBP1 pathway of the unfolded protein response. J Biol Chem. 2004; 279:17158–64.
21. Tardif KD, Waris G, Siddiqui A. Hepatitis C virus, ER stress, and oxidative stress. Trends Microbiol. 2005;13:159–63.
22. Hetz C. The unfolded protein response: controlling cell fate decisions under ER stress and beyond. Nat Rev Mol Cell Biol. 2012;13:89–102.
23. Amici C, La Frazia S, Brunelli C, Balsamo M, Angelini M, Santoro MG: Inhibition of viral protein translation by indomethacin in vesicular stomatitis virus infection: role of eIF2alpha kinase PKR. Cell Microbiol 2015, 17:1391–1404.
24. Jheng JR, Lau KS, Tang WF, Wu MS, Horng JT. Endoplasmic reticulum stress is induced and modulated by enterovirus 71. Cell Microbiol. 2010;12:796–813.
25. Walter P, Ron D. The unfolded protein response: from stress pathway to homeostatic regulation. Science. 2011;334:1081–7.
26. Gallagher CM, Garri C, Cain EL, Ang KH, Wilson CG, Chen S, Hearn BR, Jaishankar P, Aranda-Diaz A, Arkin MR. Ceapins are a new class of unfolded protein response inhibitors, selectively targeting the ATF6α branch. Elife. 2016;5:e1188e0.
27. Bhattacharyya S, Sen U, Vrati S. Regulated IRE1-dependent decay pathway is activated during Japanese encephalitis virus-induced unfolded protein response and benefits viral replication. J Gen Virol. 2014;95:71–9.
28. Ambrose RL, Mackenzie JM. ATF6 signaling is required for efficient West Nile virus replication by promoting cell survival and inhibition of innate immune responses. J Virol. 2013;87:2206–14.
29. Li G, Poulsen M, Fenyvuesvolgyi C, Yashiroda Y, Yoshida M, Simard JM, Gallo RC, Zhao RY. Characterization of cytopathic factors through genome-wide analysis of the Zika viral proteins in fission yeast. Proc Natl Acad Sci U S A. 2017;114:376–85.
30. Hetz C, Chevet E, Harding HP. Targeting the unfolded protein response in disease. Nat Rev Drug Discov. 2013;12:703–19.
31. Khajavi M, Lupski JR. Balancing between adaptive and maladaptive cellular stress responses in peripheral neuropathy. Neuron. 2008;57:329–30.
32. Yang W, Paschen W. Unfolded protein response in brain ischemia: a timely update. J Cereb Blood Flow Metab. 2016;36:2044–50.
33. Mercado G, Castillo V, Soto P, Sidhu A. ER stress and Parkinson's disease: pathological inputs that converge into the secretory pathway. Brain Res. 1648;2016:626–32.
34. Deng C, Liu S, Zhang Q, Xu M, Zhang H. Isolation and characterization of Zika virus imported to China using C6/36 mosquito cells. Virol Sin. 2016;31:1–4.
35. Liu Y, Zheng Z, Shu B, Meng J, Zhang Y, Zheng C, Ke X, Gong P, Hu Q, Wang H. SUMO modification stabilizes Enterovirus 71 polymerase 3D to facilitate viral replication. J Virol. 2016;90:10472–85.
36. Zheng Z, Li H, Zhang Z, Meng J, Mao D, Bai B, Lu B, Mao P, Hu Q, Wang H. Enterovirus 71 2C protein inhibits TNF-α-mediated activation of NF-κB by suppressing IκB kinase β phosphorylation. J Immunol. 2011;187:2202–12.
37. Lazear H, Govero J, Smith A, Platt D, Fernandez E, Miner J, Diamond M. A mouse model of Zika virus pathogenesis. Cell Host Microbe. 2016;19:1–11.
38. Rossi SL, Tesh RB, Azar SR, Muruato AE, Hanley KA, Auguste AJ, Langsjoen RM, Paessler S, Vasilakis N, Weaver SC. Characterization of a novel murine model to study Zika virus. Am J Trop Med Hygi. 2016;94:1362–9.
39. Yoshida H, Matsui T, Yamamoto A, Okada T, Mori K. XBP1 mRNA is induced by ATF6 and spliced by IRE1 in response to ER stress to produce a highly active transcription factor. Cell. 2001;107:881–91.
40. Oishi N, Duscha S, Boukari H, Meyer M, Xie J, Wei G, Schrepfer T, Roschitzki B, Boettger EC, Schacht J. XBP1 mitigates aminoglycoside-induced endoplasmic reticulum stress and neuronal cell death. Cell Death Dis. 2015;6;e1763.

41. Hirota M, Kitagaki M, Itagaki H, Aiba S. Quantitative measurement of spliced XBP1 mRNA as an indicator of endoplasmic reticulum stress. J Toxicol Sci. 2006;31:149–56.
42. Gu XW, Yan JQ, Dou HT, Liu J, Liu L, Zhao ML, Liang XH, Yang ZM. Endoplasmic reticulum stress in mouse decidua during early pregnancy. Mol Cell Endocrinol. 2016;434:48–56.
43. Isler JA, Skalet AH, Alwine JC. Human cytomegalovirus infection activates and regulates the unfolded protein response. J Virol. 2005;79:6890–9.
44. Amorim R, Temzi A, Griffin BD, Mouland AJ. Zika virus inhibits eIF2α-dependent stress granule assembly. PLoS Negl Trop Dis. 2017;11:e0005775.
45. Kilberg MS, Shan J, Su N. ATF4-dependent transcription mediates signaling of amino acid limitation. Trends Endocrinol Metab Tem. 2009;20:436–43.
46. Choy Meng S, Yusoff P, Lee Irene C, Newton Jocelyn C, Goh Catherine W, Page R, Shenolikar S, Peti W. Structural and functional analysis of the GADD34:PP1 eIF2α phosphatase. Cell Rep. 2015;11:1885–91.
47. Oyadomari S, Mori M. Roles of CHOP/GADD153 in endoplasmic reticulum stress. Cell Death Differ. 2004;11:381–9.
48. Medigeshi GR, Lancaster AM, Hirsch AJ, Briese T, Lipkin WI, Defilippis V, Fruh K, Mason PW, Nikolich-Zugich J, Nelson JA. West Nile virus infection activates the unfolded protein response, leading to CHOP induction and apoptosis. J Virol. 2007;81:10849–60.
49. Jheng J-R, Ho J-Y, Horng J-T. ER stress, autophagy, and RNA viruses. Front Microbiol. 2014;5:1–13.
50. Cui L, Dan X, Ye Q, Shuai H, Jiang Y, Liu X, Zhang N, Lei S, Qin CF, Xu Z. Zika virus disrupts neural progenitor development and leads to microcephaly in mice. Cell Stem Cell. 2016;19:120–6.
51. Gladwyn-Ng I, Cordón-Barris L, Alfano C, Creppe C, Couderc T, Morelli G, Thelen N, America M, Bessières B, Encha-Razavi F, et al. Stress-induced unfolded protein response contributes to Zika virus–associated microcephaly. Nat Neurosci. 2018;21:63–71.
52. Grootjans J, Kaser A, Kaufman RJ, Blumberg RS. The unfolded protein response in immunity and inflammation. Nat Rev Immunol. 2016;16:469–84.
53. Saeed M, Suzuki R, Watanabe N, Masaki T, Tomonaga M, Muhammad A, Kato T, Matsuura Y, Watanabe H, Wakita T. Role of the endoplasmic reticulum-associated degradation (ERAD) pathway in degradation of hepatitis C virus envelope proteins and production of virus particles. J Biol Chem. 2011;286:37264–73.
54. Booth L, Roberts JL, Ecroyd H, Tritsch SR, Bavari S, Reid SP, Proniuk S, Zukiwski A, Jacob A, Sepúlveda CS. AR-12 inhibits multiple chaperones concomitant with stimulating autophagosome formation collectively preventing virus replication. J Cell Physiol. 2016;231:2286–302.

2

Age-related deregulation of TDP-43 after stroke enhances NF-κB-mediated inflammation and neuronal damage

Sai Sampath Thammisetty[1,4], Jordi Pedragosa[2], Yuan Cheng Weng[1], Frédéric Calon[3,4], Anna Planas[2] and Jasna Kriz[1,5]* (iD)

Abstract

Background: TDP-43 has been identified as a disease-associated protein in several chronic neurodegenerative disorders and increasing evidence suggests its potentially pathogenic role following brain injuries. Normally expressed in nucleus, under pathological conditions TDP-43 forms cytoplasmic ubiquitinated inclusions in which it is abnormally phosphorylated and cleaved to generate a 35 and a 25 kDa C-terminal fragments. In the present study, we investigated age-related expression patterns of TDP-43 in neurons and glia and its role as modulator of inflammation following ischemic injury.

Methods: Wild-type and TDP-43 transgenic mice of different age groups were subjected to transient middle cerebral artery occlusion. The role of TDP-43 in modulation of inflammation was assessed using immunofluorescence, Western blot analysis, and in vivo bioluminescence imaging. Finally, post-mortem stroke human brain sections were analyzed for TDP-43 protein by immunohistochemistry.

Results: We report here an age-related increase and formation of ubiquitinated TDP-43 cytoplasmic inclusions after stroke. The observed deregulation in TDP-43 expression patterns was associated with an increase in microglial activation and innate immune signaling as revealed by in vivo bioluminescence imaging and immunofluorescence analysis. The presence of ubiquitinated TDP-43 aggregates and its cleaved TDP-35 and TDP-25 fragments was markedly increased in older, 12-month-old mice leading to larger infarctions and a significant increase in in neuronal death. Importantly, unlike the hallmark neuropathological features associated with chronic neurodegenerative disorders, the TDP-43-positive cytoplasmic inclusions detected after stroke were not phosphorylated. Next, we showed that an increase and/or overexpression of the cytoplasmic TDP-43 drives the pathogenic NF-κB response and further increases levels of pro-inflammatory markers and ischemic injury after stroke in age-dependent manner. Finally, analyses of the post-mortem stroke brain tissues revealed the presence of the cytoplasmic TDP-43 immunoreactive structures after human stroke.

Conclusion: Together, our findings suggest that the level of cytoplasmic TDP-43 increases with aging and may act as an age-related mediator of inflammation and neuronal injury after stroke. Thus, targeting cytoplasmic TDP-43 may have a therapeutic potential after stroke.

Keywords: Post-stroke inflammation, Aging, Acute neurodegeneration, Microglia, Innate immune response, Neuronal injury

* Correspondence: jasna.kriz@fmed.ulaval.ca
[1]CERVO Brain Research Centre, Université Laval, 2601 Chemin de la Canardière, Québec, QC G1J 2G3, Canada
[5]Department of Psychiatry and Neuroscience, Faculty of Medicine, Université Laval, 2601 Chemin de la Canardière, Québec, QC G1J2G3, Canada
Full list of author information is available at the end of the article

Background

Stroke is a leading cause of death and the major cause of long-lasting disabilities in industrialized countries ([1]). Indeed, patients surviving stroke will carry a major risk for development of vascular and/or Alzheimer's style dementia later in the life [2–4]. This risk is particularly elevated in elderly population as various cellular processes are altered in aging. Aging hampers the normal physiology of the cell, leading to a metabolic dysfunction, oxidative stress, inflammation, and/or DNA damage [5–7]. Growing evidence suggests that aging in the brain is associated with a progressive loss of immune homeostasis (a chronic low-level inflammation) leading to an overall increase in the pro-inflammatory cytokines including IL-1β, TNF-α [7, 8]. In keeping with previous evidence, we recently demonstrated that processes associated with aging significantly affect microglia activation patterns and innate immune signaling after stroke in both female and male mice [9, 10]. In particular, we observed a marked deregulation of Toll-like receptor 2 (TLR2) induction patterns in activated microglia followed by alterations in the innate immune downstream signaling events and larger infarctions [9, 10]. However, how aging affects immune signaling in neurons and/or microglia/neurons crosstalk in response to ischemic injury remains unclear.

In a search for proteins that may affect microglia/neuron immune crosstalk in aging brain, we focused our study on transactive response (TAR) DNA binding protein 43 (TDP-43). Generally localized in the nucleus, TDP-43 belongs to the family of heterogeneous nuclear ribonuclear proteins that are highly conserved in different species [11]. TDP-43 regulates gene expression by controlling several processes such as pre-mRNA splicing [11], mRNA stabilization [12], mRNA transport, and translation [13]. TDP-43 has been identified as a major constituent of ubiquitinated nuclear and cytoplasmic inclusions in frontotemporal lobar degeneration [14], ALS [15] and Alzheimer's disease [16, 17]. Normally, localized in the nucleus, under pathological conditions TDP-43 forms insoluble ubiquitinated inclusions in which it is abnormally phosphorylated and cleaved to generate a 35 and a 25 kDa C-terminal fragments lacking the N-terminus nuclear localization signal [15, 18]. In addition to processes associated with chronic neurodegeneration, increasing evidence suggests that deregulation of TDP-43 neurons may occur following brain injuries including single and repetitive traumatic brain injury (TBI) [19, 20], while Uchino and colleagues recently reported presence of TDP-43-positive inclusions in aging brains [21]. To date, the molecular mechanisms by which TDP-43 may induce neurodegeneration and neuronal death remain elusive. However, our previous work suggests that TDP-43 may serve as a modulator of inflammation, acting as co-activator of p65 NF-κB [22]. Here, we hypothesized that gradual age-related accumulation of cytoplasmic TDP-43 may trigger activation of NF-κB pathogenic pathways, leading to a deregulation of innate immune response and thus increasing susceptibility of neurons to ischemic injury.

The current study was designed to identify and characterize the age-related expression patterns of TDP-43 in neurons and microglia and to evaluate its role as modulator of inflammation following ischemic injury. We report here an age-related increase and long-lasting mislocalization of TDP-43 after stroke. The observed accumulation of cytoplasmic TDP-43 was associated with an increase in microglial activation and innate immune signaling seen by in vivo bioluminescence imaging and immunofluorescence analysis. The presence of ubiquitinated TDP-43 aggregates and its cleaved TDP-35 and TDP-25 fragments was markedly increased in older, 12-month-old mice, which showed larger infarctions alongside with an increase in neuronal death. We next showed that increase and/or overexpression of the cytoplasmic TDP-43 drives the NF-κB response and further increase levels of pro-inflammatory markers and ischemic injury after stroke. Overall, our results suggest that TDP-43 may act as an age-related modulator of inflammation after stroke. Based on our results, we propose that therapies targeting cytoplasmic TDP-43 may have a potential to modulate post-ischemic inflammation and to protect dying neurons in the ischemic microenvironment. Of note, the post-mortem analysis of the brains autopsied at different time points after human stroke suggests the presence of TDP-43 immunoreactive structures localized in the cytoplasm of the neurons in periphery and the core region of the ischemic lesion.

Materials and methods
Animals

The wild-type (C57Bl/6) mice of 3 and 12 month old (representing a middle aged mouse group) were selected for study. The TLR2-luc-GFP transgenic reporter mice were developed, validated, and genotyped as described previously [23]. These animals do not develop any overt phenotype and were used for in vivo bioluminescence imaging analysis of microglia activation/innate immune response. The TDP-43 A315T transgenic mice were generated, described, and genotyped as described in [24]. The TDP-43 A315T mice develop age-related cognitive deficits resembling frontotemporal dementia phenotypes. All our transgenic colonies are kept in C57Bl/6 genetic background. All experimental animals used in this study were provided with water and healthy diet and were monitored during the entire experimental protocol. The animals were held in the pathogen-free animal facility of the CERVO Brain Research Institute, 3–5 mice per cage in the controlled environment having the 12 h day and night cycles. To avoid the biological effects of sex on ischemic injury, the experiments were performed on male mice. All the experimental procedures were approved by the Laval University Animal care Ethics Committee and are in accordance with the *Guide to the Care and Use of Experimental Animals* of the Canadian Council on Animal Care.

Surgical procedure

Transient focal cerebral ischemia was induced by unilateral left middle cerebral artery occlusion (MCAO) as described [23]. Wild-type mice of around 3–12 months were selected and unilateral transient focal cerebral ischemia was induced by intraluminal filament occlusion of the left middle cerebral artery (MCA) with a 6–0 silicone-coated monofilament suture for 1 h followed by reperfusion times of 24 h, 48 h, 72 h, 5 days, and 10 days after surgery. The body temperature was maintained at 37 °C with a heating pad.

In vivo bioluminescence imaging

The images were obtained by using IVIS 200 imaging system (Caliper LS-Xenogen, Alameda, CA, USA). Twenty minutes prior to imaging session, the mice were administered with D-luciferin (150 mg/kg bw), a substrate for luciferase dissolved in 0.9% saline. The mice were then anesthetized in 2% isoflurane in 100% oxygen at a flow rate of 2 L/min, placed in a heated light-tight imaging chamber. All the animals were imaged before for baseline expression and then continued at different time points post MCAO. Images were captured using a high sensitivity CCD camera with wavelengths ranging from 300 to 600 nm and exposure time for imaging of brain was set for 1 min. The bioluminescence emission was quantified by determining the total number of photons emitted per second (p/s) using live image 2.5 acquisitions and imaging software. Region of interest measurements were used to convert surface radiance (p/s/cm^2/sr) to source flux or the total flux of photons expressed in photons/second. The data are represented as pseudo-color images indicating light intensity (red and yellow, most intense), which were superimposed over gray-scale reference photographs [25].

Protein lysate preparation and immunoblots

Cytoplasmic and nuclear fractions were obtained as per the protocol described earlier [26, 27]. Five hundred milligrams of fresh brain tissue samples were transferred to 1 ml of cell lysis buffer (10 mM HEPES, 10 mM NaCl, 1 mM KH$_2$PO$_4$, 5 mM MgCl$_2$, phosphatase, and protease inhibitors), and homogenized by applying two strokes in a glass homogenizer. The suspension was incubated for 10 min on ice and then homogenized by applying six strokes in a motorized homogenizer at 250 rpm.

Differential centrifugation was performed after restoration with 100 μl of 2.5 M sucrose. The first round of centrifugation was performed at 6300×g for 10 min at 4 °C. The pellet was collected and suspended in TSE buffer (10 mM Tris, 300 mM sucrose, 1 mM EDTA, 0.1% Non idet P-40, 10× v/w, phosphatase, and protease inhibitors pH 7.5) and homogenized with 30 strokes using a motorized Teflon potter at 250 rpm. The obtained suspension was centrifuged at 4000×g for 5 min. The resulting supernatant was discarded, and the pellet was washed with TSE buffer until the supernatant was clear. Pellet was then suspended in RIPA buffer (50 mM Tris, 1 mM EDTA, 150 mM Nacl, 0.1% SDS, 1% Non-idet P-40, 0.5% sodium deoxycholate, phosphatase, and protease inhibitors) with 2% SDS as nuclear fraction. The supernatant collected from the first round of differential centrifugation was subjected for centrifugation at 10,700 g for around 30 min and the supernatant collected was used as cytoplasmic fraction. The protein lysates from different fractions were quantified by Bradford and subjected for Western blot and co-immunoprecipitation as described previously [24].

Tissue collection and immunohistochemistry

The mice were anesthetized and perfused transcardially with phosphate buffer solution followed by 4% paraformaldehyde at pH 7.4. The brain tissue was post fixed overnight in 4% paraformaldehyde and then cryo-preserved in 30% sucrose. The following procedure was adopted for the study as described earlier [24]. The fixed brains were sliced into 25 μm sections, washed with phosphate buffer saline thrice, and blocked with 5% goat serum for 1 h. The sections were incubated over night with respective primary antibodies—rabbit polyclonal TDP-43 (Protein tech, IL, USA, 1:1000), mouse monoclonal NeuN (Millipore; 1:1000), rabbit polyclonal Iba1 (WAKO; 1:500), rat monoclonal CD11b (serotech 1:500), and caspase-3 (Cell signaling; 1:100), mouse monoclonal ubiquitin (Millipore; 1:500) followed by incubation with respective fluorescent goat Alexa Fluor 488 and 594 (1:500) secondary antibodies (Invitrogen) for 2 h at room temperature. Finally, the microscopic images were captured using confocal microscope (Zeiss) and Apotome (Zeiss Axio vision).

Infarct size

The mice were anesthetized and perfused transcardially using phosphate buffer saline followed by 4% paraformaldehyde solution (pH 7.4). The brains were then sectioned to 25-μm-thick slices and stained with cresyl violet histological stain. The mean stroke area of approximately ten sections from 3 to 12 months old were calculated after 72 h post MCAO by using ImageJ software and expressed as % stroke area.

(%Stroke area = (infarct size / total contra lateral side of the section) × 100) [28].

Cytokine array

The mouse cytokine array (Ray bio Mouse cytokine Antibody Array, C1 series, Ray bio, Inc.) was used to detect the levels of different cytokines in sham, acute, chronic stroke-operated mice. The array was performed according to the manufacturer's instructions. The protein lysates were obtained by homogenization of brains of from respective groups using 1x cell lysis buffer (provided in the kit). The protein concentration was determined for each sample and diluted to 300 μg in 1x blocking buffer. Samples for each group (three mice/group) were pooled and incubated with array membrane overnight at 4 °C. After washes, the membranes were incubated with biotin conjugated primary antibody provided in the kit overnight at 4 °C and next day following successive washes, membranes were incubated with secondary antibody provided for 2 h at room temperature. As per the ray biotech protocol, protein levels were visualized by chemiluminescence and quantified using ImageJ software. The protein levels on each array were standardized against an internal positive control on the array (Lalancette et al. 2007; Bohacek et al. 2012).

Immunohistochemistry/human tissue

As described previously [29], paraffin-embedded human brain sections of 5 μm from the frontal cortical lobe were examined to evaluate reactivity towards TDP-43 protein. The paraffin-embedded sections were deparaffinized in xylene and rehydrated in a descending series of ethanol. Endogenous peroxidases were blocked with 5% hydrogen peroxide in methanol, and antigen retrieval was carried out using sodium citrate buffer for 30 min. Sections were then blocked by using goat serum and incubated overnight with anti-TDP-43 (abnova: E2 clone 1:1000). Next, labeling was detected by using species-specific biotinylated the EnVision™ + System, Peroxidase (Dako, Agilent). Slides were cover slipped using DPX mounting medium (#06522, Sigma). For the used tissues, we obtained written consent from the families for tissue removal after death for diagnostic and research purposes at the Neurological Tissue bank of the Biobank-Hospital Clínic-Institut d'Investigacions Biomèdiques August Pi i Sunyer (IDIBAPS). We also obtained tissue from control subjects stored at this Biobank. The study had the approval of the Ethics Committee of Hospital Clínic de Barcelona (CEIm). Features of the cases are shown in Additional file 1: Table S1.

Statistical analysis

The data quantified and represented as mean ± SEM. Statistical analysis was carried using Prism 7 (Graph Pad Software, La Jolla, CA, USA). Comparison between two groups was achieved by unpaired t test and comparisons between multiple groups were done using one-way ANOVA followed by Tukey's post-hoc multiple comparison test. Statistical significance was defined when $^{***}p < 0.001$, $^{**}p < 0.01$, $^{*}p < 0.05$. In all experimental procedures, n (per group) = 5–10 animal.

Results

Increase in cytoplasmic TDP-43 and pathological TDP-35, TDP-25 fragments in the 12-month-old mice after stroke

The presence of pathological TDP-43-positive inclusions in cytoplasm and nucleus of both the neurons and glia in ALS, FTLD, and Alzheimer's has been widely established [17, 24]. Moreover, growing evidence suggests that TDP-43 may have a role in the acute neurodegeneration/neuroinflammation triggered by different types of brain injuries including TBI and stroke. To better understand the role of TDP-43 in the brain response to ischemic injury, we first characterized the expression pattern of TDP-43 by immunofluorescence staining employing anti-TDP-43 antibody in the wild-type (WT) mice that were subjected to transient MCAO followed by different reperfusion periods. While within the first 24 h after stroke TDP-43 expression was mostly limited to the nuclei, at 48 h after MCAO, few cells start to show cytoplasmic TDP-43, while at 72 h post-stroke till the latest time point analyzed (30 days), most of the cells displayed strong cytoplasmic TDP-43 immunoreactivity (Fig. 1a). Because incidence of stroke increases with aging (peaking at middle age time), we next performed MCAO on 3- and 12-month-old WT mice and asked whether TDP-43 subcellular distribution and expression patterns in control conditions and after stroke are affected by processes of aging. Normally, TDP-43 is a nuclear protein (Fig. 1b, c upper panels) and as shown in Fig. 1d, e, the expression of whole-length TDP-43 from the nuclear lysates isolated from control brains and 72 h post MCAO mice did not show significant difference between 3 and 12 month mice. Because brain injury may trigger formation of the pathological TDP-43 species including TDP-35 and TDP-25 C-terminal fragments, we next asked whether aging may contribute to a formation of pathological TDP-43 species. To address this issue, we analyzed the expression patterns of TDP-43, TDP-35, and TDP-25 fragments in the cytoplasmic lysate collected 72 h post MCAO. While ischemic injury caused mislocalization of TDP-43 into cytoplasm in both age groups (Fig. 1b, c, f), Western blot analysis revealed a significant increase in the expression of whole-length cytoplasmic TDP-43 in the ischemic brains of 12 months compared to 3-month-old mice and corresponding controls (Fig. 1f, g). The same expression pattern was observed for pathological TDP-35 and TDP-25 fragments.

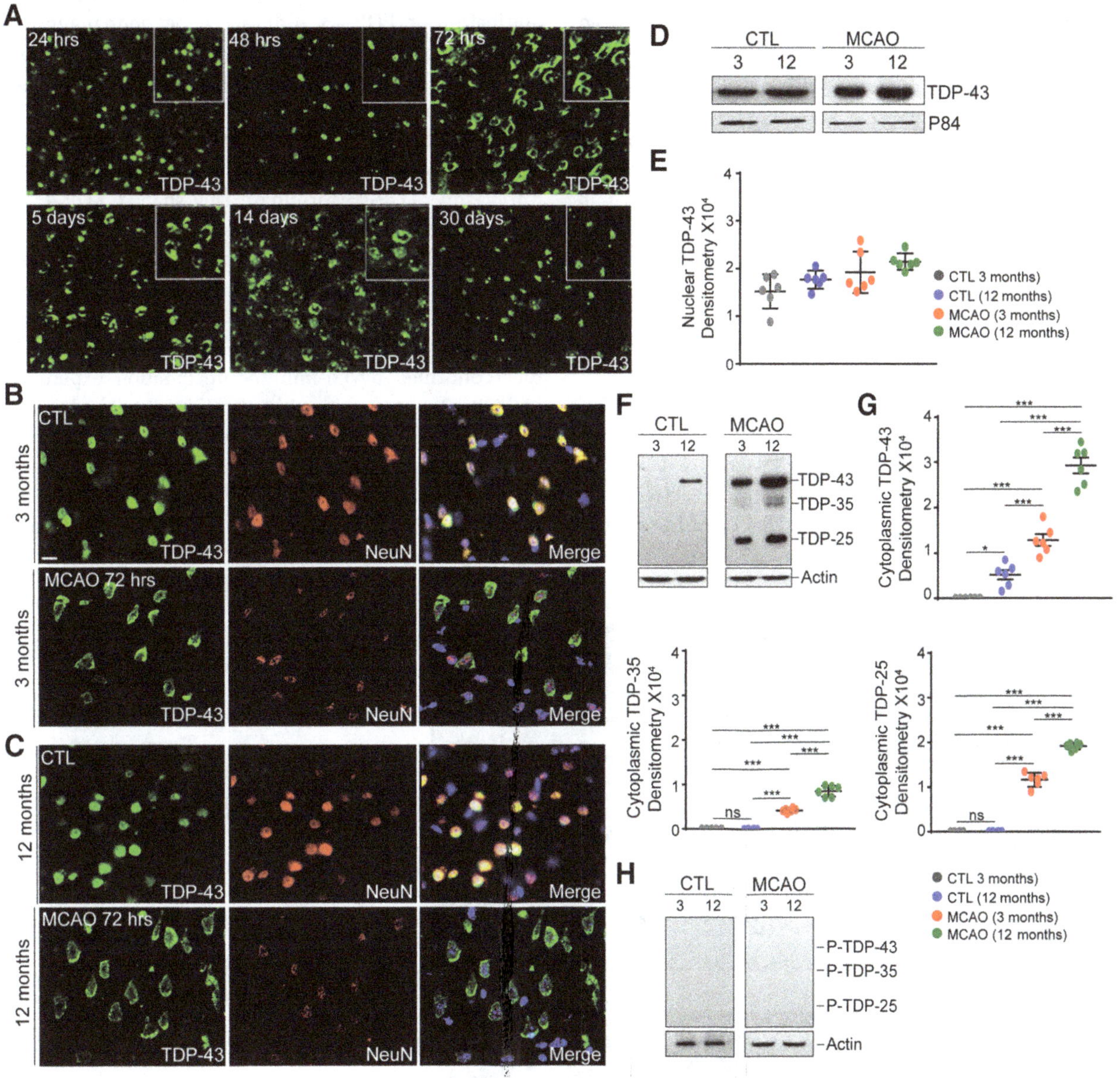

Fig. 1 Characterization of TDP-43 expression patterns in aging and stroke. **a** Immunofluorescence of the brain cortex of wild-type 3-month-old mice using TDP-43 antibody at different time points after MCAO reveals mislocalization of TDP-43 protein into cytoplasm starting 72 h after MCAO. **b** Double immunofluorescence of the brain cortex sections of 3- and **c** 12-month-old mice in control conditions CTL (upper panels) and 72 h after MCAO using TDP-43 antibody (green) and NeuN antibody (red) show nuclear localization of TDP-43 in control conditions and cytoplasmic mislocalization of TDP-43 in neuronal cells in both age groups. **d, e** Western blot of nuclear lysates from 3- and 12-month-old mice using TDP-43 antibody in control and 72 h post MCAO does not reveal any significant changes in the levels of whole length TDP-43. P84 is used as loading control. **f** Western blot of cytoplasmic lysates from 3- and 12-month-old mice using TDP-43 antibody in control and 72 h after MCAO show expression of whole length TDP-43, fragmented TDP-35, and TDP-25. **g** Western blot of cytoplasmic lysates from 3- and 12-month-old mice using phospho-TDP-43 antibody in control and 72 h after MCAO show no expression of whole length P-TDP-43, fragmented P-TDP-35, or P-TDP-25. **h** Normalized densitometry values of immunoblots from control and 72 h after MCAO reveal significant increase in the levels of whole length TDP-43, pathological TDP-35, and TDP-25 fragments in aging. Actin is used as loading control. Quantified data in the figure was presented as mean ± SEM and statistical significance between the groups was achieved using ANOVA followed by Tukey's multiple comparison test and depicted as ***p < 0.001. Scale bar represents 10 and 20 μm

As further revealed in Fig. 1f, ischemic injury in older, 12-month-old animals was associated with significantly higher increase in the expression of pathological cytoplasmic TDP-35 and TDP-25 fragments when compared to 3 month old (Fig. 1f, g). Importantly, the pathological TDP-35 and TDP-25 fragments were not detected in the cytoplasmic lysates from the brains of 3- and 12-month-old controls, non-stroked mice (Fig. 1f, g). Of note, a low amount of full-length cytoplasmic TDP-43 was detected in the brains of non-stroked 12-month-old mice. Taken together, our results suggest that cytoplasmic mislocalization of TDP-43 after stroke may represent a common mechanism of the neuronal response to ischemic injury while formation and expression of pathogenic, truncated TDP-35 and TDP-25 species suggests an age-related process. Importantly, as shown in Fig. 1h, unlike the chronic neurodegeneration, acute brain ischemia did not trigger formation of phosphorylated TDP-43 aggregates.

Formation of TDP-43-ubiquitin aggregates in neurons and TDP-43 mislocalization in microglial cells after MCAO is enhanced in older mice

The main histological feature of neurodegenerative disorders such as ALS/FTLD and to a lesser extent AD is a presence of ubiquitinated TDP-43 immunoreactive cytoplasmic inclusions in neuronal and glial cells. In order to

determine if cerebral ischemia increases the level of ubiquitination of TDP-43 in an age-dependent manner, we performed a double immunofluorescence analysis using anti-TDP-43 and anti-ubiquitin antibodies on 3- and 12-month-old control mice and 72 h after MCAO. As shown in Fig. 2a, a double immunofluorescence analysis revealed a colocalization of ubiquitin staining with the cytoplasmic TDP-43 forming a ring-shaped TDP-43/ubiquitin aggregates. The TDP-43/ubiquitin aggregates were present in the mice of both age groups (Fig. 2a); however, the number of TDP-43/ubiquitin positive inclusions seems to be higher in the ischemic brains of the 12 months mice. These results obtained by immunofluorescence were further confirmed by co-immunoprecipitation experiments of TDP-43 protein with ubiquitin (Fig. 2b). The immunoprecipitation experiments clearly demonstrated that TDP-43 is highly ubiquitinated 72 h after MCAO. The intensity of ubiquitination of TDP-43 was more pronounced in the brains of 12-month-old mice compared to the

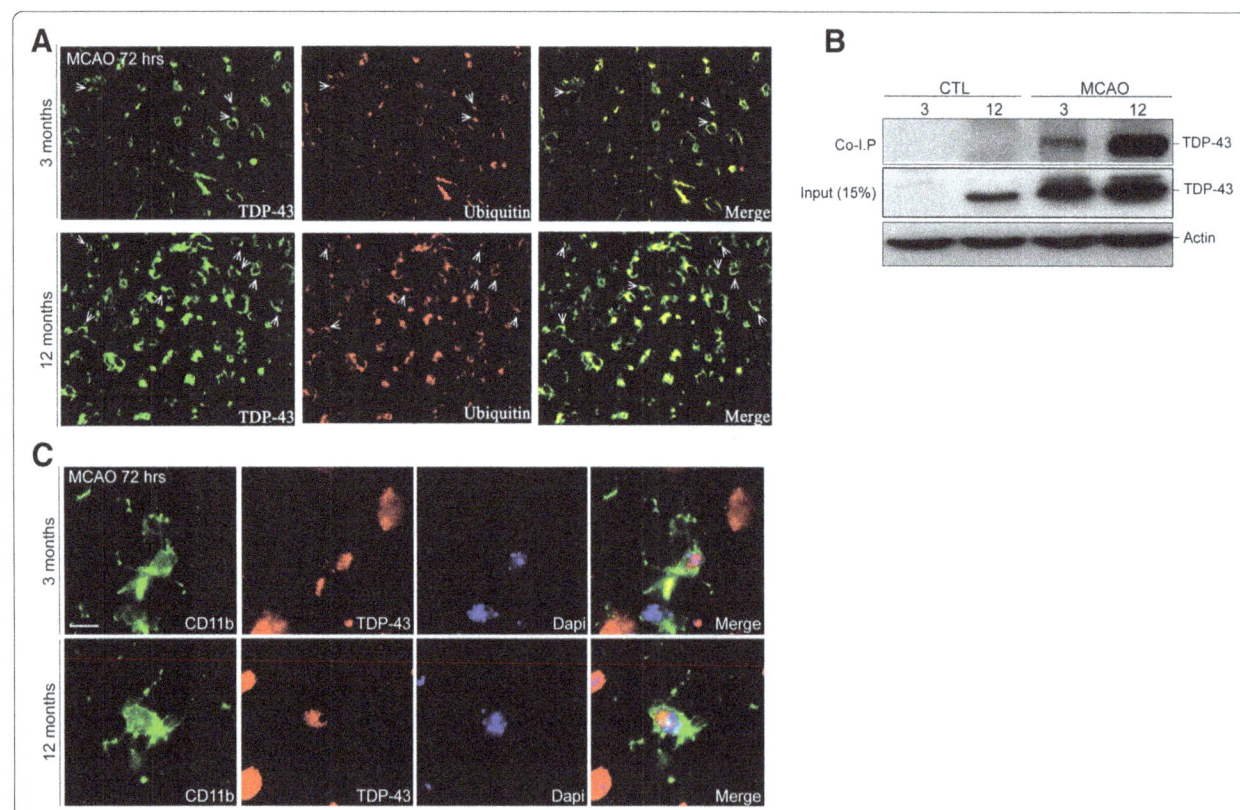

Fig. 2 Cytoplasmic TDP-43 shows ubiquitin positivity and microglia/macrophages exhibit TDP-43 mislocalization. **a** Double immunofluorescence of the brain cortex sections of 3- and 12-month-old mice 72 h after MCAO using TDP-43 antibody (green) and ubiquitin (red) reveal the formation of cytoplasmic TDP-43-ubiquinated aggregates 72 h after MCAO in 3- and 12-month-old mice. **b** Co-immunoprecipitation of ubiquitin using rabbit polyclonal TDP-43 from the cytoplasmic lysates of 3- and 12-month-old control and MCAO operated mice reveal the ubiquitination of TDP-43 after 72 h post MCAO. Note that TDP-43 ubiquitination is increased in 12-month-old transgenic mice after MCAO. Western blot of TDP-43 using rabbit polyclonal TDP-43 is shown as 15% input to confirm the presence of TDP-43 protein in the cytoplasmic lysate we used for Co-immunoprecipitation and actin is shown as loading control. **c** Double immunofluorescence of the brain cortex sections of 3- and 12-month-old mice 72 h after MCAO using TDP-43 antibody (red) and CD11b antibody (green) show mislocalization of TDP-43 in microglial cells in both age groups. Scale bar represents 10 μm

3-month-old mice 72 h after MCAO. Importantly, the control samples of both the age groups were devoid of ubiquitinated TDP-43 protein. Next, we asked whether ischemic injury triggers cytoplasmic mislocalization of TDP-43 in glial cells. As further revealed in Fig. 2c, we observed few microglial cells showing cytoplasmic TDP-43 72 h post MCAO in both age groups suggesting that deregulation of TDP-43 is not only confine to neurons after acute stroke.

Enhanced inflammatory response in aging mice following ischemic injury

Microglial activation coupled with a marked induction of Toll-like receptor 2 (TLR2) are characteristic features of the brain response to ischemic injury [23]. Our previous reports have demonstrated that overexpression of TDP-43 in transgenic mice increases expression of inflammatory markers and TLR2 in glial cells [17, 24]; thus, we hypothesized that increase in TDP-43 levels and the formation of ubiquitin/TDP-43-positive inclusions observed predominately in 12-month-old mice would favor shift of microglial profiles toward pro-inflammatory phenotype resulting in an increase of the TLR2 response after stroke. To visualize microglial activation patterns and TLR2 response after MCAO, we took advantage of the TLR2-luc/GFP reporter mouse model previously generated and validated in our laboratory (Fig. 3a) [23]. In this in vivo model system, the reporter genes luciferase and GFP are co-expressed under transcriptional control of the murine TLR2 gene promoter thus allowing visualization of the luciferase signals from the brains of living mice [23]. Importantly, our previous studies have demonstrated that the TLR2 signal induction represents a valid readout measure of microglia activation after stroke [30–32]. As shown in Fig. 3b, we analyzed and compared the TLR2 signals normalized to a baseline value after stroke in young and old mice. The quantitative analysis of the TLR2 signals after MCAO revealed a significant increase in the TLR2 signal in 12-month-old mice when compared to 3-month-old mice. The differences were more pronounced in the acute phase of the response, i.e., 48–72 h after stroke (Fig. 3a, b). That microglial cells were more activated in the ischemic brains of 12-month-old mice was further confirmed by the quantitative analysis of the standard microglial marker Iba1. As shown in Fig. 3c, Western blot analysis of brain homogenates collected from 3- and 12-month-old mice in control conditions and 72 h after MCAO showed a marked increase in Iba 1 expression levels after stroke when compared to control conditions. The expression of Iba1 was strongly induced by MCAO in both age groups. However, a significantly higher induction of Iba1 was observed in the ischemic brains of the 12-month-old mice when compared to younger mice (Fig. 3c). Importantly when comparing the non-stroke controls, a baseline

expression level of Iba1 was also significantly higher in 12-month-old controls animals when compare to younger animals. Together, these findings suggest the existence of age-dependent processes that are associated with an increase in inflammatory signaling in the brain.

We previously demonstrated that deregulation of TDP-43 observed in a mouse model of ALS/FTDL potentiates NF-κB-mediated pathogenic pathways [22]. We showed that TDP-43 may act as a co-activator of the P65 subunit of NF-κB and helps in the transcription of pro-inflammatory genes leading to release of inflammatory cytokines and causing inflammation-induced neurodegeneration [22]. The active form of P65, the phospho P65 (P-P65), can be used as an indicator of NF-κB-associated inflammation. We next examined whether NF-κB-mediated pathway is activated after stroke and whether the observed age-related increase in cytoplasmic TDP-43 is associated with an increase in P-P65. As shown in Fig. 3d, we quantified the P-P65 level in nuclear lysate from the brains of 3- and 12-month-old controls and acutely stroked mice (72 h post MCAO). The P-P65 levels were found to be significantly up-regulated in 12-month-old mice 72 h post MCAO when compared to 3-month-old mice in the same conditions (Fig. 3d). Although we observed a tendency, there was no significant difference in P-P65 level between 3- and 12-month-old control mice (Fig. 3d). To further asses the age-dependent immune profile of the brain after stroke, as previously described [33], we performed a multiplex cytokine array analysis. We measured expression levels of several pro- and anti-inflammatory cytokines in the brain. As shown in Fig. 3e, analysis of the inflammatory response in the brains of stroked mice revealed an increase in general immune response in the 12-month-old mice 72 h after MCAO. In fact, cytokine array data showed a significant increase in the levels of both the pro- and anti-inflammatory cytokines and chemokines like IL-1β, TNF-α, CCL5, GM-CSF, IL-6, IL-4, IL-10, and IL-17 in this specific group (Fig. 3e).

Larger ischemic lesions and increased neuronal death are observed in 12-month-old mice

We next investigated to what extent the observed age-related deregulation of cytokine response after stroke affects evolution of the post-stroke ischemic injury. As previously described [33] and shown in Fig. 4a, we first measured and compared the size of the ischemic lesion in 3- and 12-month-old mice. The cresyl-violet-stained sections were analyzed 72 h after MCAO. In agreement with previous results, there was a significant, 17.4% increase in the size of ischemic lesion in the 12-month-old mice when compared to 3-month-old mice (Fig. 4a, b). As further shown in Fig. 4c, d, the observed increase in brain damage was

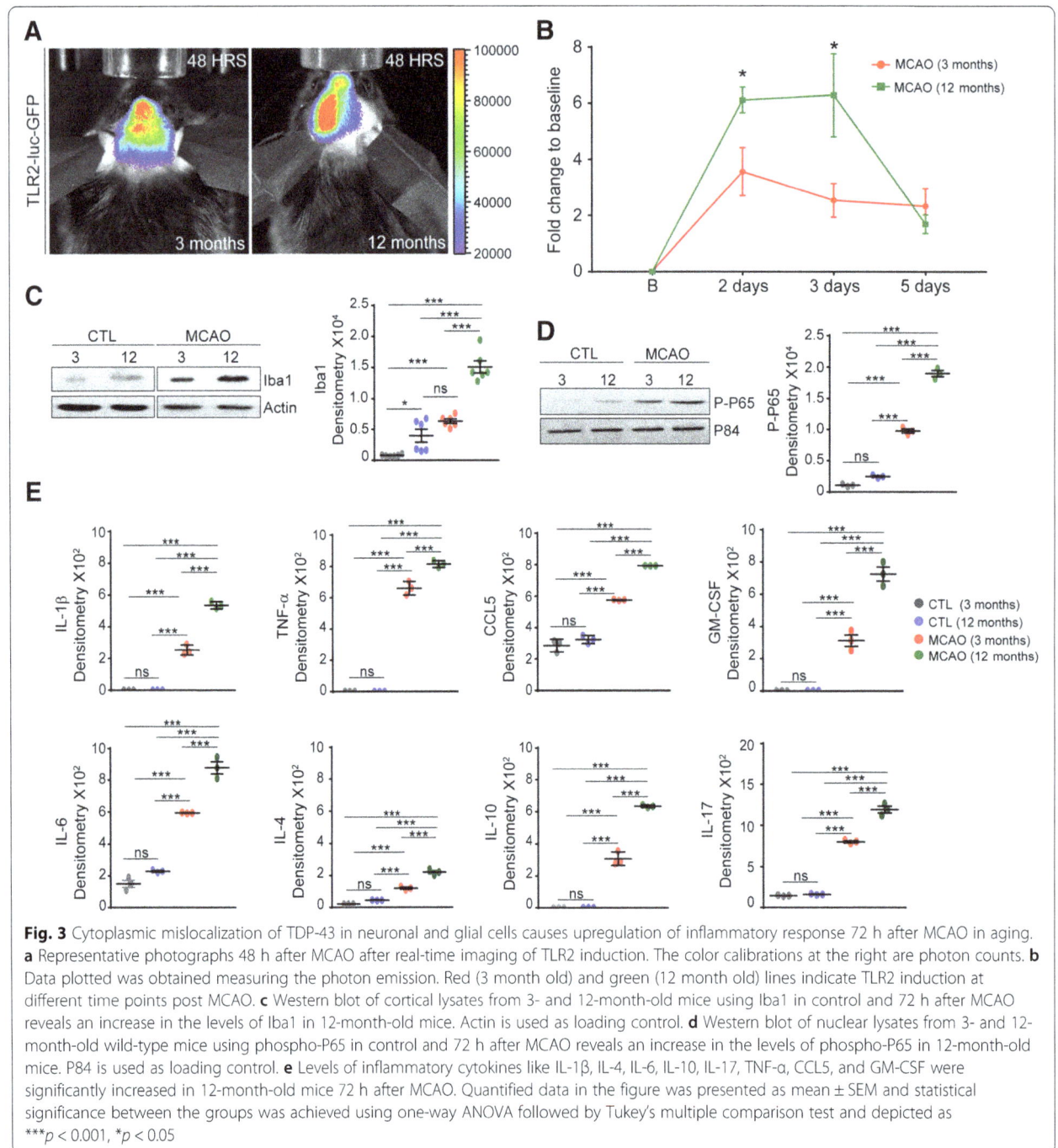

Fig. 3 Cytoplasmic mislocalization of TDP-43 in neuronal and glial cells causes upregulation of inflammatory response 72 h after MCAO in aging. **a** Representative photographs 48 h after MCAO after real-time imaging of TLR2 induction. The color calibrations at the right are photon counts. **b** Data plotted was obtained measuring the photon emission. Red (3 month old) and green (12 month old) lines indicate TLR2 induction at different time points post MCAO. **c** Western blot of cortical lysates from 3- and 12-month-old mice using Iba1 in control and 72 h after MCAO reveals an increase in the levels of Iba1 in 12-month-old mice. Actin is used as loading control. **d** Western blot of nuclear lysates from 3- and 12-month-old wild-type mice using phospho-P65 in control and 72 h after MCAO reveals an increase in the levels of phospho-P65 in 12-month-old mice. P84 is used as loading control. **e** Levels of inflammatory cytokines like IL-1β, IL-4, IL-6, IL-10, IL-17, TNF-α, CCL5, and GM-CSF were significantly increased in 12-month-old mice 72 h after MCAO. Quantified data in the figure was presented as mean ± SEM and statistical significance between the groups was achieved using one-way ANOVA followed by Tukey's multiple comparison test and depicted as ***$p < 0.001$, *$p < 0.05$

accompanied by an increase in cellular death/apoptosis. Namely, a Western blot analysis of brain tissue homogenates from the ipsilateral/ischemic region of the brain showed a significant, twofold increase in the expression levels of the cleaved caspase-3 in the ischemic brains of 12-month-old mice, 72 h after MCAO (Fig. 4d). Next, a double immunofluorescence analysis revealed that the vast majority of the cleaved caspase-3 expressing cells were positive for neuronal marker NeuN (Fig. 4e). In accordance with our

previous work [31, 34], this suggests that neurons are the principal cell type undergoing cellular stress and apoptosis after MCAO.

TDP-43 cytoplasmic mislocalization exacerbates ischemic injury and neuroinflammation after stroke

Previous evidence suggests that cytoplasmic mislocalization of TDP-43 and formation of ubiquitinated aggregates is toxic to neurons and may enhance neuroinflammation [22, 24, 35]. Here, we hypothesized

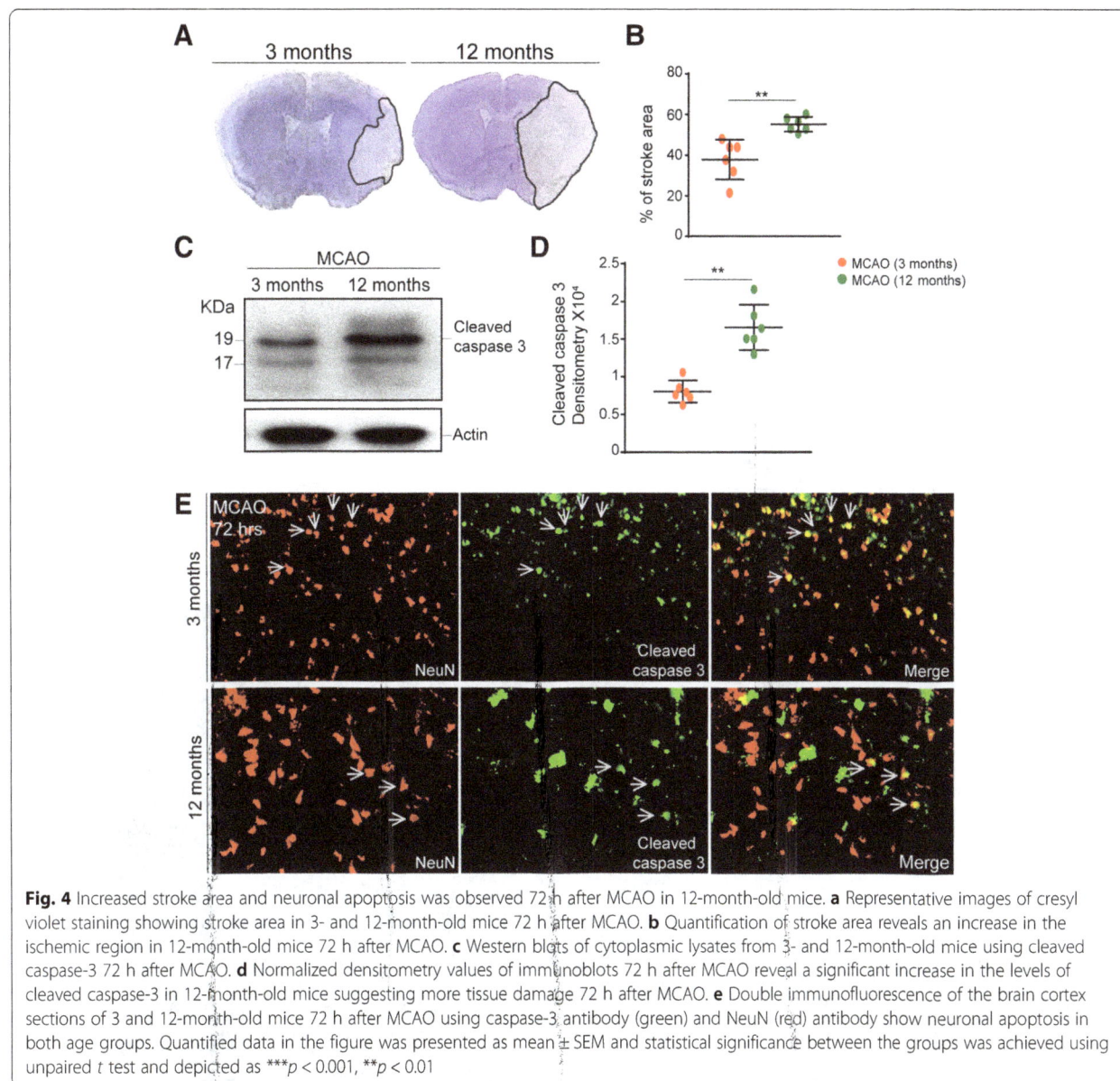

Fig. 4 Increased stroke area and neuronal apoptosis was observed 72 h after MCAO in 12-month-old mice. **a** Representative images of cresyl violet staining showing stroke area in 3- and 12-month-old mice 72 h after MCAO. **b** Quantification of stroke area reveals an increase in the ischemic region in 12-month-old mice 72 h after MCAO. **c** Western blots of cytoplasmic lysates from 3- and 12-month-old mice using cleaved caspase-3 72 h after MCAO. **d** Normalized densitometry values of immunoblots 72 h after MCAO reveal a significant increase in the levels of cleaved caspase-3 in 12-month-old mice suggesting more tissue damage 72 h after MCAO. **e** Double immunofluorescence of the brain cortex sections of 3 and 12-month-old mice 72 h after MCAO using caspase-3 antibody (green) and NeuN (red) antibody show neuronal apoptosis in both age groups. Quantified data in the figure was presented as mean ± SEM and statistical significance between the groups was achieved using unpaired t test and depicted as ***$p < 0.001$, **$p < 0.01$

that age-related increase in the cytoplasmic TDP-43 observed in the brains of 12-month-old mice in control conditions and after stroke alters the immune microenvironment and may increase the susceptibility of neurons to ischemic damage. To test our hypothesis, we took advantage or the transgenic TDP-43 mice with moderate and ubiquitous overexpression of human TDP-43 (Tg line A315T). Importantly, at young age, starting at 2–3 months, these mice show an increase in cytoplasmic/ubiquitinated TDP-43 in neurons and glial cells, corresponding (resembling) to TDP-43 expression levels and/or expression patterns in aged, 12-month-old WT mice. In keeping with our hypothesis and as shown in Fig. 5a, b, the size of ischemic lesion was significantly increased in TDP-43 transgenic mice when compared to WT aged-matched littermates. Here, it

is noteworthy that the observed increase in the size of ischemic lesion was corresponding to a size of ischemic lesion observed in 12-month-old mice (Figs. 3a and 4a). As shown by Western blot analysis, the cleaved caspase-3 expression levels were significantly increased in the ischemic brains of TDP-43 transgenic mice (Fig. 5c, d). A double immunofluorescence labeling for neuronal markers NeuN and cleaved caspase-3 revealed a marked co-localization of these two markers indicating an increase in the number of apoptotic neurons in the ischemic brains of TDP-43 transgenic mice (Fig. 5e). Next, we asked whether observed exacerbation of the ischemic injury and injury-induced neuronal apoptosis is caused by an increase in NF-κB-mediated inflammation. As described above (see Fig. 5f, g), we measured the levels of nuclear P65, an

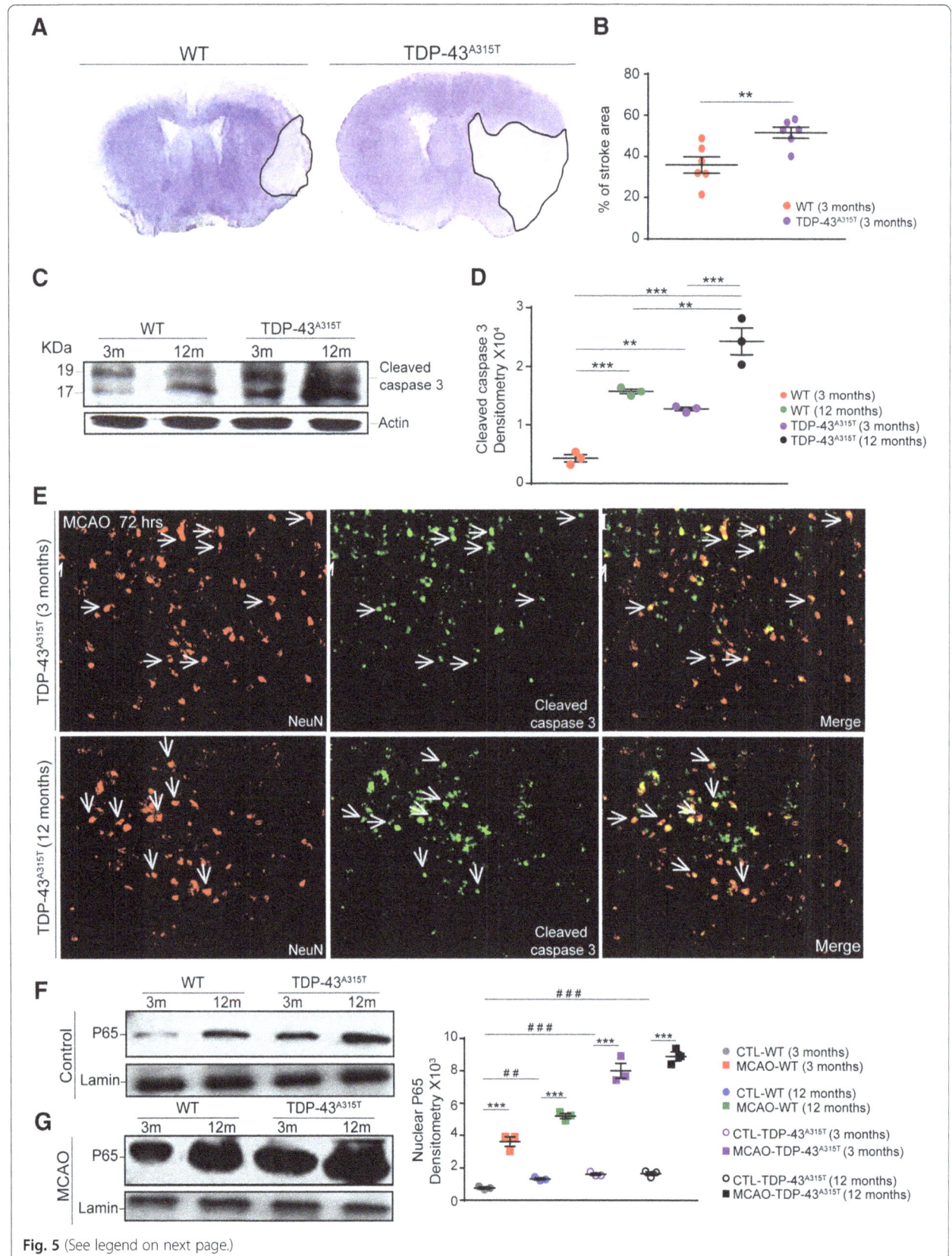

A

WT   TDP-43^A315T

B

C

KDa

WT   TDP-43^A315T
3m   12m   3m   12m

19
17

Cleaved
caspase 3

Actin

D

E

MCAO 72 hrs

TDP-43^A315T (3 months)

NeuN   Cleaved
              caspase 3   Merge

TDP-43^A315T (12 months)

NeuN   Cleaved
              caspase 3   Merge

F

Control

WT   TDP-43^A315T
3m   12m   3m   12m

P65

Lamin

G

MCAO

WT   TDP-43^A315T
3m   12m   3m   12m

P65

Lamin

Fig. 5 (See legend on next page.)

(See figure on previous page.)
Fig. 5 Overexpression of TDP-43 increases brain damage and inflammatory response after stroke. **a** Representative image of cresyl violet staining showing stroke area in 3-month-old WT and TDP-43^{A315T} 72 h after MCAO. **b** Quantification of stroke area reveals an increase in the ischemic lesion in TDP-43^{A315T} compared to WT mice. **c** Western blots of cytoplasmic lysates coming from 3- and 12-month-old WT and TDP-43^{A315T} mice using cleaved caspase-3. **d** Quantification of immunoblots 72 h after MCAO reveal a significant increase in the levels of cleaved caspase-3 in 12-month-old TDP-43^{A315T} mice when compared to the 3-month TDP-43^{A315T} or the 12-month-old WT control. **e** Double immunofluorescence of the brain cortex sections of 3- and 12-month-old TDP-43^{A315T} mice 72 h after MCAO using caspase-3 antibody (green) and NeuN (red) antibody show neuronal apoptosis in both age mice. **f** Expression of P65 by revealed by Western blot in control mice (3- and 12-month-old WT and TDP-43^{A315T}). **g** Expression of P65 by revealed by Western blot 72 h after MCAO (3- and 12-month-old WT and TDP-43^{A315T}). Normalized densitometry values of Western blot reveal a general significant increase in the levels of P65 after MCAO in either age group or mice. 3- and 12-month-old TDP-43^{A315T} show a higher P65 base level compared to the 3-month-old WT control. Quantified data in the figure was presented as mean ± SEM and statistical significance between the groups was achieved using unpaired t test and depicted as ***$p < 0.001$, **$p < 0.01$

indicator of NF-κB-associated inflammation, in nuclear lysate from the brains of 3- and 12-month-old controls and TDP-43 transgenic mice in control conditions and following stroke (72 h post MCAO). As further shown in Fig. 5f, g, the expression of nuclear P65 is significantly increased in 12-month-old WT mice when compared to young WT controls. Interestingly, as shown in Fig. 5f, g, the expression of nuclear P65 is at comparable levels between old controls and 3-month-old TDP-43 transgenic mice thus suggesting a correlation of cytoplasmic TDP-43 levels and NF-κB activation.

Increase in the cytoplasmic TDP-43 immunoreactivity in human stroke

At present, it remains unclear to what extent and/or whether TDP-43 pathology is associated with ischemic injury in human stroke. To address this issue, we performed immunohistochemistry analyses of the post-mortem post-stroke brain tissue autopsied at 1 to 5 days after stroke. The analysis was performed by focusing on two distinct region of the ischemic lesion, the peri-infarct and core region (cortical sections) and compared with corresponding controls. The analysis was performed using a human anti-TDP-43 antibody (Fig. 6a, b). As shown in Fig. 6a, control sections stained with an anti-human TDP-43 antibody displayed well-circumscribed and positively stained nuclei, while the cytoplasmic compartment was almost completely devoid of TDP-43 immunoreactivity. Interestingly, resembling the TDP-43 expression patterns following single traumatic brain injury in humans [20], the TDP-43 staining following acute ischemic stroke revealed increased immunoreactivity within the cytoplasm and in some cases extending

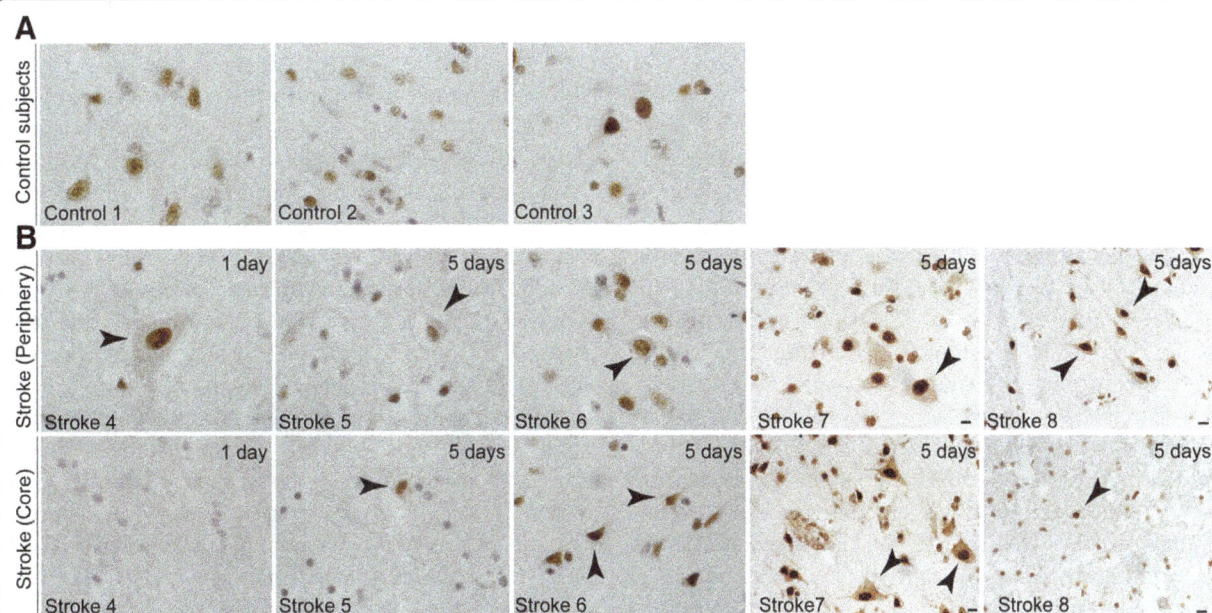

Fig. 6 TDP-43 immunoreactivity in human stroke. **a** Immunohistochemistry of a control contralateral and non-affected hemisphere of the human subjects using anti human TDP-43 antibody reveals the localization of TDP-43 in the nucleus. **b** TDP-43 immunohistochemistry on cortical sections of human subjects died 1 day (stroke 4) and 5 days (stroke 5, 6, 7, 8) after ischemic stroke reveals the localization of TDP-43 in the cytoplasm of neurons in the periphery and core regions of the ischemia, which is indicated with arrow marks in black. Scale bar represents 20 μm

into processes (Fig. 6b). The increase in the cytoplasmic TDP-43 immunoreactivity was more prominent at day 5 after stroke. Hence, ischemic stroke in humans is associated with an increase in TDP-43 immunoreactivity in the cytoplasmic compartment. However, unlike the TDP-43 expression patterns observed in the chronic TDP-43 proteinopathies, in stroke, the nuclei remain positively stained for TDP-43.

Discussion

The work presented here provides an important in vivo evidence for a pathogenic role of TDP-43 in stroke. Based on the results presented in this study, we propose here that age-related deregulation of TDP-43 exacerbates inflammation and ischemic injury and may contribute to post-stroke neurodegenerative processes. By investigating TDP-43 expression patterns after stroke in young and 12-month-old mice, we showed (i) a marked increase and accumulation of TDP-43 in cytoplasmic compartment in neurons and microglia (ii) levels of mislocalized/cytoplasmic TDP-43 and its cleaved pathogenic fragments TDP-35 and TDP-25 were more elevated in aged mice, (iii) observed deregulation of TDP-43 was associated with an increase in post-stroke inflammation and larger infarctions, (iv) overexpression of TDP-43 further exacerbated ischemic injury and markedly enhances inflammation via activation of NF-κB, and (v) mislocalization of TDP-43 into cytoplasmic compartment occurred also in human stroke.

Cerebral ischemia is characterized by a marked acute and chronic inflammatory response. We and others have shown that post-stroke inflammation may have a marked chronic component that may last several months following an initial ischemic event and may contribute to development of the chronic brain injury [23, 36]. However, the molecular mechanisms driving the long-lasting post-stroke inflammation, and potentially leading to a neurodegeneration, remain elusive. Based on the results described in the current study, we hypothesized that the age-related accumulation of TDP-43 in the cytoplasm (see Fig. 2) may drive chronic inflammation after stroke and thus contribute to ischemic injury.

To date, little is known about the role of TDP-43 in the pathogenesis of stroke. The alterations in TDP-43 expression in response to ischemic injury have been recently described by Kanazawa and colleagues in an acute rat model of ischemic injury [37]. However, the study has been limited to a 24 h after stroke time period [37]. Our findings are generally in agreement with the initial report. However, we observed a long-lasting (up to 30 days post MCAO) cytoplasmic accumulation/deregulation of TDP-43 after stroke (Fig. 1). In addition, our study extends the initial report in several ways. First, in keeping with recent report of the TDP-43 contribution

in aging, we investigated the expression patterns of the TDP-43 after stroke in two different age groups (3 and 12 month old). Importantly, our results revealed markedly increased accumulation of the cytoplasmic TDP-43 in older mice. The fact that in older mice the cytoplasmic TSP-43 was present even at the baseline levels may have significantly affected the initial brain response to ischemic injury. Indeed, the levels of pathogenic TDP-35 and TDP-25 fragments after stroke were significantly increased in 12-month-old mice when compared to young animals, thus further suggesting a strong component of aging in TDP-43 mediated pathology. As previously mentioned, TDP-43 expression is normally restricted to nucleus and has a role in the regulation of gene transcription, mRNA splicing, mRNA stability, and transport. However, in pathological conditions, TDP-43 becomes mislocalized to the cytoplasm of both neurons and glial cells and cleaved by the caspases into 35 kDa and 25 kDa fragments to form potentially pathogenic aggregates [38].

Here, we presume that cytoplasmic accumulation of TDP-43 during ischemic stroke occurred because of deregulation of its nuclear import. In fact, the C-terminal fragments of TDP-43 that are formed during aging/stress lack functional nuclear localization signal [39]. Cytoplasmic accumulation of TDP-43 protein was reported in different neurodegenerative diseases [37, 40] [17]. For example, development of many age-related pathological and biochemical changes like formation of C-terminal TDP-43 fragments, TDP-43/ubiquitin aggregates, and neuroinflammation have been reported in mouse model of ALS [41]. Indeed, in TDP-43 proteinopathies, dying neurons display the presence of ubiquitin inclusions as the ubiquitin-dependent protein degradation pathways were hampered [42]. Another important feature of TDP-43 proteinopathies is a presence of phosphoTDP-43 aggregates. Evidence suggests that casein kinase 1 phosphorylates TDP-43 to form insoluble phosphoTDP-43 aggregates in most of the TDP-43 proteinopathies [43]. To investigate the formation and presence of insoluble phosphoTDP-43 aggregates after ischemic injury and in aging, we collected urea-SDS insoluble fraction and performed immunoblots. Surprisingly, we did not detect phosphorylated TDP-43 aggregates in any of tested age groups after stroke, suggesting that TDP-43 pathology has distinct molecular signature after stroke when compared to chronic neurodegenerative TDP-43 proteinopathies.

Another hallmark of the brain response to ischemic injury and neurodegeneration is activation of glial cells. Indeed, previous studies reported TDP-43 cytoplasmic inclusions glial cells in the spinal cords of the ALS patients [15] while in vitro studies using microglia and astrocyte culture exhibits TDP-43 mislocalization in induced neuroinflammatory conditions [41]. Furthermore, our previous studies have demonstrated that binding of its N-terminal and RRM1 domains to p65, TDP-43 acts as co-activator of p65 NF-kB thus leading to enhanced activation of the NF-κB pathways [22]. Importantly, NF-κB may interact with specific proteins and DNA sequences to trigger inflammation and ischemic injury-induced neuronal apoptosis [44]. It was reported that NF-κB translocate to the nucleus from the cytoplasm in cerebral ischemic injury [45]. Indeed, in the present study, we demonstrated a TDP-43-mediated deregulation and activation of NF-κB pathway. We measured the nuclear phosphorylation levels of P65 subunit of NF-κB after stroke in both 3- and 12-month-old mice. We observed that after the ischemic injury, the phospho-P65 subunit travels to the nucleus from the cytoplasm in both groups. There was an increased amount of phospho-P65 subunit in the nucleus of 12-month-old mice compared to 3-month-old mice 72 h after MCAO. In an additional *proof-of-concept* experiments using TDP-43 A315T transgenic mice that overexpress TDP-43 in the cytoplasm, at the similar levels as 12-month-old WT mice, we observed comparable levels of nuclear phosphorylation levels of P65 subunit of NF-κB after stroke.

An important question here is how deregulation of TDP-43 affects neuronal survival and microglia-neuron crosstalk after ischemic injury. Substantial loss of nuclear TDP-43 in ischemic neurons may lead to nuclear dysfunction. Indeed, a series of in vitro experiments showed that TDP-43 depletion/silencing may cause disturbance in cell cycle leading to cell death [46]. Additional evidence suggests that TDP-25 fragments formed in the cytoplasm of neurons can gain toxic functions and thus cause tissue damage albeit the mechanism remains unknown [47]. Importantly, both of these neuropathological features were detected in ischemic brain tissue and affected neurons. Therefore, we examined whether the observed age-related TDP-43 deregulation may lead ultimately lead to more neuronal damage. Indeed, we found a significantly larger infarctions in the 12-month-old than 3-month-old mice 72 h after MCAO as well as an increased in cleaved caspase-3 levels in aging brain after 72 h post ischemia, while the analyses of the ischemic lesion in the context of TDP-43 cytoplasmic overexpression also showed direct correlation between TDP-43 expression levels and the size of the ischemic lesion. The important question that has been raised here is whether the observed deregulation in TDP-43 expression patterns is present in human stroke? Importantly, analyses of the post-mortem and post-stroke brain tissues revealed the presence of the cytoplasmic TDP-43 immunoreactive structures in human stroke resembling those observed after single brain trauma [20].

Together, our results suggest that deregulation of TDP-43 may represent a converging pathogenic pathway that drives neuroinflammation following acute brain injuries and in chronic neurodegeneration.

Conclusion

In conclusion, ischemic injury is associated with a marked and age-related deregulation of TDP-43. Further, we observed a significant increase in TDP-43-mediated modulation of NF-κB neuroinflammation leading to increase in neuronal injury and neurodegeneration after stroke. Although the stroked tissue did not display the full neuropathological feature associated with chronic TDP-43 proteinopathies, i.e., the presence of highly phosphorylated TDP-43 aggregates and complete depletion of nuclear TDP-43, we showed that ischemic injury may cause a long-lasting cytoplasmic accumulation of TDP-43. Thus, it is possible that deregulation of TDP-43 observed after the initial ischemic event may drive chronic post-stroke inflammatory response and may represent an age-related risk factor for development of neurodegenerative disorders. Based on our results, we propose that therapies targeting mislocalized/cytoplasmic TDP-43 may have a potential to attenuate post-stroke inflammation and ischemia-induced neuronal injury.

Abbreviations
CCD: Charge coupled device; CCL5: Chemokine C-C motif ligand 5; GM-CSF: Granulocyte-macrophage colony stimulating factor; MCAO: Middle cerebral artery occlusion; NF-κB: Nuclear factor kappa B; TDP-43: Transactive response (TAR) DNA binding protein 43 (TDP-43); TLR2: Toll-like receptor 2; WT: Wild type

Acknowledgements
Not applicable.

Funding
Canadian Institutes for Health Research (CIHR-No 93768) and Heart and stroke Foundation Canada (G-17-0018372) to JK, Canadian Consortium for Neurodegenerative Diseases and Aging (CCNA-Team 2) (JK). SST is recipient of Scholarship from Alzheimer Society of Canada.

Authors' contributions
SST is responsible for generation of all data. SST analyzed all the figures and wrote the manuscript. JP and AP analyzed post-mortem human brain samples. YCW is responsible for inducing stroke in mice models and genotyping data. FC helped in designing the work. JK conceived the study, participated in the experimental design, and wrote the manuscript. All the authors have read and approved the manuscript.

Competing interests

The authors declare that they have no competing interests.

Author details

[1]CERVO Brain Research Centre, Université Laval, 2601 Chemin de la Canardière, Québec, QC G1J 2G3, Canada. [2]IDIBAPS, Barcelona, Spain. [3]Research Centre of the CHUQ, Université Laval, Québec, QC G1J2G3, Canada. [4]Faculty of Pharmacy, Université Laval, Québec, QC G1J2G3, Canada. [5]Department of Psychiatry and Neuroscience, Faculty of Medicine, Université Laval, 2601 Chemin de la Canardière, Québec, QC G1J2G3, Canada.

References

1. Hankey GJ. Stroke: how large a public health problem, and how can the neurologist help? Arch Neurol. 1999;56:748–54.
2. Stephenson J. Rising stroke rates spur efforts to identify risks, prevent disease. JAMA. 1998;279:1239–40.
3. Fisher M, Bogousslavsky J. Further evolution toward effective therapy for acute ischemic stroke. JAMA. 1998;279:1298–303.
4. Savva GM, Stephan BC. Alzheimer's society vascular dementia systematic review G: epidemiological studies of the effect of stroke on incident dementia: a systematic review. Stroke. 2010;41:e41–6.
5. Houtkooper RH, Argmann C, Houten SM, Canto C, Jeninga EH, Andreux PA, Thomas C, Doenlen R, Schoonjans K, Auwerx J. The metabolic footprint of aging in mice. Sci Rep. 2011;1:134.
6. Sandu RE, Buga AM, Uzoni A, Petcu EB, Popa-Wagner A. Neuroinflammation and comorbidities are frequently ignored factors in CNS pathology. Neural Regen Res. 2015;10:1349–55.
7. Buga AM, Di Napoli M, Popa-Wagner A. Preclinical models of stroke in aged animals with or without comorbidities: role of neuroinflammation. Biogerontology. 2013;14:651–62.
8. Jiang T, Cadenas E. Astrocytic metabolic and inflammatory changes as a function of age. Aging Cell. 2014;13:1059–67.
9. Cordeau P Jr, Lalancette-Hebert M, Weng YC, Kriz J. Estrogen receptors alpha mediates postischemic inflammation in chronically estrogen-deprived mice. Neurobiol Aging. 2016;40:50–60.
10. Rahimian R, Cordeau P Jr, Kriz J. Brain response to injuries: when microglia go sexist. Neuroscience. 2018. In press. https://doi.org/10.1016/j.neuroscience.2018.02.048.
11. Wang HY, Wang IF, Bose J, Shen CK. Structural diversity and functional implications of the eukaryotic TDP gene family. Genomics. 2004;83:130–9.
12. Strong MJ, Volkening K, Hammond R, Yang W, Strong W, Leystra-Lantz C, Shoesmith C. TDP43 is a human low molecular weight neurofilament (hNFL) mRNA-binding protein. Mol Cell Neurosci. 2007;35:320–7.
13. Wang IF, Wu LS, Chang HY, Shen CK. TDP-43, the signature protein of FTLD-U, is a neuronal activity-responsive factor. J Neurochem. 2008;105:797–806.
14. Mackenzie IR, Neumann M, Bigio EH, Cairns NJ, Alafuzoff I, Kril J, Kovacs GG, Ghetti B, Halliday G, Holm IE, et al. Nomenclature and nosology for neuropathologic subtypes of frontotemporal lobar degeneration: an update. Acta Neuropathol. 2010;119:1–4.
15. Arai T, Hasegawa M, Akiyama H, Ikeda K, Nonaka T, Mori H, Mann D, Tsuchiya K, Yoshida M, Hashizume Y, Oda T. TDP-43 is a component of ubiquitin-positive tau-negative inclusions in frontotemporal lobar degeneration and amyotrophic lateral sclerosis. Biochem Biophys Res Commun. 2006;351:602–11.
16. Chang XL, Tan MS, Tan L, Yu JT. The role of TDP-43 in Alzheimer's disease. Mol Neurobiol. 2016;53:3349–59.
17. Tremblay C, St-Amour I, Schneider J, Bennett DA, Calon F. Accumulation of transactive response DNA binding protein 43 in mild cognitive impairment and Alzheimer disease. J Neuropathol Exp Neurol. 2011;70:788–98.
18. Neumann M, Sampathu DM, Kwong LK, Truax AC, Micsenyi MC, Chou TT, Bruce J, Schuck T, Grossman M, Clark CM, et al. Ubiquitinated TDP-43 in frontotemporal lobar degeneration and amyotrophic lateral sclerosis. Science. 2006;314:130–3.
19. Smith DH, Johnson VE, Stewart W. Chronic neuropathologies of single and repetitive TBI: substrates of dementia? Nat Rev Neurol. 2013;9:211–21.
20. Johnson VE, Stewart W, Trojanowski JQ, Smith DH. Acute and chronically increased immunoreactivity to phosphorylation-independent but not

21. pathological TDP-43 after a single traumatic brain injury in humans. Acta Neuropathol. 2011;122:715–26.
21. Uchino A, Takao M, Hatsuta H, Sumikura H, Nakano Y, Nogami A, Saito Y, Arai T, Nishiyama K, Murayama S. Incidence and extent of TDP-43 accumulation in aging human brain. Acta Neuropathol Commun. 2015;3:35.
22. Swarup V, Phaneuf D, Dupre N, Petri S, Strong M, Kriz J, Julien JP. Deregulation of TDP-43 in amyotrophic lateral sclerosis triggers nuclear factor kappaB-mediated pathogenic pathways. J Exp Med. 2011;208:2429–47.
23. Lalancette-Hebert M, Phaneuf D, Soucy G, Weng YC, Kriz J. Live imaging of toll-like receptor 2 response in cerebral ischaemia reveals a role of olfactory bulb microglia as modulators of inflammation. Brain. 2009;132:940–54.
24. Swarup V, Phaneuf D, Bareil C, Robertson J, Rouleau GA, Kriz J, Julien JP. Pathological hallmarks of amyotrophic lateral sclerosis/frontotemporal lobar degeneration in transgenic mice produced with TDP-43 genomic fragments. Brain. 2011;134:2610–26.
25. Cordeau P Jr, Lalancette-Hebert M, Weng YC, Kriz J. Live imaging of neuroinflammation reveals sex and estrogen effects on astrocyte response to ischemic injury. Stroke. 2008;39:935–42.
26. Guillemin I, Becker M, Ociepka K, Friauf E, Nothwang HG. A subcellular prefractionation protocol for minute amounts of mammalian cell cultures and tissue. Proteomics. 2005;5:35–45.
27. Wils H, Kleinberger G, Janssens J, Pereson S, Joris G, Cuijt I, Smits V, Ceuterick-de Groote C, Van Broeckhoven C, Kumar-Singh S. TDP-43 transgenic mice develop spastic paralysis and neuronal inclusions characteristic of ALS and frontotemporal lobar degeneration. Proc Natl Acad Sci U S A. 2010;107:3858–63.
28. Tureyen K, Vemuganti R, Sailor KA, Dempsey RJ. Infarct volume quantification in mouse focal cerebral ischemia: a comparison of triphenyltetrazolium chloride and cresyl violet staining techniques. J Neurosci Methods. 2004;139:203–7.
29. Kwong LK, Irwin DJ, Walker AK, Xu Y, Riddle DM, Trojanowski JQ, Lee VM. Novel monoclonal antibodies to normal and pathologically altered human TDP-43 proteins. Acta Neuropathol Commun. 2014;2:33.
30. Lalancette-Hebert M, Faustino J, Thammisetty SS, Chip S, Vexler ZS, Kriz J. Live imaging of the innate immune response in neonates reveals differential TLR2 dependent activation patterns in sterile inflammation and infection. Brain Behav Immun. 2017;65:312–27.
31. Lalancette-Hebert M, Swarup V, Beaulieu JM, Bohacek I, Abdelhamid E, Weng YC, Sato S, Kriz J. Galectin-3 is required for resident microglia activation and proliferation in response to ischemic injury. J Neurosci. 2012; 32:10383–95.
32. Lalancette-Hebert M, Julien C, Cordeau P, Bohacek I, Weng YC, Calon F, Kriz J. Accumulation of dietary docosahexaenoic acid in the brain attenuates acute immune response and development of postischemic neuronal damage. Stroke. 2011;42:2903–9.
33. Bohacek I, Cordeau P, Lalancette-Hebert M, Gorup D, Weng YC, Gajovic S, Kriz J. Toll-like receptor 2 deficiency leads to delayed exacerbation of ischemic injury. J Neuroinflammation. 2012;9:191.
34. Lalancette-Hebert M, Gowing G, Simard A, Weng YC, Kriz J. Selective ablation of proliferating microglial cells exacerbates ischemic injury in the brain. J Neurosci. 2007;27:2596–605.
35. Dutta K, Patel P, Rahimian R, Phaneuf D, Julien JP. Withania somnifera reverses Transactive response DNA binding protein 43 Proteinopathy in a mouse model of amyotrophic lateral sclerosis/Frontotemporal lobar degeneration. Neurotherapeutics. 2017;14:447–62.
36. Radlinska BA, Ghinani SA, Lyon P, Jolly D, Soucy JP, Minuk J, Schirrmacher R, Thiel A. Multimodal microglia imaging of fiber tracts in acute subcortical stroke. Ann Neurol. 2009;66:825–32.
37. Kanazawa M, Kakita A, Igarashi H, Takahashi T, Kawamura K, Takahashi H, Nakada T, Nishizawa M, Shimohata T. Biochemical and histopathological alterations in TAR DNA-binding protein-43 after acute ischemic stroke in rats. J Neurochem. 2011;116:957–65.
38. Buratti E, Baralle FE. The molecular links between TDP-43 dysfunction and neurodegeneration. Adv Genet. 2009;66:1–34.
39. Winton MJ, Igaz LM, Wong MM, Kwong LK, Trojanowski JQ, Lee VM. Disturbance of nuclear and cytoplasmic TAR DNA-binding protein (TDP-43) induces disease-like redistribution, sequestration, and aggregate formation. J Biol Chem. 2008;283:13302–9.
40. Giordana MT, Piccinini M, Grifoni S, De Marco G, Vercellino M, Magistrello M, Pellerino A, Buccinna B, Lupino E, Rinaudo MT. TDP-43 redistribution is an

early event in sporadic amyotrophic lateral sclerosis. Brain Pathol. 2010;20: 351–60.

41. Correia AS, Patel P, Dutta K, Julien JP. Inflammation induces TDP-43 Mislocalization and aggregation. PLoS One. 2015;10:e0140248.

42. Forman MS, Trojanowski JQ, Lee VM. TDP-43: a novel neurodegenerative proteinopathy. Curr Opin Neurobiol. 2007;17:548–55.

43. Nonaka T, Arai T, Buratti E, Baralle FE, Akiyama H, Hasegawa M. Phosphorylated and ubiquitinated TDP-43 pathological inclusions in ALS and FTLD-U are recapitulated in SH-SY5Y cells. FEBS Lett. 2009;583:394–400.

44. Akira S, Takeda K. Toll-like receptor signalling. Nat Rev Immunol. 2004;4:499–511.

45. Huang H, Zhong R, Xia Z, Song J, Feng L. Neuroprotective effects of rhynchophylline against ischemic brain injury via regulation of the Akt/ mTOR and TLRs signaling pathways. Molecules. 2014;19:11196–210.

46. Ayala YM, Misteli T, Baralle FE. TDP-43 regulates retinoblastoma protein phosphorylation through the repression of cyclin-dependent kinase 6 expression. Proc Natl Acad Sci U S A. 2008;105:3785–9.

47. Zhang YJ, Xu YF, Cook C, Gendron TF, Roettges P, Link CD, Lin WL, Tong J, Castanedes-Casey M, Ash P, et al. Aberrant cleavage of TDP-43 enhances aggregation and cellular toxicity. Proc Natl Acad Sci U S A. 2009;106:7607–12.

3

Leukemia inhibitory factor modulates the peripheral immune response in a rat model of emergent large vessel occlusion

Stephanie M. Davis[1], Lisa A. Collier[1], Edric D. Winford[2], Christopher C. Leonardo[5], Craig T. Ajmo Jr[5], Elspeth A. Foran[6], Timothy J. Kopper[3,4], John C. Gensel[3,4] and Keith R. Pennypacker[1,2*] (iD)

Abstract

Background: The migration of peripheral immune cells and splenocytes to the ischemic brain is one of the major causes of delayed neuroinflammation after permanent large vessel stroke. Other groups have demonstrated that leukemia inhibitory factor (LIF), a cytokine that promotes neural cell survival through upregulation of antioxidant enzymes, promotes an anti-inflammatory phenotype in several types of immune cells. The goal of this study was to determine whether LIF treatment modulates the peripheral immune response after stroke.

Methods: Young male (3 month) Sprague-Dawley rats underwent sham surgery or permanent middle cerebral artery occlusion (MCAO). Animals were administered LIF (125 μg/kg) or PBS at 6, 24, and 48 h prior to euthanization at 72 h. Bone marrow-derived macrophages were treated with LIF (20 ng/ml) or PBS after stimulation with interferon gamma + LPS. Western blot was used to measure protein levels of CD11b, IL-12, interferon inducible protein-10, CD3, and the LIF receptor in spleen and brain tissue. ELISA was used to measure IL-10, IL-12, and interferon gamma. Isolectin was used to label activated immune cells in brain tissue sections. Statistical analysis was performed using one-way ANOVA and Student's t test. A Kruskal-Wallis test followed by Bonferroni-corrected Mann-Whitney tests was performed if data did not pass the D'Agostino-Pearson normality test.

Results: LIF-treated rats showed significantly lower levels of the LIF receptor and interferon gamma in the spleen and CD11b levels in the brain compared to their PBS-treated counterparts. Fluorescence from isolectin-binding immune cells was more prominent in the ipsilateral cortex and striatum after PBS treatment compared to LIF treatment. MCAO + LIF significantly decreased splenic levels of CD11b and CD3 compared to sham surgery. MCAO + PBS treatment significantly elevated splenic levels of interferon inducible protein-10 at 72 h after MCAO, while LIF treatment after MCAO returned interferon inducible protein 10 to sham levels. LIF administration with interferon gamma + LPS significantly reduced the IL-12/IL-10 production ratio compared to macrophages treated with interferon gamma + LPS alone.

Conclusions: These data demonstrate that LIF promotes anti-inflammatory signaling through alterations of the IL-12/interferon gamma/interferon inducible protein 10 pathway.

Keywords: Stroke, Inflammation, Macrophages, Ischemia, Cytokines

* Correspondence: keith.pennypacker@uky.edu
[1]Department of Neurology, University of Kentucky, 741 S. Limestone BBSRB B457, Lexington, KY 40536-0905, USA
[2]Department of Neuroscience, University of Kentucky, 800 Rose St. Lexington, Lexington, KY 40536, USA
Full list of author information is available at the end of the article

Background

Permanent occlusion of the brain's major arteries, also known as emergent large vessel occlusion (ELVO), is one of the deadliest types of acute ischemic stroke and a major cause of adult disability [1–3]. Due to the size of the thrombus creating the blockage, ELVO patients are often resistant to treatment with tissue plasminogen activator (tPA), the only FDA-approved drug for the treatment of stroke. The increased use of stent retrievers for performing endovascular thrombectomy has allowed for restoration of cerebral blood flow up to 24 h after the onset of symptoms [4–6]. However, patients who are deemed ineligible for endovascular thrombectomy are left without sufficient treatment options [7]. Our laboratory has examined the inflammatory response to stroke using the permanent middle cerebral artery occlusion, which simulates ELVO.

Although neural cell death during large-vessel stroke is commonly associated with energy failure and low levels of oxygen, resulting brain damage occurs during two distinct phases of cellular damage. The acute cytotoxicity phase, which occurs minutes to hours after the onset of stroke, results in the death of cells within the ischemic core. The second phase of brain damage begins approximately 12–24 h after the onset of focal cerebral ischemia and results from systemic activation of the peripheral immune system [8, 9]. Within the ischemic brain, dying neurons and glia release compounds such as ATP, fractalkine, or other danger-associated molecular patterns, which activate microglia, the resident macrophage-like immune cells in the brain [10–13]. Once activated, microglia damage the blood-brain barrier via the release of pro-inflammatory cytokines and matrix metalloproteinases [14].

Increased permeability of the blood-brain barrier contributes to cerebral edema and renders cells in the parenchyma vulnerable to invading peripheral immune cells. These immune cells infiltrate the brain approximately 48 h after cerebral ischemia and include monocytes/macrophages, lymphocytes, and neutrophils [15–17]. Although certain populations of these immune cells, such as anti-inflammatory macrophages/microglia, may play a crucial role in phagocytosis and tissue repair, pro-inflammatory leukocytes potentiate further damage in the area surrounding the ischemic core (penumbra). In addition, peripheral B and T cells that are exposed to CNS-specific antigens may contribute towards the post-stroke adaptive immune response by antibody secretion or direct cytotoxicity [18, 19]. This secondary phase continues until approximately 96 h after the onset of stroke, when the infarct reaches its maximum volume [20, 21].

Of the peripheral immune cell populations that migrate to the brain after stroke, a substantial portion of them originate in the spleen. After stroke, elevated levels of norepinephrine and epinephrine mediate splenic contraction through the activation of α- and β-adrenoreceptors in the white pulp, where splenic leukocytes reside [22, 23]. These leukocytes are released into the peripheral circulation, although the secretion of pro-inflammatory mediators causes these cells to migrate towards the injured hemisphere and amplify the inflammatory response in the brain. Previous studies revealed inverse relationships between post-stroke spleen weights and infract volumes in addition to spleen weights and splenic CD8+ cytotoxic T cell count. These findings show that greater splenic atrophy is the result of more infiltrating immune cells, which mediate delayed neurodegeneration [24–27]. Our lab previously demonstrated that splenectomy 2 weeks prior to permanent middle cerebral artery occlusion (MCAO) had significantly increased infarct volumes after stroke [26]. Interferon gamma (IFNγ) production by T cells and natural killer (NK) cells and subsequent induction of interferon inducible protein 10 (IP-10) triggers the first step in the delayed inflammatory response [26, 28–30]. Clinical data have shown that this post-stroke splenic response not only occurs in human stroke patients, but also differs among patients of different ages and racial backgrounds [31–33].

Leukemia inhibitory factor (LIF) is a cytokine in the IL-6 family that promotes survival of neurons and glia in several animal models of neurodegenerative disease, such as amyotrophic lateral sclerosis [34, 35], multiple sclerosis [36–42], spinal cord injury [43, 44], and stroke [45–47]. Our laboratory has identified several cytoprotective mechanisms of LIF, which include the upregulation of antioxidant enzymes peroxiredoxin IV and metallothionein III in oligodendrocytes [46, 48] and superoxide dismutase 3 in neurons [47]. Other groups have shown that in the efficacy of LIF in treating animal models of neurodegenerative disease may lie in its ability to modulate the immune system in addition to its pro-survival signaling [42, 49].

Several groups have reported that LIF alters the phenotype of macrophages/microglia from a pro-inflammatory to an anti-inflammatory phenotype. While pro-inflammatory macrophages worsen tissue damage during stroke via the release of pro-inflammatory mediators (tumor necrosis factor-α, IL-12, IL-6, IL-1β, nitric oxide, etc.), anti-inflammatory cells are primarily phagocytic and release anti-inflammatory mediators. In addition, these macrophages/microglia recruit other anti-inflammatory cells such as CD4 + CCR4+ helper T lymphocytes and regulatory T cells (Tregs) to the site of injury. Duluc et al. demonstrated that LIF and IL-6, in conjunction with macrophage colony-stimulating factor cause monocytes to differentiate into IL-12^{low} IL-10^{high} tumor-associated macrophages, a specialized class of anti-inflammatory leukocytes that protect cancerous growths from NK cells [50].

Although pro-inflammatory macrophages/microglia further damage neural cells after stroke by perpetuating inflammation and producing reactive oxygen species, macrophages/microglia with an anti-inflammatory phenotype contribute to the repair process during ischemia [13, 51]. Therefore, LIF may indirectly reduce the neuroinflammation-associated damage during stroke by increasing the population of anti-inflammatory macrophages/microglia.

Previously, we showed that LIF reduces tissue damage and improves function recovery after stroke through the Akt-dependent upregulation of antioxidant enzymes in neurons and oligodendrocytes [46, 47]. The purpose of this study is to determine whether LIF alters the post-stroke splenic response by changing the phenotype of macrophages/microglia from a pro-inflammatory to an anti-inflammatory phenotype.

Methods
Animal care
Animal procedures were pre-approved by the Institutional Animal Care and Use Committee at the University of South Florida and performed according to the NIH Guide for the Care and Use of Laboratory Animals. Power analysis was used to determine the appropriate number of animals for each experiment. Sprague–Dawley rats were purchased from Envigo (Indianapolis, IN, USA). C57BL/6 mice were purchased from Jackson Laboratories (Bar Harbor, ME, USA). Animals were maintained on a 12-h light–dark cycle (07:00–19:00 h) in a climate-controlled room and allowed access to food and water ad libitum. In vivo procedures were performed on young (3 months), male rats weighing between 300 and 350 g. For in vitro experiments, bone marrow was harvested from young mice (2–3 months).

Middle cerebral artery occlusion
Permanent focal cerebral ischemia was induced using the intraluminal middle cerebral artery occlusion (MCAO) model as previously described [52]. A 40-mm monofilament was introduced through the ligated external carotid artery and advanced through the internal carotid artery. The filament was advanced until it reached the origin of the middle cerebral artery. Reduction in cerebral blood flow was confirmed using Laser Doppler (Moore Lab Instruments, Farmington, CT). Only animals experiencing ≥ 60% reduction in cerebral perfusion were included in the study. Animals subjected to the sham MCAO procedure were anesthetized and underwent exposure of the common carotid artery without subsequent occlusion of the middle cerebral artery.

Drug treatment
All animals were treated prophylactically with ketoprofen (10 mg/kg s.c.), atropine (0.25 mg/kg s.c.) with two additional doses of ketoprofen at 24 and 48 h post-MCAO. Recombinant human LIF (ProSpec, Ness Ziona, Israel) (125 μg/kg) or PBS (pH 7.4) was administered intravenously at 6, 24, and 48 h post-MCAO as previously described [46, 47]. Animals were randomly assigned to treatment groups and all lab personnel administering drugs were blinded to treatments.

Tissue collection
Rats were euthanized at 72 h post-MCAO via intraperitoneal injection of ketamine/xylazine solution (75 mg/kg and 7.5 mg/kg) [53]. Spleens were collected immediately prior to perfusion. Animals used for immunohistochemical analysis were perfused transcardially with normal saline followed by 4% paraformaldehyde in phosphate buffer. Animals used for biochemical analysis were perfused with saline but not paraformaldehyde prior to obtaining tissue. Fresh brain tissue was separated into ipsilateral and contralateral hemispheres, snap-frozen, and stored at – 80 °C until further processing. Fixed brains were cryopreserved in 20% followed by 30% sucrose solutions and cut into 30-μm sections using a cryostat. Brain tissue used in these experiments was located between + 1.7 and – 3.3 mm from the bregma.

Tissue homogenization
To obtain whole cell extracts, frozen tissue was homogenized in whole cell lysis buffer containing the following: 50 mM Tris pH 8, 150 mM NaCl, 0.1% SDS, 1% IGEP AL, 1 mM PMSF, and a Complete Mini protease inhibitor cocktail (Roche Diagnostics, Indianapolis, IN). An electric homogenizer was used to disrupt tissue, and lysates were incubated on ice for 20 min. Tissue lysates were vortexed and pipetted to break up nuclei. Protein concentrations were determined by performing a Bradford Assay according to the manufacturer's protocol (Bio-Rad, Hercules, CA). Briefly, Bradford reagent containing Coomassie blue was added to diluted protein samples and absorbance was read at 595 nm using a SmartSpec 3000 spectrophotometer (Bio-Rad). Concentrations were determined by comparing the absorbance readings against a standard curve.

Isolectin staining
Isolectin IB4 (0.05% v/v) from *Griffonia simplicifolia* conjugated to AlexaFluor® 488 dye was used to label activated macrophages and microglia in the cortical and striatal tissue of PBS- and LIF-treated rat brains according to a previously described procedure [20]. Coverslips were mounted onto slides using VECTASHIELD® medium containing 4′, 6-diamidino-2-phenylindole (DAPI) (Vector

Labs, Burlingame, CA). Images were captured using a Nikon Eclipse Ti microscope (Minato, Tokyo, Japan) interfaced with NIS Elements Imaging Software (Nikon).

3,3-Diaminobenzidine immunohistochemistry

To detect CD11b-positive cells in brain tissue, 3,3-diaminobenzidine (DAB) immunohistochemistry was performed according to a previously described protocol [54]. The following antibodies were used: mouse α-CD11b (OX42) (1:3000; Bio-Rad; Hercules, CA) and horse α-mouse (1:300; Vector-Labs; Berlingame, CA). Slides were cover slipped with DPX medium (BDH Laboratories, Poole, England) and images were acquired with a Nikon Eclipse Ti microscope interfaced with NIS Elements Imaging Software (Nikon).

DAB staining of spleen tissue was also performed according to a previously described protocol, albeit with minor modifications. Briefly, cryopreserved spleen tissue sections (30 μm) were dried at 37 °C, rehydrated with PBS (pH 7.4), and permeabilized for 1 h containing 10% goat serum, 0.3% 1 M Lysine, and 0.3% Triton-X-100. Following permeabilization, spleen sections were treated for 40 min with 3% H_2O_2 to quench endogenous peroxidase activity. Sections were incubated overnight in the following antibodies: rabbit α-LIFR (1:200; Santa Cruz; RRID:AB_2136015) and mouse α-FoxP3 (1:5000; Abcam; RRID:AB_447114). Secondary detection was achieved using goat α-rabbit and goat α-mouse biotinylated secondary antibodies (1:300; Vector Labs). Slides were mounted with DPX medium (BDH Laboratories) after dehydration with ethanol and clearing with xylenes. All images were acquired using a Nikon Eclipse Ti microscope interfaced with NIS Elements Imaging Software (Nikon).

Western blot analysis

Western blotting was used for semi-quantitative measurement of protein expression using a previously described procedure [47]. Briefly, whole cell lysates from brain and spleen tissue were run on 10% SDS-PAGE gels and transferred to nitrocellulose membranes. Membranes were blocked in Li-Cor TBS-based Blocking Buffer (Lincoln, NE) and probed with the following antibodies: rabbit α-LIFR (1:100; Santa Cruz), rabbit α-IL-12 p40 (1:100; Abbiotec RRID:AB_10636335), mouse α-CD11b (1:1000; Abcam). Membranes were incubated in IRDye 800CW goat α-rabbit antibodies (1:20,000; Li-Cor; RRID:AB_2651127) for detection of protein bands. Membranes were visualized using the Odyssey CLx Imaging System (Li-Cor). To normalize for loading, membranes containing whole cell extracts were re-probed with mouse α-β-actin (1:5000; Novus Biologicals; RRID:AB_1216153) and IRDye 680RD goat α-mouse antibodies (1:20,000; Li-Cor; RRID:AB_10956588).

Bone marrow-derived macrophage cell culture

Bone marrow-derived macrophages (BMDMs) were isolated from C57BL/6 mice (3 months of age) as previously described [55–57]. Briefly, cells were extracted from the femur and tibia and seeded at a density of $8 \times 10^5 - 1 \times 10^6$ cells/ml in Dulbecco's modified Eagle's medium (DMEM) containing 10% FBS, 1% penicillin/streptomycin, 1% HEPES, 0.001% β-mercaptoethanol, and 20% supernatant containing macrophage colony-stimulating factor from SL929 cells (gifted by Phillip Popovich from The Ohio State University) [58]. Following 7 days of in vitro differentiation, cells were re-seeded at a density of 1×10^6 cells/ml in DMEM containing 10% FBS, 1% penicillin/streptomycin, 1% HEPES, and 0.001% β-mercaptoethanol. The next day, a classically activated phenotype (M1) was induced using N2A medium containing LPS (50 ng/ml) and IFNγ (20 ng/ml). LIF (20 ng/ml) or PBS was co-administered with the LPS and IFNγ. Macrophage-conditioned media was collected 24 h after stimulation and centrifuged at 13,000 rpm at 4 °C for 10 min prior to measurement of IL-12 p40 and IL-10 via ELISA [59].

ELISA

To measure the release of IFNγ, TNFα, IL-1β, IL-6, and IL-10 in rat spleen tissue, ELISA was performed according to manufacturer's protocol using the appropriate DuoSet ELISA kits (R&D Systems, Inc., Minneapolis, MN). ELISA was also used to measure IL-12 p40 and IL-10 release in macrophage supernatants according to the manufacturer's protocol using the Mouse IL-12 p40 and IL-10 ELISA kits (Cat # EMIL12P40 and Cat # EM2IL105; Thermo Fisher Scientific, Waltham, MA).

Data analysis

Images were minimally processed in a uniform matter across treatment groups and were analyzed using ImageJ software (NIH, Bethesda, MD). The D'Agostino-Pearson test was performed to determine whether data was normally distributed. Statistical analysis for experiments containing two groups was performed using Student's t test, or the Mann-Whitney U Test if the data sets did not pass the D'Agostino-Pearson test. Welch's correction was used in the case of unequal variances. Statistical analysis for experiments containing three or more groups was performed using the one-way ANOVA followed by Fisher's Protected LSD test to determine individual differences If data did not pass the D'Agostino-Pearson test, the Kruskal-Wallis H test was used, and individual differences were detected using Bonferroni-corrected Mann-Whitney U tests. A p value equal to 0.05 or less was considered statistically significant. All reported p values are one-tailed.

Results

LIF decreases LIFR expression but does not alter spleen weight after MCAO

Western blotting was used to determine whether MCAO and LIF treatment altered levels of LIFR in the spleen at 72 h post-MCAO. At 72 h post-MCAO, there was a significant change in splenic LIFR expression among sham, PBS, and LIF-treated rats ($F_{2,21} = 3.511$; $p = 0.0484$). LIFR levels in the spleens of LIF-treated ($p = 0.0086$) but not PBS-treated rats were significantly lower than those of sham rats (Fig. 1a). When the levels of LIFR were normalized to the weight of each spleen, there was no significant difference in normalized splenic LIFR levels between sham-operated, PBS-treated, and LIF-treated rats ($H = 4.295$; $p = 0.1168$). However, there was a trend towards increased normalized LIFR levels in PBS-treated rats compared to the other treatment groups (Fig. 1b). Compared to spleens from sham-operated rats, MCAO and LIF treatment caused a significant overall change in the average spleen weight ($p = 0.0008$, $F_{2,56} = 8.143$). There was a significant decrease in spleen weight among rats treated with PBS after MCAO compared to the sham-operated rats ($p = 0.0001$). Rats treated with LIF after MCAO had significantly smaller spleen weights compared to sham-operated rats ($p = 0.0062$). There was a trend towards larger spleens among rats treated with LIF post-MCAO compared to the PBS-treated group, but this trend was not significant ($p = 0.1016$; Fig. 1c).

Splenocytes express the LIF receptor after MCAO and LIF treatment

Spleen tissue sections were stained with antibodies against LIFR in order to visualize the LIF receptor in splenocytes after sham surgery, MCAO + PBS treatment, and MCAO + LIF treatment. Punctate LIFR immunoreactivity was observed in spleens from sham-operated rats while spleens from the MCAO + PBS and MCAO + LIF groups showed more diffuse staining in splenocytes. Arrows are used to identify representative cells (Fig. 2).

Splenic CD11b expression decreases after MCAO and LIF treatment

Western blotting was used to measure CD11b protein expression in the spleens of PBS and LIF-treated rats euthanized at 72 h after MCAO. At 72 h, levels of CD11b in spleen tissue were significantly altered after MCAO and LIF treatment ($p = 0.0003$; $F_{2,21} = 12.51$). There was a significant drop in CD11b levels in the spleens of PBS-treated rats ($p = 0.002$) and LIF-treated ($p = 0.0002$) rats compared to those of sham rats (Fig. 3a). When the CD11b levels were normalized to the spleen weights of each sample, there was a significant overall change in normalized CD11b levels ($p = 0.0335$; $F_{2,21} = 4.009$) and a significant decrease in normalized

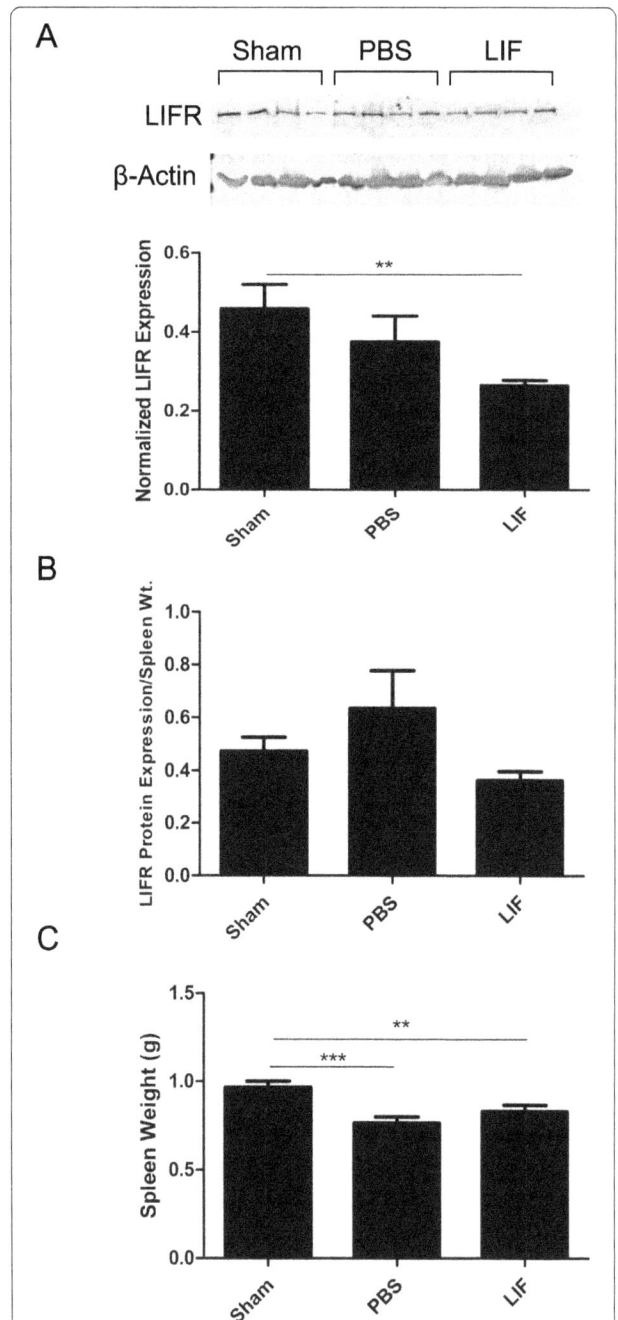

Fig. 1 LIF treatment decreases splenic LIFR but does not change spleen weight. **a** Western blotting was used to measure levels of the LIF receptor (LIFR) in the spleen 72 h after sham surgery and MCAO. There was a trend towards decreased LIFR levels after MCAO and a significant decrease in LIFR after MCAO and treatment with LIF (**$p < 0.01$). $n = 8$ animals per treatment group. **b** When LIFR protein levels were normalized to the spleen weight, there was a trend towards increased normalized LIFR in the PBS-treated group, but this increase was not significant. **c** At 72 h, spleen weights in the MCAO + PBS group (****$p < 0.0001$) and the MCAO + LIF (**$p < 0.01$) were significantly lower than the sham group. There was a trend towards a higher spleen weight in the MCAO + LIF group compared to the MCAO + PBS group, but this trend was not significant ($p = 0.1016$). $n = 18–23$ animals per treatment group

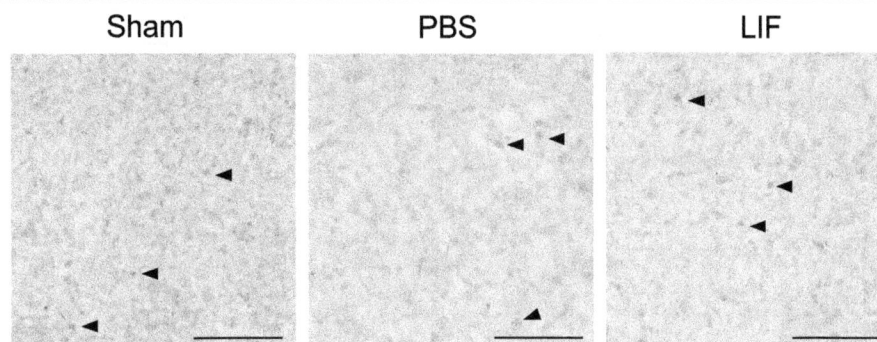

Fig. 2 LIFR+ splenocytes are observed in the spleen after MCAO and LIF treatment. DAB immunohistochemistry was used to visualize the expression of LIFR among splenocytes in tissue from sham-operated, PBS-treated, and LIF-treated cells. Although LIFR+ splenocytes were found in all three treatment groups, LIFR+ positive cells showed punctate immunoreactivity while tissue from PBS- and LIF-treated animals showed more diffuse immunoreactivity. Arrows identify representative cells. Scale bar = 50 μm

CD11b after MCAO + LIF treatment compared to sham levels ($p = 0.0043$; Fig. 3b). To determine the relationship between spleen weight and levels of CD11b in splenic tissue, Pearson r correlation analysis was performed. There was a significant positive correlation between the spleen weight at 72 h post-MCAO and sham procedure and splenic CD11b protein expression ($p = 0.0149$; Pearson $r = 0.4437$; Fig. 3c).

IL-12 p40 levels in the spleen are not altered after MCAO and LIF treatment

To measure release of IL-12 after MCAO and LIF treatment, western blotting was used to detect levels of IL-12 p40 in splenic tissue. There was no overall significant alteration in IL-12 p40 protein levels at 72 h after MCAO and LIF treatment ($p = 0.098$; $F_{2,21} = 2.600$). However, there was a strong trend towards decreased IL-12 p40 levels in the spleens of LIF-treated rats compared to PBS-treated and sham rats (Fig. 4a). When splenic IL-12 p40 levels were normalized to spleen weights, there was a trend towards increased normalized IL-12 p40 levels in the spleens of PBS-treated rats compared to LIF-treated and sham-operated rats ($F_{2,21} = 2.721$, $p = 0.0890$; Fig. 4b).

TNFα, but not IL-6 and IL-1b, are altered by MCAO + LIF treatment at 72 h after MCAO

ELISA was used to measure levels of TNFα in the spleen tissue of sham, PBS-treated, and LIF-treated rats at 72 h after MCAO. There was a significant alteration in TNFα levels at this time point ($F_{2,21} = 6.181$; $p = 0.0077$. TNFα levels were significantly lower after MCAO compared to sham levels ($p = 0.0347$) and after MCAO + LIF treatment compared to sham levels ($p = 0.0012$). However, there was no significant difference between the mean TNFα levels in the MCAO + PBS and MCAO + LIF groups ($p = 0.1038$; Fig. 5a). ELISA was also used to measure levels IL-1β and IL-6 in spleen tissue. There was a trend towards decreased IL-1β ($F_{2,20} = 3.157$; $p = 0.0644$; Fig. 5b) and

IL-6 ($F_{2,13} = 0.3225$; $p = 0.7300$; Fig. 5c) levels after MCAO + LIF treatment but this difference was not statistically significant.

Splenic IL-10 is not altered by MCAO + LIF treatment

Levels of IL-10 were measured in spleen tissue at 72 h post-MCAO using ELISA. Although there was a trend towards decreased IL-10 levels in the MCAO + PBS and MCAO + LIF groups that approached significance ($F_{2,20} = 3.437$; $p = 0.0521$), the overall difference was not statistically significant (Fig. 6).

LIF reduces CD3 immunoreactivity in the spleen

To determine whether LIF decreases development of mature T cells, western blotting was used to measure levels of CD3, a pan-T cell marker, in spleen tissue at 72 h after MCAO. At 72 h, there was a significant change in CD3 levels between spleen tissue from sham-operated, PBS-treated, and LIF-treated young rats ($F_{2,20} = 5.198$, $p = 0.0152$). There were significant decreases in overall CD3 levels in the spleens of PBS-treated ($p = 0.0405$) and LIF-treated rats compared to sham-operated rats ($p = 0.0113$; Fig. 7a). When CD3 levels were normalized to spleen weight, there was no significant difference in normalized CD3 between the three treatment groups ($F_{2,20} = 2.434$; $p = 0.1132$; Fig. 7b).

FoxP3+ immunoreactivity is observed in the spleen after MCAO + LIF treatment

Spleen sections from sham-operated, PBS-treated, and LIF-treated rats were stained with FoxP3 antibodies to identify the presence of Tregs. FoxP3+ cells were found in representative spleen sections from all three treatment groups, although FoxP3 immunoreactivity was more prominent in the representative sections from the MCAO + PBS and MCAO + LIF groups (Fig. 8).

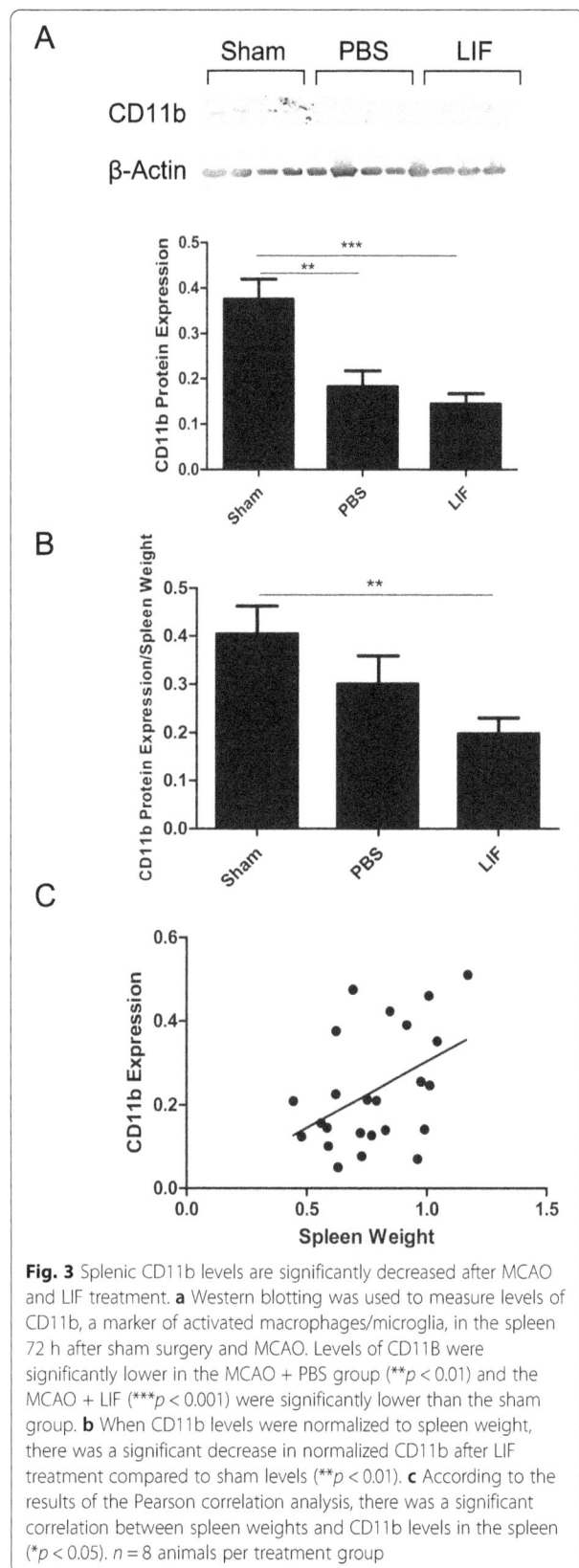

Fig. 3 Splenic CD11b levels are significantly decreased after MCAO and LIF treatment. **a** Western blotting was used to measure levels of CD11b, a marker of activated macrophages/microglia, in the spleen 72 h after sham surgery and MCAO. Levels of CD11B were significantly lower in the MCAO + PBS group (**$p < 0.01$) and the MCAO + LIF (***$p < 0.001$) were significantly lower than the sham group. **b** When CD11b levels were normalized to spleen weight, there was a significant decrease in normalized CD11b after LIF treatment compared to sham levels (**$p < 0.01$). **c** According to the results of the Pearson correlation analysis, there was a significant correlation between spleen weights and CD11b levels in the spleen (*$p < 0.05$). $n = 8$ animals per treatment group

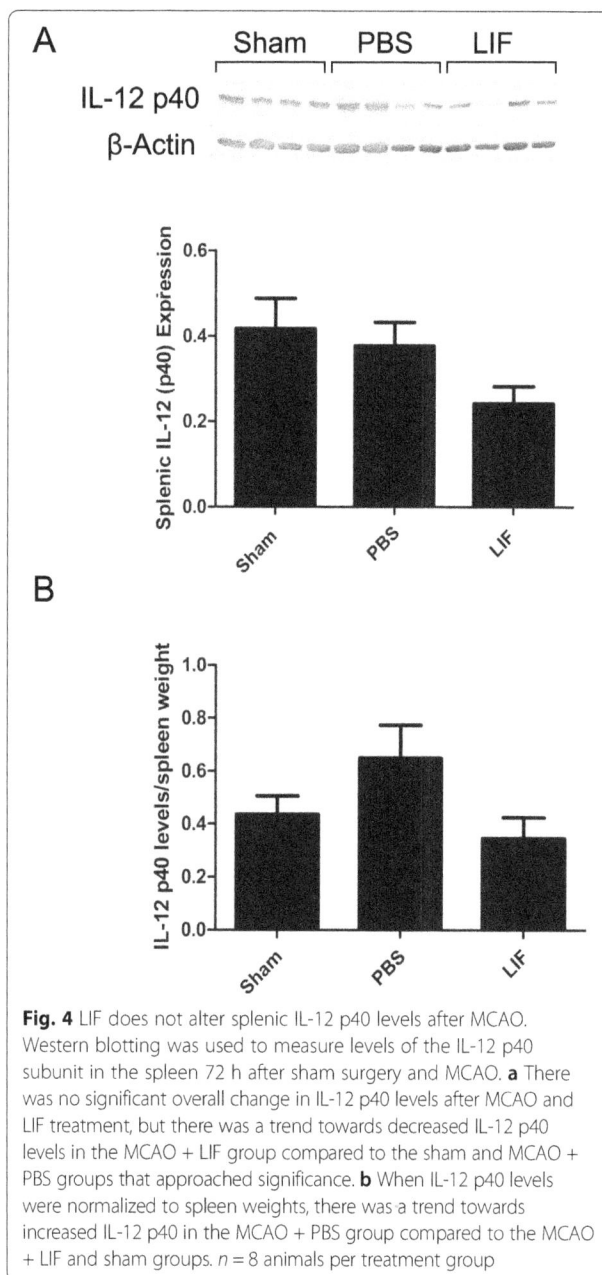

Fig. 4 LIF does not alter splenic IL-12 p40 levels after MCAO. Western blotting was used to measure levels of the IL-12 p40 subunit in the spleen 72 h after sham surgery and MCAO. **a** There was no significant overall change in IL-12 p40 levels after MCAO and LIF treatment, but there was a trend towards decreased IL-12 p40 levels in the MCAO + LIF group compared to the sham and MCAO + PBS groups that approached significance. **b** When IL-12 p40 levels were normalized to spleen weights, there was a trend towards increased IL-12 p40 in the MCAO + PBS group compared to the MCAO + LIF and sham groups. $n = 8$ animals per treatment group

IFNγ release is decreased by MCAO and LIF treatment

IFNγ levels in spleen tissue from sham, PBS-treated, and LIF-treated rats was measured using an ELISA kit and normalized to the total protein. There was a significant change in IFNγ levels in the spleen tissue of sham-operated, PBS-treated, and LIF-treated rats at 72 h post-MCAO ($F_{2,21}$ 6.365; $p = 0.0069$). There was a significant decrease in IFNγ levels in the spleens of the MCAO + PBS group ($p = 0.0364$) and the MCAO + LIF group ($p = 0.0095$) compared to the sham levels. In addition, spleen tissue from the MCAO + LIF group had significantly lower IFNγ levels compared to tissue from

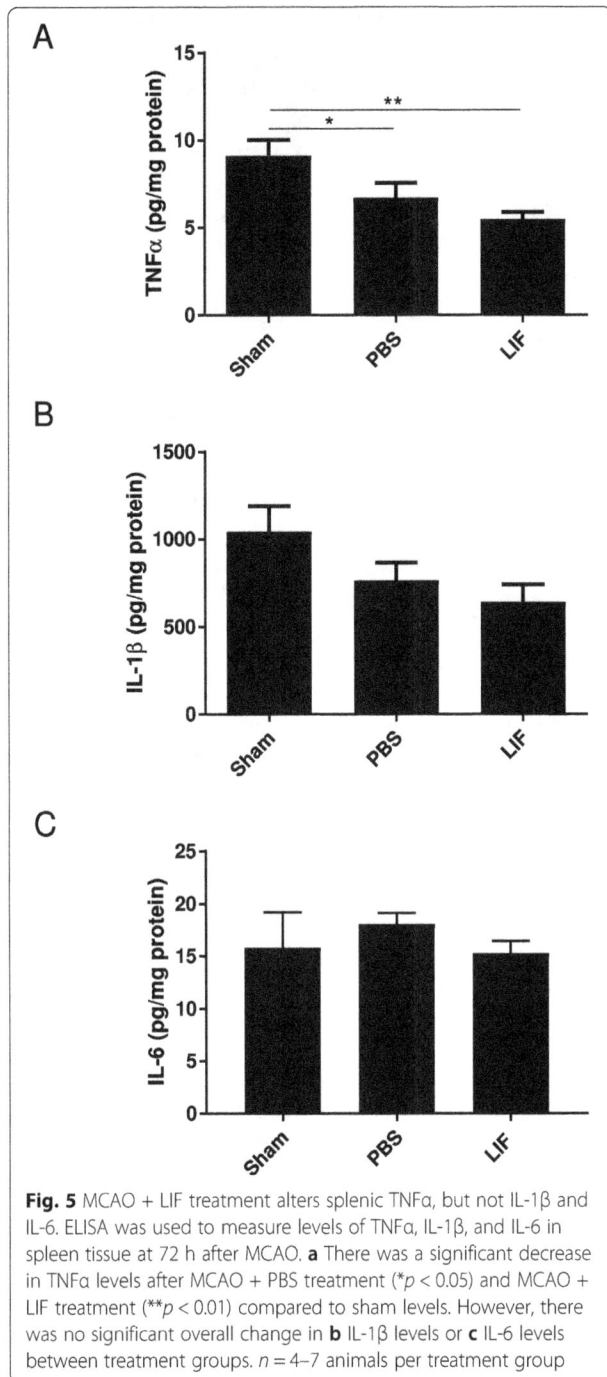

Fig. 5 MCAO + LIF treatment alters splenic TNFα, but not IL-1β and IL-6. ELISA was used to measure levels of TNFα, IL-1β, and IL-6 in spleen tissue at 72 h after MCAO. **a** There was a significant decrease in TNFα levels after MCAO + PBS treatment (*$p < 0.05$) and MCAO + LIF treatment (**$p < 0.01$) compared to sham levels. However, there was no significant overall change in **b** IL-1β levels or **c** IL-6 levels between treatment groups. $n = 4$–7 animals per treatment group

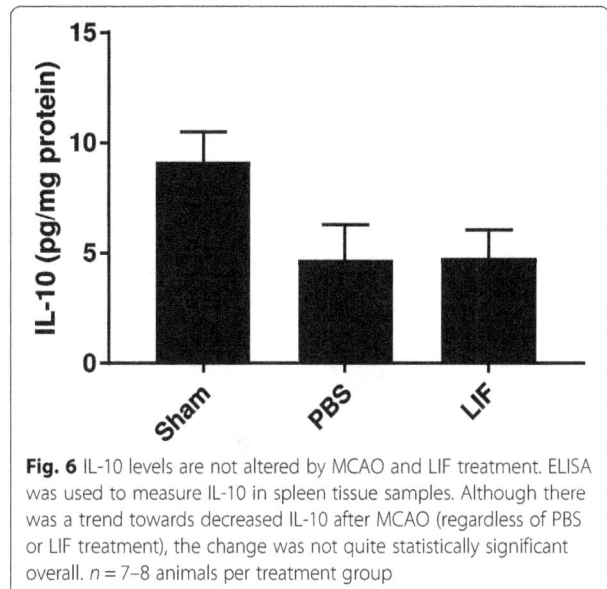

Fig. 6 IL-10 levels are not altered by MCAO and LIF treatment. ELISA was used to measure IL-10 in spleen tissue samples. Although there was a trend towards decreased IL-10 after MCAO (regardless of PBS or LIF treatment), the change was not quite statistically significant overall. $n = 7$–8 animals per treatment group

LIF treatment counteracts the increase in splenic IP-10 after MCAO

IP-10 levels were measured in splenic tissue using western blotting. At 72 h after MCAO, there was a significant alteration in IP-10 protein expression in spleen tissue ($H = 7.215$; $p = 0.0271$). Splenic IP-10 levels were significantly elevated after MCAO compared to sham levels ($p = 0.0045$). The levels of IP-10 in the spleens of LIF-treated rats were not significantly different from sham levels ($p = 1.000$), but there was a non-significant decrease in IP-10 expression compared to IP-10 expression levels of PBS-treated rats ($p = 0.1572$; Fig. 10a). When the levels of IP-10 in each tissue sample were normalized to the spleen mass, there was a significant change in normalized IP-10 levels at 72 h post-MCAO ($H = 9.065$; $p = 0.0108$). Normalized IP-10 levels remained significantly elevated compared to the sham group ($p = 0.0015$). However, treatment with LIF counteracted this upregulation of IP-10 compared to sham-operated animals (Fig. 10b).

LIF promotes anti-inflammatory phenotype in LPS/IFNγ-stimulated macrophages

Prior to stimulation with LPS + IFNγ to induce an M1 phenotype, BMDMs were treated with LIF (20 ng/ml) or PBS. Levels of IL-12 p40 and IL-10 in the supernatant were measured via ELISA. Unstimulated cells treated with LIF or PBS were used as a control. After 24 h, M1 macrophages stimulated with LIF had released significantly less IL-12 p40 compared to M1 cells treated with PBS ($t = 6.530$, df = 4, $p = 0.0014$; Fig. 11a). M1 BMDMs showed significantly elevated release of IL-10 compared to their unstimulated counterparts. Treatment with LIF prior to stimulation further elevated IL-10 release among M1 cells ($t = 2.942$, df = 4, $p = 0.0212$; Fig. 11b). LIF treatment

the MCAO + PBS rats ($p = 0.0324$; Fig. 9a). Normalizing IFNγ levels in each sample to the spleen weight also showed a significant alteration in normalized splenic IFNγ after MCAO and LIF treatment ($F_{2,21} = 5.052$, $p = 0.0162$). MCAO + PBS treatment significantly increased normalized IFNγ compared to sham levels ($p = 0.0038$), but LIF treatment significantly reduced normalized IFNγ levels compared to PBS treatment ($p = 0.0080$; Fig. 9b).

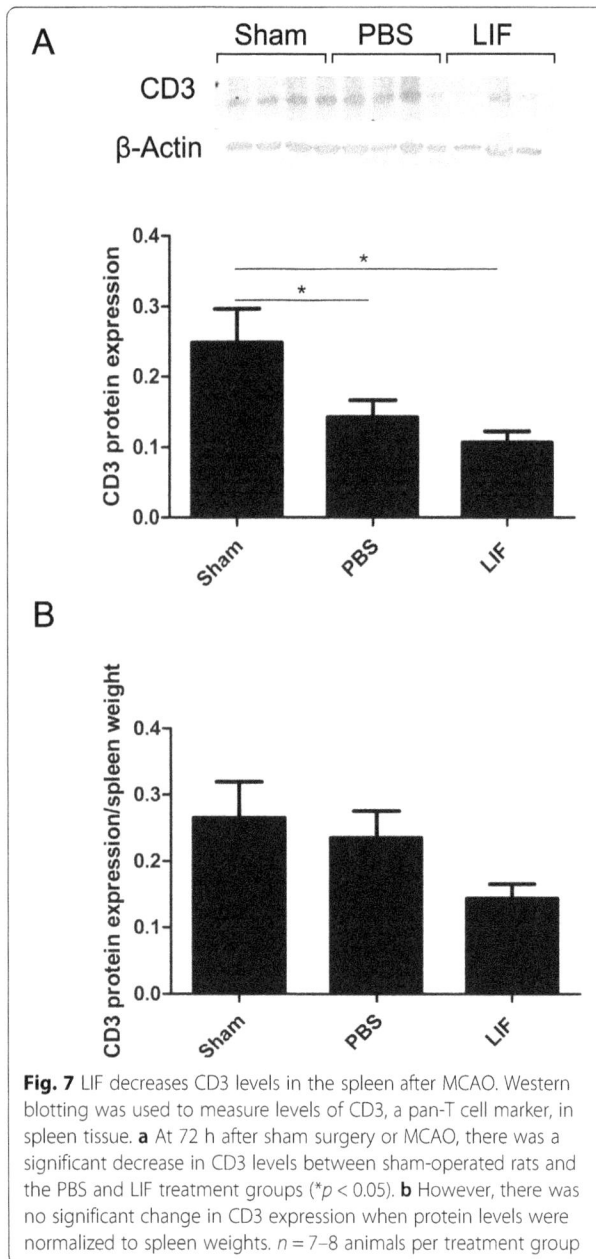

Fig. 7 LIF decreases CD3 levels in the spleen after MCAO. Western blotting was used to measure levels of CD3, a pan-T cell marker, in spleen tissue. **a** At 72 h after sham surgery or MCAO, there was a significant decrease in CD3 levels between sham-operated rats and the PBS and LIF treatment groups (*$p < 0.05$). **b** However, there was no significant change in CD3 expression when protein levels were normalized to spleen weights. $n = 7-8$ animals per treatment group

also significantly decreased the ratio of IL-12 p40 release to IL-10 release in the media compared to treatment with PBS ($t = 6.012$, df $= 4$, $p = 0.0019$; Fig. 11c).

Activated macrophages/microglia are decreased in the brains of LIF-treated rats

Activated macrophages/microglia were visualized in fixed brain tissue from PBS- or LIF-treated rats using isolectin-conjugated to AlexaFluor® 488 dye. At 72 h after MCAO, there was a less isolectin-tagged fluorescence within the cortical and striatal tissue of LIF-treated rats compared to their PBS-treated counterparts. Furthermore, representative images show that

lectin-binding cells in the striatum after LIF treatment displayed a more ramified phenotype. By contrast, lectin-binding cells in the striatum displayed an amoeboid phenotype after PBS treatment (Fig. 12a).

Antibodies against CD11b were also used to label brain sections from animals treated with PBS or LIF after MCAO. Representative images show a number of amoeboid CD11b + cells in the cortex and striatum of tissue from animals treated with PBS after MCAO. By contrast, the cortical and striatal tissue from LIF-treated rats contained more CD11b + cells with a ramified phenotype (Fig. 12b).

Western blotting was used to quantify protein levels of CD11b in homogenized brain tissue at 72 h after MCAO. Levels of CD11b in the ipsilateral tissue of PBS- and LIF-treated rats were normalized to the average CD11b levels in sham brains. There was a significant change in CD11b levels in the brain after MCAO and LIF treatment ($F_{3,18} = 7.800$; $p = 0.0015$). CD11b levels were significantly decreased in the ipsilateral hemisphere of LIF-treated rats compared to those of PBS-treated rats at 72 h after MCAO ($p = 0.0432$). Likewise, CD11b levels were significantly higher in the ipsilateral hemisphere of LIF-treated rats ($p = 0.0301$) and PBS-treated rats ($p = 0.0037$) compared to their contralateral counterparts (Fig. 12c).

Discussion

Although LIF treatment decreased protein levels of CD11b as well as the numbers of isolectin-binding cells, these results indicate that LIF exerts its primary immunomodulatory effects on splenocytes, specifically through the IL-12 p40 /IFNγ/IP-10 axis. Offner et al. previously demonstrated that induction of focal cerebral ischemia in mice stimulates the production of several pro-inflammatory cytokines from splenocytes [60]. This upregulation of cytokine production is followed by a time-dependent decrease in spleen weight due to the migration of splenocyte populations to the ischemic brain [18, 23, 26, 27].

In accordance with previously published studies, spleen size significantly decreased after MCAO compared to sham treatment, LIF-treated rats had a trend towards a larger spleen size at 72 h after MCAO. Furthermore, there was a significant downregulation in splenic LIFR protein expression in the spleens of LIF-treated rats. LIFR is degraded after prolonged stimulation with LIF in many cell types, which indicates that the splenocytes were responsive to peripherally administered LIF after stroke [61]. Although this laboratory has previously shown that the decrease in spleen size is observed as early as 24 h after stroke, this laboratory did not observe any LIF-mediated alteration in LIFR expression or spleen size prior to the 72-h time point [27].

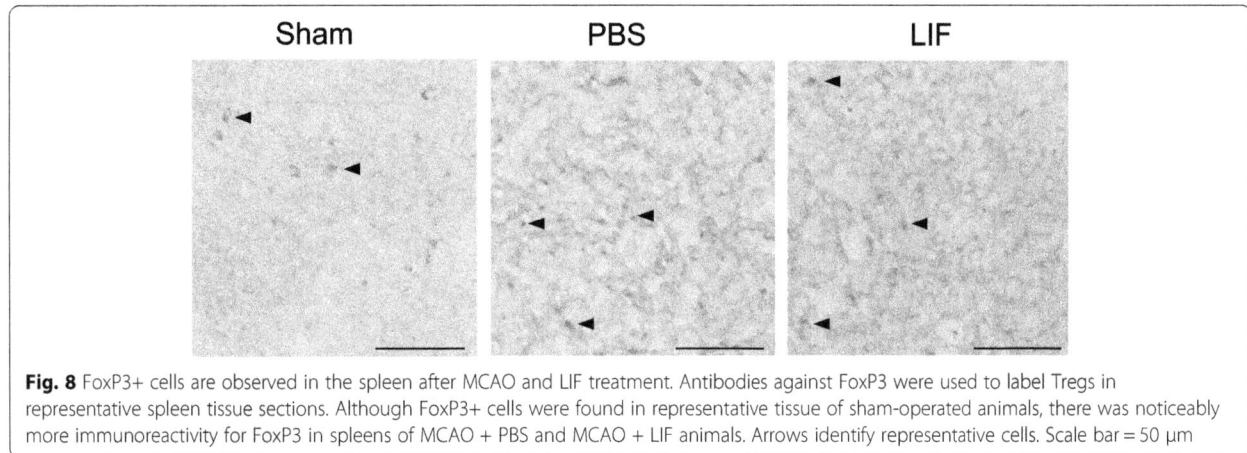

Fig. 8 FoxP3+ cells are observed in the spleen after MCAO and LIF treatment. Antibodies against FoxP3 were used to label Tregs in representative spleen tissue sections. Although FoxP3+ cells were found in representative tissue of sham-operated animals, there was noticeably more immunoreactivity for FoxP3 in spleens of MCAO + PBS and MCAO + LIF animals. Arrows identify representative cells. Scale bar = 50 μm

However, published manuscripts from this group have also shown that most prominent effects of LIF are observed at 72 h after MCAO, including improvement in motor skills, decreased tissue damage, and upregulation of antioxidant enzymes [46, 47]. Therefore, it should be expected that the prominent anti-inflammatory effects of LIF are observed at this time point.

Although this study primarily examined the effects of LIF in the spleen and brain after stroke, it is entirely possible that LIF signaling is indirectly modulating the post-stroke immune response through its actions in other tissues. Ajmo et al. previously demonstrated that the activation of adrenoreceptors in the spleen is responsible for the splenic contraction that promotes the migration of immune cells to the brain after stroke [23]. Due to its effects on the hypothalamus-pituitary-adrenal axis [62], it is possible that LIF administration is influencing the post-stroke immune response through the regulation of cortisol release [62, 63]. Furthermore, leukocytes within the peripheral circulation, including T cells, are responsible for perpetuating inflammation in rodent models of ischemic stroke [60]. Therefore, it is highly likely that systemically administered LIF is also acting on immune cells within the peripheral blood in addition to the spleen.

IL-12 is a heterodimer consisting of two subunits: the 35-kDa p35 subunit and the 40-kDa p40 submit, which is a component of the pro-inflammatory cytokine IL-23. Microglia and perivascular macrophages in brain produce IL-12/IL-23 in response to stimulation with other pro-inflammatory cytokines or damage-associated molecular patterns [19]. IL-12 p40 release from macrophages/microglia promotes further production of IL-12/IL-23 by microglia/ macrophages and perivascular dendritic cells. After the breakdown of the blood-brain barrier due to matrix metalloproteinase and cytokine production by microglia, IL-12 p40-stimulated CD8+ cytotoxic T cells, CD4+ type 1 helper T (Th1) cells, and NK cells release

IFNγ [64–66]. The results of the in vitro experiments with BMDMs demonstrate that LIF directly reduces IL-12 p40 release from pro-inflammatory macrophages. Furthermore, LIF treatment promotes in vitro release of IL-10 in BMDMs, an anti-inflammatory cytokine that counteracts IL-12 p40-mediated production of IFNγ [67].

While this upregulation of IL-10 was not observed in spleen tissue, it is possible that the migration of monocytes/macrophages into the peripheral circulation prior to 72 h after MCAO prevents us from detecting any significant change in IL-12 p40 or IL-10 in the spleen at this time point [20]. LIF treatment also did not significantly alter levels of IL-1β or IL-6, which are released primarily by monocytes/macrophages [68, 69], at this time point. However, IFNγ was significantly reduced in the spleen after LIF treatment, which demonstrates that LIF is primarily influencing the pro-inflammatory signaling generated by splenic T cells [27, 30, 53].

Our lab has demonstrated an essential role for T and NK cell-derived IFNγ in the initiation of the post-stroke splenic response. According to Seifert et al., splenic T cells upregulate IFNγ at 24 h post-MCAO. Increased IFNγ immunoreactivity in the ipsilateral hemisphere at 72 h post-MCAO corresponds with the infiltration of splenic leukocytes. A splenectomy performed 2 weeks prior to stroke onset or the administration of antibodies to neutralize IFNγ significantly reduced neurodegeneration at 96 h post-MCAO. However, administration of exogenous IFNγ restored the neuroinflammatory response in animals that underwent splenectomy [30, 53]. Following release by NK cells and T cells, IFNγ induces the production of several chemokines in macrophages/ microglia, including monocyte induced by IFNγ, interferon-inducible T cell α-chemoattractant, and IP-10 [70]. Western blot analysis showed that LIF treatment significantly reduces levels of CD3, a marker for T cells, in the spleen at 72 h post-MCAO. Although CD3 is expressed by all T cells, this reduction coupled with the

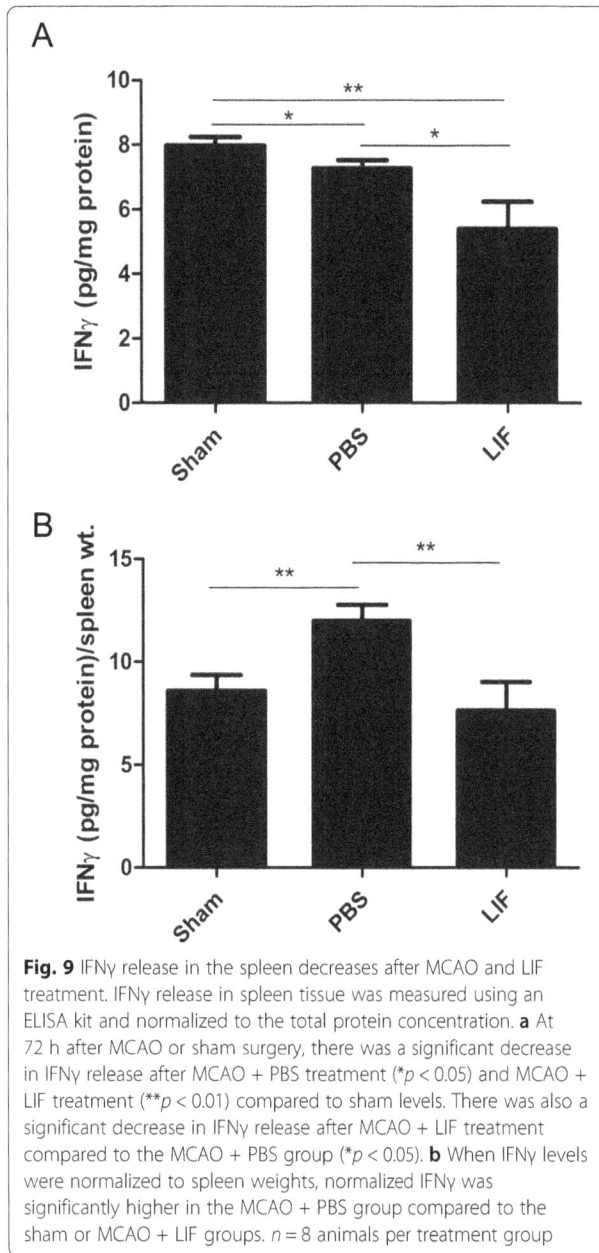

Fig. 9 IFNγ release in the spleen decreases after MCAO and LIF treatment. IFNγ release in spleen tissue was measured using an ELISA kit and normalized to the total protein concentration. **a** At 72 h after MCAO or sham surgery, there was a significant decrease in IFNγ release after MCAO + PBS treatment (*$p < 0.05$) and MCAO + LIF treatment (**$p < 0.01$) compared to sham levels. There was also a significant decrease in IFNγ release after MCAO + LIF treatment compared to the MCAO + PBS group (*$p < 0.05$). **b** When IFNγ levels were normalized to spleen weights, normalized IFNγ was significantly higher in the MCAO + PBS group compared to the sham or MCAO + LIF groups. $n = 8$ animals per treatment group

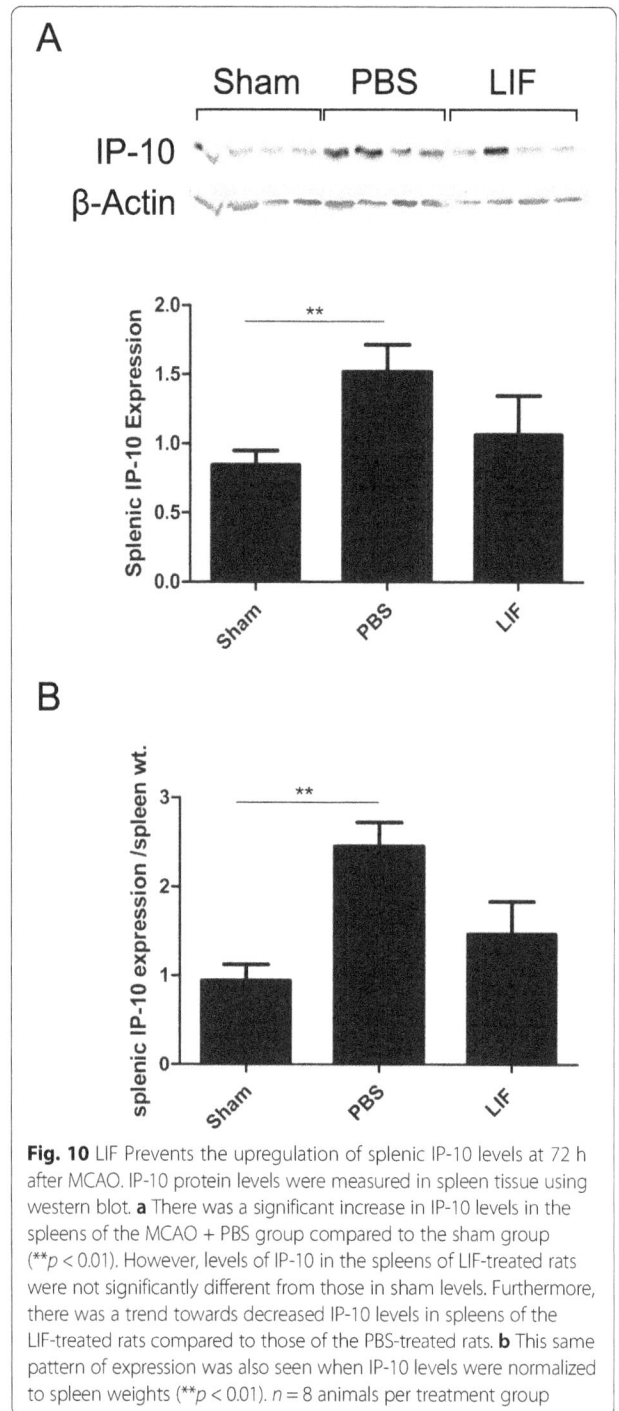

Fig. 10 LIF Prevents the upregulation of splenic IP-10 levels at 72 h after MCAO. IP-10 protein levels were measured in spleen tissue using western blot. **a** There was a significant increase in IP-10 levels in the spleens of the MCAO + PBS group compared to the sham group (**$p < 0.01$). However, levels of IP-10 in the spleens of LIF-treated rats were not significantly different from those in sham levels. Furthermore, there was a trend towards decreased IP-10 levels in spleens of the LIF-treated rats compared to those of the PBS-treated rats. **b** This same pattern of expression was also seen when IP-10 levels were normalized to spleen weights (**$p < 0.01$). $n = 8$ animals per treatment group

downregulation in IFNγ production suggest that LIF prevents the maturation of CD8+ cytotoxic T cells, which are the major producer of IFNγ after stroke [71, 72]. FoxP3-labeled spleen tissue from PBS-treated rats did not show a notable difference in immunoreactivity between PBS- and LIF-treated animals. While these results do not rule out a possible effect on CD4 + CD25 + FoxP3+ Tregs, the anti-inflammatory properties of LIF are more likely due to its abilities to suppress IFNγ production by CD8+ and CD4+ Th1 cells.

IP-10 is a chemokine that facilitates chemotaxis of pro-inflammatory CD4+ T cells to the ischemic brain via binding to CXCR3 [73]. Alternatively, IP-10, along with other IFNγ-inducible chemokines, promotes post-stroke inflammation via antagonism of the binds to the CCR3 receptor on anti-inflammatory CD4+ T cells [74]. Offner et al. first reported that IP-10 mRNA levels were increased at 22 h after transient MCAO in mice, and Seifert et al. confirmed that the IFNγ/IP-10 axis drives the migration of T cells to the brain after stroke [18, 30, 75]. In this study, splenic IP-10 levels increased after MCAO

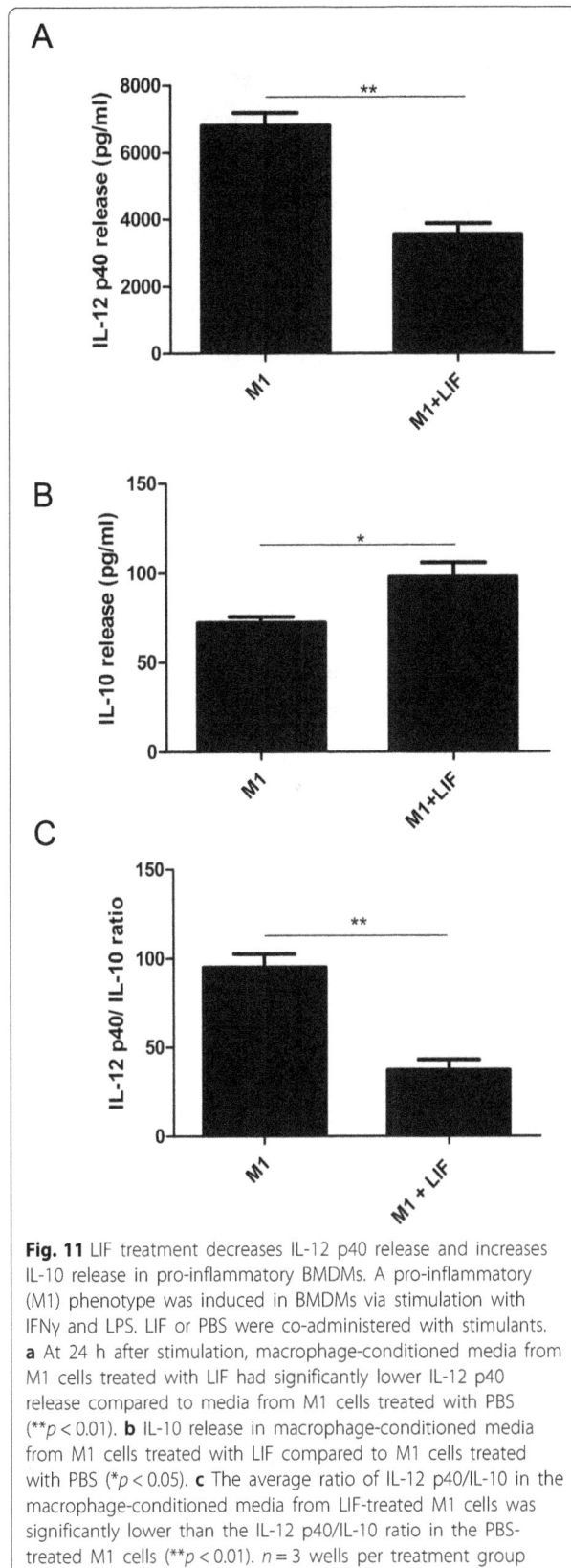

Fig. 11 LIF treatment decreases IL-12 p40 release and increases IL-10 release in pro-inflammatory BMDMs. A pro-inflammatory (M1) phenotype was induced in BMDMs via stimulation with IFNγ and LPS. LIF or PBS were co-administered with stimulants. **a** At 24 h after stimulation, macrophage-conditioned media from M1 cells treated with LIF had significantly lower IL-12 p40 release compared to media from M1 cells treated with PBS (**$p < 0.01$). **b** IL-10 release in macrophage-conditioned media from M1 cells treated with LIF compared to M1 cells treated with PBS (*$p < 0.05$). **c** The average ratio of IL-12 p40/IL-10 in the macrophage-conditioned media from LIF-treated M1 cells was significantly lower than the IL-12 p40/IL-10 ratio in the PBS-treated M1 cells (**$p < 0.01$). $n = 3$ wells per treatment group

in PBS-treated rats compared to sham-operated rats, but LIF treatment prevented the upregulation of IP-10 after MCAO. By counteracting the IFNγ-mediated increase in splenic IP-10, LIF treatment would decrease the number of pro-inflammatory immune cells migrating to the brain after stroke (Fig. 13).

Although most of the anti-inflammatory signaling promoted by LIF is occurring in the spleen, the decreased isolectin-tagged fluorescence and normalized CD11b levels in brain tissue demonstrate that LIF either decreases infiltration of monocytes/macrophages into the ischemic hemisphere or attenuates the activation of microglial cells after stroke [76]. According to Leonardo et al., the increase lectin-tagged fluorescence after permanent MCAO corresponds with increased numbers of CD11b + monocytes/macrophages into the penumbra [20]. However, we also observed that CD11b + cells in the cortical and striatal tissue of LIF-treated rats had more of a ramified phenotype, while the amoeboid phenotype was more prevalent in the tissue from PBS-treated rats. Therefore, it is possible that LIF treatment influences microglial activation in addition to monocytes/macrophages derived from the spleen. Since IP-10 is primarily responsible for facilitating chemotaxis of immune cells towards the ischemic brain, the decrease in the number of isolectin-tagged cells and CD11b levels could correspond to a smaller population of immune cells leaving the spleen [30, 77]. This explanation is further justified by the trend towards an increase in spleen weight observed after LIF treatment.

Previously released publications from our laboratory and other independent groups demonstrated that LIF promotes tissue repair and functional recovery after MCAO through Akt-dependent upregulation of protective antioxidant enzymes in neurons and oligodendrocytes. However, evidence suggests that certain Akt-inducing biological therapeutics prevent the infiltration of monocytes/macrophages and lymphocytes into the ischemic brain in addition to promoting anti-oxidation. Rowe et al. showed that administration of human umbilical cord blood (HUCB) cells at 48 h after MCAO promotes oligodendrocyte survival via the upregulation of peroxiredoxin IV and metallothionein III. In a later study by Shahaduzzaman et al., HUCB treatment after MCAO increased peroxiredoxin V expression in neurons through increased Akt signaling [78]. However, soluble factors released from HUCB cells, which include LIF, also promote anti-inflammatory signaling after stroke [46, 79]. Vendrame et al. demonstrated that intravenously injected HUCB cells migrated to the spleen during MCAO and partially counteracted the splenic immune response after stroke. Splenocytes isolated from rats treated with human umbilical cord blood cells after MCAO showed significantly decreased

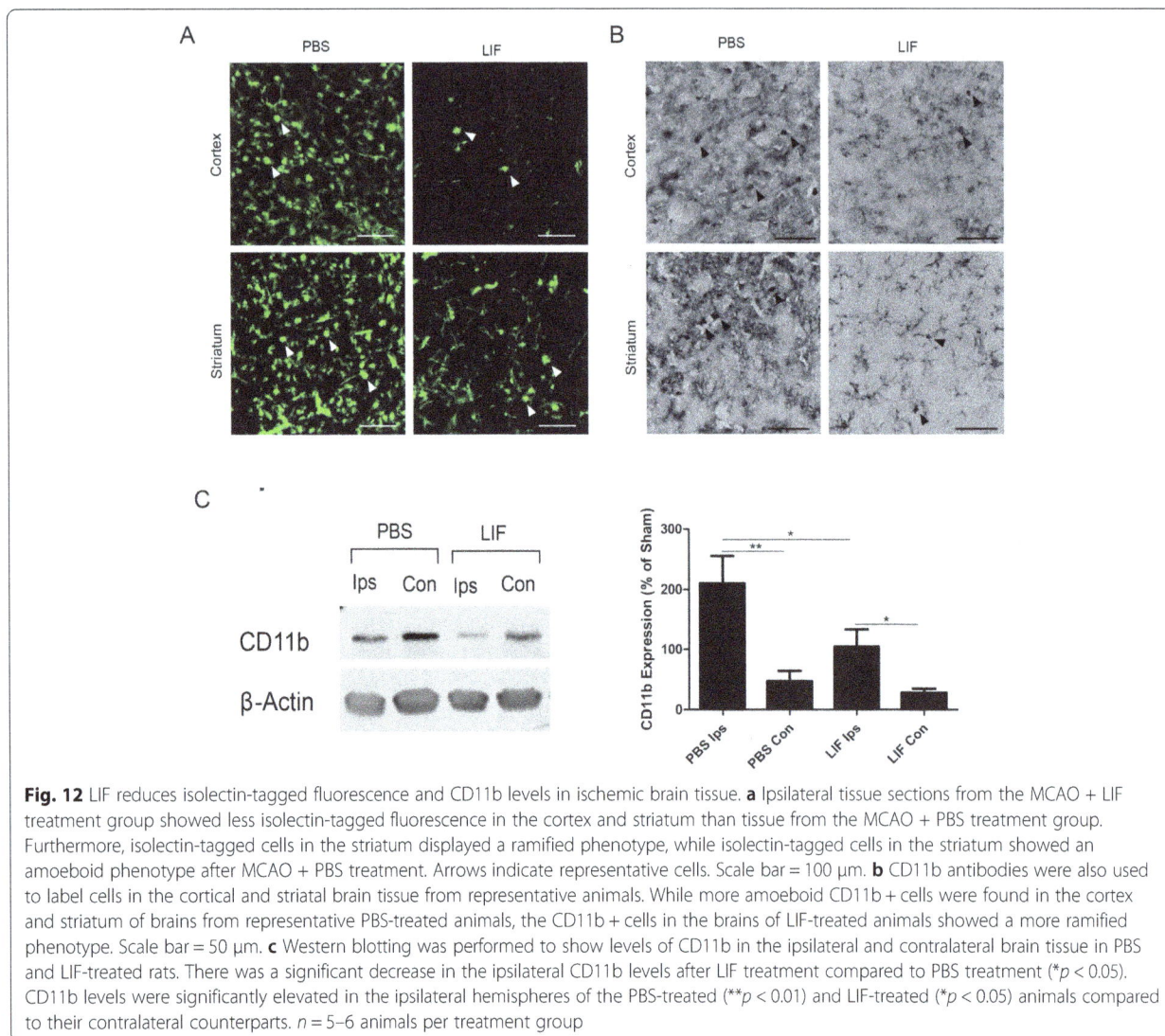

Fig. 12 LIF reduces isolectin-tagged fluorescence and CD11b levels in ischemic brain tissue. **a** Ipsilateral tissue sections from the MCAO + LIF treatment group showed less isolectin-tagged fluorescence in the cortex and striatum than tissue from the MCAO + PBS treatment group. Furthermore, isolectin-tagged cells in the striatum displayed a ramified phenotype, while isolectin-tagged cells in the striatum showed an amoeboid phenotype after MCAO + PBS treatment. Arrows indicate representative cells. Scale bar = 100 μm. **b** CD11b antibodies were also used to label cells in the cortical and striatal brain tissue from representative animals. While more amoeboid CD11b + cells were found in the cortex and striatum of brains from representative PBS-treated animals, the CD11b + cells in the brains of LIF-treated animals showed a more ramified phenotype. Scale bar = 50 μm. **c** Western blotting was performed to show levels of CD11b in the ipsilateral and contralateral brain tissue in PBS and LIF-treated rats. There was a significant decrease in the ipsilateral CD11b levels after LIF treatment compared to PBS treatment (*p < 0.05). CD11b levels were significantly elevated in the ipsilateral hemispheres of the PBS-treated (**p < 0.01) and LIF-treated (*p < 0.05) animals compared to their contralateral counterparts. n = 5–6 animals per treatment group

production of IFNγ after stimulation with concavalin-A [80]. In a subsequent study, human umbilical cord blood cell treatment after MCAO significantly attenuated the migration of pro-inflammatory isolectin-binding monocytes/macrophages into the ischemic brain [20]. Since the PI3K/Akt signaling axis promotes an anti-inflammatory phenotype in microglia/macrophages [81], it is possible that systemic LIF administration reduces inflammation among peripheral leukocytes through is transduction pathway.

Conclusion

Through this study and previously published manuscripts, this lab has demonstrated that LIF treatment after stroke promotes neuroprotection and recovery through two distinct mechanisms: Akt-dependent upregulation of antioxidant enzymes [46, 47] and modulation of the IL-12 p40/IFNγ/IP-10 signaling pathway. Future

studies dictate that these studies need to be replicated in aged rodents of both sexes, since several groups have identified sex-specific and age-dependent differences in stroke pathophysiology, specifically concerning the post-stroke immune response [82–86].

This laboratory is currently performing studies to determine the neuroprotective efficacy and anti-inflammatory action of LIF in aged (18 month) male and female rats after stroke. Preliminary results show that LIF exhibits potent anti-inflammatory signaling in the splenocytes of aged female rats after stroke. This study on aged animals also includes the use of flow cytometry to determine whether ischemic conditions alter the expression of LIFR on subpopulations of immune cells after stroke [87]. Although there are antagonists available for LIFR [88], it is very difficult to isolate the specific effects of LIFR after exogenous LIF treatment, since LIFR is also crucial for the signaling of other IL-6 family cytokines [89–91]. Therefore,

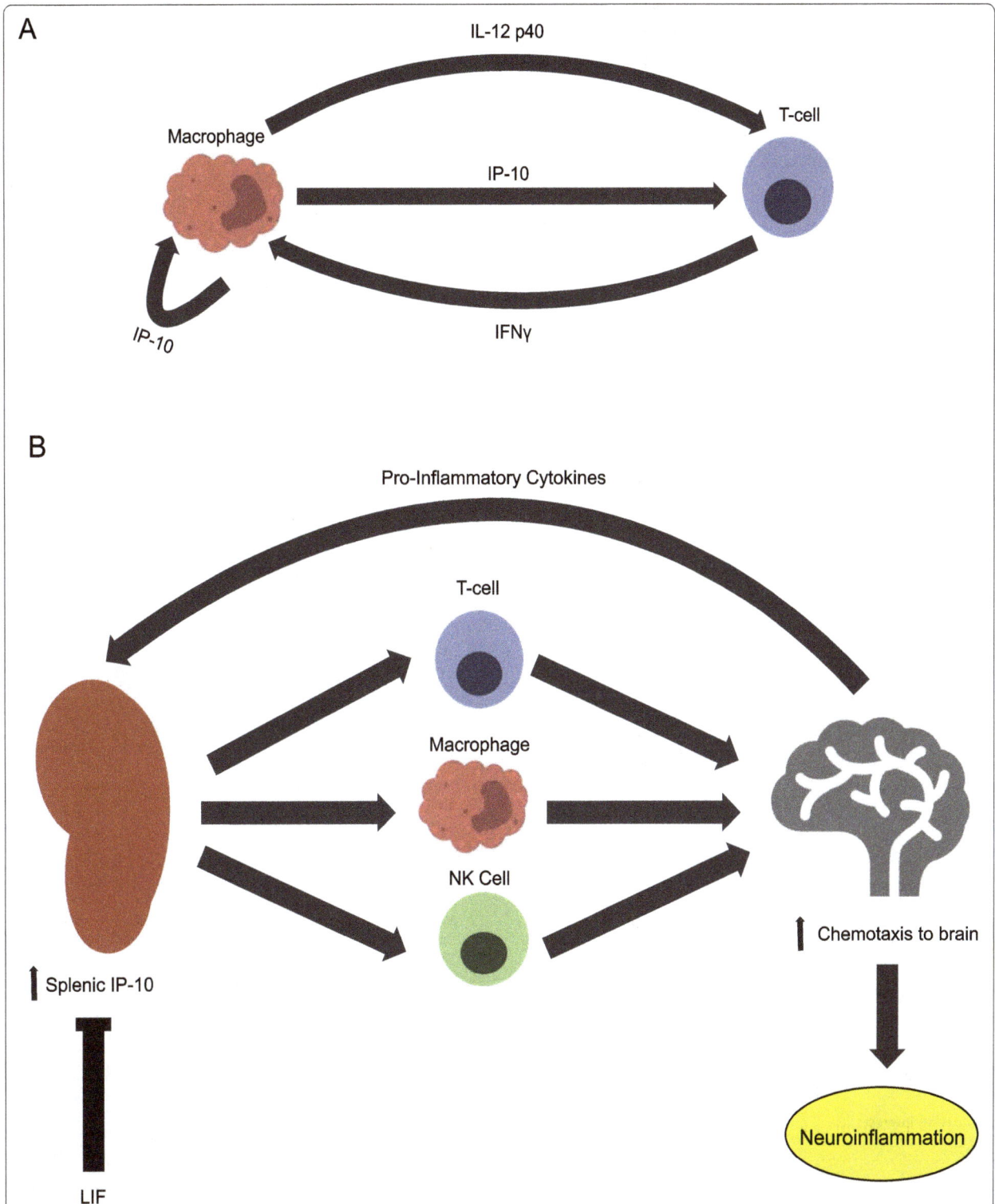

Fig. 13 The immunomodulatory effects of LIF. **a** Release of IL-12 from monocytes/macrophages activates the IL-12/IFNγ/IP-10 axis, **b** which promotes chemotaxis to the ischemic brain and increases neuroinflammation. By preventing the increase in splenic IP-10, LIF attenuates the migration of immune cells from the spleen to the ischemic brain

examining expression of LIFR among leukocyte populations might provide further insight into how LIF promotes anti-inflammatory signaling in splenocytes and peripheral blood leukocyte after stroke.

Nevertheless, these data demonstrate the need for new therapeutics that target the peripheral immune response in addition to directly promoting neuroprotection after stroke.

Abbreviations

BMDM: Bone marrow-derived macrophage; ELVO: Emergent large vessel occlusion; IFNγ: Interferon gamma; IP-10: Interferon Inducible Protein 10; LIF: Leukemia inhibitory factor; MCAO: Middle cerebral artery occlusion; NK: Natural killer; Th1: Type 1 helper T cells; Th17: IL-17+ helper T cells; tPA: Tissue plasminogen activator; Tregs: Regulatory T cells

Acknowledgements

The authors would like to acknowledge the Department of Neurology at the University of Kentucky for providing additional startup funding for experiments and equipment. The authors would also like to acknowledge Dr. Phillip Popovich for generously contributing SL929 cells, Dr. Bei Zhang for assisting with BMDM culture, and Ms. Linda Simmerman for assistance with fluorescent microscopy.

Funding

The work of K.P. is supported by internal funding from the University of Kentucky as well as the following project grants from the National Institute of Neurological Disorders and Stroke: 1R01NS091146-01, 1R56NS091146-01, and 1R21NS078517-01. The work of J.G. is also supported by funding from the National Institute for Neurological Disorders and Stroke (Project 5R01NS091582-03).

Authors' contributions

SD and KP designed all experiments for the current study except for the experiments shown in Fig. 7, which were designed, performed, and analyzed by TK and JG. Other experiments were performed and data was collected by SD, LC, TA, CC, and EF. Data analysis and interpretation was performed by SD and LC. Manuscript and figures were prepared by SD and KP. All authors were involved with revising and approving the final draft of the manuscript prior to submission.

Competing interests

The authors declare that they have no competing interests.

Author details

[1]Department of Neurology, University of Kentucky, 741 S. Limestone BBSRB B457, Lexington, KY 40536-0905, USA. [2]Department of Neuroscience, University of Kentucky, 800 Rose St. Lexington, Lexington, KY 40536, USA. [3]Department of Physiology, University of Kentucky, 800 Rose St. MS508, Lexington, KY 40536, USA. [4]Spinal Cord and Brain Injury Repair Center, University of Kentucky, 741 S. Limestone BBSRB B463, Lexington, KY 40536, USA. [5]Department of Molecular Pharmacology and Physiology, University of South Florida, 12901 Bruce B. Downs Blvd MDC 8, Tampa, FL 33612, USA. [6]Department of Molecular Medicine, University of South Florida, 12901 Bruce B. Downs Blvd MDC 7, Tampa, FL 33612, USA.

References

1. Smith WS, Lev MH, English JD, Camargo EC, Chou M, Johnston SC, Gonzalez G, Schaefer PW, Dillon WP, Koroshetz WJ. Significance of large vessel intracranial occlusion causing acute ischemic stroke and TIA. Stroke. 2009;40: 3834–40.
2. Lima FO, Furie KL, Silva GS, et al. Prognosis of untreated strokes due to anterior circulation proximal intracranial arterial occlusions detected by use of computed tomography angiography. JAMA Neurol. 2014;71:151–7.
3. Jayaraman MV, Hussain MS, Abruzzo T, Albani B, Albuquerque FC, Alexander MJ, Ansari SA, Arthur AS, Baxter B, Bulsara KR. Embolectomy for stroke with emergent large vessel occlusion (ELVO): report of the Standards and Guidelines Committee of the Society of NeuroInterventional Surgery. J Neurointerventional Surg. 2015;2015:011717 neurintsurg.
4. Campbell BC, Mitchell PJ, Kleinig TJ, Dewey HM, Churilov L, Yassi N, Yan B, Dowling RJ, Parsons MW, Oxley TJ, et al. Endovascular therapy for ischemic stroke with perfusion-imaging selection. N Engl J Med. 2015;372:1009–18.
5. Goyal M, Menon BK, van Zwam WH, Dippel DWJ, Mitchell PJ, Demchuk AM, Dávalos A, Majoie CBLM, van der Lugt A, de Miquel MA, et al. Endovascular thrombectomy after large-vessel ischaemic stroke: a meta-analysis of individual patient data from five randomised trials. Lancet. 2016;387:1723–31.
6. Menon B, Brown S, Almekhlafi M, Dippel D, Campbell B, Mitchell P, Hill M, Demchuk A, Jovin T, Davalos A, et al. 6 Efficacy of endovascular thrombectomy in patients with M2 segment middle cerebral artery occlusions: meta-analysis of data from the HERMES collaboration. J NeuroInterventional Surg. 2018;10:A139–40.
7. McMeekin P, White P, James MA, Price CI, Flynn D, Ford GA. Estimating the number of UK stroke patients eligible for endovascular thrombectomy. Eur Stroke J. 2017;2:319–26.
8. Rothstein JD, Dykes-Hoberg M, Pardo CA, Bristol LA, Jin L, Kuncl RW, Kanai Y, Hediger MA, Wang Y, Schielke JP. Knockout of glutamate transporters reveals a major role for astroglial transport in excitotoxicity and clearance of glutamate. Neuron. 1996;16:675–86.
9. Bano D, Nicotera P. Ca2+ signals and neuronal death in brain ischemia. Stroke. 2007;38:674–6.
10. Streit W, Graeber M, Kreutzberg G. Functional plasticity of microglia: a review. Glia. 1988;1:301–7.
11. Davalos D, Grutzendler J, Yang G, Kim JV, Zuo Y, Jung S, Littman DR, Dustin ML, Gan WB. ATP mediates rapid microglial response to local brain injury in vivo. Nat Neurosci. 2005;8:752–8.
12. Marsh BJ, Williams-Karnesky RL, Stenzel-Poore MP. Toll-like receptor signaling in endogenous neuroprotection and stroke. Neuroscience. 2009; 158:1007–20.
13. Patel AR, Ritzel R, McCullough LD, Liu F. Microglia and ischemic stroke: a double-edged sword. Internatl J of Phys Pathophys Pharm. 2013;5:73–90.
14. Clark AW, Krekoski CA, Bou SS, Chapman KR, Edwards DR. Increased gelatinase a (MMP-2) and gelatinase B (MMP-9) activities in human brain after focal ischemia. Neurosci Lett. 1997;238:53–6.
15. Akopov SE, Simonian NA, Grigorian GS. Dynamics of polymorphonuclear leukocyte accumulation in acute cerebral infarction and their correlation with brain tissue damage. Stroke. 1996;27:1739–43.
16. Barone FC, Feuerstein GZ. Inflammatory mediators and stroke: new opportunities for novel therapeutics. J Cereb Blood Flow Metab. 1999;19: 819–34.
17. Vendrame M, Cassady J, Newcomb J, Butler T, Pennypacker KR, Zigova T, Sanberg CD, Sanberg PR, Willing AE. Infusion of human umbilical cord blood cells in a rat model of stroke dose-dependently rescues behavioral deficits and reduces infarct volume. Stroke. 2004;35:2390–5.
18. Hurn PD, Subramanian S, Parker SM, Afentoulis ME, Kaler LJ, Vandenbark AA, Offner H. T- and B-cell-deficient mice with experimental stroke have reduced lesion size and inflammation. J Cereb Blood Flow Metab. 2007;27: 1798–805.
19. Iadecola C, Anrather J. The immunology of stroke: from mechanisms to translation. Nat Med. 2011;17:796–808.

20. Leonardo CC, Hall AA, Collier LA, Ajmo CTJ, Willing AE, Pennypacker KR. Human umbilical cord blood cell therapy blocks the morphological change and recruitment of CD-11b-expressing isolectin-binding proinflammatory cells after middle cerebral artery occlusion. J Neurosci Res. 2010;88:1213–22.

21. Leonardo CC, Musso J, Das M, Rowe DD, Collier LA, Mohapatra S, Pennypacker KR. CCL20 is associated with neurodegeneration following experimental traumatic brain injury and promotes cellular toxicity in vitro. Transl Stroke Res. 2012;3:357–63.

22. Myers MG, Norris JW, Hachniski VC, Sole MJ. Plasma norepinephrine in stroke. Stroke. 1981;12:200–4.

23. Ajmo CT Jr, Collier LA, Leonardo CC, Hall AA, Green SM, Womble TA, Cuevas J, Willing AE, Pennypacker KR. Blockade of adrenoreceptors inhibits the splenic response to stroke. Exp Neurol. 2009;218(1):47–55.

24. Chen H, Chopp M, Zhang RL, Bodzin G, Chen Q, Rusche JR, Todd RF 3rd. Anti-CD11b monoclonal antibody reduces ischemic cell damage after transient focal cerebral ischemia in rat. Ann Neurol. 1994;35:458–63.

25. Vendrame M, Gemma C, De Mesquita D, Collier L, Bickford PC, Sanberg CD, Sanberg PR, Pennypacker KR, Willing AE. Anti-inflammatory effects of human cord blood cells in a rat model of stroke. Stem Cells Dev. 2005;14:595–604.

26. Ajmo CT Jr, Vernon DO, Collier L, Hall AA, Garbuzova-Davis S, Willing A, Pennypacker KR. The spleen contributes to stroke-induced neurodegeneration. J Neurosci Res. 2008;86:2227–34.

27. Seifert HA, Hall AA, Chapman CB, Collier LA, Willing AE, Pennypacker KR. A transient decrease in spleen size following stroke corresponds to splenocyte release into systemic circulation. J Neuroimmune Pharm. 2012;7:1017–24.

28. Schoenborn JR, Wilson CB. Regulation of interferon-γ during innate and adaptive immune responses. In: Advances in Immunology. Boston: Academic Press; 2007;96:41–101.

29. Mosser DM, Edwards JP. Exploring the full spectrum of macrophage activation. Nature Rev Immuno. 2008;8:958–69.

30. Seifert HA, Collier LA, Chapman CB, Benkovic SA, Willing AE, Pennypacker KR. Pro-inflammatory interferon gamma signaling is directly associated with stroke induced neurodegeneration. J Neuroimmune Pharmacol. 2014;9:679–89.

31. Vahidy FS, Parsha KN, Rahbar MH, Lee MK, Bui TT, Nguyen C, Barreto AD, Bambhroliya AB, Sahota P, Yang B, et al. Acute splenic responses in patients with ischemic stroke and intracerebral hemorrhage. J Cereb Blood Flow Met. 2015;36(6):1012–21.

32. Vahidy FS, Rahbar MH, Lee M, Parsha KN, Sahota P, Nguyen CB, Bui T, Barreto AD, Bambhroliya AB, Aronowski J, et al. Spleen contraction in patients with ischemic stroke and brain hemorrhage: validating animal studies. Stroke. 2015;46:A166.

33. Zha A, Vahidy F, Randhawa J, Parsha K, Bui T, Aronowski J, Savitz SI. Association between splenic contraction and the systemic inflammatory response after acute ischemic stroke varies with age and race. Transl Stroke Res. 2018;9(5):484–92.

34. Kurek JB, Radford AJ, Crump DE, Bower JJ, Feeney SJ, Austin L, Byrne E. LIF (AM424), a promising growth factor for the treatment of ALS. J Neurol Sci. 1998;160(1):S106–13.

35. Azari MF, Galle A, Lopes EC, Kurek J, Cheema SS. Leukemia inhibitory factor by systemic administration rescues spinal motor neurons in the SOD1 G93A murine model of familial amyotrophic lateral sclerosis. Brain Res. 2001;922:144–7.

36. Butzkueven H, Zhang JG, Soilu-Hanninen M, Hochrein H, Chionh F, Shipham KA, Emery B, Turnley AM, Petratos S, Ernst M, et al. LIF receptor signaling limits immune-mediated demyelination by enhancing oligodendrocyte survival. Nat Med. 2002;8:613–9.

37. Butzkueven H, Emery B, Cipriani T, Marriott MP, Kilpatrick TJ. Endogenous leukemia inhibitory factor production limits autoimmune demyelination and oligodendrocyte loss. Glia. 2006;53:696–703.

38. Linker RA, Kruse N, Israel S, Wei T, Seubert S, Hombach A, Holtmann B, Luhder F, Ransohoff RM, Sendtner M. Leukemia inhibitory factor deficiency modulates the immune response and limits autoimmune demyelination: a new role for neurotrophic cytokines in neuroinflammation. J Immunol. 2008; 180:2204–13.

39. Marriott MP, Emery B, Cate HS, Binder MD, Kemper D, Wu Q, Kolbe S, Gordon IR, Wang H, Egan G, et al. Leukemia inhibitory factor signaling modulates both central nervous system demyelination and myelin repair. Glia. 2008;56:686–98.

40. Slaets H, Dumont D, Vanderlocht J, Noben JP, Leprince P, Robben J, Hendriks J, Stinissen P, Hellings N. Leukemia inhibitory factor induces an antiapoptotic response in oligodendrocytes through Akt-phosphorylation and up-regulation of 14-3-3. Proteomics. 2008;8:1237–47.

41. Rittchen S, Boyd A, Burns A, Park J, Fahmy TM, Metcalfe S, Williams A. Myelin repair in vivo is increased by targeting oligodendrocyte precursor cells with nanoparticles encapsulating leukaemia inhibitory factor (LIF). Biomaterials. 2015;56:78–85.

42. Janssens K, Van den Haute C, Baekelandt V, Lucas S, van Horssen J, Somers V, Van Wijmeersch B, Stinissen P, Hendriks JJ, Slaets H, Hellings N. Leukemia inhibitory factor tips the immune balance towards regulatory T cells in multiple sclerosis. Brain Behav Immun. 2015;45:180–8.

43. Kerr BJ, Patterson PH. Leukemia inhibitory factor promotes oligodendrocyte survival after spinal cord injury. Glia. 2005;51:73–9.

44. Azari MF, Profyris C, Karnezis T, Bernard CC, Small DH, Cheema SS, Ozturk E, Hatzinisiriou I, Petratos S. Leukemia inhibitory factor arrests oligodendrocyte death and demyelination in spinal cord injury. J Neuropathol Exp Neurol. 2006;65:914–29.

45. Suzuki S, Yamashita T, Tanaka K, Hattori H, Sawamoto K, Okano H, Suzuki N. Activation of cytokine signaling through leukemia inhibitory factor receptor (LIFR)/gp130 attenuates ischemic brain injury in rats. J Cereb Blood Flow Metab. 2005;25:685–93.

46. Rowe DR, Collier LA, Seifert HA, Chapman CB, Leonardo CC, Willing AE, Pennypacker KR. Leukemia inhibitory factor promotes functional recovery and oligodendrocyte survival in rat models of focal ischemia. Eur J Neurosci. 2014;40:3111–9.

47. Davis SM, Collier LA, Leonardo CC, Seifert HA, Ajmo CT, Pennypacker KR. Leukemia inhibitory factor protects neurons from ischemic damage via upregulation of superoxide dismutase 3. Mol Neurobiol. 2017;54:608–22.

48. Rowe D: Secreted factors from human umbilical cord blood cells protect oligodendrocytes from ischemic insult. 2011.

49. Janssens K, Slaets H, Hellings N. Immunomodulatory properties of the IL-6 cytokine family in multiple sclerosis. Annals N Y Acad Scie. 2015;1351:52–60.

50. Duluc D, Delneste Y, Tan F, Moles MP, Grimaud L, Lenoir J, Preisser L, Anegon I, Catala L, Ifrah N, et al. Tumor-associated leukemia inhibitory factor and IL-6 skew monocyte differentiation into tumor-associated macrophage-like cells. Blood. 2007;110:4319–30.

51. Merrill JE, Ignarro LJ, Sherman MP, Melinek J, Lane TE. Microglial cell cytotoxicity of oligodendrocytes is mediated through nitric oxide. J Immunol. 1993;151:2132–41.

52. Ajmo CT Jr, Vernon DO, Collier L, Pennypacker KR, Cuevas J. Sigma receptor activation reduces infarct size at 24 hours after permanent middle cerebral artery occlusion in rats. Curr Neurovasc Res. 2006;3:89–98.

53. Seifert HA, Leonardo CC, Hall AA, Rowe DD, Collier LA, Benkovic SA, Willing AE, Pennypacker KR. The spleen contributes to stroke induced neurodegeneration through interferon gamma signaling. Metab Brain Dis. 2012;27:131–41.

54. Hall AA, Guyer AG, Leonardo CC, Ajmo CT Jr, Collier LA, Willing AE, Pennypacker KR. Human umbilical cord blood cells directly suppress ischemic oligodendrocyte cell death. J Neurosci Res. 2009;87:333–41.

55. Gensel JC, Nakamura S, Guan Z, van Rooijen N, Ankeny DP, Popovich PG. Macrophages promote axon regeneration with concurrent neurotoxicity. J Neurosci. 2009;29:3956–68.

56. Gensel JC, Zhang B. Macrophage activation and its role in repair and pathology after spinal cord injury. Brain Res. 1619;2015:1–11.

57. Zhang B, Bailey WM, Braun KJ, Gensel JC. Age decreases macrophage IL-10 expression: implications for functional recovery and tissue repair in spinal cord injury. Exp Neurol. 2015;273:83–91.

58. Burgess AW, Metcalf D, Kozka I, Simpson R, Vairo G, Hamilton J, Nice E. Purification of two forms of colony-stimulating factor from mouse L-cell-conditioned medium. J Biol Chem. 1985;260:16004–11.

59. Kigerl KA, Gensel JC, Ankeny DP, Alexander JK, Donnelly DJ, Popovich PG. Identification of two distinct macrophage subsets with divergent effects causing either neurotoxicity or regeneration in the injured mouse spinal cord. J Neurosci. 2009;29:13435–44.

60. Offner H, Subramanian S, Parker SM, Afentoulis ME, Vandenbark AA, Hurn PD. Experimental stroke induces massive, rapid activation of the peripheral immune system. J Cereb Blood Flow Metab. 2006;26:654–65.

61. Blanchard F, Duplomb L, Wang Y, Robledo O, Kinzie E, Pitard V, Godard A, Jacques Y, Baumann H. Stimulation of leukemia inhibitory factor receptor degradation by extracellular signal-regulated kinase. J Biol Chem. 2000;275:28793–801.

62. Woods AM, McIlmoil CJ, Rankin EN, Packer AA, Stevens JC, Macievic JA, Brown AB, Porter JP, Judd AM. Leukemia inhibitory factor protein and receptors are expressed in the bovine adrenal cortex and increase cortisol and decrease adrenal androgen release. Domest Anim Endocrinol. 2008;35:217–30.

63. Schulze J, Vogelgesang A, Dressel A. Catecholamines, steroids and immune alterations in ischemic stroke and other acute diseases. Aging Dis. 2014;5:327.

64. Heufler C, Koch F, Stanzl U, Topar G, Wysocka M, Trinchieri G, Enk A, Steinman RM, Romani N, Schuler G. Interleukin-12 is produced by dendritic cells and mediates T helper 1 development as well as interferon-γ production by T helper 1 cells. Eur J Immunol. 1996;26:659–68.

65. Zhu J, Paul WE. CD4 T cells: fates, functions, and faults. Blood. 2008;112: 1557–69.

66. Konoeda F, Shichita T, Yoshida H, Sugiyama Y, Muto G, Hasegawa E, Morita R, Suzuki N, Yoshimura A. Therapeutic effect of IL-12/23 and their signaling pathway blockade on brain ischemia model. Biochem Biophys Res Commun. 2010;402:500–6.

67. D'andrea A, Aste-Amezaga M, Valiante NM, Ma X, Kubin M, Trinchieri G. Interleukin 10 (IL-10) inhibits human lymphocyte interferon gamma-production by suppressing natural killer cell stimulatory factor/IL-12 synthesis in accessory cells. J Exp Med. 1993;178:1041–8.

68. te Velde AA, Huijbens R, Heije K, de Vries JE, Figdor CG. Interleukin-4 (IL-4) inhibits secretion of IL-1 beta, tumor necrosis factor alpha, and IL-6 by human monocytes. Blood. 1990;76:1392–7.

69. Neuner P, Urbanski A, Trautinger F, Möller A, Kirnbauer R, Kapp A, Schöpf E, Schwarz T, Luger TA. Increased IL-6 production by monocytes and keratinocytes in patients with psoriasis. J Investig Dermatol. 1991;97:27–33.

70. Luster AD. The role of chemokines in linking innate and adaptive immunity. Curr Opin Immunol. 2002;14:129–35.

71. Arumugam TV, Granger DN, Mattson MP. Stroke and T-cells. NeuroMolecular Med. 2005;7:229–42.

72. Yilmaz G, Arumugam TV, Stokes KY, Granger DN. Role of T lymphocytes and interferon-γ in ischemic stroke. Circulation. 2006;113:2105–12.

73. Agostini C, Calabrese F, Rea F, Facco M, Tosoni A, Loy M, Binotto G, Valente M, Trentin L, Semenzato G. Cxcr3 and its ligand CXCL10 are expressed by inflammatory cells infiltrating lung allografts and mediate chemotaxis of T cells at sites of rejection. Am J Pathol. 2001;158:1703–11.

74. Loetscher P, Pellegrino A, Gong JH, Mattioli I, Loetscher M, Bardi G, Baggiolini M, Clark-Lewis I. The ligands of CXC chemokine receptor 3, I-TAC, Mig, and IP10, are natural antagonists for CCR3. J Biol Chem. 2001;276:2986–91.

75. Offner H, Subramanian S, Parker SM, Wang C, Afentoulis ME, Lewis A, Vandenbark AA, Hurn PD. Splenic atrophy in experimental stroke is accompanied by increased regulatory T cells and circulating macrophages. J Immunol. 2006;176:6523–31.

76. Streit WJ, Kreutzberg GW. Lectin binding by resting and reactive microglia. J Neurocytol. 1987;16:249–60.

77. Zhang Y, Gao Z, Wang D, Zhang T, Sun B, Mu L, Wang J, Liu Y, Kong Q, Liu X, et al. Accumulation of natural killer cells in ischemic brain tissues and the chemotactic effect of IP-10. J Neuroinflammation. 2014;11:79.

78. Shahaduzzaman M, Mehta V, Golden JE, Rowe DD, Green S, Tadinada R, Foran E, Sanberg PR, Pennypacker KR, Willing AE. Human umbilical cord blood cells induce neuroprotective change in gene expression profile in neurons afterilschemia through activation of Akt pathway. Cell Transplant. 2015; (Epub ahead of press).

79. Rowe DD, Leonardo CC, Recio JA, Collier LA, Willing AE, Pennypacker KR. Human umbilical cord blood cells protect oligodendrocytes from brain ischemia through Akt signal transduction. J Biol Chem. 2012;287:4177–87.

80. Vendrame M, Gemma C, Pennypacker KR, Bickford PC, Davis Sanberg C, Sanberg PR, Willing AE. Cord blood rescues stroke-induced changes in splenocyte phenotype and function. Exp Neurol. 2006;199:191–200.

81. Wang G, Shi Y, Jiang X, Leak RK, Hu X, Wu Y, Pu H, Li W-W, Tang B, Wang Y. HDAC inhibition prevents white matter injury by modulating microglia/macrophage polarization through the GSK3β/PTEN/Akt axis. Proc Natl Acad Sci. 2015;112:2853–8.

82. Dotson AL, Wang J, Saugstad J, Murphy SJ, Offner H. Splenectomy reduces infarct volume and neuroinflammation in male but not female mice in experimental stroke. J Neuroimmunol. 2015;278:289–98.

83. Bodhankar S, Lapato A, Chen Y, Vandenbark AA, Saugstad JA, Offner H. Role for microglia in sex differences after ischemic stroke: importance of M2. Metab Brain Dis. 2015;30:1515–29.

84. Dotson AL, Wang J, Chen Y, Manning D, Nguyen H, Saugstad JA, Offner H. Sex differences and the role of PPAR alpha in experimental stroke. Metab Brain Dis. 2016;31:539–47.

85. Dotson AL, Offner H. Sex differences in the immune response to experimental stroke: implications for translational research. J Neurosci Res. 2017;95:437–46.

86. Bravo-Alegria J, McCullough LD, Liu F. Sex differences in stroke across the lifespan: the role of T lymphocytes. Neurochem Int. 2017;107:127–37.

87. Davis SM, Collier LA, Martha SR, Powell DK, Pennypacker KR. Abstract WMP77: anti-inflammatory signaling by leukemia inhibitory factor is suppressed in aged animals after stroke. Am Heart Assoc. 2018.

88. Mohamet L, Heath JK, Kimber S. Determining the LIF-sensitive period for implantation using a LIF-receptor antagonist. Reproduction. 2009;138:827–36.

89. Ip NY, Nye SH, Boulton TG, Davis SM, Taga T, Li Y, Birren SJ, Yasukawa K, Kishimoto T, Anderson DJ, et al. CNTF and LIF act on neuronal cells via shared signaling pathways that involve the IL-6 signal transducing receptor component gp130. Cell. 1992;69:1121–32.

90. Arce V, Garces A, de Bovis B, Filippi P, Henderson C, Pettmann B, deLapeyrière O. Cardiotrophin-1 requires LIFRβ to promote survival of mouse motoneurons purified by a novel technique. J Neurosci Res. 1999;55:119–26.

91. Blanchard F, Wang Y, Kinzie E, Duplomb L, Godard A, Baumann H. Oncostatin M regulates the synthesis and turnover of gp130, leukemia inhibitory factor receptor alpha, and oncostatin M receptor beta by distinct mechanisms. J Biol Chem. 2001;276:47038–45.

4

Ibuprofen prevents progression of ataxia telangiectasia symptoms in ATM-deficient mice

Chin Wai Hui[1†], Xuan Song[1†], Fulin Ma[1], Xuting Shen[1,2] and Karl Herrup[1*] (iD)

Abstract

Background: Inflammation plays a critical role in accelerating the progression of neurodegenerative diseases, such as Alzheimer's disease (AD) and ataxia telangiectasia (A-T). In A-T mouse models, LPS-induced neuroinflammation advances the degenerative changes found in cerebellar Purkinje neurons both in vivo and in vitro. In the current study, we ask whether ibuprofen, a non-steroidal anti-inflammatory drug (NSAID), can have the opposite effect and delay the symptoms of the disease.

Methods: We tested the beneficial effects of ibuprofen in both in vitro and in vivo models. Conditioned medium from LPS stimulated primary microglia (LM) applied to cultures of dissociated cortical neurons leads to numerous degenerative changes. Pretreatment of the neurons with ibuprofen, however, blocked this damage. Systemic injection of LPS into either adult wild-type or adult $Atm^{-/-}$ mice produced an immune challenge that triggered profound behavioral, biochemical, and histological effects. We used a 2-week ibuprofen pretreatment regimen to investigate whether these LPS effects could be blocked. We also treated young presymptomatic $Atm^{-/-}$ mice to determine if ibuprofen could delay the appearance of symptoms.

Results: Adding ibuprofen directly to neuronal cultures significantly reduced LM-induced degeneration. Curiously, adding ibuprofen to the microglia cultures before the LPS challenge had little effect, thus implying a direct effect of the NSAID on the neuronal cultures. In vivo administration of ibuprofen to $Atm^{-/-}$ animals before a systemic LPS immune challenge suppressed cytological damage. The ibuprofen effects were widespread as microglial activation, p38 phosphorylation, DNA damage, and neuronal cell cycle reentry were all reduced. Unfortunately, ibuprofen only slightly improved the LPS-induced behavioral deficits. Yet, while the behavioral symptoms could not be reversed once they were established in adult $Atm^{-/-}$ animals, administration of ibuprofen to young mutant pups prevented their symptoms from appearing.

Conclusion: Inflammatory processes impact the normal progression of A-T implying that modulation of the immune system can have therapeutic benefit for both the behavioral and cellular symptoms of this neurodegenerative disease.

Keywords: Ataxia telangiectasia, Ibuprofen, Anti-inflammatory, Microglia, Purkinje cell

* Correspondence: herrup@ust.hk
†Chin Wai Hui and Xuan Song contributed equally to this work.
[1]Division of Life Science and State Key Laboratory of Molecular Neurobiology, Hong Kong University of Science and Technology, Clear Water Bay, Kowloon, Hong Kong
Full list of author information is available at the end of the article

Background

Ataxia telangiectasia (A-T) is a neurodegenerative disease of childhood with a prevalence between 1 in 40,000 and 1 in 100,000 people worldwide. It results from the mutation of a single gene, A-T mutated (ATM), whose gene product is a large kinase of the PI3K family. A-T symptoms include a progressive neuronal loss, ataxia, cancer susceptibility, hypersensitivity to ionizing radiation, immunodeficiency, and sterility [1–3]. The particular type of immunodeficiency found in A-T is life-threatening for nearly one third of A-T patients because of the resulting increase in susceptibility to infections, particularly of the lung [4]. In the context of a neurodegenerative disease, the co-occurrence of these immune problems is noteworthy since the immune and nervous system maintain extensive communication through the entire lifespan [5, 6]. The development of the central nervous system (CNS) can be significantly altered by immune challenges, and in the adult, unchecked inflammatory signals and the resulting cytokine imbalances usually lead to fatigue, impaired cognition, as well as slower healing and recovery after nerve injury [7–12]. Chronic inflammation is found in many age-related disorders, where it raises the susceptibility to cardiovascular difficulties, asthma, and cancer [13]. Many late-onset neurodegenerative diseases are also associated with a long-term inflammatory process, and in vitro studies suggest that this process involves the release of a large profile of pro-inflammatory cytokines [14, 15] and reactive oxygen species (ROS) [16, 17]. In A-T patients, sustained immune challenges, including bacterial infections and chronic inflammation, greatly contribute to the development of disease pathology [18, 19]. Furthermore, reports from clinical trials have shown that glucocorticoids, powerful anti-inflammatory hormones, are able to ameliorate the symptoms of A-T [20, 21]. The finding of peripheral immune deficiency in A-T patients is well established and highlights the contribution of the immune system to the symptoms of A-T. The contribution of the immune system, in particular, the microglia of the brain's innate immune system, to the neurological and neuropathological abnormalities of A-T remains less certain.

Previous studies in experimental systems have shown that microglia have a significant impact on the process of neurodegeneration in A-T in both mouse and Drosophila models [22, 23]. Studies from our lab have found that systemic LPS administration triggers exaggerated neuronal damage in both short (1 week) [24] and long (1 month) [25] time frames. In this study, we investigated the effect of ibuprofen, a non-selective non-steroidal anti-inflammatory drug (NSAID). NSAIDs are regarded as non-selective COX inhibitors to reduce neuroinflammation, promote neuronal survival, and improve cognitive function in rodent models of different neurodegenerative conditions—Alzheimer's disease (AD), traumatic brain injury, and exaggerated

excitotoxicity [26–28]. Epidemiological studies suggest that they are protective in human AD [29] and are of significant benefit in mouse models of AD if they are administered before symptoms appear [29, 30]. Unfortunately, prospective AD clinical trials showed little efficacy in subjects with mild dementia, but two human studies have shown that ibuprofen is able to modify the progression of mild AD [31] and can directly block LPS-induced microglial activation and impairments of spatial working memory [32]. These human studies have been replicated in mouse models of AD [30, 33–35] with the exception of the 5XFAD mouse [36].

Here, we report that in vitro ibuprofen pretreatment offers significant protection. In vivo $Atm^{-/-}$ animals pretreated with ibuprofen for 2 weeks are less vulnerable to LPS-induced motor dysfunction, have less Purkinje cell damage, and show reduced microglial activation. In the absence of an exogenous immune challenge, ibuprofen treatment of young presymptomatic $Atm^{-/-}$ animals improved multiple classic histopathological features of the $Atm^{-/-}$ brain. These data support a potential role for ibuprofen in preventing the development of neuropathological symptoms in A-T. While ibuprofen did not improve the motor performance of the $Atm^{-/-}$ mice in the treatment regimen we used, it proved to be effective in preventing new pathological signs from developing. Taken together, our data suggest that administration of the NSAID ibuprofen can impact the progression of A-T at both the cellular and organismal level.

Methods and materials

Atm-deficient mice

A breeding colony of mice with a targeted disruption of the Atm gene Atm^{tm1Awb} [37] was obtained from The Jackson Laboratory (Bar Harbor, ME). Generation of mutants was achieved through the mating of heterozygous $Atm^{+/-}$ males and $Atm^{+/-}$ females. The mice were maintained on a 129/SvJ genetic background. Genotyping was performed on extracted tail DNA using PCR techniques that were described previously [37]. All animal experimental protocols were approved both by the Animal Ethics Committee at HKUST and their care that was in accord with the institutional and Hong Kong guidelines.

Injections with lipopolysaccharide

Lipopolysaccharide (LPS, *Escherichia coli* serotype 055:B5) was purchased from Sigma-Aldrich (L2880, St. Louis, MO, USA), dissolved in distilled water, and stored at − 20 °C. Adult mice (3-month-old) of $Atm^{+/+}$ and $Atm^{-/-}$ genotypes were given daily intraperitoneal injections of LPS (1 mg/kg for a period of 4 days) in keeping with our previous protocol [24]. A control group was treated on the same schedule with injection of filtered saline only. Mice were killed on the fifth day, 24 h after the last injection. Mice in both groups were monitored carefully for signs of sickness or distress during the entire period. Following sacrifice, the brains were dissected and the tissues prepared as described below.

Ibuprofen oral administration

Commercial ibuprofen was purchased from CVS pharmacy and kept at room temperature. Two treatment groups were established. In the first group, the dose of ibuprofen used (62.5 mg/kg) [38] was orally administrated to P10 mice of $Atm^{+/+}$ and $Atm^{-/-}$ genotypes once per day for 2 weeks to investigate whether ibuprofen could block the development of the A-T symptoms that normally appear during this early postnatal period. A control group of the same age was untreated. Mice were killed as above immediately after receiving the last oral suspension. A second group of 3-month-old adult animals ($Atm^{+/+}$ and $Atm^{-/-}$ genotypes) were administrated ibuprofen (0.5 mg/ml of drinking water, calculated based on the amount of water consumed by mice and administration dose as mentioned above) for 2 weeks to investigate whether ibuprofen could prevent the progression of A-T symptoms. Mice then received daily intraperitoneal injections of LPS (1 mg/kg) for 4 days with or without oral administration of ibuprofen (62.5 mg/kg). Mice were killed on the fifth day, 24 h after the last injection. During the treatment, mice were monitored carefully.

Rotarod test

After treatment with LPS or/and ibuprofen, mice were subjected to rotarod testing without initial training to measure motor coordination but not motor learning. Mice were placed on the rotating rod for 1 min then tested for coordination by measuring the time they were able to remain on the rod as the rotation speed accelerated (4–40 rpm with an acceleration of 4 rpm/10s). The experimental groups were randomized in different positions while running on the rods. The rotarod software (ANY-maze Behavior Tracking Software; Stoelting Co., Wood Dale, IL) calculates the number of times the animal complete an entire rotation of 360° during the observation period.

Open field test

The open field test is used to determine gross locomotor activity and exploration habits. Mice were introduced singly into a square arena (50 × 50 cm) bounded by tall walls with a defined (but invisible) center area of 25 × 25 cm. Mice were allowed to acclimate to the testing room overnight before training. Mice were placed in the center of the square arena and allowed to freely move for 10 min while being tracked by an automated tracking system (Stoelting ANY-maze, Wood Dale, U.S.A). After 4 to 5 days of treatment with LPS or/and ibuprofen administration, the mice were tested every 2 days. Mice

were killed immediately after the third test on the fifth day (Fig. 3c). The experimental groups were randomized in different open field platforms.

Tissue preparation and histology

Animals were deeply anesthetized with Avertin (0.02 cc/g body weight) and perfused with cold PBS for 3 min. After perfusion, the brain was dissected out and bisected along the midline. Half of the brain was stored at – 80 °C for future use. Half was fixed in 4% paraformaldehyde (PFA, Sigma-Aldrich) at 4 °C overnight. After washing twice with PBS, the brain was transferred to 30% sucrose solution and incubated at 4 °C overnight for cryoprotection. Brains were then embedded in OCT and frozen quickly in powdered dry ice. Ten micron cryostat sections were cut and allowed to air dry on pre-coated *SuperPlus* glass slides.

Primary microglia cell culture and preparation of LPS conditioned medium

Primary microglia were isolated from C57BL/6J mice using our established protocol [39]. Briefly, a mixed glial cell population was obtained from P2–P5 pups and was cultured for 2 weeks in DMEM medium supplemented with 10% FBS and 1% pen/strep. Pure microglia were obtained by shaking at 37 °C for 4 h. LPS conditioned medium (LM) was prepared by incubating microglia cells at a density of 50,000 per well in a 24-well plate in Neurobasal medium containing 10 μg/ml LPS for 2 days. In another group, ibuprofen (200 μM) was added to the microglial cultures for 6 h and before treating them with 10 μg/ml LPS for 2 days. A control group was treated in Neurobasal medium without LPS (MM). After the two-day treatment, the medium was obtained and centrifuged to remove cells and debris, then used for neuronal treatment within 24 h. Microglial cells were washed by PBS once and lysed for further studies. THP-1 cells were cultured in RPMI 1640 medium with 10% FBS and 0.05 mM β-mercaptoethanol for routine passage. β-mercaptoethanol was removed from the medium when cells were treated with stimulus.

Primary cortical neuronal culture

Embryonic cortical neurons were isolated by standard procedures [40]. All cultures were grown for a minimum of 13 days in vitro (DIV) before any treatment. Cultures were then pretreated with ibuprofen (80, 120, and 200 μM) or DMSO for 24 h after which MM or LM (12.5% volume/volume) was added for another 48 h. For histological studies, cells were washed with PBS and fixed in 4% PFA for 15 min. After rinsing in PBS, cells were stored in 0.1% PFA if longer-term storage was required.

Antibodies for histological and Western studies

PCNA, p38, phospho-p38 (Thr180/Tyr182), ERK, phospho-ERK (Thr202/Tyr204), JNK, phospho-JNK (Thr183/Tyr185), NFκB p105/50, NFκB p65, phospho-NFκB p65 (Ser536), RelB, Akt, phospho-Akt (Ser473), and phospho-Akt (Thr308) antisera were purchased from Cell Signaling Technology (Danvers, MA, USA); CD45, Iba-1, GFAP, γ-H2AX, HDAC4, MAP2, GAPDH, 8-oxoguanine, and Ki67 antisera were purchased from Abcam (Cambridge, MA, USA); and cyclin A1 and c-Rel antisera were purchased from Santa Cruz Biotechnology (Dallas, Texas, USA). Secondary antisera conjugated with fluorescent Alexa dye 488 and 647 and Cy3 were purchased from Life Technologies and Jackson ImmunoResearch (West Grove, PA, USA). HRP-conjugated secondary antibodies were purchased from Cell Signaling Technology and Life Technologies.

Annexin V/propidium iodide apoptotic assay

Apoptotic and necrotic events in cell culture were assayed by annexin V/propidium iodide (V13245, Life Technologies) following the manufacturer's protocol. In brief, coverslips were washed with cold PBS and immediately incubated with working solution containing propidium iodide and Alexa Fluor® 488 annexin V diluted in an annexin-binding buffer for 15 min. After washing with annexin-binding buffer, coverslips were mounted with anti-fading fluorescence media from Vector Laboratories (Burlingame, CA, USA).

Immunocytochemistry and immunofluorescence

Immunocytochemistry was performed on mouse brain cryosections or PFA fixed cells according to standard methods [25]. Briefly, sections or cells were blocked in PBS containing 0.3% Triton X-100 and 10% donkey serum for 1 h in room temperature. They were then incubated in the same solution with primary antibodies overnight at 4 °C and immersed in fluorescent secondary antibodies for 1 h at room temperature. After counterstaining with DAPI for 5 min, all sections were mounted with anti-fading fluorescence media (Vector Laboratories) under a glass coverslip. All coverslips were mounted on glass slides. Experiments were the results of triplicate cultures established on separate days.

Cell counting and Iba1/GFAP analysis

The method for cell counting was described previously [24]. Briefly, five fields were randomly chosen at × 200 final magnification on an Olympus fluorescent microscope and every neuron was counted in the images from immunohistochemistry and immunocytochemistry. The percentage of the positive PCs and cultured neurons with markers of interest were counted and expressed as a fraction of the total MAP2-positive PCs/neurons. For cell counting in the frontal cortex, total MAP2-labeled neurons within layers II to V that co-localized with markers of interest were counted at the same magnification. Iba1 and GFAP signals were analyzed in three images/animal using ImageJ software (National Institutes of Health). The threshold value was set at ~ 40 in the measurement tool, and the percentages of Iba1/GFAP occupied areas in each image were measured. Iba1 and GFAP staining factors were normalized to the untreated $Atm^{+/+}$ group and expressed in a normalized ratio.

Quantitative real-time PCR

Microglia, THP-1 cells, and mouse cerebellar tissues were lysed in buffer containing 3% β-mercapethanol; total RNA was then extracted and reverse-transcribed as previously described [40]. Real-time PCR was performed using SYBR Premix Ex Taq (Takara Biotechnology) in the 7500 Real-Time PCR System (Applied Biosystems, Life Technologies). ROX II was applied as the reference dye. The sets of primers used are listed in Tables 1 and 2. Expression levels of *Gapdh* or *18SRNA* were used for normalization.

Western blot analysis

Western blots were performed on mouse cerebellar tissues according to standard methods [40]. Tissue lysates were prepared in RIPA lysis buffer (Millipore, Billerica, MA, U.S.A) containing protease and phosphatase inhibitors (Roche, Grenzacherstrasse, Basel, Schweiz). Protein samples were separated by gel electrophoresis, transferred to nitrocellulose membrane (Bio-Rad), and blocked with 5% albumin bovine serum (Sigma-Aldrich) or 5% milk (Bio-Rad). After incubation with primary antibodies at room temperature overnight and then secondary antibodies at room temperature for 1 h, protein signals were visualized using ECL substrate reagents (Thermo Scientific, Waltham, MA, USA). The intensities of the bands were quantified by ImageJ and normalized to the GAPDH level.

ELISA

ELISA kits against TNFα (#DY410) and IL1β (#DY401) were purchased from R&D systems. Cerebellar protein

Table 1 Primer for *Mus musculus*

	Forward	Reverse
Ym1	cagctgggatcttcctacca	attctgcattccagcaaagg
Trem2	ctggaaccgtcaccatcact	aggctagaggtgacccacag
Il1β	gccacctttttgacagtgatgag	aaggtccacgggaaagacac
Tnfa	aggcactcccccaaaagatg	ccacttggtggtttgtgagtg
iNOS	acagggagaaagcgcaaaac	gaacattctgtgctgtcccag
Il6	agacaaagccagagtccttcag	tgtgactccagcttatctcttgg
Ccl2	gctgtagttttttgtcaccaagctc	agtgcttgaggtggttgtgg
Il12	ctcacccttaggacccagga	ctcacccttaggacccagga
Gapdh	ggagaaacctgccaagtatga	ggtcctcagtgtagcccaag

Table 2 Primer pairs for *Homo sapiens*

	Forward	Reverse
NFκB1 (P50/P105)	cctggatgactcttgggaaa	tcagccagctgtttcatgtc
RelA (P65)	ggcgagaggagcacagatac	ctgatagcctgctccaggtc
COX2	ctgttgcggagaaaggagtc	tcatggaagatgcattggaa
IL1β	cagccaatcttcattgctca	gcatcttcctcagcttgtcc
TNFα	tccttcagacaccctcaacc	aggccccagtttgaattctt
IL6	aaagaggcactggcagaaaa	caggggtggttattgcatct
IL8	ggtgcagtttgccaaggag	ttccttggggtccagacaga
CD45	ggcagacaccagaattggtt	gggagaaagggagtggaaag
CD11B	agaacaacatgcccagaacc	gcggtcccatatgacagtct
SOCS3	caagaagccaaccaggagag	gttcagcattcccgaagtgt
18SRNA	tgcatgtctaagtacgcacggcc	gatagggcagacgttcgaatggg

lysate was diluted in 1:10, and protein levels of TNFα and IL1β were determined according to the manufacturer's protocol. Both forms of IL-1 β, pro-IL-1 β, and cleaved-IL-1β were detected by the ELISA kit. However, the signals were more specific to the cleaved form. Quantification was performed based on the cleaved form of IL-1 β.

Statistics

Student's unpaired *t test* and two-way ANOVA with Bonferroni post hoc test (Prism, GraphPad software, Version 7) were used to determine the differences in values between different groups. $p < 0.05$ was considered statistically significant. These are the symbols used for significance in the figures: */#: $p < 0.05$, **/##: $p < 0.01$, ***/###: $p < 0.001$.

Study approval

All animals were housed at the Animal and Plant Care Facility of Hong Kong University of Science and Technology. All procedures involving animals were approved by the Department of Health, Hong Kong. In the writing of the article, every effort has been made to follow the ARRIVE guidelines (https://www.nc3rs.org.uk/arrive-guidelines).

Results

Microglia-mediated immune challenge contributes to the neuronal damage in vitro

Previous studies in our lab have found that an LPS (lipopolysaccharide) immune challenge significantly exaggerates neuronal damage in both the short and long-term [24, 25]. To replicate this effect in an in vitro system, we established enriched cultures of microglia from wild-type mice, applied LPS (lipopolysaccharide) directly to the cultures (10 μg/ml for 48 h), harvested the medium, and applied it to separate cultures of the neuron. This treatment was effective as the LPS-conditioned medium (LM) caused the exposed neuronal cells to undergo a marked

morphological change (Fig. 1). In addition, the neurons demonstrated enhanced stress. They showed significant cell loss as measured by decreased MAP2 counts and increased cell cycle activity as measured by both enhanced Ki67 and cyclin D staining. This was not an effect of residual LPS in the LM; direct treatment of neuronal cultures with 10 μg/ml LPS (Table 3) failed to induce any of these symptoms of neuronal damage. A measurable neuronal response was also seen with conditioned medium from un-stimulated microglial cultures (MM), as high concentrations of MM (12.5%) induced a slight degree of damage to the cultured neurons [41]. Nonetheless, neurotoxicity was significantly exaggerated when microglia were pretreated with LPS; this shows that under a specific immune challenge, more harmful substances were released into the medium [42]. To more closely mimic the chemistry of the human immune response, we repeated these experiments with the human THP-1 monocyte cell line instead of primary mouse microglia [43–45]. This treatment also upregulated the expression of pro-inflammatory genes (Additional file 1: Figure S1). Further, just as with the medium from primary mouse microglial cells, both unstimulated (TM) and LPS-stimulated (LM) conditioned media from THP-1 cells caused neurotoxicity and ectopic cell cycle reentry (Additional file 2: Figure S2A-N).

Given the fact that direct application of LPS does not damage cells in neuronal cultures, these data demonstrate that it is the products of microglia, responding to the LPS challenge, that cause the damage. To determine the nature of the neurodegeneration caused by conditioned media, neurons were stained with annexin V/propidium iodide [46]. With these reagents, apoptotic cells fluoresce green while cells that die by non-apoptotic means show red plus green fluorescence. Live cells show little or no fluorescence (Fig. 2j–o). In cultures treated only with MM, cells were only lightly labeled with annexin V (green) suggesting that the deaths were largely apoptotic events. No obvious cell death of any kind was identified in control groups (Fig. 2j). Under 12.5% LM treatment, however, most cells showed strong green plus red signals (Fig. 2l). This suggests that LM kills neurons via a non-apoptotic, possibly necrotic process (see also Fig. 1).

Ibuprofen attenuates inflammatory stress and cell death

To determine whether ibuprofen could be effective at reducing the complex inflammatory stress caused by activation of the innate immune system, DIV14 cortical neurons were pretreated with ibuprofen 24 h before the MM or LM challenge. Cells were then stained with cell cycle markers to assess neuronal stress. ANOVA revealed a significant effect of ibuprofen treatment on ectopic cell cycle reentry with significant conditioned medium cross ibuprofen interaction. (Fig. 1 and Additional file 2: Figure S2A–N)

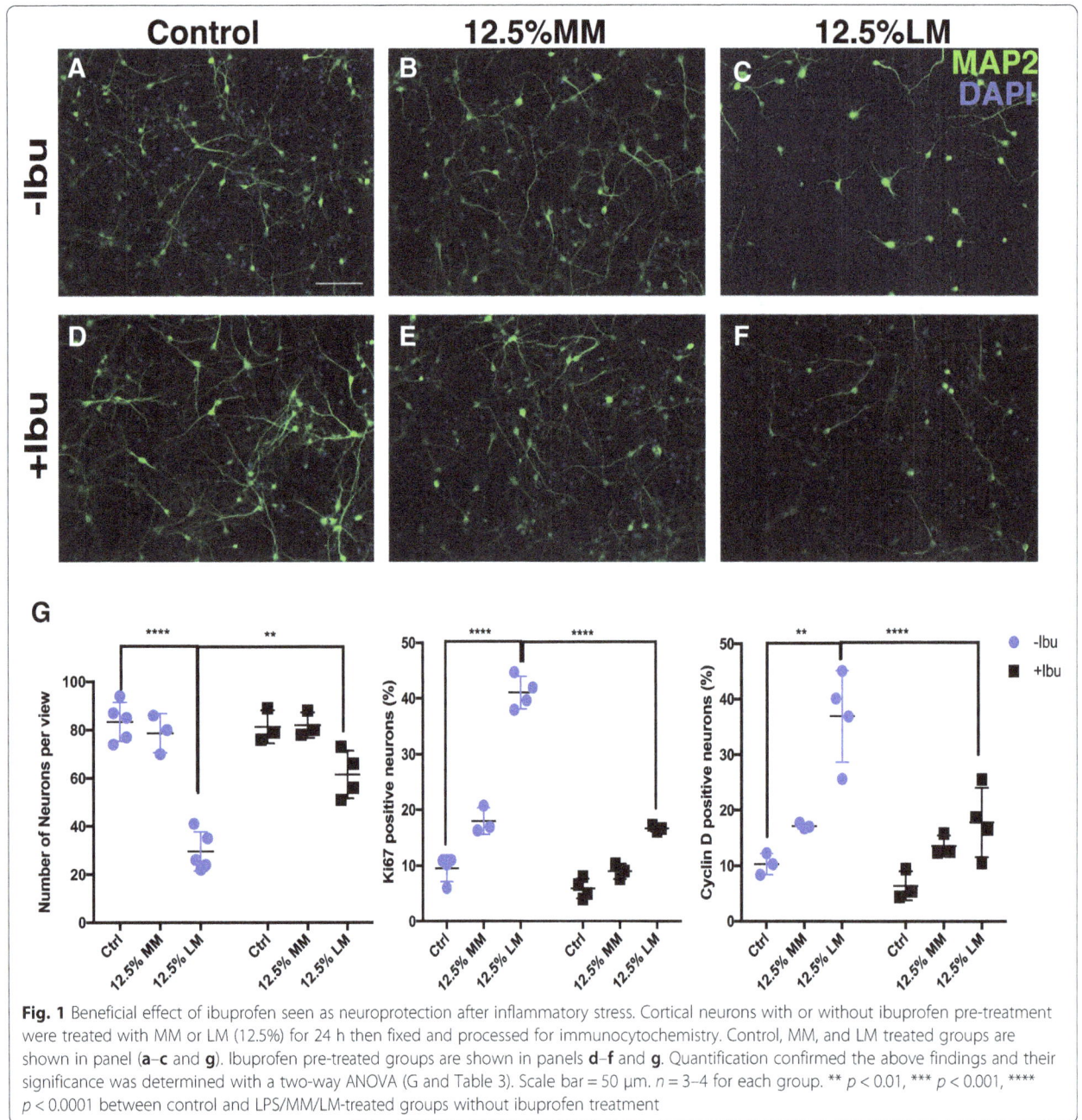

Fig. 1 Beneficial effect of ibuprofen seen as neuroprotection after inflammatory stress. Cortical neurons with or without ibuprofen pre-treatment were treated with MM or LM (12.5%) for 24 h then fixed and processed for immunocytochemistry. Control, MM, and LM treated groups are shown in panel (**a**–**c** and **g**). Ibuprofen pre-treated groups are shown in panels **d**–**f** and **g**. Quantification confirmed the above findings and their significance was determined with a two-way ANOVA (G and Table 3). Scale bar = 50 μm. n = 3–4 for each group. ** $p < 0.01$, *** $p < 0.001$, **** $p < 0.0001$ between control and LPS/MM/LM-treated groups without ibuprofen treatment

Ibuprofen treatment alone did not induce any significant changes in control cultures or neuronal cultures subjected to direct LPS treatment (Fig. 1 and data not shown). In the more complex environment of LM conditioned medium, however, post hoc tests showed that ibuprofen treatment suppressed LPS-induced neuronal cell cycle events (CCEs) (Fig. 1g, Additional file 2: Figure S2I–N and Table 3). Notably, 120 μM ibuprofen significantly reduced neuronal apoptosis as measured by the annexin V/PI signal (Fig. 2m–o). Thus, when applied directly to neurons, ibuprofen has a significant neuroprotective effect against LM-induced neuroinflammation.

Interestingly, ibuprofen pretreatment of the microglial themselves did not block their activation by LPS nor their ability to produce neurotoxic material in their medium (Fig. 2a–i). LPS induced a substantial morphological change from a resting ramified state to a more amoeboid-like active stage. To our surprise, however, pretreating the microglia with ibuprofen for 12 h (Fig. 2c, d, g, h) did not block the effect of LPS and had little impact on the activation of the immune pathway in microglia (Fig. 2e–i). After LPS stimulation, the percentage of cells with an activated NF-κB pathway, as measured by the translocation of p65 from the

Table 3 Two-way ANOVAs analysis for cyclin D and Ki67 counts in all treatment groups

	Cyclin D p value	Ki67 p value
Control vs LPS	**< 0.05**	> 0.05
Control vs 12.5% LM	**< 0.001**	**< 0.0001**
12.5% LM vs 12.5% LM		
+ 200 µM ibuprofen	**< 0.0001**	**< 0.0001**
Control vs 6.25% LM	**< 0.001**	**< 0.001**
6.25% LM Vs 6.25% LM		
+ 200 µM ibuprofen	**< 0.001**	**< 0.001**
Control vs 6.25% MM	**< 0.05**	> 0.05
6.25% MM Vs 6.25% MM		
+ 200 µM ibuprofen	> 0.05	> 0.05
Control vs 12.5% MM	**< 0.05**	**< 0.05**
12.5% MM Vs 12.5% MM		
+ 200 µM ibuprofen	**< 0.05**	**< 0.05**

Samples that are statistically significant were shown in boldface in the table

cytoplasm to the nucleus, significantly increased, but pretreatment with ibuprofen failed to block this response. We speculate that, given the long-term nature of our assay, these results are most likely due to the chronic versus acute nature of the inflammatory response that we measured [47]. Our data therefore demonstrate that ibuprofen can provide immunoprotection to neurons if applied directly and this effect is independent of any direct effect of ibuprofen on LPS-stimulated microglia.

Ibuprofen improves LPS-induced symptoms in $Atm^{-/-}$ mice

In vivo ATM deficiency exacerbates the neuronal damage induced by LPS-triggered bouts of neuroinflammation [24]. To test the effects of ibuprofen on this response, we administered LPS by i.p. injection to 3-month-old $Atm^{+/+}$ and $Atm^{-/-}$ mice for 4 days. Mice from all treatment groups were then subjected to behavioral testing. Two days after its initiation, ANOVA revealed significant effects of the LPS treatment (distance traveled: $[F(1, 27) = 12.12, p = 0.0017]$, body rotation: $[F(1, 27) = 8.91, p = 0.0114]$) and genotype (distance traveled: $[F(1, 27) = 20.35, p = 0.0001]$, body rotation: $[F(1, 27) = 36.37, p < 0.0001]$). LPS injection led to reduced motor behavior as seen by both reduced total travel distance ($Atm^{+/+}$: $p < 0.05$; $Atm^{-/-}$: $p < 0.01$—Fig. 3a) and reduced number of body rotations (Fig. 3b). The LPS-induced behavioral deficiency, observed at day three, remained stable at day five in the wild-type ($Atm^{+/+}$) animals, but continued to decline in the $Atm^{-/-}$ mutant mice (distance traveled: $[F(1, 27) = 14.48, p = 0.0007]$, post hoc test: $p < 0.01$; body rotation: $[F(1, 27) = 23.35, p = 0.0004]$, post hoc test: $p < 0.01$) (Fig. 3a–b). Thus, an LPS challenge

worsens many of the AT neurological phenotypes and exacerbates the subtle motor deficiency of the AT mouse model.

We then tested whether ibuprofen might have beneficial effects in blunting an LPS-induced inflammatory challenge in vivo. The experimental procedure is diagrammed in Fig. 3c. Three-month-old $Atm^{+/+}$ and $Atm^{-/-}$ animals were administered ibuprofen (0.5 mg/ml in their drinking water) for 2 weeks. Animals were subjected to rotarod and open field tests after 1 week of ibuprofen treatment. One week later, we began a daily regimen of intraperitoneal injections of LPS (1 mg/kg) for 4 days. During this final phase, we tested mice in the open field every 2 days. We confirmed the compromised motor performance of the $Atm^{-/-}$ animals on the rotarod (Fig. 3d—$[F(1, 64) = 7.80, p = 0.0069]$, post hoc test: $p < 0.05$ by ANOVA) and open-field tests (Fig. 3a—$[F(1, 27) = 14.05, p = 0.0009]$, post hoc test: $p < 0.05$) and showed that LPS injection further degraded the performance of both mutant and wild-type animals in the open field test. Unfortunately, a 2-week ibuprofen treatment of $Atm^{+/+}$ mice was unable to block the LPS effect, consistent with its modest long-term effect on the microglial reaction. Although the motor behavior performance of $Atm^{-/-}$ animals continued to decline, ibuprofen led to a modest lessening of the LPS-induced deterioration (Fig. 3e). There was little effect of the NSAID on the baseline behavior of $Atm^{-/-}$ mice (Fig. 3d, e) although open field behavior improved slightly on day five.

Ibuprofen promotes anti-inflammatory and anti-oxidative effects in ATM-deficient conditions

While the behavioral deficits were largely refractory to change, we found important anti-inflammatory and anti-oxidative effects of ibuprofen at the cellular level. At this resolution, the effects of chronic LPS treatment on brain microglia were apparent, as assessed by Iba1 staining and morphology (Fig. 4i). LPS administration significantly induced microglia activation in both wild-type and $Atm^{-/-}$ mice. We quantified the Iba1 staining factor by measuring the area occupied by Iba1-positive glia and dividing by the total area of the image. The deep cerebellar nuclei (DCN) represent the final output of the cerebellar circuitry and the hyperexcitability of this region leads to cerebellar ataxia when there is a loss of inhibitory inputs from cortical Purkinje cells [48]. We therefore focused our analysis on this region. ANOVA revealed a significant effect of LPS treatment on both genotypes ($Atm^{+/+}$: $[F(1, 12) = 33.46, p < 0.0001]$, $Atm^{-/-}$: $[F(1, 12) = 125.93, p < 0.0001]$) but the effect of ibuprofen was seen only in $Atm^{-/-}$ animals $[F(1, 12) = 19.61, p = 0.0008]$. Iba1 microglial staining increased after LPS injection, and this reaction could be suppressed by ibuprofen treatment in both genotypes

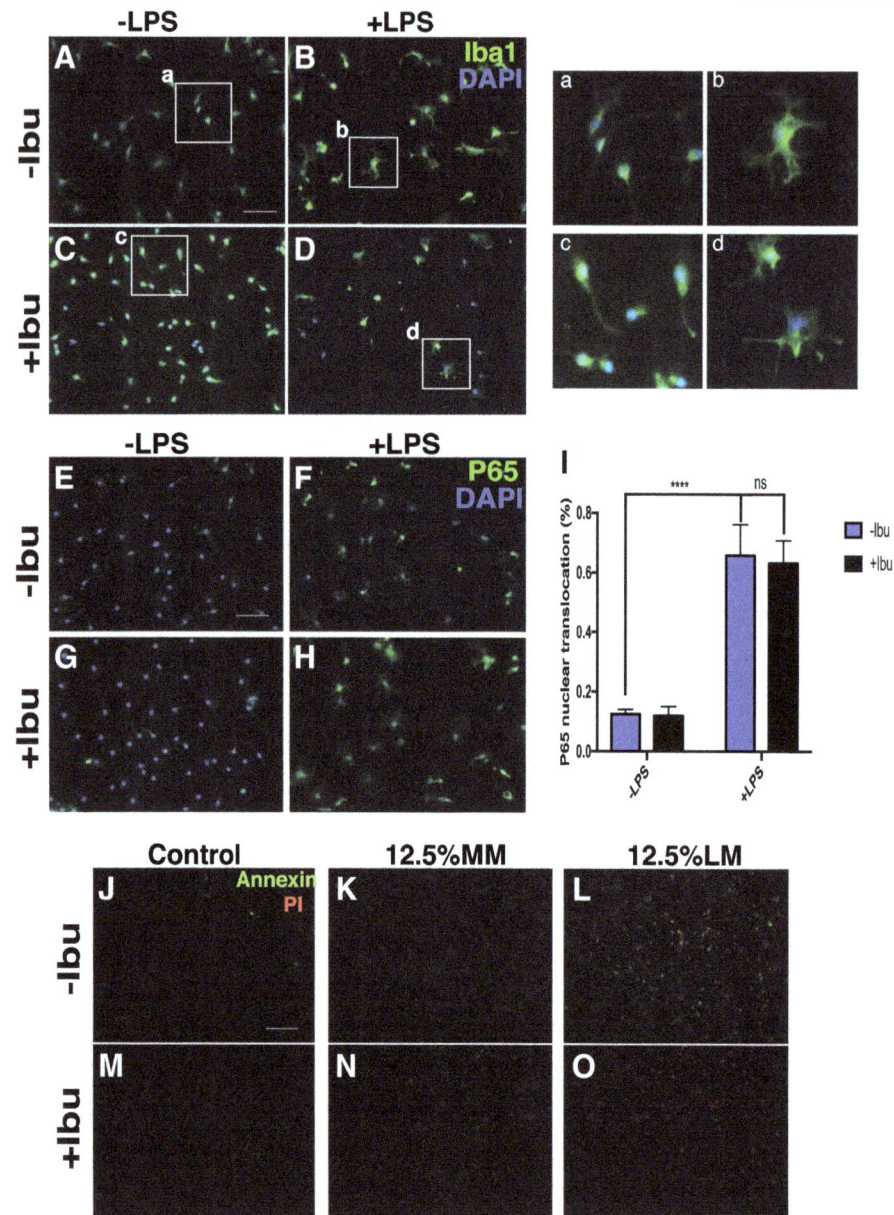

Fig. 2 a, b LPS challenge dramatically changes the morphology of microglia and induces the activation of the NF-κB pathway (**e, f**, and **i**). **c, d, g–i** Ibuprofen did not block the activation of microglia after LPS stimulation. **j–o** Both annexin V and PI signals accumulated in neuronal culture when treated with LM. Ibuprofen pretreatment significantly blocked both apoptotic and necrotic processes. Scale bar = 50 μm. $n = 4$ for each group. ** $p < 0.01$, *** $p < 0.001$, **** $p < 0.0001$

(Fig. 4a–d, i). This effect reached significance only in $Atm^{-/-}$ animals pre-treated with ibuprofen. Examined before the immune stimulus, $Atm^{-/-}$ cerebellar astrocytes showed evidence of reduced activation as assessed by GFAP immunostaining (Fig. 4j). LPS was able to activate astrocytes in the $Atm^{-/-}$ mutant cerebellum ([$F(1, 10) = 21.67$, $p < 0.0001$], post hoc test: $p < 0.001$) but not in $Atm^{+/+}$ animals, consistent with our previous work [24]. Even in $Atm^{-/-}$ mutants, however, ibuprofen failed to reduce the astrocytic response to LPS (Fig. 4e–h, j).

In chronic inflammatory situations lasting days, rather than hours, TNFα exposure has a neuroprotective role while chronic IL1β stimulates neurodegeneration in $Atm^{-/-}$ cerebellum [25]. To determine the effects of ibuprofen treatment on these two cytokines, ELISA was performed on whole cerebellar lysates. LPS and ATM deficiency alone each showed a trend towards reduced TNFα in the cerebellum (Fig. 4k). A decrease in ATM-deficient cells would be consistent with our previous observations and could partially explain how

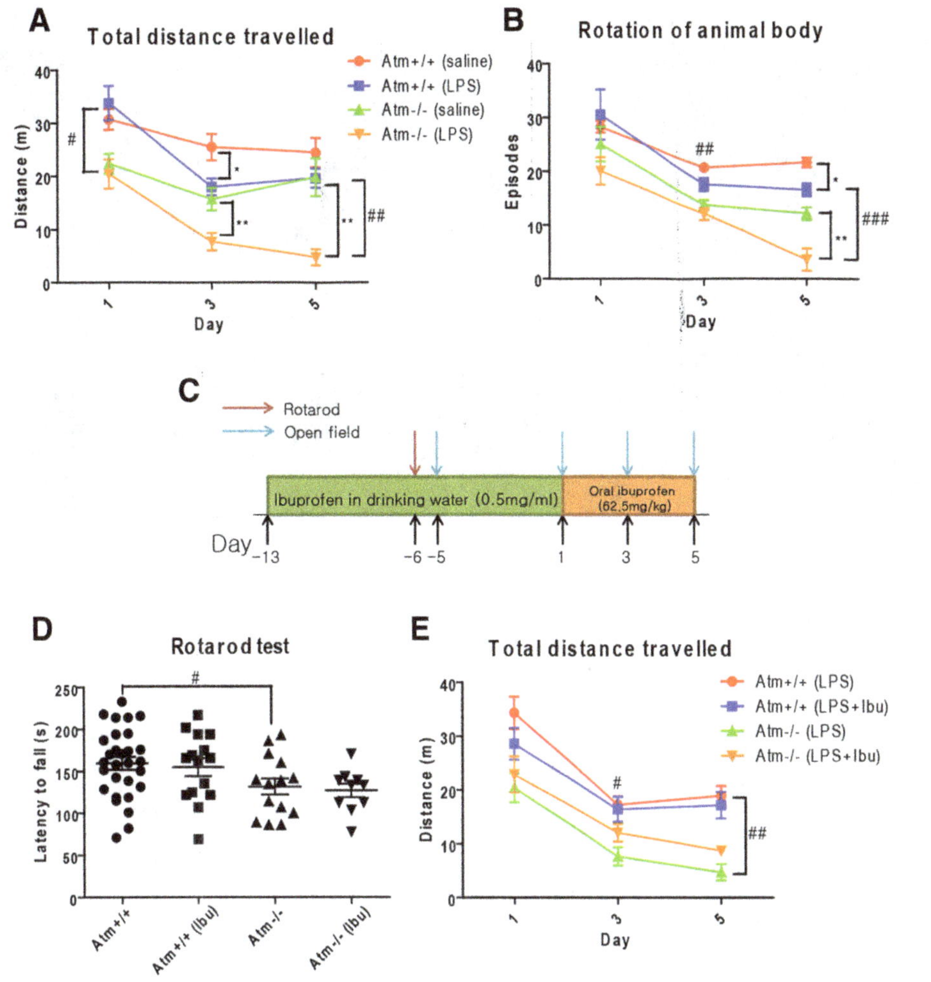

Fig. 3 Rotarod and open field test on $Atm^{+/+}$ and $Atm^{-/-}$ animals with 2-week ibuprofen administration followed by 4-day LPS injection. $Atm^{-/-}$ animal traveled less distance (A) on day 1 before LPS administration. After LPS injection, both genotypes showed a significant loss of motor activity as measured by distance traveled (**a**) and rotation (**b**) on day 3 although some recovery was noted at day 5. $n = 6$–10 for each group. **c** Experimental timeline for ibuprofen experiment. **d** ATM deficiency significantly reduced rotarod performance of $Atm^{-/-}$ animal and ibuprofen failed to improve it. **e** Similar results were observed in open field tests; ibuprofen failed to improve reduced motor activities in LPS injected $Atm^{-/-}$ animals. $n = 8$–11 for each group. Two-way ANOVA was used for analyzing differences in genotype and ibuprofen treatment within an individual day. * $p < 0.05$, ** $p < 0.01$ between saline and LPS groups within the same genotype; # $p < 0.05$, ## $p < 0.01$, ### $p < 0.001$ between $Atm^{+/+}$ and $Atm^{-/-}$ groups with the same treatment

inflammation and ATM deficiency accelerate cerebellar damage [24]. We note that the ibuprofen pretreatment regimen failed to change even the trend in TNFα levels in both $Atm^{+/+}$ and $Atm^{-/-}$ cerebella (Fig. 4k).

Recent studies have demonstrated that peripheral immune cells also contribute to neurodegeneration in several CNS disorders [49–52]. This led us to look for infiltration of proliferating monocytes using CD45 immunohistochemistry. LPS significantly increased monocyte infiltration (Additional file 3: Figure S3A, C, E, G) in the cerebellum from both genotypes. The expression of $Ym1$ and $Trem2$, two genes associated with the inhibition of inflammation and restoration of homeostasis [53, 54], were upregulated in both genotypes after LPS challenge ($Trem2$: $Atm^{+/+}$:

$[F(1, 8) = 118.67, p < 0.0001]$, post hoc test: $p < 0.001$; $Atm^{-/-}$: $[F(1, 8) = 230.22, p < 0.0001]$, post hoc test: $p < 0.001$) ($Ym1$: $[Atm^{+/+}$: $F(1, 8) = 9.44, p = 0.0153]$, post hoc test: $p < 0.05$; $Atm^{-/-}$: $[F(1, 8) = 8.97, p = 0.0172]$, post hoc test: $p < 0.05$)) (Additional file 2: Figure S2I and J). Ibuprofen treatment suppressed the LPS-induced monocyte infiltration and further upregulated $Trem2$ expression in the remaining CNS monocytes in $Atm^{-/-}$ cerebellum ($[F(1, 8) = 23.98, p = 0.0012]$, post hoc test: $p < 0.001$) (Additional file 2: Figure S2C, D, G, H, J), suggesting a possible mechanism for the anti-inflammatory effect of ibuprofen in neurodegenerative disease.

Immunohistochemistry was performed to assess the anti-oxidative effect of ibuprofen. As shown in Fig. 5a, c,

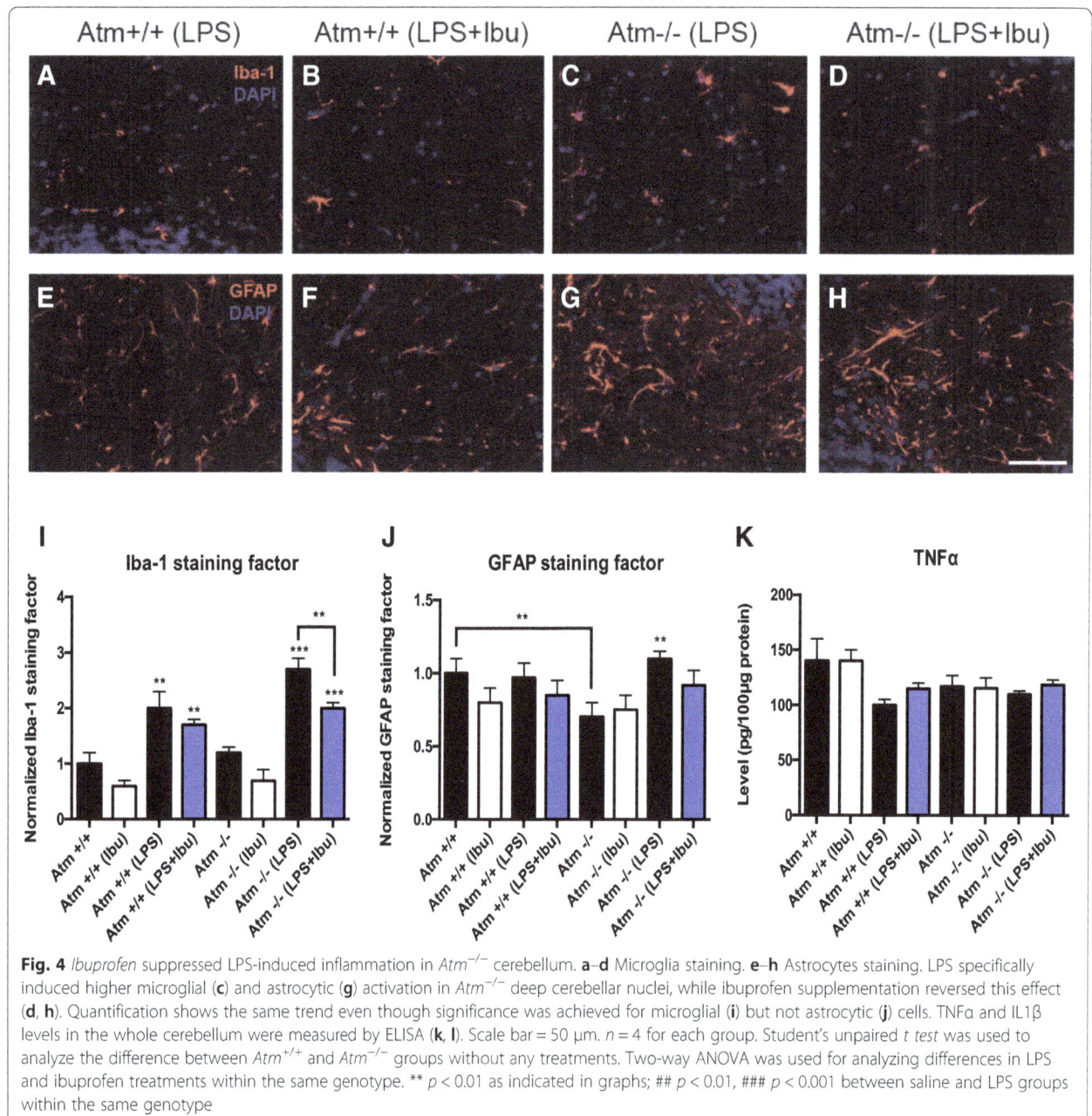

Fig. 4 *Ibuprofen* suppressed LPS-induced inflammation in *Atm*$^{-/-}$ cerebellum. **a–d** Microglia staining. **e–h** Astrocytes staining. LPS specifically induced higher microglial (**c**) and astrocytic (**g**) activation in *Atm*$^{-/-}$ deep cerebellar nuclei, while ibuprofen supplementation reversed this effect (**d**, **h**). Quantification shows the same trend even though significance was achieved for microglial (**i**) but not astrocytic (**j**) cells. TNFα and IL1β levels in the whole cerebellum were measured by ELISA (**k**, **l**). Scale bar = 50 μm. n = 4 for each group. Student's unpaired *t test* was used to analyze the difference between *Atm*$^{+/+}$ and *Atm*$^{-/-}$ groups without any treatments. Two-way ANOVA was used for analyzing differences in LPS and ibuprofen treatments within the same genotype. ** $p < 0.01$ as indicated in graphs; ## $p < 0.01$, ### $p < 0.001$ between saline and LPS groups within the same genotype

Atm$^{-/-}$ cells contain higher levels of DNA oxidation as measured by 8-Oxo-2′-deoxyguanosine (8-oxo-dG), and LPS administration drives up both the total 8-oxo-dG signal intensity as well as the percentage of 8-oxo-dG positive neurons in both wildtype and *Atm*$^{-/-}$ mice (Fig. 5a, c, e). Interestingly, not only did the total intensity of 8-oxo-dG increase in the LPS treated mice but also its nuclear localization. The nature of the cytoplasmic signal is not clear, but the enhanced levels of oxidized DNA in the cell nucleus is further evidence of the significant oxidative stress in the cells experience in these conditions and may help explain the appearance of neuronal cell cycle reentry [55] (Fig. 5a, b, d). Ibuprofen

was able to blunt the LPS-induced DNA oxidation in both wildtype and ATM-deficient mice, suggesting its neuroprotective effects might be due to its function as an antioxidant. The in vivo effect was incomplete, however, as the rescue was only partial (Fig. 5). Our in vitro analysis confirmed the anti-oxidative effect of ibuprofen (Additional file 2: Figure S2O). LM treatment dramatically increased the intensity of 8-oxo-dG in cultured neurons while MM had little effect. Pre-incubation with ibuprofen significantly reduced the oxidative stress induced by LM in neuronal culture. Thus, ibuprofen alleviates the inflammatory stress caused by an LPS challenge and further

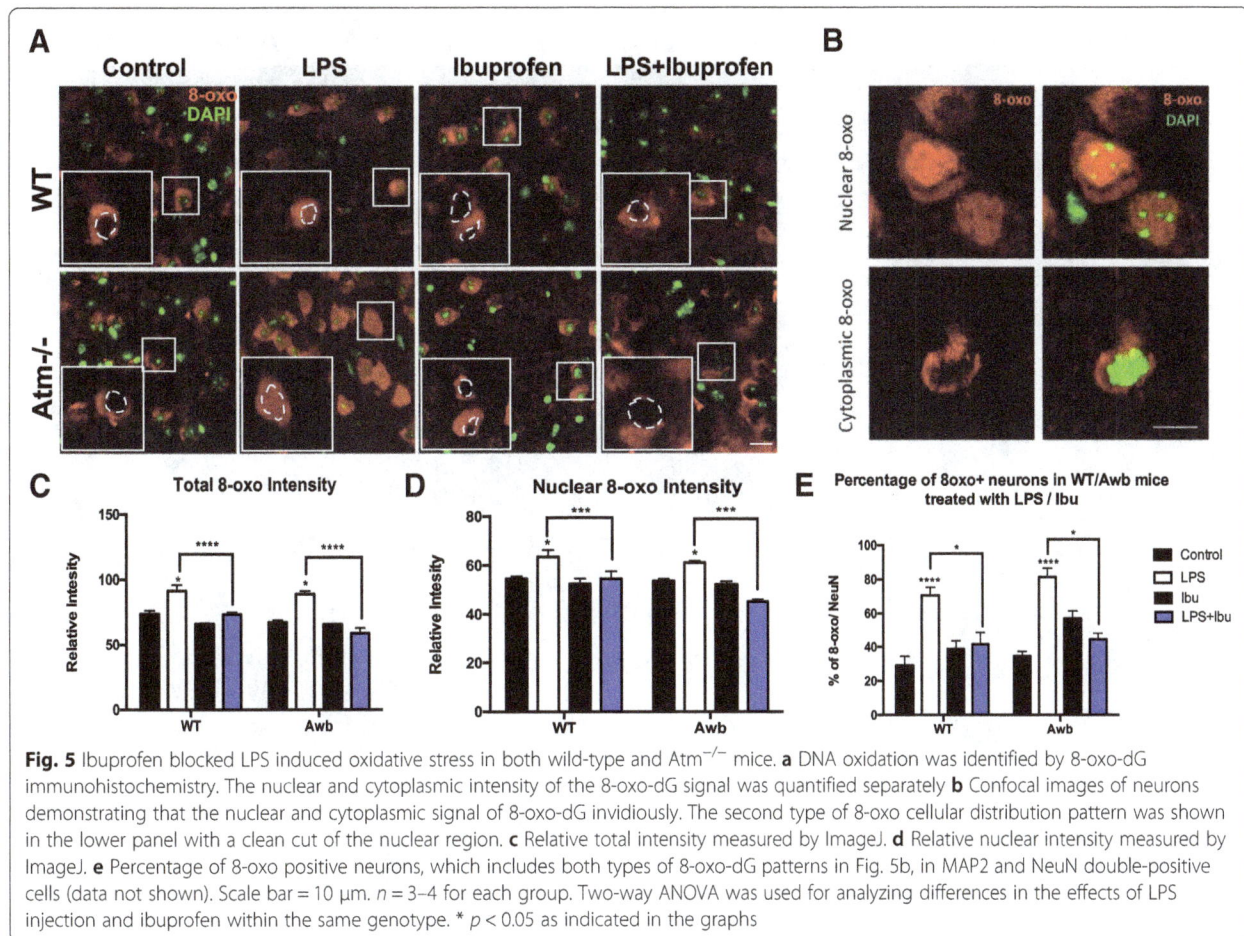

Fig. 5 Ibuprofen blocked LPS induced oxidative stress in both wild-type and Atm$^{-/-}$ mice. **a** DNA oxidation was identified by 8-oxo-dG immunohistochemistry. The nuclear and cytoplasmic intensity of the 8-oxo-dG signal was quantified separately **b** Confocal images of neurons demonstrating that the nuclear and cytoplasmic signal of 8-oxo-dG invidiously. The second type of 8-oxo cellular distribution pattern was shown in the lower panel with a clean cut of the nuclear region. **c** Relative total intensity measured by ImageJ. **d** Relative nuclear intensity measured by ImageJ. **e** Percentage of 8-oxo positive neurons, which includes both types of 8-oxo-dG patterns in Fig. 5b, in MAP2 and NeuN double-positive cells (data not shown). Scale bar = 10 μm. $n = 3$–4 for each group. Two-way ANOVA was used for analyzing differences in the effects of LPS injection and ibuprofen within the same genotype. * $p < 0.05$ as indicated in the graphs

mitigates the neuronal cell loss in both wild-type and $Atm^{-/-}$ mice.

Ibuprofen reduces cellular pathology in Atm$^{-/-}$ cerebellum

To monitor the neuropathological correlates of these changes, 10 μm brain sections were immunoassayed with markers of cell cycle, DNA damage, and epigenetic and oxidative stress. Two-way ANOVA analysis revealed the main effects of LPS treatment on cyclin A ($Atm^{+/+}$: [$F(1, 23) = 28.49$, $p < 0.0001$]), γ-H2AX ($Atm^{+/+}$: [$F(1, 23) = 60.97$, $p < 0.0001$], $Atm^{-/-}$: [$F(1, 17) = 8.86$, $p = 0.0089$]) and HDAC4 ($Atm^{+/+}$: [$F(1, 23) = 15.68$, $p = 0.0006$], $Atm^{-/-}$: [$F(1, 17) = 8.49$, $p = 0.0097$]), and of ibuprofen treatment on cyclin A ($Atm^{-/-}$: [$F(1, 17) = 6.04$, $p = 0.0251$]), γ-H2AX ($Atm^{-/-}$: [$F(1, 17) = 6.69$, $p = 0.0198$]), and HDAC4 ($Atm^{-/-}$: [$F(1, 17) = 11.68$, $p = 0.0033$]). Consistent with our previous data [24], at baseline, $Atm^{-/-}$ PCs had significantly higher neuronal cell cycle events ($p < 0.05$) (Fig. 6m), DNA damage ($p < 0.01$) (Fig. 6n), and nuclear localization of HDAC4 ($p < 0.001$) (Fig. 6o) than $Atm^{+/+}$ PCs. Unfortunately, ibuprofen had no significant therapeutic effect on these three established

phenotypes. As reported, LPS-induced immune challenge increased the three markers in both $Atm^{+/+}$ and mutant PCs [24] (Fig. 6m–o). Unlike the unstimulated mice, however, if given before the LPS treatment, ibuprofen significantly blunted the increase in three markers. Post hoc analysis showed that ibuprofen significantly reduced cyclin A ($p < 0.001$), γ-H2AX ($p < 0.01$), and nuclear HDAC4 ($p < 0.001$) in $Atm^{-/-}$ Purkinje cells after LPS administration (Fig. 6m–o). These results indicate that ibuprofen counteracts the negative synergy between the Atm genotype and the neuroinflammatory environment, reducing the vulnerability of $Atm^{-/-}$ Purkinje cells to LPS-induced damage.

Ibuprofen suppresses LPS- and ATM deficiency-induced p38 phosphorylation

LPS-induced neuronal damage is correlated with the activation of the MAPK, Akt, and NFκB pathways [25]. This led us to ask whether ibuprofen was able to suppress these changes. Whole cerebellar lysates were prepared, followed by Western blots with antisera to proteins involved in above three pathways. LPS, with or without ibuprofen, stimulated no obvious activation

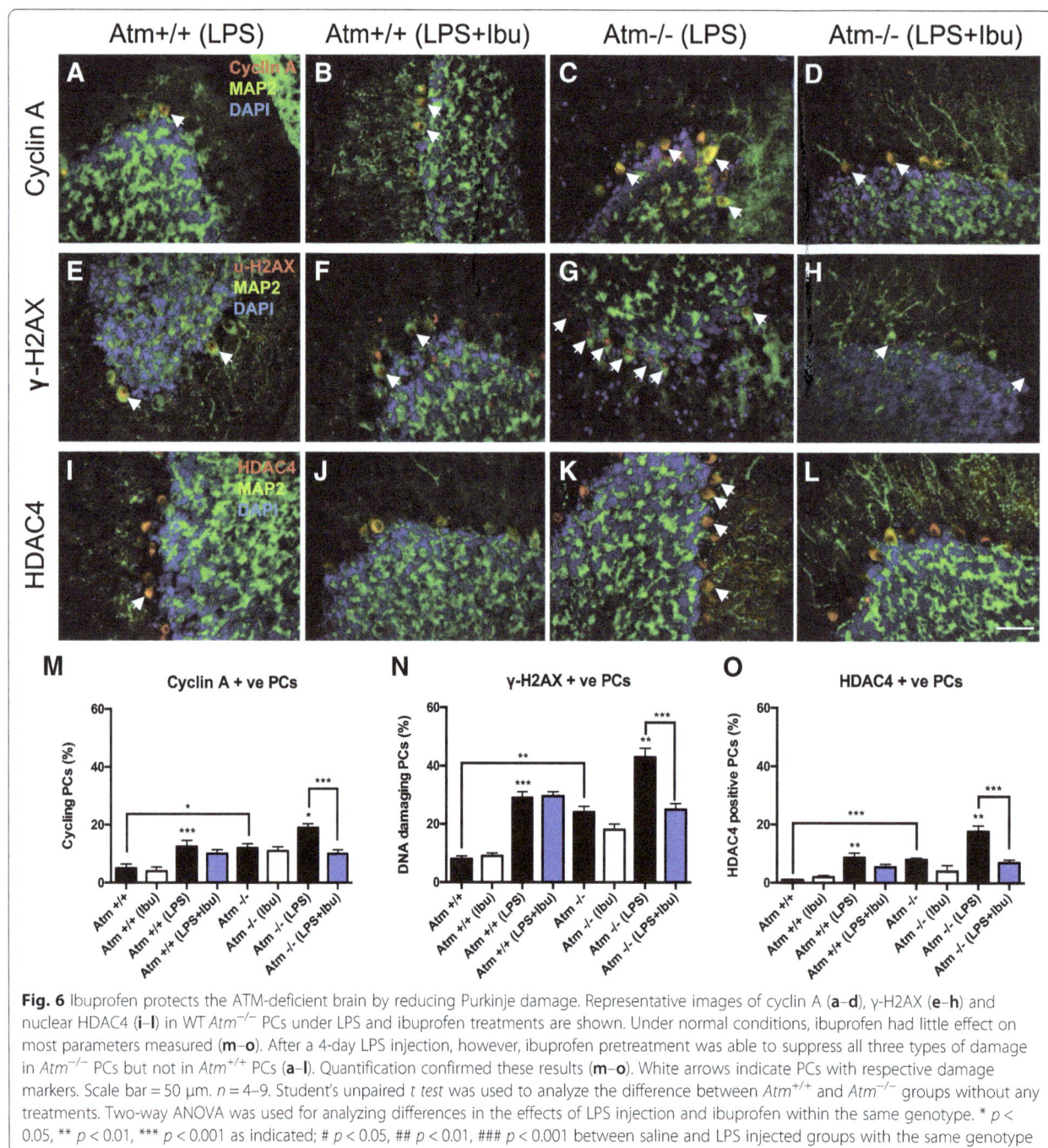

Fig. 6 Ibuprofen protects the ATM-deficient brain by reducing Purkinje damage. Representative images of cyclin A (**a–d**), γ-H2AX (**e–h**) and nuclear HDAC4 (**i–l**) in WT $Atm^{-/-}$ PCs under LPS and ibuprofen treatments are shown. Under normal conditions, ibuprofen had little effect on most parameters measured (**m–o**). After a 4-day LPS injection, however, ibuprofen pretreatment was able to suppress all three types of damage in $Atm^{-/-}$ PCs but not in $Atm^{+/+}$ PCs (**a–l**). Quantification confirmed these results (**m–o**). White arrows indicate PCs with respective damage markers. Scale bar = 50 μm. $n = 4–9$. Student's unpaired t test was used to analyze the difference between $Atm^{+/+}$ and $Atm^{-/-}$ groups without any treatments. Two-way ANOVA was used for analyzing differences in the effects of LPS injection and ibuprofen within the same genotype. * $p < 0.05$, ** $p < 0.01$, *** $p < 0.001$ as indicated; # $p < 0.05$, ## $p < 0.01$, ### $p < 0.001$ between saline and LPS injected groups with the same genotype

(phosphorylation) of ERK or Akt pathways in whole cerebella extracts of either genotype (Additional file 4: Figure S4). As PCs represent less than 1% of the total number of cells in the cerebellum, whole cell lysates might obscure differences that were taking place only in this one cell type. We therefore turned to immunohistochemistry to investigate the levels of phospho-p38 specifically in PCs. In this way, we found that both ATM deficiency and LPS injection in wild-type mice induced p38 activation in PCs (Fig. 7c, e and Additional file 5:

Figure S5). In $Atm^{-/-}$ mice, LPS injection did not show any combinatorial effect. Unexpectedly, p38 induction in $Atm^{-/-}$ animals trended lower after LPS injection (Fig. 7g and Additional file 5: Figure S5). Two-way ANOVA revealed significant differences in LPS ($Atm^{+/+}$: [$F(1, 8) = 66.27$, $p < 0.0001$], $Atm^{-/-}$: [$F(1, 8) = 13.20$, $p = 0.0068$]) and ibuprofen treatments ($Atm^{+/+}$: [$F(1, 8) = 44.00$, $p = 0.0002$], $Atm^{-/-}$: [$F(1, 8) = 296.98$, $p < 0.0001$]) in both genotypes. Ibuprofen was able to block the LPS-induced increase in p38 phosphorylation and surprisingly was equally effective

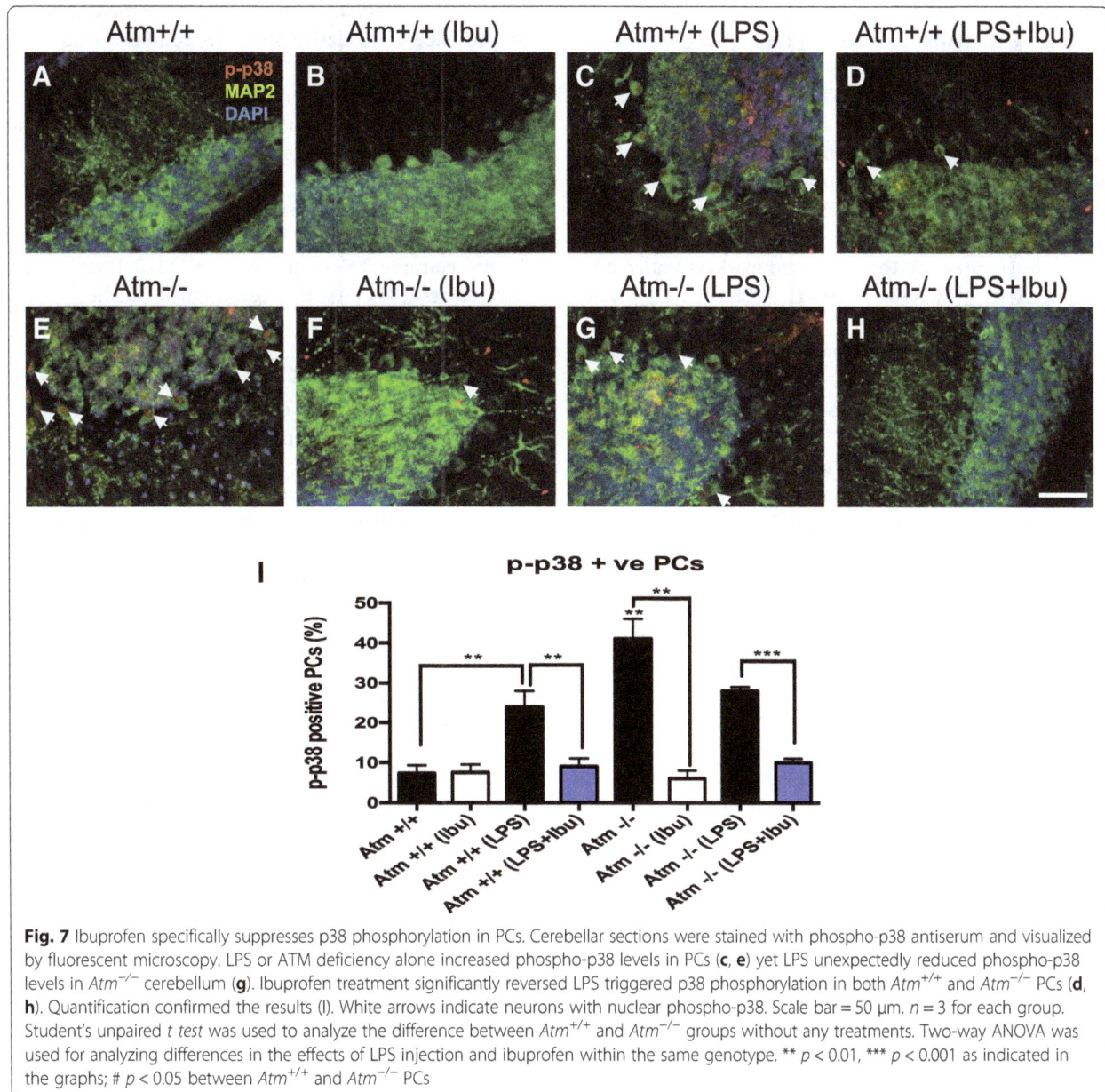

Fig. 7 Ibuprofen specifically suppresses p38 phosphorylation in PCs. Cerebellar sections were stained with phospho-p38 antiserum and visualized by fluorescent microscopy. LPS or ATM deficiency alone increased phospho-p38 levels in PCs (**c, e**) yet LPS unexpectedly reduced phospho-p38 levels in $Atm^{-/-}$ cerebellum (**g**). Ibuprofen treatment significantly reversed LPS triggered p38 phosphorylation in both $Atm^{+/+}$ and $Atm^{-/-}$ PCs (**d, h**). Quantification confirmed the results (I). White arrows indicate neurons with nuclear phospho-p38. Scale bar = 50 μm. $n = 3$ for each group. Student's unpaired t test was used to analyze the difference between $Atm^{+/+}$ and $Atm^{-/-}$ groups without any treatments. Two-way ANOVA was used for analyzing differences in the effects of LPS injection and ibuprofen within the same genotype. ** $p < 0.01$, *** $p < 0.001$ as indicated in the graphs; # $p < 0.05$ between $Atm^{+/+}$ and $Atm^{-/-}$ PCs

at reducing the ATM-dependent activation of p38 in PCs (Fig. 7 b, d, f, h and Additional file 5: Figure S5). Quantification of the immunohistochemistry confirmed these results ($Atm^{+/+}$: $p < 0.01$; $Atm^{-/-}$: $p < 0.001$) (Fig. 7i). These data thus suggest that ibuprofen mainly delays the A-T progression at least in part through the suppression of p38 activation in the cerebellum.

Early ibuprofen treatment delays the initiation of A-T symptoms

All of the above studies were performed in adult $Atm^{-/-}$ mice with established pathology and defined motor symptoms. We note that even at this relatively late disease stage, ibuprofen is still beneficial. We next asked whether ibuprofen might perhaps have more significant protective effects if it were applied before the first appearance of symptoms. To test this, wild-type and $Atm^{-/-}$ mice were administratid ibuprofen orally for 2 weeks starting at age P10, an age before the earliest signs of PC distress are apparent [56]. After 2 weeks of treatment, the animals were killed by perfusion and their brains embedded in OCT for sectioning on a cryostat. Immunostaining was performed to access the level of neuronal damage. We found significant effects of genotype (PCNA: [$F(1, 14) = 54.19$, $p < 0.0001$; cyclin A: [$F(1, 14) = 21.23$, $p = 0.0004$]) and ibuprofen treatment (cyclin A: [$F(1, 14) = 10.82$, $p = 0.0054$]) in the damage markers by two-way ANOVA. Post hoc test revealed that ibuprofen blocked the developmental appearance of ectopic cell cycling in the $Atm^{-/-}$ Purkinje cells (PCNA: $p < 0.01$, cyclin A: $p < 0.001$— Fig. 8a, b). By contrast, DNA damage was induced in $Atm^{-/-}$ Purkinje cells ($[F(1, 14) = 26.64, p = 0.0001]$, post hoc test: $p < 0.01$) but not significantly reduced under ibuprofen treatment (Fig. 8c). No change was found in HDAC4 localization (Fig. 8d). The same phenomenon was observed in $Atm^{-/-}$ neocortical neurons where we found a significant effect of ibuprofen in suppressing these damage markers under post hoc analysis (PCNA: $p < 0.05$; cyclin A: $p < 0.05$; γ-H2AX: $p < 0.01$—Fig. 8e–g). In wild-type brains, ibuprofen had no effect, perhaps because there was little to no signal to begin with, (Fig. 8a–h). Of note, we found that HDAC4 translocation to the nucleus was not obvious in 1-month-old $Atm^{-/-}$ animals. This suggests that, although it will develop as an important phenotype by 3 months of age (Fig. 6 plus reference [57]), it is less prominent in the developing $Atm^{-/-}$ brain.

Discussion

The immune and nervous systems interact extensively—with each affecting the behavior of the other for both good and bad. ATM deficiency, in humans and in mice, illustrates this point well. By morphological criteria, brain microglial cells are activated in humans, $Atm^{-/-}$ mice, and a recently developed $Atm^{-/-}$ rat model and display a more severe pro-inflammatory syndrome [58, 59]. The innate immune system in ATM deficiency also appears to be hypersensitive to exogenous challenges [60, 61]. The exaggerated loss of motor function after LPS treatment of $Atm^{-/-}$ mice and the correlated changes seen in our immunohistochemistry findings suggest that this hypersensitivity leads to neuronal cell stress as seen in the accumulation of neuronal cell cycle events, evidence of DNA damage, and the nuclear localization of HDAC4 in Purkinje neurons.

Recent developments make it likely that the involvement of ATM in this chronic activation of the immune system is due in part to the presence of DNA damage. Accumulated cytoplasmic DNA, presumably enhanced after DNA damage, can trigger an innate immune response [58, 59, 62, 63]. .In our model, increased oxidative stress, produced during the immune challenge, induces DNA damage in the nucleus. In the absence of ATM function, DNA repair is compromised which leads to DNA fragments accumulating in the cytoplasm. This would then serve as a "danger" signal that would initiate an immune response via the viral DNA sensor STING or other factors [59]. Thus, an immune challenge exacerbates the oxidative stress in a cell leading to more DNA damage and an increased cellular reliance on ATM function.

Anti-oxidative effect as the main protective mechanism

The presence of oxidative stress in conditions of ATM deficiency is clear and our data suggest that it is in fact the ability of ibuprofen to function as an anti-oxidant that serves as the major source of its ability to blunt the effects of an immune challenge both in vivo and in vitro. Previous findings and our own results have shown that LPS induces cytokine expression [14, 15] and triggers the release of reactive oxygen products [16, 17] in primary cultured microglia, human THP-1 cells, and macrophages [34]. As the conditioned medium from LPS-stimulated microglia (LM) contains a "cocktail" of cytokines and ROS, it is likely that these works together to cause neuronal damage. As expected, LPS increased the neurotoxic effect of the medium from unstimulated microglia (MM) and ibuprofen was able to rescue this damage. Similar to our findings (Fig. 2 and Additional file 1: Figure S1), several groups have shown that ibuprofen fails to significantly inhibit inflammation in the cultured innate immune cells and in the monocyte-neuronal co-culture system with acute inflammation [64, 65]. Indeed, in one case study of a patient with acute endotoxemia, ibuprofen was actually found to cause significant increases of circulating pro-inflammatory TNF-α and IL-6 [66]. .Importantly, in a series of related observations, long-term ibuprofen treatment and the resulting inhibition of COX activity enhanced rather than suppressed the inflammatory phenotype of macrophages [47]. As a result, the anti-inflammatory features of ibuprofen are affected by the dose, duration of incubation, and the cell types used for the experiment, an important feature to keep in mind when clinical studies are designed.

Evidence for the role of oxidative damage in the action of ibuprofen can also be found in the response of neuronal cultures challenged by exposure to medium from LPS-stimulated cells (LM). Ibuprofen reduced the number of neurons showing signs of oxidative stress and cellular damage if it was administered directly to the neurons before they were exposed to LM (Figs. 1 and 2 and Additional file 2: Figure S2). This neuroprotective effect may be due in part to the anti-oxidative properties of ibuprofen (Fig. 5 and Additional file 2: Figure S2) as described previously [34]. Oxidative stress is believed to induce neuronal apoptosis and/or necrosis-like cell death which does not involve caspase activation [67]. The data in Fig. 2 shows that LM enhances the PI signal of our cell death marker indicating the neuronal deaths are most likely necrosis-like events. Also, ibuprofen pre-treatment is able to reduce PI signal in LM treated neurons, suggesting a reduction in intracellular superoxide anion production from neurons and the anti-oxidative feature of ibuprofen [67]. The previous study showed that, even as a DNA damage repair protein, ATM can also be activated by intracellular oxidative stress. Normal

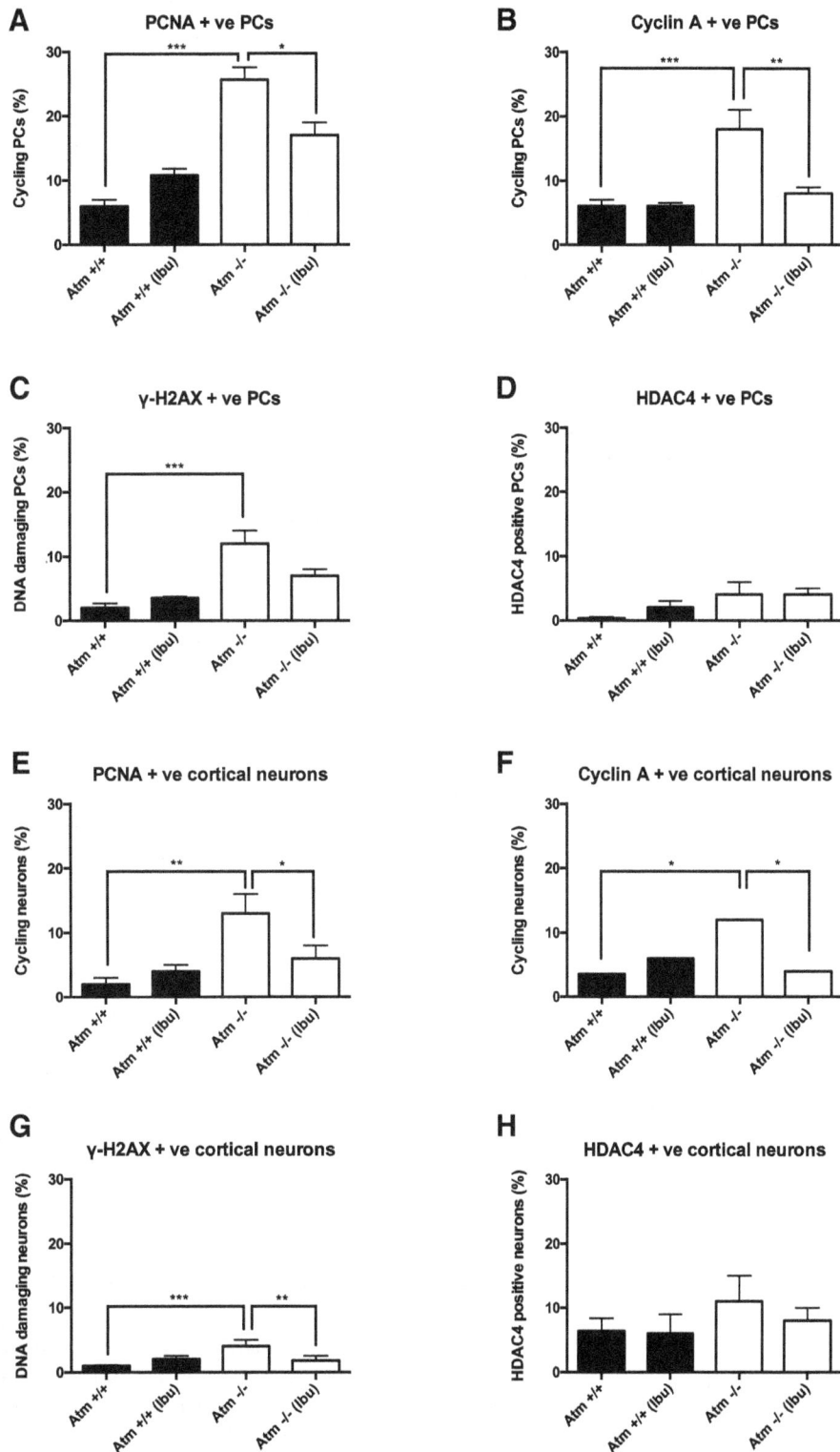

Fig. 8 Ibuprofen reduces early cellular damage in $Atm^{-/-}$ animals. Ibuprofen prevented cell cycle reentry (**a–b**) and DNA damage (**c**) in $Atm^{-/-}$ PCs; the pattern of nuclear translocation of HDAC4 remained unchanged (**d**). Similar results were observed in $Atm^{-/-}$ cortical neurons as measured by neuronal cell cycle activity (**e–f**), DNA damage (**g**) and nuclear HDAC4 expression (**h**). Ibuprofen alone did not induce any changes in $Atm^{+/+}$ cerebellum (**a–d**) or cortex (**e–h**). $n = 4$–5 for each group. Two-way ANOVA was used for analyzing differences in genotype and ibuprofen treatment. * $p < 0.05$, ** $p < 0.01$, *** $p < 0.001$

function and activity of ATM is significantly crucial for keeping the redox balance in the cytoplasm [68, 69]. During the LPS challenge, immune cells like microglia and THP-1 cells produce substances that serve as reactive oxidants and greatly contribute to the neuronal cell damage. Ibuprofen pretreatment relieves the oxidative stress in the microenvironment and contributes to the homeostasis in the central nerves system. These data are consistent with work from Wilkinson et al. that ibuprofen can directly protect neurons from oxidative stress [34].

Ibuprofen can prevent but not reverse the progression of A-T symptoms

The question that naturally arises from these findings is whether reducing this innate immune system hypersensitivity might have therapeutically beneficial effects. We previously showed in a series of studies in mouse models of Alzheimer's disease (AD) that increasing inflammation with a broad-spectrum LPS challenge advances the timing of AD symptoms while oral NSAIDs (ibuprofen or naproxen) retard it [33]. We were encouraged by these earlier findings to test whether a regimen of NSAID administration might also prove beneficial in a mouse model of A-T. As ibuprofen can directly block LPS-induced dendritic loss and reduce spine density [51], we tested whether it might also suppress inflammation-induced A-T symptoms either in vitro or in vivo.

Based on our earlier work in mouse models of Alzheimer's disease (AD) [33], we hypothesized that ibuprofen might prevent the emergence of A-T symptoms. This hypothesis has largely proved correct. Indeed, the similarities in the response to ibuprofen of the A-T and AD models are striking, despite the fact that they are two very different neurodegenerative diseases. In parallel with the findings in the AD mice, neither the cellular nor the behavioral symptoms of adult A-T animals are reversed with NSAID therapy. PC stress fails to improve following ibuprofen treatment, and there is no obvious improvement in behavioral test performance—either coordination as measured on the rotarod or open field behavior.

Yet, ibuprofen can blunt the effects of additional immune/oxidative challenges. Similar to AD animals with ibuprofen supplementation [33, 49, 52, 70, 71], mature A-T animals treated with ibuprofen are less vulnerable to LPS-induced motor dysfunction; more modest benefits were observed for LPS-treated $Atm^{+/+}$ (Fig. 4c–e). These results indicate that ibuprofen can suppress new or accelerated symptom appearance during an inflammatory challenge, but once symptoms are established, it cannot reverse the previous damage. This is exactly the situation found when the impact of ibuprofen is tested on the chronic inflammation found in AD model mice.

It is interesting to note that while ibuprofen does not reverse the behavioral symptoms of mature $Atm^{-/-}$ cerebellum, it nonetheless reduces the microglial morphological response (Fig. 4), tissue oxidation (Fig. 5), and several types of PC damage (Fig. 6). These results are consistent with other groups who found that neuronal abnormalities could be reversed by ibuprofen through anti-inflammatory and anti-oxidative effects [26–28, 34] and is in line with our tissue culture findings showing that ibuprofen applied directly to neurons blocks the effects of LM; but if applied to the microglia themselves, it has little effect. The anti-inflammatory component of the effect of ibuprofen on cerebellar Purkinje cells should be viewed in the context, cerebellar microglia have different immune responses from those in cerebral cortex and hippocampus [72], and in this difference may lie the regional variability that accompanies the clinical picture in AD as well as A-T. Thus, A-T has its most dramatic effects in the cerebellum, and neuronal damage in AD is most obvious in entorhinal cortex and hippocampus. Further support for this concept comes from bioinformatics reports showing that cerebellar microglial cells have different clusters of expressed genes compared to cortical microglia. The classical (LPS) and alternative (interleukin 4) activated pathways in cerebellar microglia are also different from those observed in other brain regions [73]. An additional contributor to this regional variation might be the fact that the cerebellum has the smallest numbers of microglia and astrocytes in vivo [74].

Early ibuprofen treatment reverses the development of A-T symptoms

More dramatic than the protection offered against new LPS-induced symptoms in adult animals is our finding that ibuprofen prevents the development of symptoms during the natural history of the Atm^{tm1Awb} mouse A-T model. Normally, cellular symptoms such as elevated cell cycle events appear between postnatal day 10 and 20 in the mouse [56]. But beginning at P10, 2 weeks of oral ibuprofen administration totally blocked the appearance of disease symptoms in both cerebellum and cortex. These data have potentially important clinical relevance as they suggest that ibuprofen might block or retard the development A-T pathology in pre-symptomatic children. The data lead to the hypothesis that under normal conditions, established disease symptoms cannot be improved by NSAID treatment, but before they appear or worsen, an individual suffering with ATM deficiency might benefit from this simple therapeutic approach. At the very least, as we have suggested previously [24], aggressive anti-inflammatory treatment during the course of A-T could have significant benefit. More speculative for the moment, but potentially more exciting, our experiments with the pre-symptomatic ATM-deficient mice suggest that early intervention in children might postpone the onset of disease symptoms for an unknown period of time. Taken together with our current findings, the data argue that ibuprofen should be considered as a therapeutic agent in preventing the initiation of A-T.

Conclusions

The current study shows that the severity of the symptoms of A-T is closely correlated with the level of neuro-inflammation and oxidative stress in the CNS. We find that the common NSAID, ibuprofen, is able to partially prevent the exacerbated behavioral deficits induced by an acute immune system challenge and can suppress several cellular deficits observed in LPS-stressed $Atm^{-/-}$ mice. The data suggest that the actions of ibuprofen include both anti-inflammatory and anti-oxidative effects. Based on our findings, we propose that early ibuprofen treatment may help to prevent or delay the progression of A-T in human patients.

Additional files

Additional file 1: Figure S1. Gene expression profile of microglia and THP-1 cells under LPS challenge and ibuprofen pretreatment. THP-1 cells were treated with ibuprofen (0, 3, 10, 40, 80, 200 μM) for 6 h and then challenged with LPS for 48 h. Gene expression of $TNF\alpha$ (D), $IL1\beta$ (E), $IL6$ (F), $COX2$ (G) and $IL8$ (H), $SOCS3$ (I), $CD45$ (J), $CD11b$ (K), $P50$ (L) and $P65$ (M) was assessed by PCR. (A). Microglia were treated with LPS for 48 h and then assessed by qPCR. (B). qPCR analysis of microglia treated with LPS and ibuprofen. $N = 3–4$ for each group. Student's unpaired t test was used to analyze the difference between vehicle and LPS treated groups. Two-way ANOVA was used for analyzing differences in LPS and ibuprofen treatments. *, $p < 0.05$, **, $p < 0.01$, ***, $p < 0.001$ between LPS group and control group without ibuprofen pretreatment. (PDF 208 kb)

Additional file 2: Figure S2. (A-N). Ibuprofen pretreatment of THP-1 cells partially rescued LPS-induced neuronal damage. (A-H). Conditioned medium from ibuprofen pretreated THP-1 cells was harvested and applied to DIV14 cultured neurons. Ibuprofen has positive effect on neuronal survival and partially attenuated the appearance of CCEs as measured either by EdU or Ki67. $n = 3$ for each group. Two-way ANOVA was used for analyzing ibuprofen effect within each TM/LM treatment. (O). Oxidative stress in the cultured neuron was measured by 8-oxoguanine. LM from primary cultured microglia was then applied to neuronal culture. It significant increase the level of 8-oxoguanine while ibuprofen alleviate the oxidative stress in the culture system. Scale bar = 50 μm. $n = 3$ for each group (PDF 3439 kb)

Additional file 3: Figure S3. Ibuprofen stimulated formation of tissue-repairing monocytes in cerebellum. LPS stimulated monocyte infiltration while ibuprofen suppressed this invasion (C, D, G, H). Although ibuprofen failed to further stimulate $Ym1$ expression (I), it specifically induced $Trem2$ expression in monocytes infiltrating the $Atm^{-/-}$ cerebellum (J). Scale bar = 50 μm. $n = 3$ for each group. Two-way ANOVA was used for analyzing differences in LPS and ibuprofen treatments within the same genotype. ***, $p < 0.001$ between groups with and without ibuprofen treatment in LPS injected $Atm^{-/-}$ cerebellum; #, $p < 0.05$, ##, $p < 0.01$, ###, $p < 0.001$ groups with and without LPS treatment in the same genotype. (TIF 2427 kb)

Additional file 4: Figure S4. Akt, MAPK and NFκB pathways were investigated in cerebellar lysates by immunoblotting (A, B). Ibuprofen failed to affect ERK, JNK, Akt or p65 phosphorylation during an LPS challenge (C, E, F, G and data not shown). It reduced p38 phosphorylation only in $Atm^{+/+}$ cerebellum (D). $n = 4$ for each group.

Two-way ANOVA was used for statistical analysis. *, $p < 0.05$ compared to $Atm^{+/+}$ saline group. (PDF 771 kb)

Additional file 5: Figure S5. Ibuprofen specifically suppresses p38 phosphorylation in PCs. Cerebellar sections were stained with phospho-p38 antiserum and visualized by fluorescent microscopy. LPS or ATM deficiency alone increased phospho-p38 levels in PCs (C, E) yet LPS unexpectedly reduced phospho-p38 levels in $Atm^{-/-}$ cerebellum (G). Ibuprofen treatment significantly reversed LPS triggered p38 phosphorylation in both $Atm^{+/+}$ and $Atm^{-/-}$ PCs (D, H). (PDF 3474 kb)

Abbreviations
AD: Alzheimer's disease; A-T: Ataxia telangiectasia; ATM: Ataxia telangiectasia-mutated; CCE: Cell cycle event; CNS: Central nervous system; DCN: Deep cerebellar nuclei; LM: LPS-stimulated microglia conditioned medium; LM: LPS-stimulated THP-1 cell conditioned medium; LPS: Lipopolysaccharide; MM: Unstimulated microglia conditioned medium; NSAID: Non-steroidal anti-inflammatory drug; PC: Purkinje cell; ROS: Reactive oxygen species; TM: Unstimulated THP-1 cell conditioned medium

Acknowledgements
We express our sincere thanks to the technicians in core animal facility from Hong Kong University of Science and Technology for the routine management in mouse colonies. We also gratefully thank Prof. Nancy Ip for providing the THP-1 cell line used in the current study.

Funding
This work was supported by the National Key Basic Research Program of China (2013CB530900), The Research Grants Council, HKSAR (HKUST GRF660813 and GRF 16101315), the BrightFocus Foundation, A-T Children's Project, and by the US NIH (NS71022). The support of The Hong Kong University of Science and Technology (R9321) is also gratefully acknowledged.

Authors' contributions
CWH, XS, and KH conceived and designed the experiments. CWH XS, XTS, and FLM performed the experiments. CWH, XS, XTS, FLM, and KH analyzed the data. CWH, XS, XTS, and KH wrote the paper. All authors read and approved the final manuscript.

Authors' information
Information for all the co-authors is listed in the title page.

Competing interests
The authors declare that they have no competing interests.

Author details
[1]Division of Life Science and State Key Laboratory of Molecular Neurobiology, Hong Kong University of Science and Technology, Clear Water Bay, Kowloon, Hong Kong. [2]Present address: School of Biomedical Sciences, The University of Hong Kong, Pokfulam, Hong Kong.

References

1. Lavin MF, Shiloh Y. The genetic defect in ataxia-telangiectasia. Annu Rev Immunol. 1997;15:177–202.
2. Chun HH, Gatti RA. Ataxia-telangiectasia, an evolving phenotype. DNA Repair (Amst). 2004;3:1187–96.
3. Biton S, Barzilai A, Shiloh Y. The neurological phenotype of ataxia-telangiectasia: solving a persistent puzzle. DNA Repair (Amst). 2008;7:1028–38.
4. Gatti RA, Becker-Catania S, Chun HH, Sun X, Mitui M, Lai CH, Khanlou N, Babaei M, Cheng R, Clark C, et al. The pathogenesis of ataxia-telangiectasia. Learning from a Rosetta stone. Clin Rev Allergy Immunol. 2001;20:87–108.
5. Heppner FL, Ransohoff RM, Becher B. Immune attack: the role of inflammation in Alzheimer disease. Nat Rev Neurosci. 2015;16:358–72.
6. Milatovic D, Zaja-Milatovic S, Montine KS, Shie FS, Montine TJ. Neuronal oxidative damage and dendritic degeneration following activation of CD14-dependent innate immune response in vivo. J Neuroinflammation. 2004;1:20.
7. Steinman L. Elaborate interactions between the immune and nervous systems. Nat Immunol. 2004;5:575–81.
8. Veres TZ, Rochlitzer S, Braun A. The role of neuro-immune cross-talk in the regulation of inflammation and remodelling in asthma. Pharmacol Ther. 2009;122:203–14.
9. Matt SM, Johnson RW. Neuro-immune dysfunction during brain aging: new insights in microglial cell regulation. Curr Opin Pharmacol. 2015;26:96–101.
10. Austin PJ, Berglund AM, Siu S, Fiore NT, Gerke-Duncan MB, Ollerenshaw SL, Leigh SJ, Kunjan PA, Kang JW, Keay KA. Evidence for a distinct neuro-immune signature in rats that develop behavioural disability after nerve injury. J Neuroinflammation. 2015;12:96.
11. Morris G, et al. The neuro-immune pathophysiology of central and peripheral fatigue in systemic immune-inflammatory and neuro-immune diseases. Mol Neurobiol. 2016;53(2):1195-219.
12. Gutierrez-Fernandez F, Pinto-Gonzalez M, Gonzalez-Perez O. Neuro-immune interactions in the postnatal ventricular-subventricular zone. J Stem Cells. 2014;9:53–64.
13. Ermakov AV, Konkova MS, Kostyuk SV, Izevskaya VL. Oxidized extracellular DNA as a stress signal in human cells. Oxidative Med Cell Longev. 2013;2013:649747.
14. Schildberger A, Rossmanith E, Eichhorn T, Strassl K, Weber V. Monocytes, peripheral blood mononuclear cells, and THP-1 cells exhibit different cytokine expression patterns following stimulation with lipopolysaccharide. Mediat Inflamm. 2013;2013:697972.
15. Chanput W, Mes J, Vreeburg RA, Savelkoul HF, Wichers HJ. Transcription profiles of LPS-stimulated THP-1 monocytes and macrophages: a tool to study inflammation modulating effects of food-derived compounds. Food Funct. 2010;1:254–61.
16. Sarna LK, Wu N, Hwang SY, Siow YL, O K. Berberine inhibits NADPH oxidase mediated superoxide anion production in macrophages. Can J Physiol Pharmacol. 2010;88:369–78.
17. Zhang X, Cao J, Jiang L, Zhong L. Suppressive effects of hydroxytyrosol on oxidative stress and nuclear factor-kappaB activation in THP-1 cells. Biol Pharm Bull. 2009;32:578–82.
18. Bhatt JM, Bush A. Microbiological surveillance in lung disease in ataxia telangiectasia. Eur Respir J. 2014;43:1797–801.
19. Staples ER, McDermott EM, Reiman A, Byrd PJ, Ritchie S, Taylor AM, Davies EG. Immunodeficiency in ataxia telangiectasia is correlated strongly with the presence of two null mutations in the ataxia telangiectasia mutated gene. Clin Exp Immunol. 2008;153:214–20.
20. Menotta M, Biagiotti S, Bianchi M, Chessa L, Magnani M. Dexamethasone partially rescues ataxia telangiectasia-mutated (ATM) deficiency in ataxia telangiectasia by promoting a shortened protein variant retaining kinase activity. J Biol Chem. 2012;287:41352–63.
21. Zannolli R, Buoni S, Betti G, Salvucci S, Plebani A, Soresina A, Pietrogrande MC, Martino S, Leuzzi V, Finocchi A, et al. A randomized trial of oral betamethasone to reduce ataxia symptoms in ataxia telangiectasia. Mov Disord. 2012;27:1312–6.
22. Kuljis RO, Xu Y, Aguila MC, Baltimore D. Degeneration of neurons, synapses, and neuropil and glial activation in a murine Atm knockout model of ataxia-telangiectasia. Proc Natl Acad Sci U S A. 1997;94:12688–93.
23. Petersen AJ, Rimkus SA, Wassarman DA. ATM kinase inhibition in glial cells activates the innate immune response and causes neurodegeneration in Drosophila. Proc Natl Acad Sci U S A. 2012;109:E656–64.
24. Yang Y, Hui CW, Li J, Herrup K. The interaction of the atm genotype with inflammation and oxidative stress. PLoS One. 2014;9:e85863.
25. Hui CW, Herrup K. Individual cytokines modulate the neurological symptoms of ATM deficiency in a region specific manner (1, 2, 3). eNeuro. 2015;2:ENEURO-0032.
26. Cakala M, Malik AR, Strosznajder JB. Inhibitor of cyclooxygenase-2 protects against amyloid beta peptide-evoked memory impairment in mice. Pharmacol Rep. 2007;59:164–72.
27. Gopez JJ, Yue H, Vasudevan R, Malik AS, Fogelsanger LN, Lewis S, Panikashvili D, Shohami E, Jansen SA, Narayan RK, Strauss KI. Cyclooxygenase-2-specific inhibitor improves functional outcomes, provides neuroprotection, and reduces inflammation in a rat model of traumatic brain injury. Neurosurgery. 2005;56:590–604.
28. Scali C, Giovannini MG, Prosperi C, Bellucci A, Pepeu G, Casamenti F. The selective cyclooxygenase-2 inhibitor rofecoxib suppresses brain inflammation and protects cholinergic neurons from excitotoxic degeneration in vivo. Neuroscience. 2003;117:909–19.
29. Vlad SC, Miller DR, Kowall NW, Felson DT. Protective effects of NSAIDs on the development of Alzheimer disease. Neurology. 2008;70:1672–7.
30. Choi JK, Carreras I, Aytan N, Jenkins-Sahlin E, Dedeoglu A, Jenkins BG. The effects of aging, housing and ibuprofen treatment on brain neurochemistry in a triple transgene Alzheimer's disease mouse model using magnetic resonance spectroscopy and imaging. Brain Res. 2014;1590:85–96.
31. Babiloni C, Frisoni GB, Del Percio C, Zanetti O, Bonomini C, Cassetta E, Pasqualetti P, Miniussi C, De Rosas M, Valenzano A, et al. Ibuprofen treatment modifies cortical sources of EEG rhythms in mild Alzheimer's disease. Clin Neurophysiol. 2009;120:709–18.
32. Jin DQ, Sung JY, Hwang YK, Kwon KJ, Han SH, Min SS, Han JS. Dexibuprofen (S(+)-isomer ibuprofen) reduces microglial activation and impairments of spatial working memory induced by chronic lipopolysaccharide infusion. Pharmacol Biochem Behav. 2008;89:404–11.
33. Varvel NH, Bhaskar K, Kounnas MZ, Wagner SL, Yang Y, Lamb BT, Herrup K. NSAIDs prevent, but do not reverse, neuronal cell cycle reentry in a mouse model of Alzheimer's disease. J Clin Invest. 2009;119:3692–702.
34. Wilkinson BL, Cramer PE, Varvel NH, Reed-Geaghan E, Jiang Q, Szabo A, Herrup K, Lamb BT, Landreth GE. Ibuprofen attenuates oxidative damage through NOX2 inhibition in Alzheimer's disease. Neurobiol Aging. 2012;33:197 e121–132.
35. Dong Z, Yan L, Huang G, Zhang L, Mei B, Meng B. Ibuprofen partially attenuates neurodegenerative symptoms in presenilin conditional double-knockout mice. Neuroscience. 2014;270:58–68.
36. Hillmann A, Hahn S, Schilling S, Hoffmann T, Demuth HU, Bulic B, Schneider-Axmann T, Bayer TA, Weggen S, Wirths O. No improvement after chronic ibuprofen treatment in the 5XFAD mouse model of Alzheimer's disease. Neurobiol Aging. 2012;33:833 e839–850.
37. Barlow C, Hirotsune S, Paylor R, Liyanage M, Eckhaus M, Collins F, Shiloh Y, Crawley JN, Ried T, Tagle D, Wynshaw-Boris A. Atm-deficient mice: a paradigm of ataxia telangiectasia. Cell. 1996;86:159–71.
38. Yan Q, Zhang J, Liu H, Babu-Khan S, Vassar R, Biere AL, Citron M, Landreth G. Anti-inflammatory drug therapy alters beta-amyloid processing and deposition in an animal model of Alzheimer's disease. J Neurosci. 2003;23:7504–9.
39. Lee J-K, Tansey MG. Microglia isolation from adult mouse brain. Methods Mol Biol. 2013;1041:17–23.
40. Hui CW, Zhang Y, Herrup K. Non-neuronal cells are required to mediate the effects of neuroinflammation: results from a neuron-enriched culture system. PLoS One. 2016;11:e0147134.
41. Combs CK, Johnson DE, Cannady SB, Lehman TM, Landreth GE. Identification of microglial signal transduction pathways mediating a neurotoxic response to amyloidogenic fragments of beta-amyloid and prion proteins. J Neurosci. 1999;19:928–39.
42. Wu Q, Combs C, Cannady SB, Geldmacher DS, Herrup K. Beta-amyloid activated microglia induce cell cycling and cell death in cultured cortical neurons. Neurobiol Aging. 2000;21:797–806.
43. Ang Z, Er JZ, Tan NS, Lu J, Liou YC, Grosse J, Ding JL. Human and mouse monocytes display distinct signalling and cytokine profiles upon stimulation with FFAR2/FFAR3 short-chain fatty acid receptor agonists. Sci Rep. 2016;6:34145.
44. Ingersoll MA, Spanbroek R, Lottaz C, Gautier EL, Frankenberger M, Hoffmann R, Lang R, Haniffa M, Collin M, Tacke F, et al. Comparison of gene expression profiles between human and mouse monocyte subsets. Blood. 2010;115:e10–9.

45. Chanput W, Mes JJ, Wichers HJ. THP-1 cell line: an in vitro cell model for immune modulation approach. Int Immunopharmacol. 2014;23:37–45.

46. Pietkiewicz S, Schmidt JH, Lavrik IN. Quantification of apoptosis and necroptosis at the single cell level by a combination of imaging flow cytometry with classical Annexin V/propidium iodide staining. J Immunol Methods. 2015;423:99–103.

47. Na YR, Yoon YN, Son D, Jung D, Gu GJ, Seok SH. Consistent inhibition of cyclooxygenase drives macrophages towards the inflammatory phenotype. PLoS One. 2015;10:e0118203.

48. Shakkottai VG, Chou CH, Oddo S, Sailer CA, Knaus HG, Gutman GA, Barish ME, LaFerla FM, Chandy KG. Enhanced neuronal excitability in the absence of neurodegeneration induces cerebellar ataxia. J Clin Invest. 2004;113:582–90.

49. Carnevale D, Mascio G, Ajmone-Cat MA, D'Andrea I, Cifelli G, Madonna M, Cocozza G, Frati A, Carullo P, Carnevale L, et al. Role of neuroinflammation in hypertension-induced brain amyloid pathology. Neurobiol Aging. 2012; 33:205 e219–229.

50. Huang ZJ, Hsu E, Li HC, Rosner AL, Rupert RL, Song XJ. Topical application of compound ibuprofen suppresses pain by inhibiting sensory neuron hyperexcitability and neuroinflammation in a rat model of intervertebral foramen inflammation. J Pain. 2011;12:141–52.

51. Milatovic D, Gupta RC, Yu Y, Zaja-Milatovic S, Aschner M. Protective effects of antioxidants and anti-inflammatory agents against manganese-induced oxidative damage and neuronal injury. Toxicol Appl Pharmacol. 2011;256:219–26.

52. Meunier J, Borjini N, Gillis C, Villard V, Maurice T. Brain toxicity and inflammation induced in vivo in mice by the amyloid-beta forty-two inducer aftin-4, a roscovitine derivative. J Alzheimers Dis. 2015;44:507–24.

53. Jiang T, Zhang YD, Chen Q, Gao Q, Zhu XC, Zhou JS, Shi JQ, Lu H, Tan L, Yu JT. TREM2 modifies microglial phenotype and provides neuroprotection in P301S tau transgenic mice. Neuropharmacology. 2016;105:196–206.

54. Cherry JD, Olschowka JA, O'Banion MK. Neuroinflammation and M2 microglia: the good, the bad, and the inflamed. J Neuroinflammation. 2014;11:98.

55. Herrup K, Yang Y. Cell cycle regulation in the postmitotic neuron: oxymoron or new biology? Nat Rev Neurosci. 2007;8:368.

56. Yang Y, Herrup K. Loss of neuronal cell cycle control in ataxia-telangiectasia: a unified disease mechanism. J Neurosci. 2005;25:2522–9.

57. Li J, Chen J, Ricupero CL, Hart RP, Schwartz MS, Kusnecov A, Herrup K. Nuclear accumulation of HDAC4 in ATM deficiency promotes neurodegeneration in ataxia telangiectasia. Nat Med. 2012;18:783–90.

58. Quek H, Luff J, Cheung KG, et al. Rats with a missense mutation in Atm display neuroinflammation and neurodegeneration subsequent to accumulation of cytosolic DNA following unrepaired DNA damage. J Leukoc Biol. https://doi.org/10.1189/jlb.4VMA0716-316R.

59. Quek H, Luff J, Cheung KG, et al. A rat model of ataxia-telangiectasia: evidence for a neurodegenerative phenotype. Hum Mol Genet. 2017;26(1): 109–23. https://doi.org/10.1093/hmg/ddw371.

60. McGrath-Morrow SA, Collaco JM, Crawford TO, Carson KA, Lefton-Greif MA, Zeitlin P, Lederman HM. Elevated serum IL-8 levels in ataxia telangiectasia. J Pediatr. 2010;156:682–4 e681.

61. Westbrook AM, Schiestl RH. Atm-deficient mice exhibit increased sensitivity to dextran sulfate sodium-induced colitis characterized by elevated DNA damage and persistent immune activation. Cancer Res. 2010;70:1875–84.

62. Härtlova A, Erttmann SF, et al. DNA damage primes the type i interferon system via the cytosolic dna sensor sting to promote anti-microbial innate immunity. Immunity. 2015;42(2):332–43.

63. Bo Hu, Chengcheng Jin et.al: The DNA-sensing AIM2 inflammasome controls radiation-induced cell death and tissue injury. Science 2016; 354(6313):765-768.

64. Lee M, Suk K, Kang Y, McGeer E, McGeer PL. Neurotoxic factors released by stimulated human monocytes and THP-1 cells. Brain Res. 2011;1400:99–111.

65. Hohsfield LA, Ammann CG, Humpel C. Inflammatory status of transmigrating primary rat monocytes in a novel perfusion model simulating blood flow. J Neuroimmunol. 2013;258:17–26.

66. Spinas GA, Bloesch D, Keller U, Zimmerli W, Cammisuli S. Pretreatment with ibuprofen augments circulating tumor necrosis factor-alpha, interleukin-6, and elastase during acute endotoxinemia. J Infect Dis. 1991;163:89–95.

67. Valencia A, Moran J. Reactive oxygen species induce different cell death mechanisms in cultured neurons. Free Radic Biol Med. 2004;36:1112–25.

68. Ditch S, Paull TT. The ATM protein kinase and cellular redox signaling: beyond the DNA damage response. Trends Biochem Sci. 2012;37(1):15–22. https://doi.org/10.1016/j.tibs.2011.10.002.

69. Guo Z, Kozlov S, Lavin MF, Person MD, Paull TT. ATM Activation by oxidative stress. Science. 2010;330(6003):517–21. https://doi.org/10.1126/science. 1192912.

70. Ghosal K, Stathopoulos A, Pimplikar SW. APP intracellular domain impairs adult neurogenesis in transgenic mice by inducing neuroinflammation. PLoS One. 2010;5:e11866.

71. Lim GP, Yang F, Chu T, Chen P, Beech W, Teter B, Tran T, Ubeda O, Ashe KH, Frautschy SA, Cole GM. Ibuprofen suppresses plaque pathology and inflammation in a mouse model for Alzheimer's disease. J Neurosci. 2000;20: 5709–14.

72. Pinato L, da Silveira C-MS, Franco DG, Campos LMG, Cecon E, Fernandes PACM, Bittencourt JC, Markus RP. Selective protection of the cerebellum against intracerebroventricular LPS is mediated by local melatonin synthesis. Brain Struct Funct. 2015;220:827–40.

73. Grabert K, Michoel T, Karavolos MH, Clohisey S, Baillie JK, Stevens MP, Freeman TC, Summers KM, McColl BW. Microglial brain region-dependent diversity and selective regional sensitivities to ageing. Nat Neurosci. 2016;19:504–16.

74. Savchenko VL, McKanna JA, Nikonenko IR, Skibo GG. Microglia and astrocytes in the adult rat brain: comparative immunocytochemical analysis demonstrates the efficacy of lipocortin 1 immunoreactivity. Neuroscience. 2000;96:195–203.

5

Omega-3 polyunsaturated fatty acid attenuates traumatic brain injury-induced neuronal apoptosis by inducing autophagy through the upregulation of SIRT1-mediated deacetylation of Beclin-1

Xiangrong Chen[1], Zhigang Pan[1], Zhongning Fang[1], Weibin Lin[1], Shukai Wu[1], Fuxing Yang[1], Yasong Li[1], Huangde Fu[2*], Hongzhi Gao[1*] and Shun Li[3*]

Abstract

Background: Enhancing autophagy after traumatic brain injury (TBI) may decrease the expression of neuronal apoptosis-related molecules. Autophagy-mediated neuronal survival is regulated by the sirtuin family of proteins (SIRT). Omega-3 polyunsaturated fatty acids (ω-3 PUFA) are known to have antioxidative and anti-inflammatory effects. We previously demonstrated that ω-3 PUFA supplementation attenuated neuronal apoptosis by modulating the neuroinflammatory response through SIRT1-mediated deacetylation of the HMGB1/NF-κB pathway, leading to neuroprotective effects following experimental traumatic brain injury (TBI). However, no studies have elucidated if the neuroprotective effects of ω-3 PUFAs against TBI-induced neuronal apoptosis are modulated by SIRT1-mediated deacetylation of the autophagy pathway.

Methods: The Feeney DM TBI model was adopted to induce TBI rats. Modified neurological severity scores, the rotarod test, brain water content, and Nissl staining were employed to determine the neuroprotective effects of ω-3 PUFA supplementation. Immunofluorescent staining and western blot analysis were used to detect Beclin-1 nuclear translocation and autophagy pathway activation. The impact of SIRT1 deacetylase activity on Beclin-1 acetylation and the interaction between cytoplasmic Beclin-1 and Bcl-2 were assessed to evaluate the neuroprotective effects of ω-3 PUFAs and to determine if these effects were dependent on SIRT1-mediated deacetylation of the autophagy pathway in order to gain further insight into the mechanisms underlying the development of neuroprotection after TBI.

(Continued on next page)

* Correspondence: 13265040480@163.com; hongzhi_gao@hotmail.com; morelee@163.com
[2]Department of Neurosurgery, Affiliated Hospital of YouJiang Medical University for Nationalities, Baise 533000, Guangxi Province, China
[1]Department of Neurosurgery, The Second Affiliated Hospital, Fujian Medical University, Quanzhou 362000, Fujian Province, China
[3]Department of Neurosurgery, Affiliated Hospital of North Sichuan Medical College, Sichuan Province, Nanchong 637000, China

(Continued from previous page)

Results: ω-3 PUFA supplementation protected neurons against TBI-induced neuronal apoptosis via enhancement of the autophagy pathway. We also found that treatment with ω-3 PUFA significantly increased the NAD+/NADH ratio and SIRT1 activity following TBI. In addition, ω-3 PUFA supplementation increased Beclin-1 deacetylation and its nuclear export and induced direct interactions between cytoplasmic Beclin-1 and Bcl-2 by increasing SIRT1 activity following TBI. These events led to the inhibition of neuronal apoptosis and to neuroprotective effects through enhancing autophagy after TBI, possibly due to elevated SIRT1.

Conclusions: ω-3 PUFA supplementation attenuated TBI-induced neuronal apoptosis by inducing the autophagy pathway through the upregulation of SIRT1-mediated deacetylation of Beclin-1.

Keywords: Traumatic brain injury, Omega-3 polyunsaturated fatty acid, Apoptosis, Autophagy

Introduction

Traumatic brain injury (TBI) is a major cause of disability and death in adolescence. It has been suggested that mitigating brain damage and promoting nerve functional recovery following TBI would alleviate the burden to patients and to society [1]. TBI-induced secondary injury is a complicated pathophysiological process that includes microglial activation, inflammatory responses, oxidative stress, and abnormal mitochondrial activities, all of which affect neurological function [2–4]. Damaged mitochondria release excess reactive oxygen species (ROS) after TBI, which lead to lipid peroxidation and cytotoxicity resulting in further oxidative stress and mitochondrial dysfunction [5–7]. Mitochondrial dysfunction in turn damages membrane permeability, causing excess release of mitochondrial apoptosis-associated proteins, which all promote caspase-dependent neuronal apoptosis [8]. This process involves the upregulation of caspase-3, the pro-apoptotic factor B cell lymphoma (Bcl)-2-associated X protein (Bax), and the inhibition of the anti-apoptotic protein, Bcl-2 [5].

The relationship between autophagy and apoptosis in the neurologic system is very complex and not fully understood. Considerable evidence suggests that autophagy can inhibit apoptosis based on diverse mechanisms, including that increasing autophagy removes damaged mitochondria or inactivation proteins [5, 9, 10]. As reviewed by Fernandez, sequestering of unfolded protein which are initiators of endoplasmic reticulum stress by autophagy can also reduce apoptosis [11]. Oxidative stress-induced autophagy selectively degrades oxidized substances and damages organelles to reduce oxidative injury, maintains normal mitochondrial function, and balances the intracellular microenvironment [10, 12, 13]. Other factors involved in autophagy may be due to the molecular interactions between autophagy and apoptotic processes. Enhancing autophagy after TBI may decrease the expressions of neuronal apoptosis-related downstream molecules, including cleaved caspase-3, Bcl-2, and Bax, resulting in the dissociation of the Bcl-2/Beclin-1 complexes [14–16]. Our previous study [17] also showed that the upregulation of autophagy could

attenuate TBI-induced oxidative stress and apoptosis, suggesting a protective role of autophagy after TBI. Therefore, identifying neuroprotective mechanisms that are involved in autophagy-mediated neuronal apoptosis may provide novel therapeutic strategies for TBI.

Autophagy-related genes (ATGs) perform important roles in autophagy, which control major steps in the autophagic pathway, such as growth of autophagic membranes, recognition of autophagic cargoes, and fusion of autophagosomes with lysosomes [18–20]. Beclin-1, also known as BECN1, is the homolog of the mammalian yeast protein, ATG6. As an important factor in autophagy regulation, Beclin-1 can induce the formation of pre-autophagosomal structures to promote the generation of autophagic vacuoles [21–23]. Beclin-1 interacts with several binding partners and exerts multiple-biological effects, including cell metabolism, apoptosis, and autophagy [16]. The suppression of Beclin-1 impairs the autophagy-associated post-translational processing of ATG8 (microtubule-associated protein 1 light chain 3, LC3) [24]. Interaction with phosphatidylinositide 3-kinase (PI3K) can lead to upregulation of autophagy, while interactions with Bcl-2 can result in inhibition of apoptosis [18].

Recent research has demonstrated that the deacetylation of ATGs by the sirtuin (SIRT) family of proteins is necessary for the induction of autophagosome formation [25–27]. SIRT1 is an nicotinamide adenine dinucleotide (NAD+)-dependent class III histone deacetylase and has been shown to regulate autophagy through the deacetylation of ATGs, which in turn plays major roles in regulating metabolism, DNA damage repair, and stress resistance [24, 26]. Furthermore, Beclin-1 expression levels are related acetylation of its lysine residues [26, 29]. Acetylation of Beclin-1 can lead to inhibition of autophagic responses, while deacetylation of Beclin-1 at lysine residues 430 and 437 by SIRT1 influences autophagosome maturation and subsequent biological effects [29]. These findings suggest that Beclin-1 may be a novel deacetylation target of SIRT1, which in turn elevates the autophagy pathway through Beclin-1 deacetylation [28].

Omega-3 polyunsaturated fatty acids (ω-3 PUFA), including eicosapentaenoic acid and docosahexaenoic acid, are known to be biologically active compounds with antioxidative and anti-inflammatory effects; all of which influence the pathogenesis of many diseases, including Alzheimer's disease [29], acute pancreatitis [30], Parkinson's disease [31], and cerebral ischemia [32]. We previously reported that ω-3 PUFA supplementation inhibited the neuroinflammatory response and neuronal apoptosis by regulating the HMGB1/ NF-κB signaling pathway [33]. In addition, SIRT1 levels were upregulated after ω-3 PUFA supplementation [33, 34]. We also demonstrated that ω-3 PUFA supplementation attenuates neuronal apoptosis by modulating the neuroinflammatory response through SIRT1-mediated deacetylation of the HMGB1/NF-κB pathway, leading to neuroprotective effects following experimental TBI [33]. Other research has also demonstrated that ω-3 PUFA supplementation regulates oxidative stress and inflammation by the autophagy pathway [34–36]; although the mechanism of ω-3 PUFA-mediated autophagy pathway regulation still needs further clarification. The interaction between apoptosis and autophagy provides novel therapeutic strategies for TBI [10, 37]. Post-translational modifications like lysine deacetylations and deacetylation of Beclin-1 by SIRT1 influence autophagy and autophagy-mediated neuronal survival [26, 28], which raises the possibility that neuronal apoptosis may be attenuated by modulating SIRT1-mediated deacetylation of Beclin-1 after ω-3 PUFA supplementation. Thus, in the present study, the neuroprotective effects of ω-3 PUFAs against TBI-induced neuronal apoptosis were studied. In addition, the potential molecular mechanisms focusing on the autophagy pathway and SIRT1-mediated Beclin-1 deacetylation were also investigated.

Materials and methods
Animals
All animal experiments were approved by the Fujian Provincial Medical University Experimental Animal Ethics Committee (Fuzhou, China) and were performed under strict supervision. Adult male Sprague-Dawley rats, ranging between 230 and 260 g, were purchased from the Experimental Animal Facility in Fujian Medical University and housed in a temperature (23 ± 2 °C) and light (12 h light/dark cycle) controlled room with ad libitum access to food and water.

Experimental model and drug administration
All rats were randomly assigned into a sham group, a sham+ω-3 PUFA supplementation group (sham+ω-3 group), a TBI group, and a TBI+ω-3 group. After

injury, the groups were further divided into four subgroups: a 1-day group, a 3-day group, a 7-day group, and a 14-day group (n = 12 each). Six rats in each group were sacrificed for neurological evaluation and histological studies; the remaining six rats were used for molecular studies. TBI was induced in anesthetized (50 mg/kg sodium pentobarbital; intraperitoneally) rats as described previously [33]. Briefly, a midline incision was made over the skull, and a 5-mm craniotomy was drilled through the skull 2 mm caudal to the left coronal suture and 2 mm from the midline without disturbing the dura. TBI was induced using a weight-drop hitting device (ZH-ZYQ, Electronic Technology Development Co., Xuzhou, China) with a 4.5-mm-diameter cylinder bar weighing 40 g from a height of 20 cm. Bone wax was used to seal the hole, and the scalp was sutured. All procedures were the same for each group except in the sham group, in which no weight was dropped. Approximately 30 min after TBI, the TBI+ω-3 group was intraperitoneally injected with ω-3 PUFA (2 ml/kg, diluted in dimethyl sulfoxide; Sigma, St. Louis, MO, USA) once per day for 7 consecutive days [33]. To inhibit autophagy or the SIRT1 pathway, 25 ul/kg 3-methyladenine (3-MA, 1 mmol/l, diluted in dimethyl sulfoxide; Sigma) or 25 ul/kg sirtinol (2 mmol/l, diluted in dimethyl sulfoxide; Sigma) was administered into the right lateral ventricle 24 h after intraperitoneal ω-3 PUFA injection once per day for 3 consecutive days, in order to clarify the mechanisms of ω-3 PUFA-mediated neuroprotection [38]. The remaining groups were injected with the same dose of dimethyl sulfoxide as a control.

Measurement of neurological impairment scores and the rotarod test
Neurological deficit was calculated using the neurological impairment score. Rats were subjected to exercise (muscular state and abnormal action), sensation (visual, tactile, and balance), and reflex examinations and assigned a modified neurological severity score (mNSS) [33] that was recorded when a task failed to be completed or when the corresponding reflex was lost. The mNSS score was graded on a scale of 0–18, where a total score of 18 points indicated severe neurological deficits and a score of 0 indicated normal performance, 13–18 points indicated severe injury, 7–12 indicated mean-moderate injury, and 1–6 indicated mild injury. Neurological function was measured at different time points by investigators who were blinded to group information.

The rotarod protocol was modified slightly from that in a previous report [39]. Briefly, rats underwent a 2-day testing phase with a rotarod (IITC Life Science, Woodland Hills, CA, USA), which gradually accelerated from 5 to 45 rpm over 5 min. During the procedure, the latency to fall was recorded as the time before rats fell off or gripped the rod for two successive revolutions from day 1 after TBI. The mean latency was measured at different time points by investigators who were blinded to the experimental groups.

Measurement of brain water content

Brain water content was calculated using the wet weight-dry weight method [33]. Animals were sacrificed after the mNSS test, and their cortices were removed at the edge of the bone window (200 ± 20 mg). Filter paper was used to remove excess blood and cerebrospinal fluid. The wet weight was measured, and the brains were dried in an oven at 100 °C for 24 h until a constant weight was achieved, at which point the dry weight was measured. The % brain water content was calculated as: (wet weight – dry weight)/wet weight × 100%.

Nissl staining

Formaldehyde-fixed specimens were embedded in paraffin and cut into 4-μm-thick sections that were deparaffinized with xylene and rehydrated in a graded series of alcohol. Samples were treated with Nissl staining solution for 5 min. Damaged neurons were shrunken or contained vacuoles, whereas normal neurons had a relatively large, full soma, and round, large nuclei. Average intensities or cell counts were calculated from the same sections in six rats per group with Image-Pro Plus 7.0 by investigators who were blinded to the experimental groups.

Immunohistochemical analysis

Formaldehyde-fixed specimens were embedded in paraffin and cut into 4-μm-thick sections that were deparaffinized with xylene and rehydrated in a graded series of alcohol. Antigen retrieval was carried out by microwaving in citric acid buffer. Sections were incubated with an antibody against SIRT1 (1:100; Cell Signaling Technology, Danvers, MA, USA), washed, and then incubated with secondary antibody for 1 h at room temperature. The negative control was prepared without the addition of the anti-SIRT1 antibody. A total of five sections from each animal were used for quantification, and the signal intensity was evaluated as follows [36]: 0, no positive cells; 1, very few positive cells; 2, moderate number of positive cells; 3, large number of positive cells; and 4, the highest number of positive cells.

Immunofluorescence analysis

Formaldehyde-fixed specimens were embedded in paraffin and cut into 4-μm-thick sections that were deparaffinized with xylene and rehydrated in a graded series of alcohol, followed by antigen retrieval. Sections were incubated overnight at 4 °C with antibodies against LC3 (1:200, Abcam, Cambridge, UK), NeuN (1:100; Boster Biotech, Wuhan, China), and Beclin-1 (1:200; Cell Signaling Technology). After washing, the sections were incubated with secondary antibodies for 1 h at room temperature. Cell nuclei were stained with 4′,6-diamidino-2-phenylindole. Immunopositive cells in five selected fields were counted under a microscope (Leica, Wetzlar, Germany) at × 400 magnification by investigators who were blinded to the experimental groups.

Terminal deoxynucleotidyl transferase dUTP nick-end labeling (TUNEL) assay

Apoptotic cells were detected using a TUNEL kit (Roche Diagnostics, Indianapolis, IN, USA) according to the manufacturer's instructions. Indicators of apoptosis included a shrunken cell body, irregular shape, nuclear condensation, and brown diaminobenzidine staining, as observed by microscopy at × 400 magnification. The final average percentage of TUNEL-positive cells of the six sections was regarded as the data for each sample.

Primary culture of rat hippocampal neurons

Rat brain tissues were homogenized and digested in preheated 0.25% trypsin-EDTA solution. The cells were resuspensed in Dulbecco's modified Eagle's medium (DMEM, low glucose) and cultured in DMEM medium (high glucose) supplemented with 10% FBS in 6-well cell culture plates at 37 °C in a 5% CO_2 atmosphere.

SIRT1 siRNA transfection and autophagy flux analysis

After 3 days, hippocampal neuron cells were transiently transfected with either siRNA control or the SIRT1 siRNA set in confocal petri dishes, using Lipo 2000 (Invitrogen, USA) according to the manufacturer's instructions. Both specific and control siRNAs were purchased from KeyGEN Biotech (Nanjing, China). Within 48 h, the cells were treated with mRFP-GFP-LC3 adenovirus with polybrene at a MOI = 30 and incubated for 36 h. The adenovirus was obtained from Hannbio (Shanghai, China). The cells were treated with 50 uM ω-3 PUFA and then washed with two time with 10 mM PBS, pH 7.4. Finally, cells were fixed with 4% paraformaldehyde at room temperature for 30 min and sealed with 50% glycerin/PBS. LC3 expression detection was carried on a confocal microscope (PerkinElmer, UltraView ERS). The mRFP-GFP-LC3 puncta number in the sample groups was quantified usingImage Pro Plus 6.0. and GraphPad 7.0.

Nuclear and cytoplasmic protein extraction

The tissue samples were subjected to subcellular fractionation using the cytoplasmic and nuclear protein extraction kit (KGP150, KeyGEN Biotech, Nanjing, China), using hypotonic lysis buffer (20 mM HEPES (pH 7.4), 2 mM EGTA, 2 mM MgCl2) to extract the cytosolic protein and hypertonic lysis buffer (20 mM Tris/HCl, pH 7.6, 100 mM NaCl, 20 mM KCl, 1.5 mM MgCl 2, 0.5% Nonidet P-40, and protease inhibitors) to extract the nuclear protein. The protein concentration of the lysates was determined separately via western blot by stripping the polyvinylidene difluoride (PVDF) membranes and re-probing them with laminB1 (Cell Signaling Technology) as the nuclear control and β-actin (Boster Biotech) as the cytosolic control.

Western blotting

Proteins were extracted with radioimmunoprecipitation assay lysis buffer (sc-24948; Santa Cruz Biotechnology). Proteins (30 μg) were separated by sodium dodecyl sulfate-polyacrylamide gel electrophoresis (SDS-PAGE) and transferred to a PVDF membrane that was probed with primary antibodies against B cell lymphoma (Bcl)-2 (1:400), Bax (1:200), LC3-1(1:400) and P62 (1:400), (all from Abcam); HO-1 (1:200), NQO1 (1:200), and UGT1A1 (1:200) (all from Santa Cruz Biotechnology Inc); and cleaved caspase-3 (1:200), Beclin-1 (1:200), ATG-3 (1:400), and ATG-7 (1:400; all from Cell Signaling Technology), followed by incubation with appropriate secondary antibodies. Immunoreactivity was visualized with the ECL Western Blotting Detection System (Millipore, Billerica, MA, USA). Gray value analysis was conducted with the UN-Scan-It 6.1 software (Silk Scientific Inc., Orem, UT, USA). Expression levels were normalized against β-actin (1:5000, Boster Biotech) or laminin B1 (1:3000, Cell Signaling Technology).

Immunoprecipitation (IP)

Lesioned cortices were processed with IP lysis Buffer (KGP701, KeyGEN Biotech), and subsequent homogenates were incubated with 1 μg of Beclin-1 antibody (Cell Signaling Technology) overnight at 4 °C. A 10-μl volume of protein A agarose beads (Roche, Mannheim, Germany) was added to the sample lysate for 2 h incubation at 4 °C. After IP and centrifugation, agarose beads were washed three times with lysis buffer and the homogenate were separated by

SDS-PAGE and transferred to a PVDF membrane to detectBeclin-1 expression. PVDF membranes were then stripped and reprobed with an acetyl-lysine antibody. Total acetylation levels were measured with a pan-acetyl-lysine site-specific antibody, which was purchased from Immunechem (ICP0380, KeyGEN Biotech).

Activity assay

The 2′,7′-dichlorodihydrofluorescein diacetate assay was applied to detect ROS concentrations in lesioned cortices according to the manufacturer's instructions (Yeasen Biotech Co., Ltd., Nanjing, China). Fluorescence signals were detected using a fluorescence microplate system (Enspire 2300, PerkinElmer, Norwalk, CT, USA) with a wavelength of 498 nm. The NAD +/NADH ratio was measured using the NAD+/NADH QuantificationColorimetricKit (Yusen Biotech, Shanghai, China) according to the manufacturer's instructions. The absorbance at 450 nm of the mixture was measured by a microplate reader (2030 ARVO).

Statistical analysis

All statistical analyses were performed using SPSS 18.0 statistical software (SPSS Inc., Chicago, IL, USA). The results were expressed as mean ± standard deviation. Statistical differences among the groups were assessed by one-way ANOVA and post hoc multiple comparisons were performed using Student-Newman-Keuls tests. Values of $p < 0.05$ were considered statistically significant.

Results

Neuroprotective effects of ω-3 PUFA supplementation on TBI

The neurological function scores of the sham and sham+ω-3 PUFA groups were unaltered at all time points (scored 1–3). However, neurological function was severely impaired 1 day after TBI (12.59 ± 0.78); from day 3 after TBI, rats in the TBI+ω-3 PUFA group showed significantly better neurological functions than rats in the TBI group (10.31 ± 0.43 vs 12.03 ± 0.53, $p < 0.05$) (Fig. 1c). In addition, rats in the TBI+ω-3 PUFA group showed significantly improved rotarod performances than rats in the TBI group from day 7 after TBI (72.01 ± 8.21 vs 53.11 ± 7.13, $p < 0.05$) (Fig. 1d).

Brain water content is an important predictor of TBI prognosis [33]. Compared with the sham group, the water content of brain tissue was higher (81.92% ± 0.72%) in the TBI group 3 days after injury ($p < 0.05$). The water content of the TBI+ω-3 PUFA group was markedly lower than that of the TBI group (80.26% ± 0.61% vs 81.92% ± 0.72%, $p < 0.05$; Fig. 1e).

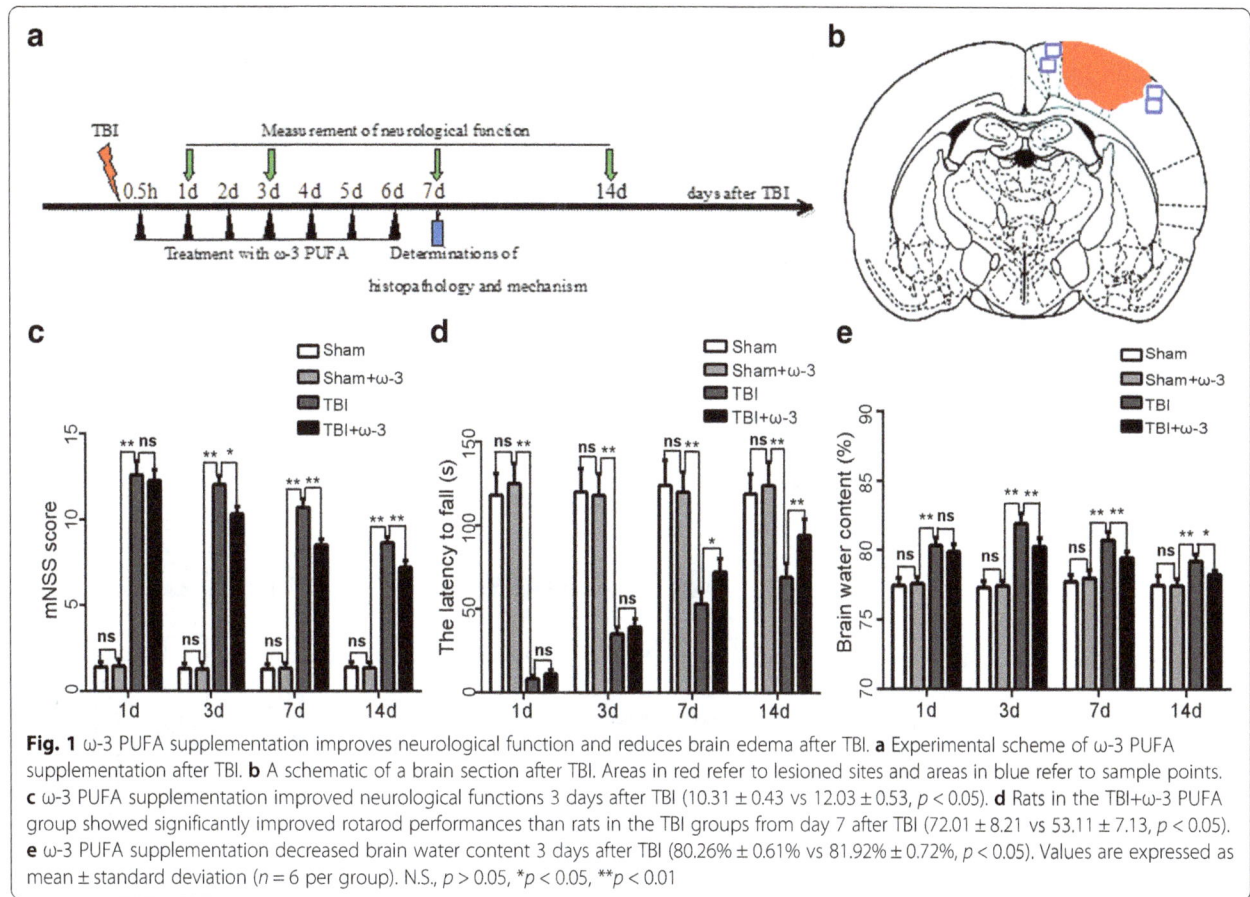

Fig. 1 ω-3 PUFA supplementation improves neurological function and reduces brain edema after TBI. **a** Experimental scheme of ω-3 PUFA supplementation after TBI. **b** A schematic of a brain section after TBI. Areas in red refer to lesioned sites and areas in blue refer to sample points. **c** ω-3 PUFA supplementation improved neurological functions 3 days after TBI (10.31 ± 0.43 vs 12.03 ± 0.53, $p < 0.05$). **d** Rats in the TBI+ω-3 PUFA group showed significantly improved rotarod performances than rats in the TBI groups from day 7 after TBI (72.01 ± 8.21 vs 53.11 ± 7.13, $p < 0.05$). **e** ω-3 PUFA supplementation decreased brain water content 3 days after TBI (80.26% ± 0.61% vs 81.92% ± 0.72%, $p < 0.05$). Values are expressed as mean ± standard deviation ($n = 6$ per group). N.S., $p > 0.05$, *$p < 0.05$, **$p < 0.01$

ω-3 PUFA supplementation protects neurons against TBI-induced neuronal apoptosis

Nissl staining was used to identify apoptotic neurons in lesioned cortices [33]. The sham group and the sham+ω-3 PUFA group showed a very low apoptotic fraction of neurons. The percentage of apoptotic cells was higher in the TBI group than in the sham group 7 days after TBI ($p < 0.05$); while the apoptotic fraction was significantly lower in the TBI+ω-3 PUFA than in the TBI group (39.19 ± 4.72% vs 73.42 ± 9.36%, $p < 0.05$; Fig. 2a, b). Western blot analyses revealed that TBI resulted in the upregulation of apoptotic factors in the cortex 7 days after TBI; however, compared to the TBI group, cleaved caspase-3 and Bax levels were decreased, whereas the anti-apoptotic factor, Bcl-2, was increased in the TBI+ω-3 PUFA group ($p < 0.05$: Fig. 2c). TUNEL staining further demonstrated that TUNEL-positive neurons were significantly decreased in the TBI+ω-3 group 7 days after TBI compared with the TBI group (47.72% ± 6.90% vs 81.41% ± 9.78%, $p < 0.05$) (Fig. 2d). These results suggest that ω-3 PUFA supplementation inhibits neuronal apoptosis and exerts a neuroprotective effect after TBI.

ω-3 PUFA supplementation protects neurons via enhancement of autophagy

Numerous studies have shown that enhancing autophagy may decrease the expression of neuronal apoptosis-related downstream molecules, thereby exerting neuroprotection after TBI [40]. Therefore, changes in autophagy activity after TBI were measured in each of the groups. Immunofluorescence staining and western blot analysis showed that compared with the TBI group, expression levels of autophagic markers (LC3-II, Beclin-1, ATG-3, and ATG-7) were dramatically increased in the TBI+ω-3 PUFA group 7 day after TBI ($p < 0.05$; Fig. 3a, b). The ω-3 PUFA group showed a suppression of autophagy at late stages compared with the early stage suppression of the control group, while SIRT1 siRNA or autophagy inhibitor reversed ω-3 PUFA-mediated increases in autophagy ($p < 0.05$; Fig. 4a, b). Western blot showed a significant increase in LC3 expression and a decrease in p62 levels in the ω-3 PUFA treatment group, which suggested a fluent autophagy degradation was mediated by the fusion of autophagosomes and lysosomes. However, the SIRT1 siRNA or autophagy inhibitor group showed an increase in p62

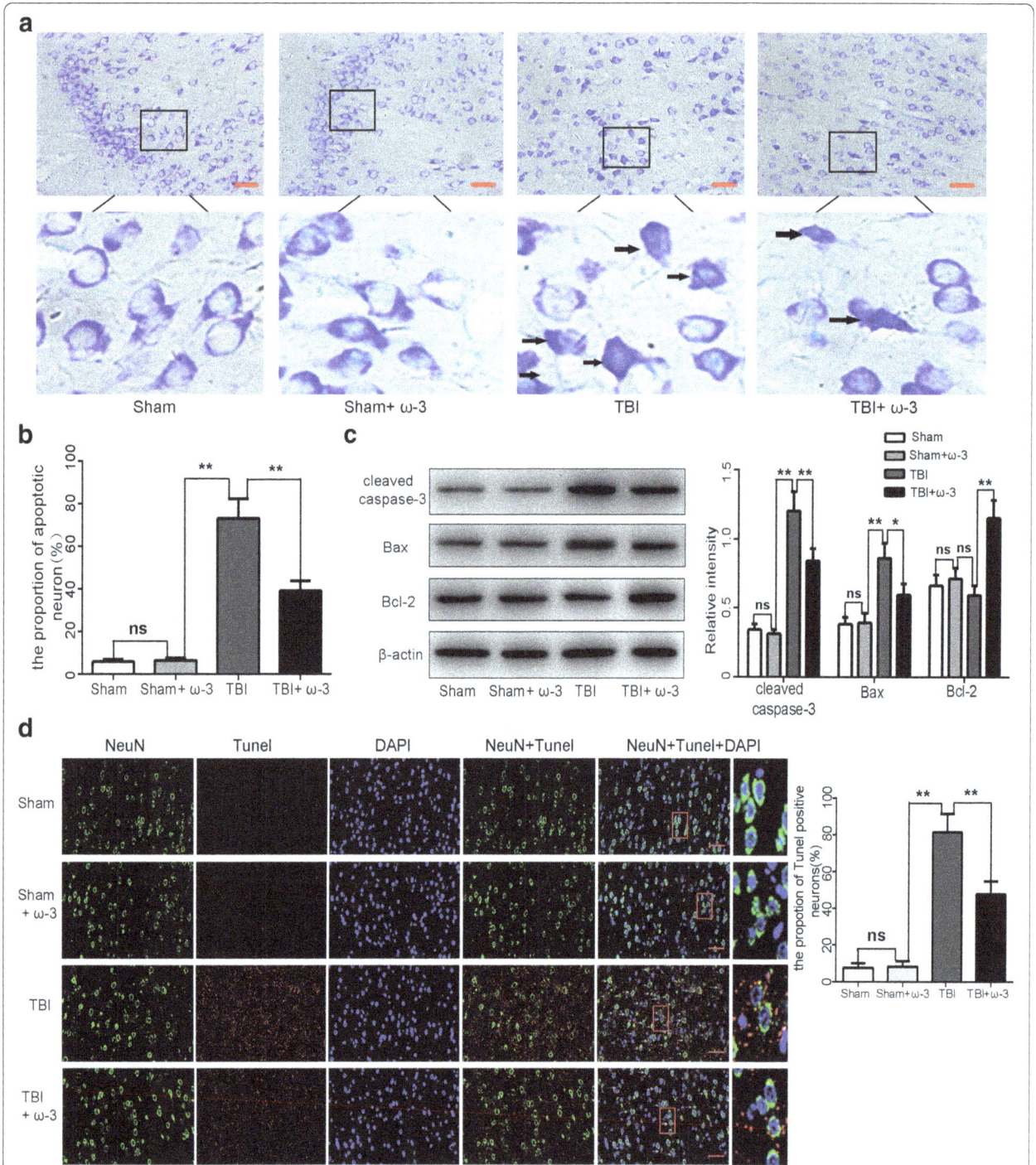

Fig. 2 ω-3 PUFA supplementation protects neurons against TBI-induced neuronal apoptosis in the lesioned cortex 7 day after TBI. **a, b** The sham group and the sham+ω-3 PUFA group had very low fractions of apoptotic neurons. The percentage of apoptotic cells was higher in the TBI group than in the sham group ($p < 0.05$); the apoptotic fraction was significantly lower in the TBI+ω-3 PUFA group than in the TBI group (39.19% ± 4.72% vs 73.42% ± 9.36%, $p < 0.05$). Representative photomicrographs of Nissl-stained neurons are shown; arrows indicate apoptotic neurons. **c** Western blot analyses revealed that TBI resulted in the upregulation of apoptotic factors in the cortex; however, compared with the TBI group, cleaved caspase-3 and Bax levels were decreased, whereas the anti-apoptotic factor, Bcl-2, was increased in TBI+ω-3 PUFA group ($p < 0.05$). **d** TUNEL staining demonstrated that TUNEL-positive neurons were significantly decreased in the TBI+ω-3 group compared with the TBI group (47.72% ± 6.90% vs 81.41% ± 9.78%, $p < 0.05$). Representative photomicrographs of TUNEL-positive neurons are shown (×400); arrows indicate apoptotic neurons. Values are expressed as mean ± standard deviation ($n = 6$ per group). N.S., $p > 0.05$, *$p < 0.05$, **$p < 0.01$. Scale bars = 50 μm

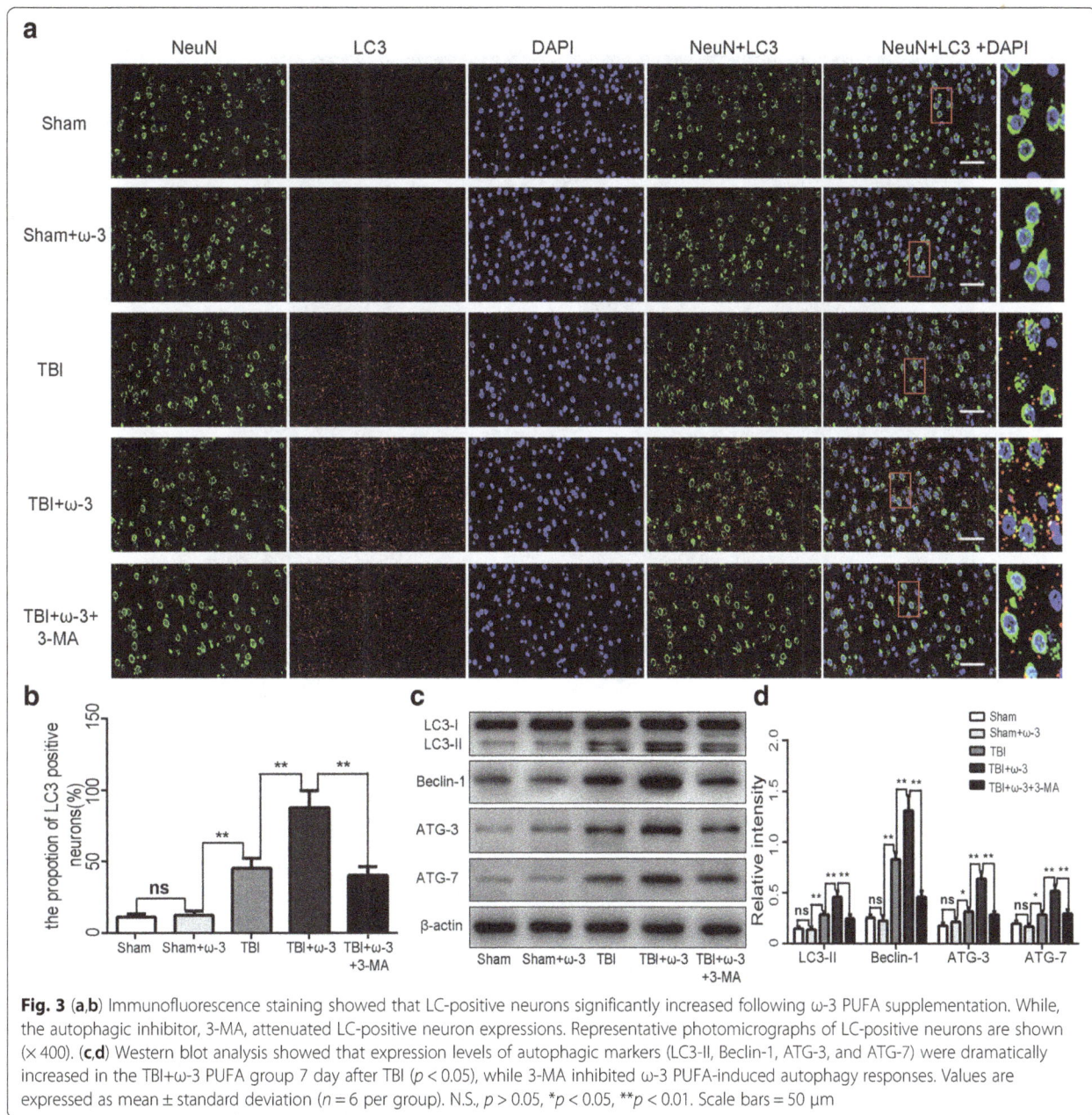

Fig. 3 (**a,b**) Immunofluorescence staining showed that LC-positive neurons significantly increased following ω-3 PUFA supplementation. While, the autophagic inhibitor, 3-MA, attenuated LC-positive neuron expressions. Representative photomicrographs of LC-positive neurons are shown (× 400). (**c,d**) Western blot analysis showed that expression levels of autophagic markers (LC3-II, Beclin-1, ATG-3, and ATG-7) were dramatically increased in the TBI+ω-3 PUFA group 7 day after TBI ($p < 0.05$), while 3-MA inhibited ω-3 PUFA-induced autophagy responses. Values are expressed as mean ± standard deviation ($n = 6$ per group). N.S., $p > 0.05$, *$p < 0.05$, **$p < 0.01$. Scale bars = 50 μm

levels but no significant increases in LC3 expression ($p < 0.05$; Fig. 4c).

To address the effects of ω-3 PUFA on oxidative stress, ROS production and expression of the antioxidative factors HO-1, NQO1, and UGT1A1 were measured. Data showed that the ROS levels increased approximately 3.1-fold in the TBI group compared with that in the sham group ($p < 0.05$; Fig. 5a, b). ω-3 PUFA supplementation decreased ROS activity ($p < 0.05$; Fig. 5a), while it significantly increased the levels of HO-1, NQO1, and UGT1A1 in lesioned cortices ($p < 0.05$; Fig. 5b). 3-MA treatment reversed ω-3 PUFA-mediated inhibition of neuronal apoptosis and

attenuated the neuroprotective effects associated with ω-3 PUFA treatment ($p < 0.05$; Fig. 5c, d).

ω-3 PUFA supplementation enhances autophagy via promoting nuclear export of Beclin-1 in lesioned cortices

Although Beclin-1 is expressed in both the nucleus and cytoplasm, it is generally acknowledged that the cytosolic localization of Beclin-1 is a prerequisite its prominent role in autophagy [41, 42]. Western blot and immunofluorescence staining analyses demonstrated that the expression of Beclin-1 in the cytosol, nuclei, and in total protein was increased 7 days after TBI and that ω-3 PUFA supplementation effectively

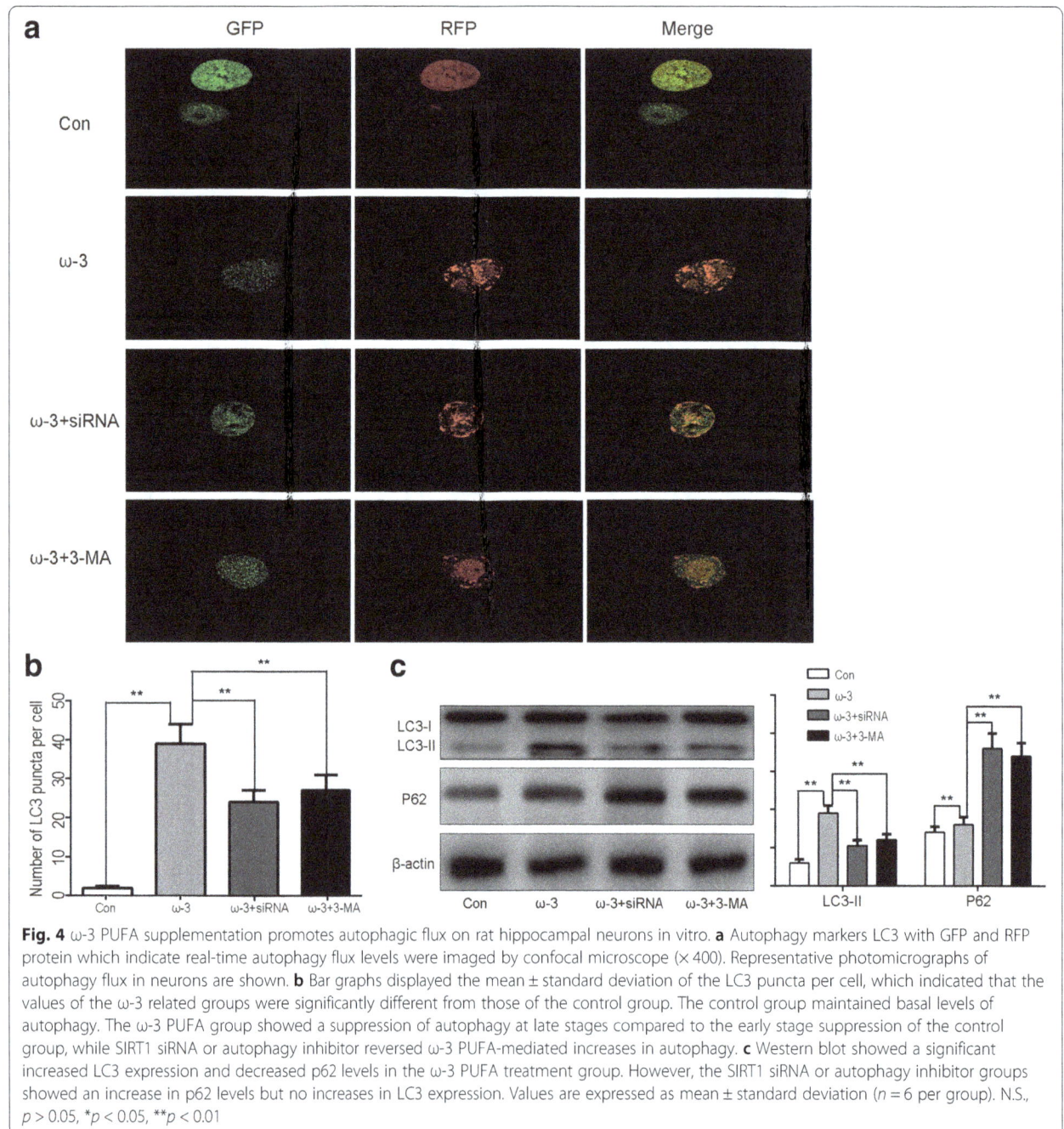

Fig. 4 ω-3 PUFA supplementation promotes autophagic flux on rat hippocampal neurons in vitro. **a** Autophagy markers LC3 with GFP and RFP protein which indicate real-time autophagy flux levels were imaged by confocal microscope (× 400). Representative photomicrographs of autophagy flux in neurons are shown. **b** Bar graphs displayed the mean ± standard deviation of the LC3 puncta per cell, which indicated that the values of the ω-3 related groups were significantly different from those of the control group. The control group maintained basal levels of autophagy. The ω-3 PUFA group showed a suppression of autophagy at late stages compared to the early stage suppression of the control group, while SIRT1 siRNA or autophagy inhibitor reversed ω-3 PUFA-mediated increases in autophagy. **c** Western blot showed a significant increased LC3 expression and decreased p62 levels in the ω-3 PUFA treatment group. However, the SIRT1 siRNA or autophagy inhibitor groups showed an increase in p62 levels but no increases in LC3 expression. Values are expressed as mean ± standard deviation ($n = 6$ per group). N.S., $p > 0.05$, *$p < 0.05$, **$p < 0.01$

increased Beclin-1 expression in the cytosol and in total protein of cells ($p < 0.05$), but not in nuclear protein ($p > 0.05$; Fig. 6a, b). In agreement with these findings, we found less cytoplasmic redistribution of nuclear Beclin-1 in the presence of the autophagy inhibitor, 3-MA, after TBI (Fig. 6a, b).

Interaction between Beclin-1 and Bcl-2 can result in inhibition of apoptosis [14–16]. Given that the overall activity of cytoplasmic Bcl-2/Beclin-1 complexes is regulated by nuclear export of Beclin-1, we examined the interaction between cytoplasmic Beclin-1 and

Bcl-2 to determine the anti-apoptotic effects of ω-3 PUFA supplementation after TBI. Results from the co-IP assay confirmed that ω-3 PUFA supplementation significantly increased interactions between cytoplasmic Beclin-1 and Bcl-2 after the TBI, while 3-MA treatment reversed these increases (Fig. 6c).

ω-3 PUFA supplementation elevates SIRT1 expression and deacetylase activity

SIRTs are a family of deacetylases that require NAD+ as a cofactor for the deacetylation reaction [38, 43].

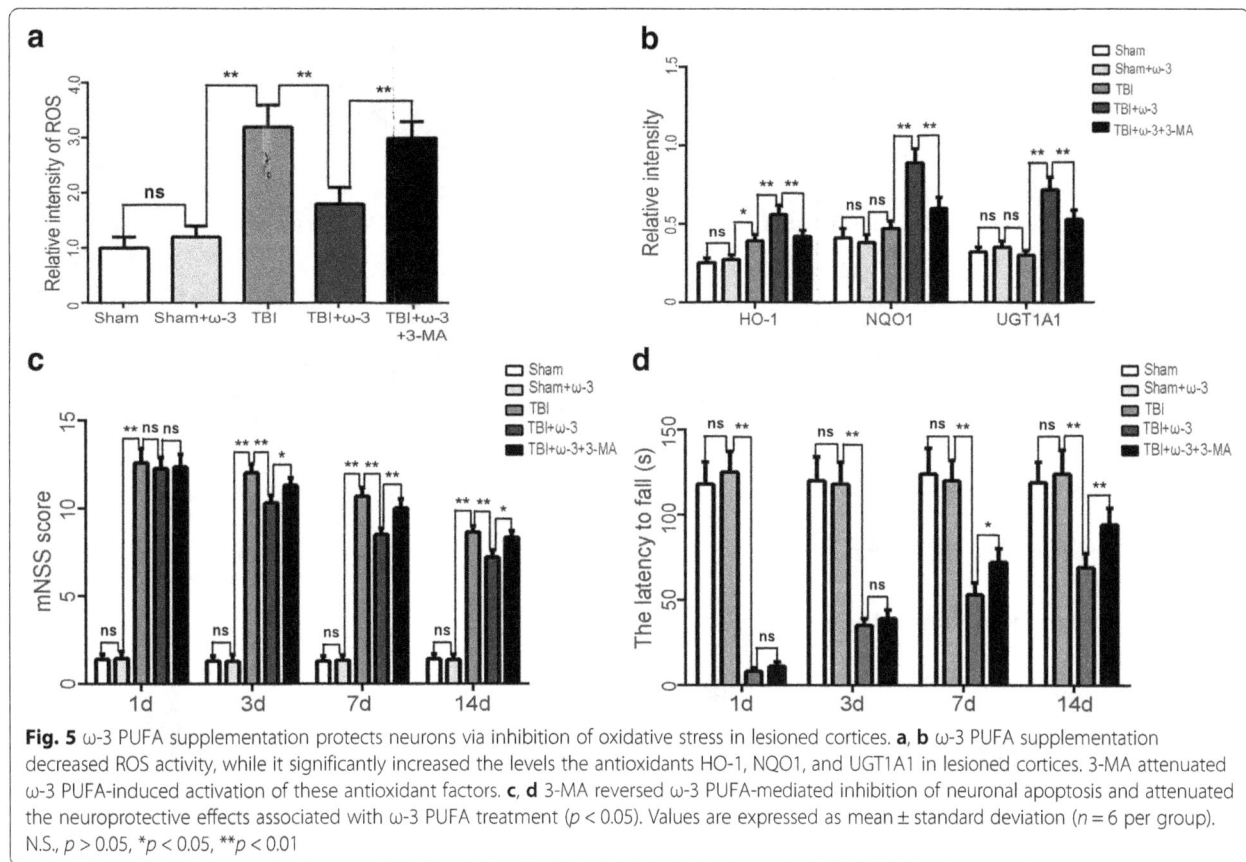

Fig. 5 ω-3 PUFA supplementation protects neurons via inhibition of oxidative stress in lesioned cortices. **a, b** ω-3 PUFA supplementation decreased ROS activity, while it significantly increased the levels the antioxidants HO-1, NQO1, and UGT1A1 in lesioned cortices. 3-MA attenuated ω-3 PUFA-induced activation of these antioxidant factors. **c, d** 3-MA reversed ω-3 PUFA-mediated inhibition of neuronal apoptosis and attenuated the neuroprotective effects associated with ω-3 PUFA treatment ($p < 0.05$). Values are expressed as mean ± standard deviation ($n = 6$ per group). N.S., $p > 0.05$, *$p < 0.05$, **$p < 0.01$

Consistent with our previous study, similar results were obtained by immunohistochemistry. SIRT1 immunoreactivity from lesioned cortices was significantly increased after ω-3 PUFA supplementation ($p < 0.05$; Fig. 7a). SIRT1 protein levels were also upregulated after ω-3 PUFA supplementation 7 days after TBI ($p < 0.05$; Fig. 7b). As SIRT1 is a NAD+-dependent histone deacetylase that affects NAD+ metabolism [44, 45], we also measured the NAD+/NADH ratio to detect SIRT1 activity. Treatment with ω-3 PUFA significantly increased the NAD+/NADH ratio ($p < 0.05$; Fig. 7c).

ω-3 PUFA supplementation increases Beclin-1 deacetylationby elevating SIRT1 activity

Post-translational modifications such as acetylation are critical for Beclin-1 transcription and nuclear export. Deacetylation of Beclin-1 can lead to elevation of autophagic responses [26]. We therefore next focused on the molecular mechanism of Beclin-1 deacetylation and its role in driving nucleus-to-cytoplasm redistribution of Beclin-1 and subsequent autophagosome biogenesis. IP analysis showed that Beclin-1 deacetylation was increased after ω-3 PUFA supplementation compared with the TBI group ($p < 0.05$; Fig. 8a). Nuclear export of Beclin-1 and autophagy activation induced by ω-3

PUFA supplementation were reversed by pharmacological inhibition of SIRT1 (sirtinol) (Fig. 8b, c), suggesting that the enhancement of autophagy by ω-3 PUFA was dependent on SIRT1 activity.

Discussion

Accumulating evidence has demonstrated the benefits of ω-3 PUFA or its constituents against TBI-induced neural damage and secondary pathological processes [46–48]. We previously reported that ω-3 PUFA supplementation attenuates the inflammatory response by modulating microglial polarization through SIRT1-mediated deacetylation of the HMGB1/NF-κB pathway, leading to neuroprotective effects following experimental TBI [33]. Taken together with our previously reported findings, the current study also demonstrated that ω-3 PUFA supplementation reduced brain edema and improved neurological function in lesioned cortices by inhibiting neuronal apoptosis. As a dietary supplement, ω-3 PUFA may be a suitable therapeutic candidate against trauma-induced mechanical injury and secondary neuronal apoptosis and may also provide novel therapeutic approaches for TBI.

TBI-induced secondary injury is a complicated pathophysiological process that affects neurological

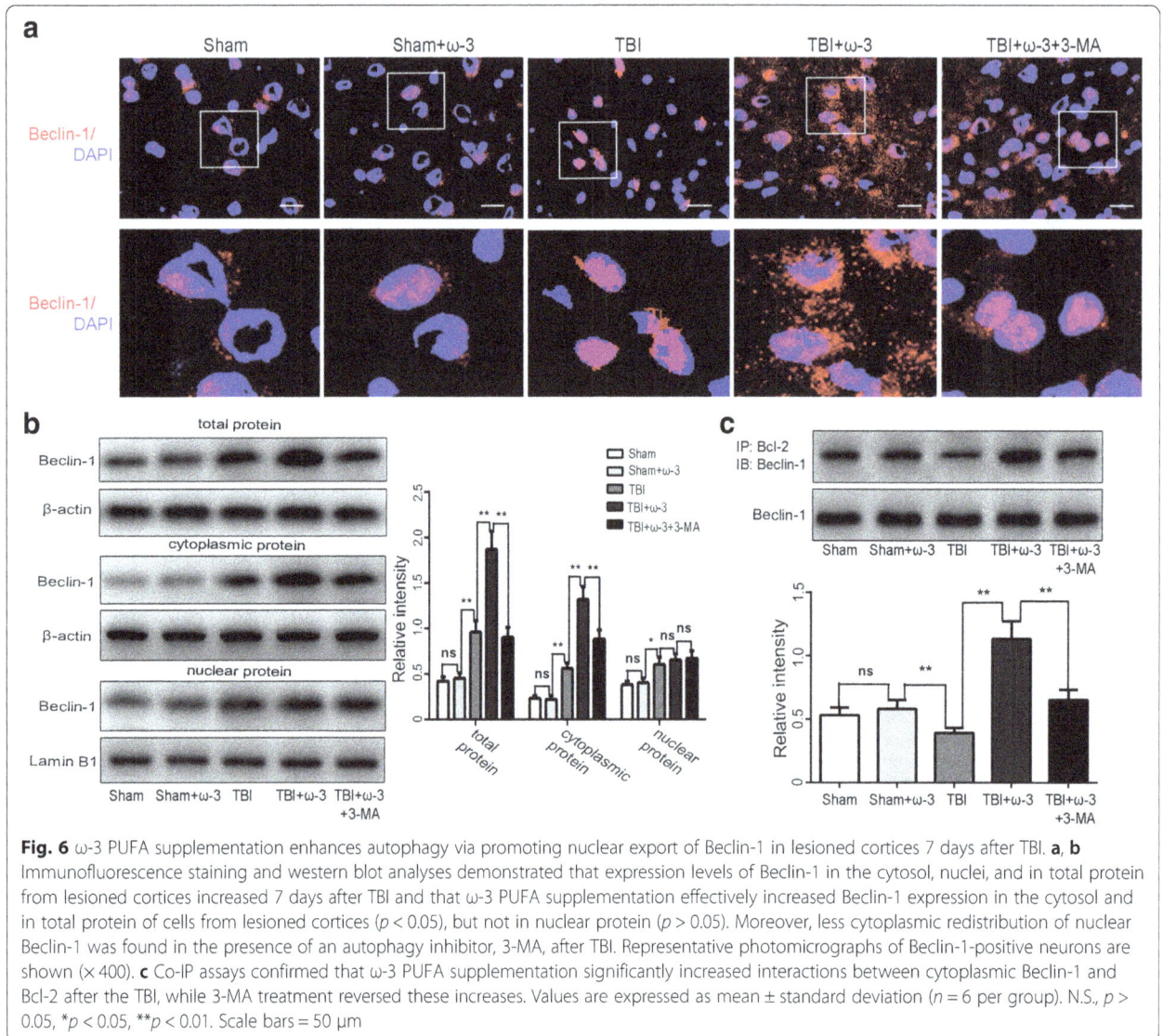

Fig. 6 ω-3 PUFA supplementation enhances autophagy via promoting nuclear export of Beclin-1 in lesioned cortices 7 days after TBI. **a, b** Immunofluorescence staining and western blot analyses demonstrated that expression levels of Beclin-1 in the cytosol, nuclei, and in total protein from lesioned cortices increased 7 days after TBI and that ω-3 PUFA supplementation effectively increased Beclin-1 expression in the cytosol and in total protein of cells from lesioned cortices ($p < 0.05$), but not in nuclear protein ($p > 0.05$). Moreover, less cytoplasmic redistribution of nuclear Beclin-1 was found in the presence of an autophagy inhibitor, 3-MA, after TBI. Representative photomicrographs of Beclin-1-positive neurons are shown (× 400). **c** Co-IP assays confirmed that ω-3 PUFA supplementation significantly increased interactions between cytoplasmic Beclin-1 and Bcl-2 after the TBI, while 3-MA treatment reversed these increases. Values are expressed as mean ± standard deviation ($n = 6$ per group). N.S., $p > 0.05$, *$p < 0.05$, **$p < 0.01$. Scale bars = 50 μm

function [2–4]. Damaged mitochondria release excess ROS after TBI, which lead to oxidative stress and mitochondrial dysfunction [5–7]. Oxidative stress is critical for neurodegeneration after TBI and is also related to neuronal apoptosis [15]. In response, oxidative stress-induced autophagy selectively degrades oxidized substances and damaged organelles to reduce oxidative injury, maintain normal mitochondrial function, and balance the intracellular microenvironment [10, 12, 13]. In our study, ROS production and the expression of antioxidative factors were significantly increased after TBI. ω-3 PUFA supplementation decreased ROS production and enhanced the expression of these antioxidative factors. Upregulation of autophagy has been found to reduce TBI-induced oxidative stress and apoptosis, suggesting a protective role of autophagy after TBI [9]. In the current study, compared with the TBI group, Beclin-1-positive neurons were increased after ω-3 PUFA supplementation and the expression of other autophagic markers were also dramatically increased, suggesting that ω-3 PUFA supplementation improves autophagy in neurons after TBI. Furthermore, the inhibition of neuronal apoptosis induced by ω-3 PUFA supplementation was reversed by pharmacological inhibition of autophagy, suggesting that autophagy plays a critical role in ω-3 PUFA-mediated neuroprotection after TBI.

Nuclear proteins may be important components of the autophagic machinery acting as reserves for cytoplasm proteins, which are exported to the cytoplasm during the maturation of autophagosomes [41, 42]. In our study, ω-3 PUFA supplementation also facilitated Beclin-1 nuclear export. Supporting this possibility, we found less cytoplasmic redistribution of nuclear Beclin-1 in the presence of the autophagy inhibitor after TBI, suggesting that ω-3 PUFA supplementation

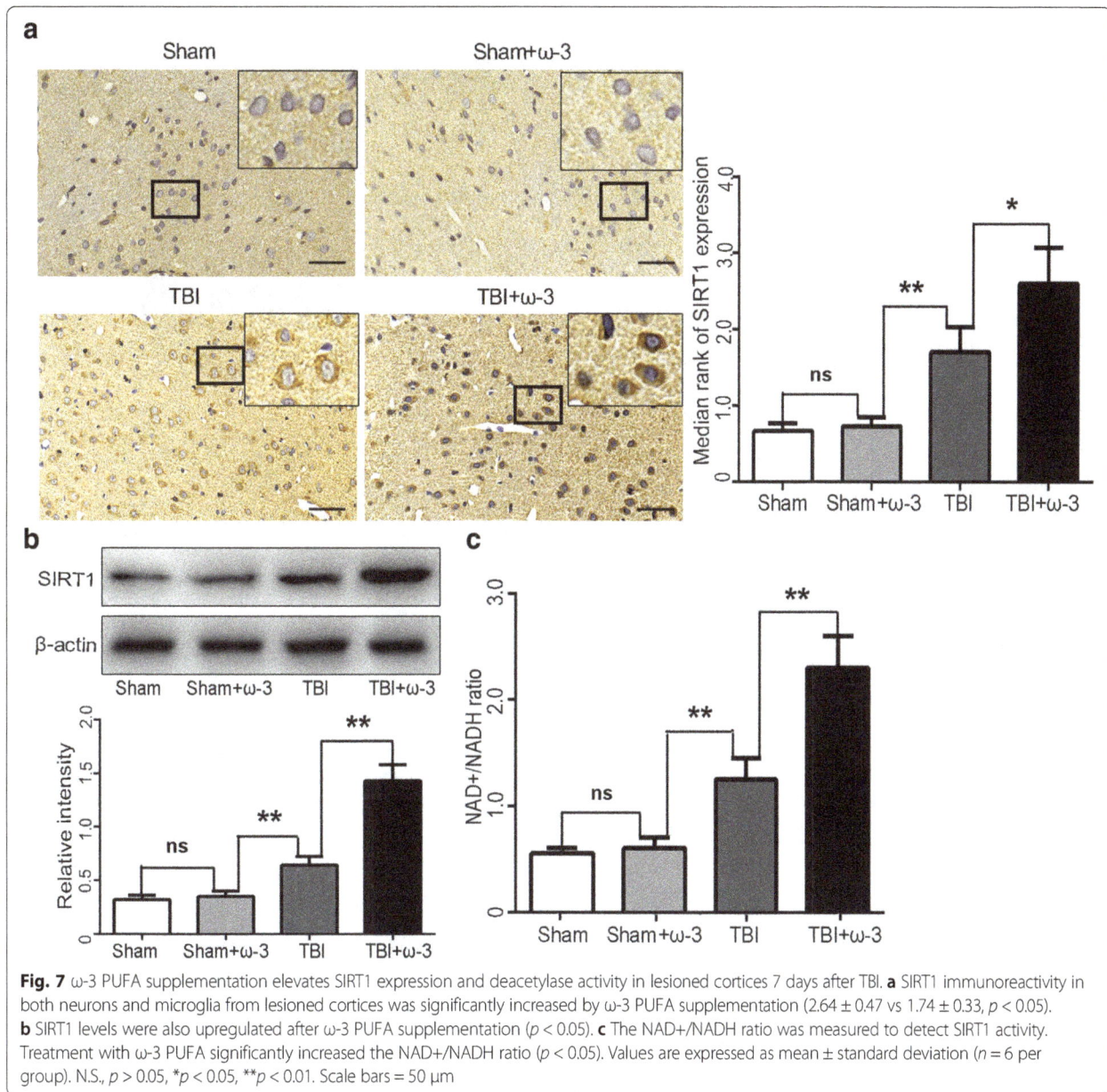

Fig. 7 ω-3 PUFA supplementation elevates SIRT1 expression and deacetylase activity in lesioned cortices 7 days after TBI. **a** SIRT1 immunoreactivity in both neurons and microglia from lesioned cortices was significantly increased by ω-3 PUFA supplementation (2.64 ± 0.47 vs 1.74 ± 0.33, $p < 0.05$). **b** SIRT1 levels were also upregulated after ω-3 PUFA supplementation ($p < 0.05$). **c** The NAD+/NADH ratio was measured to detect SIRT1 activity. Treatment with ω-3 PUFA significantly increased the NAD+/NADH ratio ($p < 0.05$). Values are expressed as mean ± standard deviation ($n = 6$ per group). N.S., $p > 0.05$, *$p < 0.05$, **$p < 0.01$. Scale bars = 50 µm

can activate the autophagy pathway by promoting the nuclear export of Beclin-1. Beclin-1 interacts with several binding partners and exerted multiple-biological effects, including cell metabolism, apoptosis, and autophagy [15, 18]. Bcl-2 and Bax, important apoptotic regulators tested in this study, are also regulated by Beclin-1. Additionally, caspase-mediated cleavage of ATGs and Beclin-1 can switch autophagy to apoptosis [15, 16]. Given that the overall activity of cytoplasmic Bcl-2/Beclin-1 complexes is regulated by nuclear export of Beclin-1, we examined the interaction between cytoplasmic Beclin-1 and Bcl-2 to determine the anti-apoptotic effects of ω-3 PUFA supplementation after TBI. Results from the co-IP

assay confirmed that ω-3 PUFA supplementation significantly increased interactions between cytoplasmic Beclin-1 and Bcl-2 after TBI. These results indicate that ω-3 PUFA supplementation exerts neuroprotective effects and enhances autophagy after TBI, possibly by enhancing the nuclear export of Beclin-1.

Post-translational modifications like lysine deacetylations by SIRT1 regulate autophagy-mediated neuronal survival, supporting the idea that neuronal apoptosis is attenuated by SIRT1-mediated deacetylation of the autophagy pathway [25, 26, 49]. Deacetylation at Beclin-1 lysine residues by SIRT1 influences autophagosome maturation [26]. Our previous study [33] confirmed that SIRT1 activity was involved in

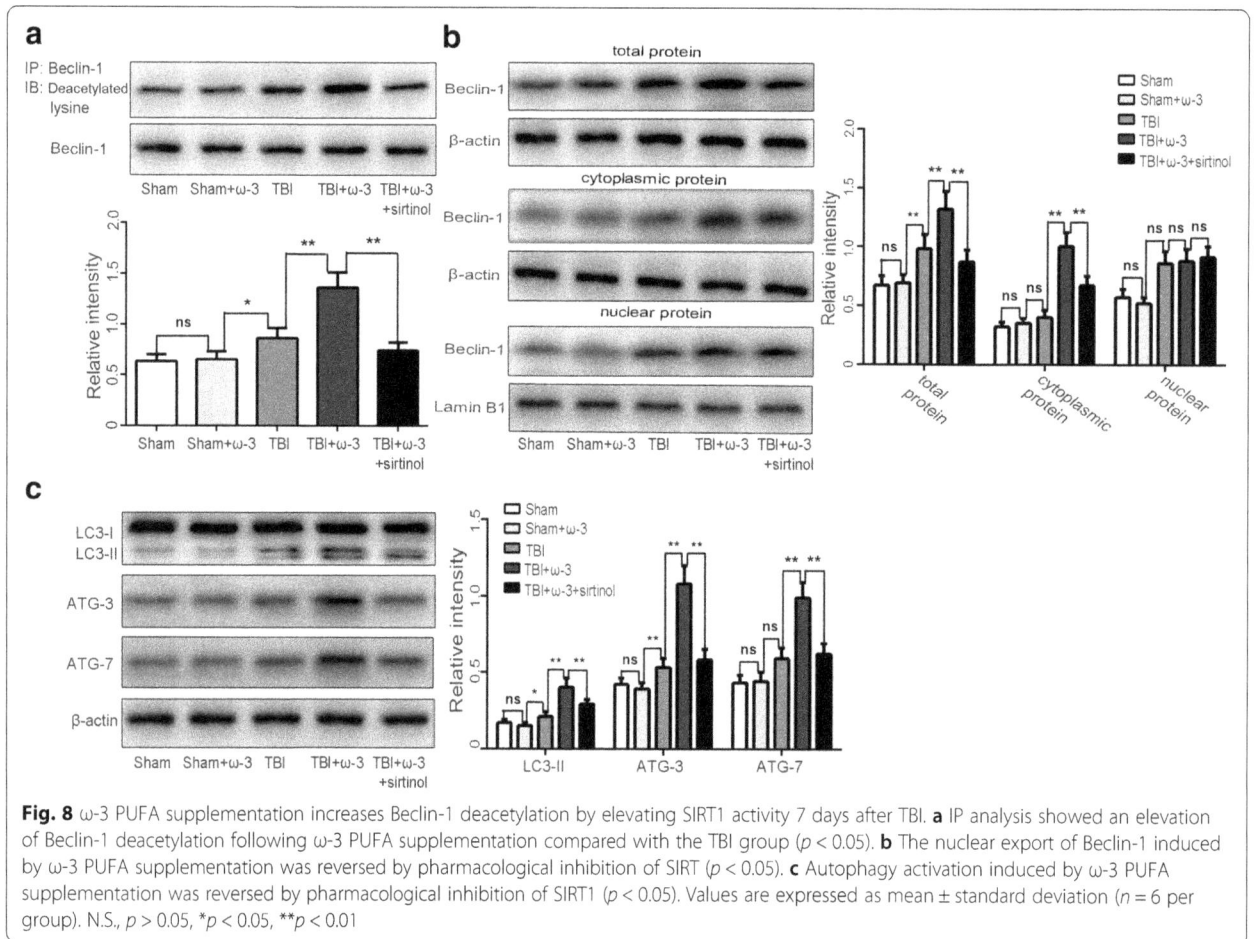

Fig. 8 ω-3 PUFA supplementation increases Beclin-1 deacetylation by elevating SIRT1 activity 7 days after TBI. **a** IP analysis showed an elevation of Beclin-1 deacetylation following ω-3 PUFA supplementation compared with the TBI group ($p < 0.05$). **b** The nuclear export of Beclin-1 induced by ω-3 PUFA supplementation was reversed by pharmacological inhibition of SIRT ($p < 0.05$). **c** Autophagy activation induced by ω-3 PUFA supplementation was reversed by pharmacological inhibition of SIRT1 ($p < 0.05$). Values are expressed as mean ± standard deviation ($n = 6$ per group). N.S., $p > 0.05$, *$p < 0.05$, **$p < 0.01$

inflammatory mechanisms after TBI. In addition, SIRT1 levels were upregulated after ω-3 PUFA supplementation, indicating that ω-3 PUFA inhibited neuronal apoptosis in a SIRT1 deacetylation-mediated-dependent manner [33]. Our IP analysis further showed that Beclin-1 acetylation was decreased in acetyl-lysine immunoprecipitate fractions after ω-3 PUFA supplementation compared with the TBI group. The nuclear export of Beclin-1 and autophagy activation induced by ω-3 PUFA supplementation was reversed by pharmacological inhibition of SIRT1. In agreement with these findings, SIRT1 siRNA neurons showed a suppression of autophagy at early stages compared to the late stage suppression of ω-3 PUFA treatment in vitro. Overall, these results indicate that ω-3 PUFA supplementation attenuates neuronal apoptosis and exerts neuroprotective effects by enhancing autophagy after TBI and is likely dependent on elevated SIRT1 levels. Because TBI-induced secondary injury is a complicated pathophysiological process, future studies involving the interaction between the apoptosis, autophagy, and neuroinflammation should be investigated to elucidate the mechanisms involved

in the neuroprotective effects of ω-3 PUFA against TBI-induced neuronal apoptosis.

Conclusion

In summary, ω-3 PUFA supplementation inhibited neuronal apoptosis and exerted neuroprotective effects through enhancing the autophagy pathway after TBI. Moreover, ω-3 PUFA increased Beclin-1 deacetylation and its nuclear export and induced direct interactions between cytoplasmic Beclin-1 and Bcl-2 by increasing SIRT1 activity following TBI; subsequently leading to inhibition of neuronal apoptosis. These results indicate that ω-3 PUFA supplementation attenuates TBI-induced neuronal apoptosis by inducing the autophagy pathway through the upregulation of SIRT1-mediated deacetylation of Beclin-1.

Abbreviations
3-MA: 3-Methyladenine; ATG: Autophagy-related gene; Bax: Bcl-2-associated X protein; Bcl-2: B cell lymphoma-2; HO-1: Heme oxygenase-1; IP: Immunoprecipitation; LC3: Microtubule-associated protein 1 light chain 3; mNSS: Modified neurological severity scores; NQO1: NAD(P)Hquinone oxidoreductase 1; PI3K: Phosphatidylinositol 3-kinase; PVDF: Polyvinylidene difluoride; ROS: Reactive oxygen species; SDS-PAGE: Sodium dodecyl sulfate-polyacrylamide gel electrophoresis; SIRT: Sirtuin; TBI: Traumatic brain injury; TUNEL: Terminal deoxynucleotidyl transferase dUTP nick-end labeling; ω-3 PUFA: Omega-3 polyunsaturated fatty acid

Acknowledgements
We would like to thank Dr. Hongzhi Gao (Department of Central Laboratory, the Second Affiliated Hospital, Fujian Medical University) for his advice and expert technical support. Sincere appreciation is also given to the teachers and our colleagues from the Second Affiliated Hospital of Fujian Medical University, who participated in this study with great cooperation.

Funding
This work was supported by grants from the funds for Fujian Province Scientific Foundation (no. 2015J01443) and Fujian Province Science and technology innovation Foundation (no. 2017Y9201) from Dr. Xiangrong Chen; Sichuan Provincial Department of Education (no. 18ZA0205) and the Health and Family Planning Commission of Sichuan Province (no. 17PJ174) from Dr. Shun Li.

Authors' contributions
XC contributed to the conception and design and writing of the manuscript. ZP, ZF, SW, and WL supported several experiments, acquisition of data, analysis, and interpretation of data. FY and YL contributed to the statistical analysis and revision of the manuscript. XC, HF, HG, and SL contributed to the technical support, obtaining of funding, conception and design, and revision of the manuscript. All authors read and approved the final manuscript.

Competing interests
The authors declare that they have no competing interests.

References
1. Zhang R, Liu Y, Yan K, Chen L, Chen XR, Li P, Chen FF, Jiang XD. Anti-inflammatory and immunomodulatory mechanisms of mesenchymal stem cell transplantation in experimental traumatic brain injury. J Neuroinflammation. 2013;10:106.
2. Hopp S, Nolte MW, Stetter C, Kleinschnitz C, Siren AL, Albert-Weissenberger C. Alleviation of secondary brain injury, posttraumatic inflammation, and brain edema formation by inhibition of factor XIIa. J Neuroinflammation. 2017;14:39.
3. Sinha SP, Avcu P, Spiegler KM, Komaravolu S, Kim K, Cominski T, Servatius RJ, Pang KC. Startle suppression after mild traumatic brain injury is associated with an increase in pro-inflammatory cytokines, reactive gliosis and neuronal loss in the caudal pontine reticular nucleus. Brain Behav Immun. 2017;61:353–64.
4. McKee CA, Lukens JR. Emerging roles for the immune system in traumatic brain injury. Front Immunol. 2016;7:556.
5. Ding K, Xu J, Wang H, Zhang L, Wu Y, Li T. Melatonin protects the brain from apoptosis by enhancement of autophagy after traumatic brain injury in mice. Neurochem Int. 2015;91:46–54.

6. Roth TL, Nayak D, Atanasijevic T, Koretsky AP, Latour LL, McGavern DB. Transcranial amelioration of inflammation and cell death after brain injury. Nature. 2014;505:223–8.
7. Fischer MT, Sharma R, Lim JL, Haider L, Frischer JM, Drexhage J, Mahad D, Bradl M, van Horssen J, Lassmann H. NADPH oxidase expression in active multiple sclerosis lesions in relation to oxidative tissue damage and mitochondrial injury. Brain. 2012;135:886–99.
8. Gao Y, Zhuang Z, Gao S, Li X, Zhang Z, Ye Z, Li L, Tang C, Zhou M, Han X, et al. Tetrahydrocurcumin reduces oxidative stress-induced apoptosis via the mitochondrial apoptotic pathway by modulating autophagy in rats after traumatic brain injury. Am J Transl Res. 2017;135:886–99.
9. Zhang L, Wang H, Fan Y, Gao Y, Li X, Hu Z, Ding K, Wang Y, Wang X. Fucoxanthin provides neuroprotection in models of traumatic brain injury via the Nrf2-ARE and Nrf2-autophagy pathways. Sci Rep-Uk. 2017;7:46763.
10. Lin C, Chao H, Li Z, Xu X, Liu Y, Hou L, Liu N, Ji J. Melatonin attenuates traumatic brain injury-induced inflammation: a possible role for mitophagy. J Pineal Res. 2016;61:177–86.
11. Fernandez A, Ordonez R, Reiter RJ, Gonzalez-Gallego J, Mauriz JL. Melatonin and endoplasmic reticulum stress: relation to autophagy and apoptosis. J Pineal Res. 2015;59:292–307.
12. Levine B, Kroemer G. Autophagy in the pathogenesis of disease. Cell. 2008; 132:27–42.
13. Szatmari-Toth M, Kristof E, Vereb Z, Akhtar S, Facsko A, Fesus L, Kauppinen A, Kaarniranta K, Petrovski G. Clearance of autophagy-associated dying retinal pigment epithelial cells - a possible source for inflammation in age-related macular degeneration. Cell Death Dis. 2016;7:e2367.
14. Liu CL, Chen S, Dietrich D, Hu BR. Changes in autophagy after traumatic brain injury. J Cereb Blood Flow Metab. 2008;28:674–83.
15. Marquez RT, Xu L. Bcl-2:Beclin 1 complex: multiple, mechanisms regulating autophagy/apoptosis toggle switch. Am J Cancer Res. 2012;2:214–21.
16. Ciechomska IA, Goemans GC, Skepper JN, Tolkovsky AM. Bcl-2 complexed with Beclin-1 maintains full anti-apoptotic function. Oncogene. 2009;28: 2128–41.
17. Chen X, Wang H, Zhou M, Li X, Fang Z, Gao H, Li Y, Hu W. Valproic acid attenuates traumatic brain injury-induced inflammation in vivo: involvement of autophagy and the Nrf2/ARE signaling pathway. Front Mol Neurosci. 2018;11:117.
18. Schmitz KJ, Ademi C, Bertram S, Schmid KW, Baba HA. Prognostic relevance of autophagy-related markers LC3, p62/sequestosome 1, Beclin-1 and ULK1 in colorectal cancer patients with respect to KRAS mutational status. World J Surg Oncol. 2016;14:189.
19. Dupont N, Nascimbeni AC, Morel E, Codogno P. Molecular mechanisms of noncanonical autophagy. Int Rev Cell Mol Biol. 2017;328:1–23.
20. Frudd K, Burgoyne T, Burgoyne JR. Oxidation of Atg3 and Atg7 mediates inhibition of autophagy. Nat Commun. 2018;9:95.
21. Pant K, Saraya A, Venugopal SK. Oxidative stress plays a key role in butyrate-mediated autophagy via Akt/mTOR pathway in hepatoma cells. Chem Biol Interact. 2017;273:99–106.
22. Park SE, Yi HJ, Suh N, Park YY, Koh JY, Jeong SY, Cho DH, Kim CS, Hwang JJ. Inhibition of EHMT2/G9a epigenetically increases the transcription of Beclin-1 via an increase in ROS and activation of NF-kappaB. Oncotarget. 2016;7:39796–808.
23. Jin S, Tian S, Chen Y, Zhang C, Xie W, Xia X, Cui J, Wang RF. USP19 modulates autophagy and antiviral immune responses by deubiquitinating Beclin-1. EMBO J. 2016;35:866–80.
24. He R, Peng J, Yuan P, Xu F, Wei W. Divergent roles of BECN1 in LC3 lipidation and autophagosomal function. Autophagy. 2015;11:740–7.
25. Huang R, Xu Y, Wan W, Shou X, Qian J, You Z, Liu B, Chang C, Zhou T, Lippincott-Schwartz J, et al. Deacetylation of nuclear LC3 drives autophagy initiation under starvation. Mol Cell. 2015;57:456–66.
26. Sun T, Li X, Zhang P, Chen W, Zhang H, Li D, Deng R, Qian X, Jiao L, Ji J, et al. Acetylation of Beclin 1 inhibits autophagosome maturation and promotes tumour growth. Nat Commun. 2015;6:7215.
27. Contreras AU, Mebratu Y, Delgado M, Montano G, Hu CA, Ryter SW, Choi AMK, Lin Y, Xiang J, Chand H, et al. Deacetylation of p53 induces autophagy by suppressing Bmf expression. J Cell Biol. 2013;201:427–37.
28. Qiu G, Li X, Wei C, Che X, He S, Lu J, Wang S, Pang K, Fan L. The prognostic role of SIRT1-autophagy axis in gastric cancer. Dis Markers. 2016;2016:6869415.
29. Serini S, Calviello G. Reduction of oxidative/nitrosative stress in brain and its involvement in the neuroprotective effect of n-3 PUFA in Alzheimer's disease. Curr Alzheimer Res. 2016;13:123–34.

30. Wang B, Wu X, Guo M, Li M, Xu X, Jin X, Zhang X. Effects of ω-3 fatty acids on toll-like receptor 4 and nuclear factor-κB p56 in lungs of rats with severe acute pancreatitis. World J Gastroentero. 2016;22:9784–93.

31. Delattre AM, Carabelli B, Mori MA, Kempe PG, Rizzo DSL, Zanata SM, Machado RB, Suchecki D, Andrade DCB, Lima M, et al. Maternal omega-3 supplement improves dopaminergic system in pre- and postnatal inflammation-induced neurotoxicity in Parkinson's disease model. Mol Neurobiol. 2017;54:2090–106.

32. Chang CY, Kuan YH, Li JR, Chen WY, Ou YC, Pan HC, Liao SL, Raung SL, Chang CJ, Chen CJ. Docosahexaenoic acid reduces cellular inflammatory response following permanent focal cerebral ischemia in rats. J Nutr Biochem. 2013;24:2127–37.

33. Chen X, Wu S, Chen C, Xie B, Fang Z, Hu W, Chen J, Fu H, He H. Omega-3 polyunsaturated fatty acid supplementation attenuates microglial-induced inflammation by inhibiting the HMGB1/TLR4/NF-κB pathway following experimental traumatic brain injury. J Neuroinflammation. 2017;14:143.

34. Inoue T, Tanaka M, Masuda S, Ohue-Kitano R, Yamakage H, Muranaka K, Wada H, Kusakabe T, Shimatsu A, Hasegawa K, et al. Omega-3 polyunsaturated fatty acids suppress the inflammatory responses of lipopolysaccharide-stimulated mouse microglia by activating SIRT1 pathways. Biochim Biophys Acta. 2017;1862:552–60.

35. Gwon DH, Hwang TW, Ro JY, Kang YJ, Jeong JY, Kim DK, Lim K, Kim DW, Choi DE, Kim JJ. High endogenous accumulation of omega-3 polyunsaturated fatty acids protect against ischemia-reperfusion renal injury through AMPK-mediated autophagy in Fat-1 mice. Int J Mol Sci. 2017;18:2081.

36. Shen L, Yang Y, Ou T, Key CC, Tong SH, Sequeira RC, Nelson JM, Nie Y, Wang Z, Boudyguina E, et al. Dietary PUFAs attenuate NLRP3 inflammasome activation via enhancing macrophage autophagy. J Lipid Res. 2017;58:1808–21.

37. Vlahakis A, Lopez MN, Powers T. Mitochondrial respiration links TOR complex 2 signaling to calcium regulation and autophagy. Autophagy. 2017;13:1256–7.

38. Zhang X, Wu Q, Wu L, Ye Z, Jiang T, Li W, Zhuang Z, Zhou M, Zhang X, Hang C. Sirtuin 1 activation protects against early brain injury after experimental subarachnoid hemorrhage in rats. Cell Death and Disease. 2016;7:e2416.

39. Yang X, Wu Q, Zhang L, Feng L. Inhibition of histone deacetylase 3 (HDAC3) mediates ischemic preconditioning and protects cortical neurons against ischemia in rats. Front Mol Neurosci. 2016;9:131.

40. Tang C, Shan Y, Hu Y, Fang Z, Tong Y, Chen M, Wei X, Fu X, Xu X. FGF2 attenuates neural cell death via suppressing autophagy after rat mild traumatic brain injury. Stem Cells Int. 2017;2017:2923182.

41. Balan M, Pal S. A novel CXCR3-B chemokine receptor-induced growth-inhibitory signal in cancer cells is mediated through the regulation of Bach-1 protein and Nrf2 protein nuclear translocation. J Biol Chem. 2014;289:3126–37.

42. Grishchuk Y, Ginet V, Truttmann AC, Clarke PG, Puyal J. Beclin 1-independent autophagy contributes to apoptosis in cortical neurons. Autophagy. 2011;7:1115–31.

43. Xie XQ, Zhang P, Tian B, Chen XQ. Downregulation of NAD-dependent deacetylase SIRT2 protects mouse brain against ischemic stroke. Mol Neurobiol. 2016;54:7251–61.

44. Wang T, Yang B, Ji R, Xu W, Mai K, Ai Q. Omega-3 polyunsaturated fatty acids alleviate hepatic steatosis-induced inflammation through Sirt1-mediated nuclear translocation of NF-kappaB p65 subunit in hepatocytes of large yellow croaker (Larmichthys crocea). Fish Shellfish Immunol. 2017;71:76–82.

45. Ma Y, Nie H, Chen H, Li J, Hong Y, Wang B, Wang C, Zhang J, Cao W, Zhang M, et al. NAD(+)/NADH metabolism and NAD(+)-dependent enzymes in cell death and ischemic brain injury: current advances and therapeutic implications. Curr Med Chem. 2015;22:1239–47.

46. Harvey LD, Yin Y, Attarwala IY, Begum G, Deng J, Yan HQ, Dixon CE, Sun D. Administration of DHA reduces endoplasmic reticulum stress-associated inflammation and alters microglial or macrophage activation in traumatic brain injury. Asn Neuro. 2015;7:1759091415618969.

47. Kurtys E, Eisel UL, Verkuyl JM, Broersen LM, Dierckx RA, de Vries EF. The combination of vitamins and omega-3 fatty acids has an enhanced anti-inflammatory effect on microglia. Neurochem Int. 2016;99:206–14.

48. Pu H, Guo Y, Zhang W, Huang L, Wang G, Liou AK, Zhang J, Zhang P, Leak RK, Wang Y, et al. Omega-3 polyunsaturated fatty acid supplementation improves neurologic recovery and attenuates white matter injury after experimental traumatic brain injury. J Cereb Blood Flow Metab. 2013;33:1474–84.

49. Hariharan N, Maejima Y, Nakae J, Paik J, DePinho RA, Sadoshima J. Deacetylation of FoxO by Sirt1 plays an essential role in mediating starvation-induced autophagy in cardiac myocytes. Circ Res. 2010;107:1470–82.

6

α1-antitrypsin mitigates NLRP3-inflammasome activation in amyloid β$_{1-42}$- stimulated murine astrocytes

Taraneh Ebrahimi[1], Marcus Rust[1], Sarah Nele Kaiser[1], Alexander Slowik[2], Cordian Beyer[2], Andreas Rembert Koczulla[3], Jörg B. Schulz[1,4], Pardes Habib[1†] and Jan Philipp Bach[1*†] (iD)

Abstract

Background: Neuroinflammation has an essential impact on the pathogenesis and progression of Alzheimer's disease (AD). Mostly mediated by microglia and astrocytes, inflammatory processes lead to degeneration of neuronal cells. The NLRP3-inflammasome (NOD-like receptor family, pyrin domain containing 3) is a key component of the innate immune system and its activation results in secretion of the proinflammatory effectors interleukin-1β (IL-1β) and interleukin-18 (IL-18). Under physiological conditions, cytosolic NLRP3-inflammsome is maintained in an inactive form, not able to oligomerize. Amyloid β$_{1-42}$ (Aβ$_{1-42}$) triggers activation of NLRP3-inflammasome in microglia and astrocytes, inducing oligomerization and thus recruitment of proinflammatory proteases. NLRP3-inflammasome was found highly expressed in human brains diagnosed with AD. Moreover, NLRP3-deficient mice carrying mutations associated with familial AD were partially protected from deficits associated with AD.

The endogenous protease inhibitor α1-antitrypsin (A1AT) is known for its anti-inflammatory and anti-apoptotic properties and thus could serve as therapeutic agent for NLRP3-inhibition. A1AT protects neurons from glutamate-induced toxicity and reduces Aβ$_{1-42}$-induced inflammation in microglial cells. In this study, we investigated the effect of Aβ$_{1-42}$-induced NLRP3-inflammasome upregulation in primary murine astrocytes and its regulation by A1AT.

Methods: Primary cortical astrocytes from BALB/c mice were stimulated with Aβ$_{1-42}$ and treated with A1AT. Regulation of NLRP3-inflammasome was examined by immunocytochemistry, PCR, western blot and ELISA. Our studies included an inhibitor of NLRP3 to elucidate direct interactions between A1AT and NLRP3-inflammasome components.

Results: Our study revealed that A1AT reduces Aβ$_{1-42}$-dependent upregulation of NLRP3 at the mRNA and protein levels. Furthermore, A1AT time-dependently mitigated the expression of caspase 1 and its cleavage product IL-1β in Aβ$_{1-42}$-stimulated astrocytes.

Conclusion: We conclude that Aβ$_{1-42}$-stimulation results in an upregulation of NLRP3, caspase 1, and its cleavage products in astrocytes. A1AT time-dependently hampers neuroinflammation by downregulation of Aβ$_{1-42}$-mediated NLRP3-inflammasome expression and thus may serve as a pharmaceutical opportunity for the treatment of Alzheimer's disease.

Keywords: Neuroinflammation, NLRP3, NALP3, Inflammasome, Alzheimer's disease, Amyloid β, Alpha 1-antitrypsin, Astrocytes

* Correspondence: jbach@ukaachen.de
†P Habib and J P Bach contributed equally to this work.
[1]Department of Neurology, RWTH Aachen University, Aachen, Germany
Full list of author information is available at the end of the article

Background

Alzheimer's disease (AD) is the most common form of dementia with more than 40 million patients affected worldwide [1]. By 2050, the number is expected to quadruple [2]. Age is the most important risk factor [3], because the incidence of AD doubles every 5 years after the age of 65 years [3]. There is no causal treatment so far. To date, almost all biologicals or secretase inhibitors have failed in clinical trials which emphasize the need for further research into novel therapeutic options. Treatment of patients, even with early symptoms, only starts when the disease pathology has progressed and neural tissue has irreversibly been damaged for years. Therefore, current trials focus on patients with prodromal disease signs [4–11].

Following the amyloid hypothesis, accumulation of extracellular $A\beta_{1-42}$-oligomers is one of the earliest and driving factors for pathogenesis of AD [12, 13]. The majority of in vitro studies investigated the effect of $A\beta_{1-42}$ after an incubation time of 24–72 h [14–16]. Current scientific literature reveals less data about a possible damaging effect of $A\beta_{1-42}$-stimulation on the central nervous system (CNS) after short-term stimulation of only a few hours [14].

Besides $A\beta_{1-42}$, AD is mainly characterized by hyperphosphorylation of tau and neuroinflammation mediated by microglia and astrocytes, causing neuronal cell death [17–21]. A key component of the innate immune system is the NOD-like receptor family, pyrin domain-containing 3 (NLRP 3) [22, 23]. Though ubiquitously expressed in CNS, NLRP3 is found highly expressed in Alzheimer's patients' brains [22–24]. Under physiological conditions, an inactive form of NLRP3 is located in the cytoplasm [14, 25]. However, in the absence of activating signals, the NLRP3-inflammasome is not able to oligomerize [25]. After NLRP3-receptors recognize danger signals released by damaged cells and pathogens [26], NLRP3, the adaptor protein ASC (apoptosis-associated speck-like protein containing a CARD) and pro-caspase 1 form a subcellular multiprotein complex, known as NLRP3-inflammasome [22, 23, 27]. Subsequently, pro-caspase 1 is activated by autoproteolysis and catalyzes the cleavage of the precursors pro-IL-1β and pro-IL-18 [27]. Mostly induced by microglia and astrocytes, secretion of pro-inflammatory cytokines IL-1β and IL-18 drives inflammatory responses and causes neuronal damaging [27–29].

Inflammasomes are linked to neurodegenerative diseases: activated NLRP3 was observed in Parkinson's disease in the midbrain and cerebrospinal fluid [30–33]. Furthermore, in an experimental ischemic stroke model, NLRP3-deficiency was protective against ischemic neuronal damage [34].

In a cellular model of Alzheimer's disease, Halle et al. 2008 first described that activation of NLRP3-inflammasome is induced by $A\beta_{1-42}$ in microglia, leading to an overexpression of the pro-inflammatory cytokine IL-1β [14]. Moreover, $A\beta_{1-42}$ activates the NLRP3-inflammasome in astrocytes [35]. Alike microglia, as a part of the CNS immune response, reactive astrocytes surround amyloid deposits and perform phagocytosis [35–37]. Most studies investigated $A\beta_{1-42}$-mediated inflammatory processes in microglia and little is known about inflammasome activation in $A\beta_{1-42}$-stimulated astrocytes [14, 15, 24, 38–40]. Since inflammation occurs as one of the first cellular and molecular responses after cell stress, short-term effects of $A\beta$-stimulation in astrocytes need further characterization. Aside from cell culture models, also in human models of AD high expression of NLRP3-inflammasome was found. More precise, an upregulation of NLRP3 expression in peripheral monocytes from individuals with AD was identified [16]. Moreover, in frontal cortex and hippocampus lysates from AD patients increased amounts of cleaved caspase 1 were detected [24]. Interestingly, NLRP3 deficient mice carrying genes associated with familial AD were protected from spatial memory deficits [24].

Therefore, a potent inhibition of the NLRP3-inflammasome could be a new therapeutic approach. The protease inhibitor α1-antitrypsin (A1AT) is known for its anti-inflammatory and anti-apoptotic properties in both hepatic and lung cells [41–44]. Conveniently, A1AT is therapeutically used in patients with A1AT-deficiency and therefore well-established as a pharmaceutical agent. Recently, we demonstrated that A1AT also protected neurons from glutamate-induced toxicity [45] and reduced $A\beta_{1-42}$-induced inflammation in microglial cells [15]. In addition, we found that A1AT inhibited calpain and stabilized calcium-homeostasis [15]. This study investigated the regulation of NLRP3-inflammasome by A1AT in $A\beta_{1-42}$-stimulated murine astrocytes. In order to elucidate a direct interaction between A1AT and the NLRP3-inflammasome, we have included an inhibitor of NLRP3. MCC950 is a highly potent and specific inhibitor of NLRP3, without affecting AIM2, NLRC4, or NLRP4 [46–49]. Recent data revealed that MCC950 stimulated $A\beta$-phagocytosis in vitro, and reduced $A\beta$-accumulation in a mouse model of AD, which was associated with improved cognitive function [50].

Methods

Primary cortical murine astrocyte culture

Postnatal (P0 to P2) cortical astrocyte culture preparation from BALB/c mice (Charles River) was performed as previously described by Habib et al. 2014 [51]. Preparation was conducted in accordance with animal welfare policy of University Hospital Aachen and the government of the State of North Rhine-Westphalia, Germany (no. 84.02.04.2015.A292). Briefly, after brain dissection meninges and blood vessels were removed, cortex was isolated, homogenized, and dissolved in Dulbecco's phosphate-buffered saline (DPBS, Life Technologies, USA) containing 1% (*v/v*) trypsin and 0.02% (*v/v*) EDTA. The cell suspension was filtered through a 50 μm nylon mesh. After centrifugation (1400 rpm, 5 min), pellets were re-suspended in Gibco™ Dulbeccos's modified Eagle medium (DMEM, Life Technologies, USA) and seeded on flasks in DMEM with additional 10% fetal bovine serum (FBS, PAA, Austria) and 0.5% penicillin-streptomycin (Invitrogen, USA). All flasks and plates were coated by poly-L-ornithine (PLO, Sigma-Aldrich, Germany) prior to cell seeding. Cells were kept in a humidified incubator at 37 °C and 5% CO_2. After cell confluence was about 80%, flasks were shaken for 2 h (150 rpm, 37 °C) to remove microglia and oligodendrocytes from astrocytes. Additionally, before each subcultivation the 2 h machine shaking was repeated, the contaminating cells were transferred to the medium and then removed.

For subcultivation, cells were trypsinized with 2.5% (*v/v*) trypsin diluted in PBS/EDTA and seeded on new flasks in a 1:3 ratio. Medium was refreshed every second day. Subcultivation was performed when cells reached a confluence of about 80%. At passage 2, astrocytes were seeded on experimental plates 48 h prior to stimulation. 24 h before stimulation medium was changed to phenol red-free Gibco™ Roswell Park Memorial Institute (RPMI 1640, Life Technologies, USA) with additional 5% FBS and 0.5% penicillin-streptomycin (Fig. 1a).

Astrocyte culture purity was examined by immunocytochemistry (ICC) using anti-GFAP-antibody (glial fibrillary acidic protein), anti-Iba1-antibody (ionized calcium binding adaptor molecule 1), anti-Olig2-antibody (oligodendrocyte transcription factor 2) and Hoechst (33342, Trihydrochloride, Trihydrate, Invitrogen, USA) for

nucleus staining. A detailed list of antibodies used for ICC is illustrated in Table 1. The average of astrocyte purity was 95%, less than 5% of the cells were microglia, under 0.5% of the cells remained undefined (Additional file 1: Figure S2B).

Preparation of A1AT, amyloid β₁₋₄₂, LPS, and MCC950

A1AT originated from Prolastin (Grifols, Barcelona, Spain). 1000 mg of the powder were dissolved in 25 mL ultrapure water to obtain a concentration of 40 mg/mL. The solution was aliquoted and stored at − 80 °C.

To generate Amyloid β_{1-42} oligomers, we used the procedure described by Kayed et al. [52] and Gold et al. [15]. Briefly, 300 μg $A\beta_{1-42}$ (Bachem, Bubendorf, Switzerland) were dissolved in 90 μL hexafluoroisopropanol, 210 μL ultrapure water and diluted with 900 μL 100 mM NaCl, 50 mM Tris (pH 7.4). The solution was stirred for 48 h on a magnetic stirrer at room temperature. Next, the tube was weighed again, and weight difference was adjusted with 100 mM NaCl 50 mM Tris (pH 7.4). The $A\beta_{1-42}$ concentration of this solution was 56 mM. After centrifugation (16,000×*g*, 10 min), the supernatant was used for cell culture experiments. A negative control containing all ingredients but $A\beta_{1-42}$ was established to evaluate possible solvent effects on astrocytes. Lipopolysaccharides (LPS) from *Escherichia coli* (Sigma-Aldrich, Germany) were used at a concentration of 1 μg/mL, as an extra stimulus for maximum cell stimulation. Stimulation time of all reagents was 3 h and 6 h. In order to reveal the short-term inflammasome regulation after $A\beta_{1-42}$ and to understand the mechanism of early inflammation in AD, we decided for short term stimulation of cells.

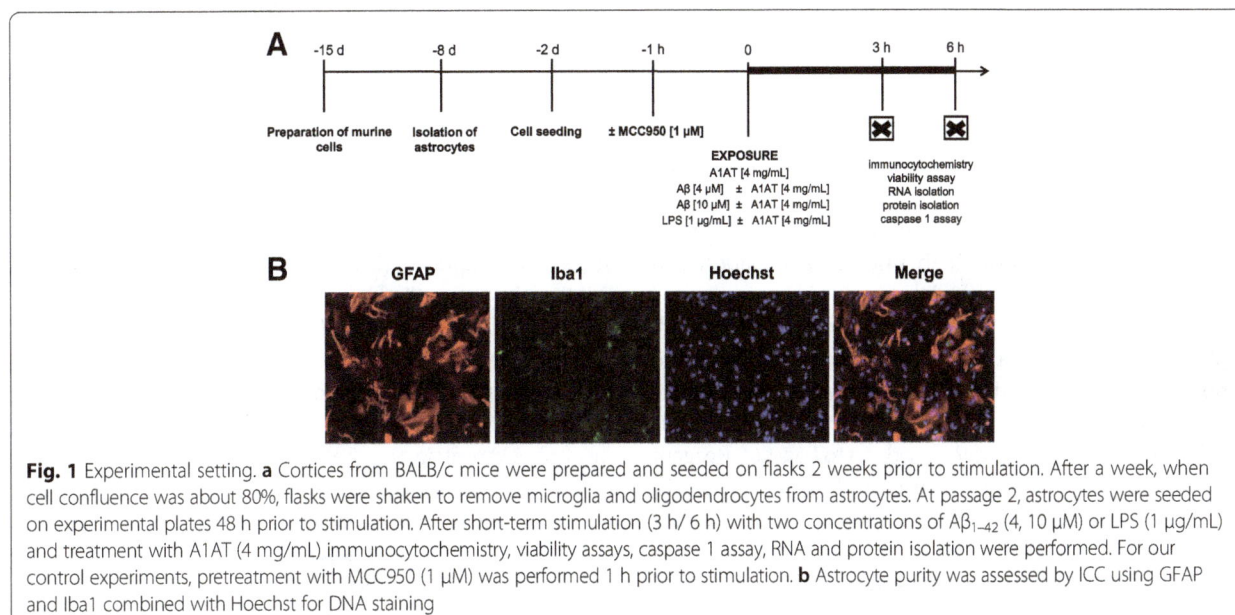

Fig. 1 Experimental setting. **a** Cortices from BALB/c mice were prepared and seeded on flasks 2 weeks prior to stimulation. After a week, when cell confluence was about 80%, flasks were shaken to remove microglia and oligodendrocytes from astrocytes. At passage 2, astrocytes were seeded on experimental plates 48 h prior to stimulation. After short-term stimulation (3 h/ 6 h) with two concentrations of Aβ₁₋₄₂ (4, 10 μM) or LPS (1 μg/mL) and treatment with A1AT (4 mg/mL) immunocytochemistry, viability assays, caspase 1 assay, RNA and protein isolation were performed. For our control experiments, pretreatment with MCC950 (1 μM) was performed 1 h prior to stimulation. **b** Astrocyte purity was assessed by ICC using GFAP and Iba1 combined with Hoechst for DNA staining

Table 1 Antibodies for immunocytochemistry

Antibody	Company	Order no.	Host	Dilution
Anti-goat 488	Life Technologies, USA	A11055	Donkey	1:500
Anti-goat 594	Life Technologies, USA	A11058	Donkey	1:500
Anti-mouse 488	Life Technologies, USA	A21202	Donkey	1:500
Anti-mouse 594	Life Technologies, USA	A21203	Donkey	1:500
Anti-rabbit 488	Life Technologies, USA	A21206	Donkey	1:500
Anti-rabbit 594	Life Technologies, USA	A21207	Donkey	1:500
GFAP	EnCor Biotechnology, USA	RPCA-GFAP	Rabbit	1:1000
Iba 1	Abcam, UK	ab107159	Goat	1:200
Iba 1	Millipore, USA	MABN92	Mouse	1:600
Iba 1	Wako, Japan	019–19,741	Rabbit	1:1000
NLRP3	Adipogen, USA	AG-20B-0014	Mouse	1:333
Olig2	Millipore, USA	MABN50	Mouse	1:1000
Olig2	Millipore, USA	AB9610	Rabbit	1:500

Primary and secondary antibodies used for immunocytochemical staining are listed

MCC950 (Adipogen, USA) was diluted in DMSO (dimethylsulfoxid, Sigma-Aldrich, Germany) and used in a concentration of 1 μM. MCC950 incubated 1 h before further treatment, according to previous studies by Coll et al. [46]. Then, treatment with A1AT, Amyloid β_{1-42}, and LPS was performed for 3 h and 6 h.

Cells were kept in the incubator at 37 °C and 5% CO_2.

Dose-dependency studies

A dose-dependency study with increasing concentrations of A1AT [1, 2, 4, 8, 10, and 12 mg/mL] and Aβ_{1-42} [1, 2, 4, 8, 10, and 12 μM] was performed to determine the sublethal concentration for primary astrocytes. Lactate dehydrogenase (LDH) and Cell Titer-Blue (CTB) assay were used to assess cell viability after 3 h stimulation.

Cell viability

LDH-release

CytoTox 96® Non-Radioactive Cytotoxicity Assay (Promega, USA) was performed according to the manufacturer's protocol to measure release of lactate dehydrogenase (LDH) as a marker of cellular viability. Astrocytes were seeded on a 96-well plate 48 h prior to stimulation and were finally stimulated with Aβ_{1-42} or LPS, and treated with A1AT. After 3 h/6 h incubation time, 50 μL of each well was transferred to a fresh 96-well plate. In addition to a no-treatment-cell control, a no-cell control, one positive control containing LDH and a control containing astrocytes lysed with Triton X-100 were used. CytoTox 96® Reagent (Promega, USA) was added to each well, and the absorbance was recorded at 490 nm by Infinite® M200 (Tecan, Switzerland). Data are presented as percentage of maximum LDH release (100%), which was determined by astrocytes lysed with 1% Triton X-100.

CTB assay

CellTiter-Blue® Cell Viability Assay (Promega, USA) was performed according to manufacturer's protocol to assess metabolic activity of the cells. Astrocytes were seeded on a 96-well plate 48 h prior to stimulation and finally stimulated with Aβ_{1-42} or LPS and treated with A1AT. After 3 h and 6 h incubation time, CellTiter-Blue® Reagent (Promega, USA) was added to each well. After 2.5–3 h, a color switch (reduction of resazurin) was observed and fluorescence was recorded at $560_{Ex}/590_{Em}$ by Infinite® M200 (Tecan, Switzerland).

Semi-quantitative and quantitative real-time PCR

After 3 h/6 h of stimulation, medium was removed and peqGOLD TriFast™ (Peqlab, Germany) was added to cells. RNA was isolated using phenol-chloroform extraction method as previously described [53]. Afterwards, RNA concentration was measured by NanoDrop® ND-1000 (Thermo Fisher Scientific, USA). RNA purity was examined using 260/280 ratio, which was at 2.0 ± 0.1. Samples were diluted with ultrapure water to attain same RNA concentration in each sample. For DNA transcription, samples were transcribed by moloney murine leukemia virus (M-MLV) reverse transcriptase (Invitrogen™, USA) using random primer (Invitrogen™, USA). Semi-quantitative PCR with 30–32 cycles was performed to assess cDNA transcription success, starting with reference genes primer HPRT (hypoxanthine phosphoribosyltransferase 1), GAPDH (glycerinaldehyd-3-phosphate-dehydrogenase), and Hsp90 (heat shock protein 90). Table 2 contains all primers used for PCR. Positive control contained mouse cortex and negative control contained ultrapure water. A Thermocycler Mastercycler ep gradient S (Eppendorf, Germany) was used with the following settings: 3 min at 95 °C, 40 s at 95 °C, 40 s at respective annealing temperature

Table 2 Primers for PCR

Primer	Sequence	Bp	AT
ASC	Forward: CTTGTCAGGGGATGAACTCAAAA Reverse: GCCATACGACTCCAGATAGTAGC	154	60
Casp1	Forward: CCGTGGAGAGAAACAAGGAGT Reverse: CCCCTGACAGGATGTCTCCA	180	62
GAPDH	Forward: TGTGTCCGTCGTGGATCTGA Reverse: CCTGCTTCACCACCTTCTTGA	77	65
HPRT	Forward: GCTGGTGAAAAGGACCTCT Reverse: CACAGGACTAGAACACCTGC	249	61
Hsp90	Forward: TACTACTACTCGGCTTTCCCGT Reverse: TCGAATCTTGTCCAGGGCATC	192	64
IL-1β	Forward: CAGCTCATATGGGTCCGACA Reverse: CTGTGTCTTTCCCGTGGACC	251	61
IL-18	Forward: SGCCTGTGTTCGAGGATATGACT Reverse: CCTTCACAGAGAGGGTCACAG	122	62
NLRP3	Forward: CCTGGGGGGACTTTGGAATCA Reverse: GATCCTGACAACACGCGGA	113	65

List of primers, respective sequences, base pairs (bp) and annealing temperature in °C (AT) used for sq-PCR and q-RT-PCR

(Table 2), and 45 s at 72 °C, 45 s at 72 °C. Nucleic acids were detected after application on 3% agarose gel containing Midori Green Advance (Biozym, Germany) for DNA staining and electrophoresis (25 min, 125 V constant, 400 mA). Gels were then photographed in E-box VX2 (Peqlab, Germany).

For quantitative real-time PCR, a dilution series containing all samples was established, starting from 100% with dilution factor 2. Then, samples were diluted 1:10 with ultrapure water. Master mixture included SensiMix™ SYBR and Fluorescein (Bioline, USA), ultrapure water and primer (Table 2). CFX Connect™ Real-Time PCR Detection System (Bio-Rad, USA) was used. The following settings were adjusted: 10 min at 95 °C, 15 s at 95 °C, 30 s at respective annealing temperature (40 cycles), 30 s at 72 °C, and 5 s at 72 °C. The software quantified DNA products by melting curve analysis. An addition gel electrophoresis was performed to control the size of the amplified DNA products. First, the expression of reference genes was measured. All following target gene expressions were normalized to reference genes HPRT, GAPDH, and Hsp90. Using the qbase+ software (Biogazelle, Belgium), the relative quantification was calculated by the ΔΔCt-method and data were expressed as relative amount of the three housekeeping genes, respectively, by using the multiple reference gene normalization method. Untreated cell controls were set to 1.

Immunocytochemistry

Immunocytochemistry (ICC) was performed as previously described by Habib et al. 2014 [51]. Astrocytes were seeded on cover slips on a 24-well plate. After stimulation, cells were fixed with 3.7% paraformaldehyde, lysed with Triton X-100, blocked with blocking buffer, and incubated with primary antibody. A negative control was established by incubating the cover slip only with blocking buffer without primary antibody. On the next day, the secondary antibody was applied and incubated for 2 h. After washing the cover slips, nuclei were stained by Hoechst (33342, Trihydrochloride, Trihydrate, Invitrogen, USA). A detailed list of antibodies used for ICC can be found in Table 1. Fluorescence images were taken with Leica DM6000 B (Leica Microsystems, Germany). For each experiment, the identical microscope settings were selected. Fluorescence intensity was measured using ImageJ (USA),

Western blot

Samples were generated from cell lysate and supernatant. Pierce™ BCA Protein Assay Kit (Thermo Fisher Scientific, USA) was used according to manufacturer's protocol to measure protein concentration. The absorbance was recorded at 562 nm by Tecan Infinite® M200 reader (Tecan, Switzerland). Western blot was performed as previously described by Dang et al. 2011 [54, 55]. Briefly, after astrocytes were stimulated for 3 h/ 6 h, the lysis and extraction buffer as well as protease inhibitors were added. The buffer consists of 10 mM HEPES (PromoCell, Germany), 1.5 mM MgCl2 (Sigma-Aldrich, Germany), 10 mM KCl, 0.5 mM DTT, and 0.05% NP-40 (pH = 7.9.).

Samples were heated for 5 min at 95 °C, loaded on gels, and electrophoresis was performed (10 min at 80 V, 1 h at 140 V). PVDF membranes (Trans-Blot® Turbo™ RTA Mini PVDF Transfer Kit, Bio-Rad, USA) were activated with methanol, and then blotting was performed by Trans-Blot® Turbo™ Transfer System (Bio-Rad, USA) (22 min, 14 V). Blotting success was verified by incubating the membrane with methanol and Ponceau S. The membrane was incubated with the primary antibody overnight; on the next day, the secondary antibody was added after washing the membrane. Table 3 reveals the antibodies used. Chemiluminescence detection system was performed using Pierce™ ECL Western Blotting Substrate (Thermo Fisher Scientific, USA). Densitometric analysis was performed using ImageJ Software (USA).

ELISA

Samples were generated from supernatant. Pierce™ BCA Protein Assay Kit (Thermo Fisher Scientific, USA) was used according to manufacturer's protocol to measure protein concentration. The absorbance was recorded at 562 nm by Tecan Infinite® M200 reader (Tecan, Switzerland). Murine IL-1β Standard ABTS ELISA (PeproTech, USA) was performed according to manufacturer's protocol. Capture antibody was incubated on a 96-well plate overnight. Wells were blocked for 1 h then incubated overnight with standard and samples in triplicate. Next, detection antibody was incubated for 2 h. Avidin-HRP conjugate was incubated for 30 min, afterwards ABTS was added. The color

Table 3 Antibodies for western blotting

Antibody	Company	Order no.	Host	Dilution
Anti-mouse	Sigma-Aldrich, Germany	A4416	Goat	1:4000
Anti-rabbit	Bio-Rad, USA	170–6515	Goat	1:5000
ASC (N15)-R	Santa Cruz, USA	sc-22514-R	Rabbit	1:1000
Caspase 1	Adipogen	20B0042C100	Mouse	1:1000
Caspase 1 p10	Santa Cruz, USA	sc-514	Rabbit	1:1000
Caspase 1 p20	Bioss	bs-6368R	Rabbit	1:500
IL-1β	Abcam, UK	ab9722	Rabbit	1:1000
IL-1β	Cell Signaling Technology, USA	12242S	Mouse	1:1000
IL-18	Abcam, UK	Ab71495	Rabbit	1:1000
IL-18	Santa Cruz, USA	sc-7954	Rabbit	1:1000
NLRP3	Bioss, USA	bs-10021R	Rabbit	1:1000
β-actin	Santa Cruz, USA	sc-47,778	Mouse	1:5000

List of primary and secondary antibodies used for western blotting. Antibodies were diluted in 5% milk

development was recorded at 405 nm by Tecan Infinite® M200 reader (Tecan, Switzerland).

Caspase 1 assay

FAM-FLICA® Caspase-1 Assay Kit (ImmunoChemistry Technologies, USA) was performed according to the manufacturer's protocol to detect caspase 1 activity after 3 h and 6 h stimulation time. FLICA was incubated for 1 h at 37 °C. Hoechst 33342 (1:10000) was used for nuclear staining, cells then were fixed with 3.7% paraformaldehyde. Fluorescence images were taken with Leica DM6000 B (Leica Microsystems, Germany); for each experiment, the exact same microscope settings were adjusted. The number of caspase 1 active cells was counted and set in relation to the total amount of counted astrocytes per well. For each treatment group, 100 cells/well in 5 wells were counted.

Data analysis

All experiments were performed at least three times in triplicate. All data are presented as arithmetic mean ± standard deviation of the mean. Prior to the analysis the residuals of data were tested for normal distribution with the Shapiro-Wilk normality test using JMP® (Version 10, SAS Institute Inc., Cary, NC, USA, 1989–2007). Secondly, equal variance was tested with the Bartlett test. In case that one of these tests was significant, a Box-Cox transformation was performed, and the test for normality and equal variance were repeated with the new calculated values. Finally, a one-way ANOVA was applied followed by the Tukey-HSD post-hoc test for intergroup differences. When transformation of data failed to convert non-normal into normal distributed data, rank data were calculated and used for one-way ANOVA analysis, which results in the Kruskal-Wallis non-parametric analysis followed by the Tukey-HSD post-hoc test. Statistical

significance was set at p value ≤ 0.05 (*/a ≤ 0.05, **/aa ≤ 0.01, ***/aaa ≤ 0.001).

Results

After primary astrocytes were stimulated according to work flow (Fig. 1a), culture purity of 95% astrocytes on average was examined by ICC, less than 5% of the remaining cells were microglia (Fig. 1b, Additional file 2: Figure S1 and Additional file 1: Figure S2).

Amyloid β$_{1-42}$ had a dose-dependent cytotoxic effect on astrocytes

First, we incubated astrocytes with Aβ$_{1-42}$ for 3 h to assess the short-term effect on cell viability. A concentration range of frequently used doses between 1 μM and 12 μM was selected [14, 15]. Aβ$_{1-42}$ induced a concentration-depended release of LDH into the medium, reaching 50% release and a significant difference compared to the control condition at a concentration of 12 μM (Additional file 3: Figure S3A). In comparison, the stimulation with LPS (1 μg/mL) led to a LDH-release of about 60%. The metabolic activity of Aβ$_{1-42}$-stimulated primary astrocytes (Cell Titer-Blue-assay) revealed no significant dose-dependent differences (Additional file 4: Figure S4A). To rule out cytotoxic effects, the further studies were performed with sublethal doses of Aβ$_{1-42}$ at 4 μM and 10 μM.

To examine a possible cytotoxic effect of A1AT, dose-dependency studies were performed. 3 h incubation of astrocytes with increasing concentrations of 1 mg/mL to 12 mg/mL of A1AT did not affect LDH release (Additional file 3: Figure S3B), also CTB assay showed no influence on metabolic activity of astrocytes (Additional file 4: Figure S4B).

Moreover, co-exposure of astrocytes with Aβ$_{1-42}$ (4 μM and 10 μM) and A1AT (1 mg/mL) had no impact on LDH release (Fig. 2a, c, Additional file 3: Figure S3C)

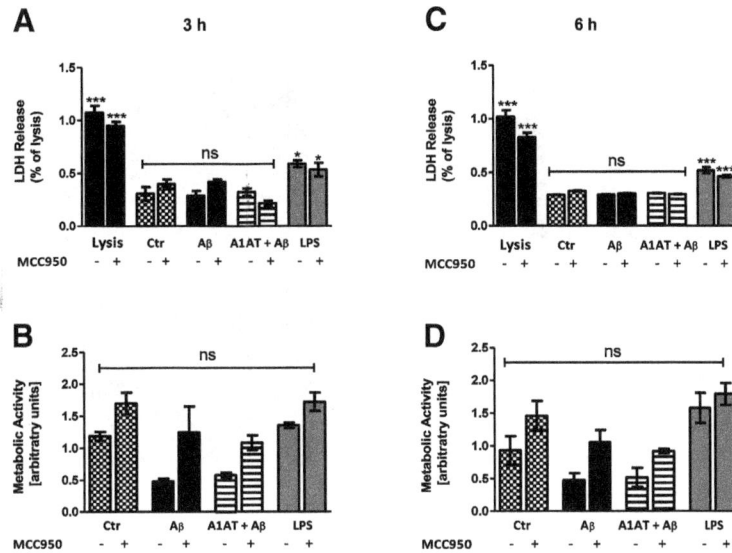

Fig. 2 Effect of Aβ$_{1-42}$ stimulation and A1AT treatment ± MCC950 on cell viability at 3 h and 6 h. Treatment with Aβ$_{1-42}$ [4 μM], A1AT [4 mg/mL], and MCC950 [1 μM] did not affect LDH-release at 3 h and 6 h stimulation, whereas LPS-stimulation [1 μg/mL] significantly increased LDH-release (**a**, **c**). Cell lysis defined maximal (100%; 1.0) release of LDH. MTT-assay (**b**, **d**) revealed a trend towards decrease in cell metabolism after 3 h and 6 h Aβ$_{1-42}$-stimulation, which was not significant. Treatment with MCC950 led to an increase of cell metabolism in each treatment group at 3 h and 6 h, which was not significant. $^{*/a}p < 0.05$; $^{**/aa}p < 0.01$; $^{***/aaa}p < 0.001$, ns not significant compared to untreated cell control (ctr)

or cell metabolism (Fig. 2b, d, Additional file 4: Figure S4C). In contrast, A1AT exposure of LPS-stimulated astrocytes significantly reduced LDH release (Additional file 3: Figure S3C).

A1AT prevented Aβ$_{1-42}$-induced upregulation of NLRP3 mRNA and protein

We next evaluated the expression of NLRP3 in the given experimental settings. Stimulation of astrocytes with Aβ$_{1-42}$-oligomers significantly increased NLRP3 mRNA-expression by three-fold (Aβ$_{1-42}$, 4 μM) or four-fold (Aβ$_{1-42}$, 10 μM) in comparison to untreated controls (Fig. 3a, Fig. 4c, d). Co-treatment with 4 mg/mL A1AT almost completely blocked this increase (Fig. 3a, Fig. 4c, d). Western blot analysis revealed a significant higher protein expression of NLRP3 in Aβ$_{1-42}$-stimulated astrocytes compared to untreated controls (Fig. 3b, c, Fig. 4a, b). Co-treatment with A1AT significantly prevented this increase in NLRP3 protein expression (Fig. 3c, Fig. 4a, b). These results were confirmed by ICC. Staining with GFAP-, NLRP3-antibody and Hoechst revealed significantly higher fluorescence intensity of NLRP3-stained astrocytes stimulated with 10 μM of Aβ$_{1-42}$ (Fig. 3d, e, microscope settings were identical for each experiment). Fluorescence intensity of Aβ$_{1-42}$-stimulated cells significantly declined with co-treatment by A1AT (Fig. 3e).

To exclude that NLRP3-upregulation was due to microglia contamination, ICC-staining using Iba1- and NLRP3-antibody was performed (Additional file 5:

Figure S5). Indeed, NLRP3 was expressed by the few present microglia. But as Additional file 1: Figure S2 and Additional file 5: Figure S5 show, the amount of microglia was so low, that their impact on NLRP3-expression is negligible.

Aβ$_{1-42}$-stimulation and A1AT-treatment did not regulate ASC expression

The NLRP3-inflammasome consists of active NLRP3 (LRR, NACHT, PYD, CARD) as well as the adaptor protein ASC and pro-caspase 1. In primary astrocytes, treatment with 4 μM or 10 μM Aβ$_{1-42}$ or 4 mg/mL A1AT did not result in changes of ASC mRNA or protein expression at 3 h and 6 h stimulation time (Fig. 5).

A1AT abrogated Aβ$_{1-42}$-induced upregulation of caspase 1 and the pro-inflammatory cytokine IL-1β

Next, we analyzed caspase 1, IL-1β and IL-18 expression. Whereas 3 h treatment of primary astrocytes with 4 μM of Aβ$_{1-42}$ did not result in an increase of caspase 1 mRNA expression, treatment with 10 μM of Aβ$_{1-42}$ led to a significant increase of caspase 1 mRNA expression (Fig. 6a, Additional file 6: Figure S6A). Co-treatment with 4 mg/mL A1AT blocked the increase of caspase 1 expression significantly (Additional file 6: Figure S6A). Repeating this experiment, this time performing a 6-h stimulation, revealed that Aβ$_{1-42}$ significantly increased mRNA levels of caspase 1 in astrocytes (Fig. 6b). Co-treatment with A1AT blocked this increase in caspase 1 mRNA (Fig. 6b).

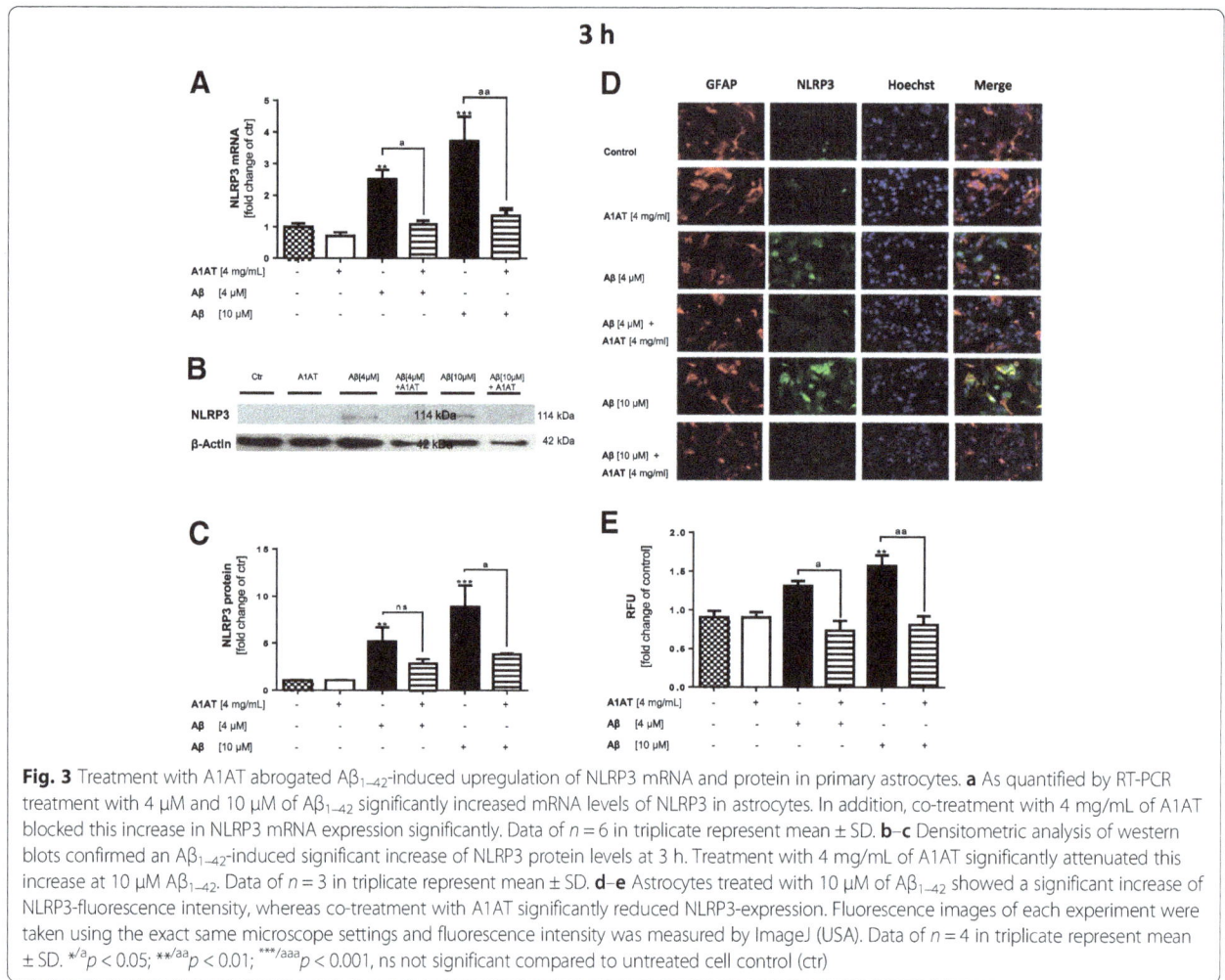

Fig. 3 Treatment with A1AT abrogated Aβ$_{1-42}$-induced upregulation of NLRP3 mRNA and protein in primary astrocytes. **a** As quantified by RT-PCR treatment with 4 μM and 10 μM of Aβ$_{1-42}$ significantly increased mRNA levels of NLRP3 in astrocytes. In addition, co-treatment with 4 mg/mL of A1AT blocked this increase in NLRP3 mRNA expression significantly. Data of $n = 6$ in triplicate represent mean ± SD. **b–c** Densitometric analysis of western blots confirmed an Aβ$_{1-42}$-induced significant increase of NLRP3 protein levels at 3 h. Treatment with 4 mg/mL of A1AT significantly attenuated this increase at 10 μM Aβ$_{1-42}$. Data of $n = 3$ in triplicate represent mean ± SD. **d–e** Astrocytes treated with 10 μM of Aβ$_{1-42}$ showed a significant increase of NLRP3-fluorescence intensity, whereas co-treatment with A1AT significantly reduced NLRP3-expression. Fluorescence images of each experiment were taken using the exact same microscope settings and fluorescence intensity was measured by ImageJ (USA). Data of $n = 4$ in triplicate represent mean ± SD. */^{a}$p < 0.05$; **/^{aa}$p < 0.01$; ***/^{aaa}$p < 0.001$, ns not significant compared to untreated cell control (ctr)

FAM-FLICA® Caspase-1 Assay, measuring active caspase-1 enzyme, showed that treatment with Aβ$_{1-42}$ significantly induced the number of caspase 1 positive cells (Fig. 7). Co-treatment with 4 mg/mL of A1AT significantly blocked this increase of caspase 1-positive cells (Fig. 7).

In the next step, pro-inflammatory cytokines cleaved by caspase 1 were assessed. Stimulation of astrocytes with 4 μM and 10 μM of Aβ$_{1-42}$ increased mRNA expression of IL-1β (Fig. 8a, b, Additional file 6: Figure S6B). Co-treatment with A1AT significantly reduced mRNA expression of IL-1β (Fig. 8a, b, Additional file 6: Fig. 6b). In contrast, IL-18 gene expression was not affected by either of the treatments at 3 h stimulation time (Fig. 8c, Additional file 6: Figure S6C). However, 6 h stimulation with Aβ$_{1-42}$ significantly increased mRNA levels of IL-18 in astrocytes, but A1AT did not block this effect (Fig. 8d).

Furthermore, western blot revealed a significant upregulation of the IL-1β-precursor in Aβ$_{1-42}$-treated cells (Fig. 9a, b). Co-treatment with A1AT blocked the effect (Fig. 9a, b). Analysis of IL-1β protein by ELISA revealed a similar effect of increased levels after Aβ$_{1-}$ $_{42}$-stimulation, which was significant at 6 h, but not at 3 h (9C-D). A1AT-treatment significantly prevented this increase time-dependently after 6 h stimulation (Fig. 9d).

MCC950 reduced caspase 1 activity and IL-1β protein expression

In order to elucidate a direct interaction between A1AT and the NLRP3-inflammasome, all studies were repeated including MCC950—a selective inhibitor of NLRP3. MCC950 had no impact on cell viability (Fig. 2a, c), but led to an increase of cell metabolism in each treatment group at 3 h and 6 h, though not significant (Fig. 2b, d). In western blot, MCC950 did not change protein levels of NLRP3 (Fig. 4a, b). Treatment with MCC950 did not alter gene expression of NLRP3, ASC, caspase 1, IL-1β, and IL-18 (Figs. 4c, d, 5E–F, 6a, b, 8a, d).

MCC950 significantly mitigated caspase 1 activity (Fig. 7) and significantly decreased IL-1β in Aβ-stimulated astrocytes examined by ELISA (Fig. 9c, d). Further, there is a trend towards a decrease of IL-1β-protein levels in the presence of MCC950 in nearly all treatment groups,

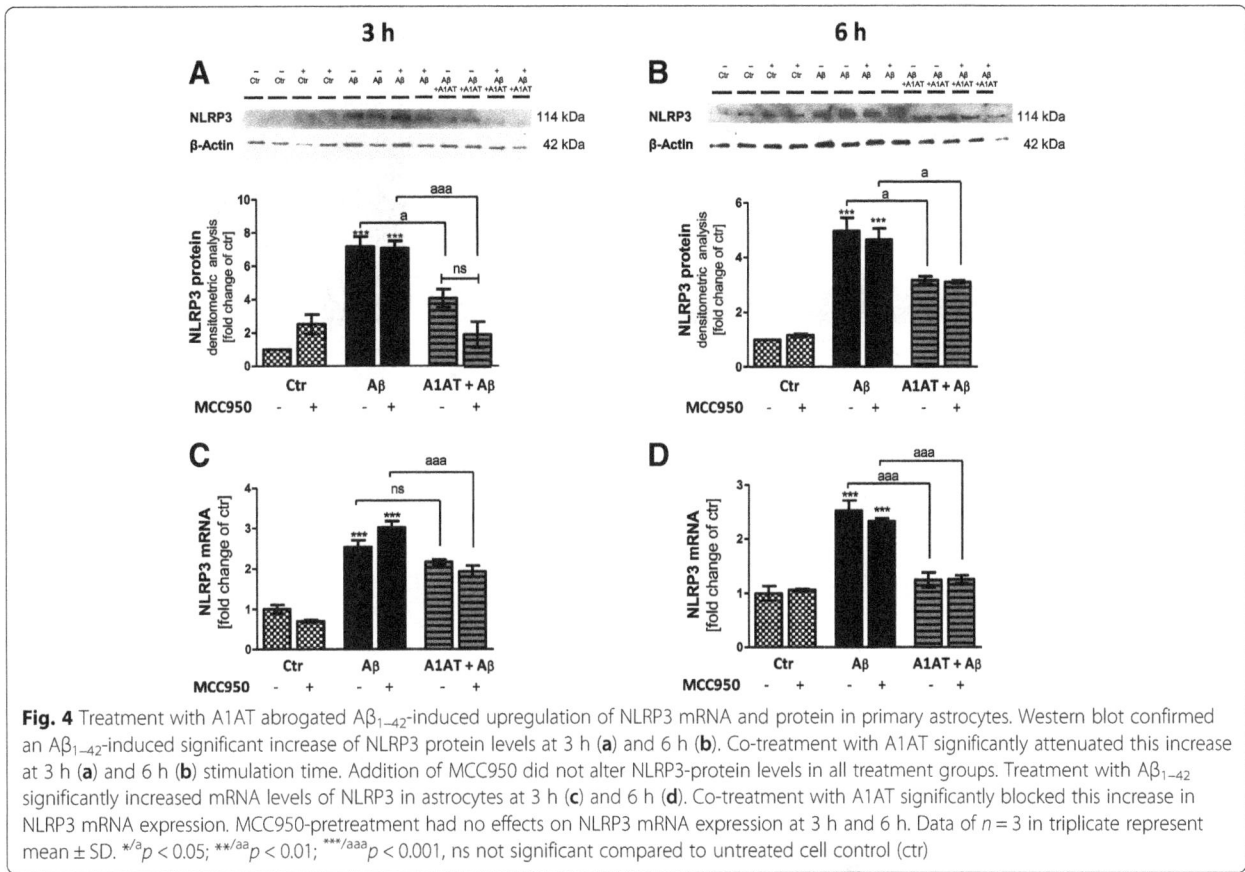

Fig. 4 Treatment with A1AT abrogated Aβ$_{1–42}$-induced upregulation of NLRP3 mRNA and protein in primary astrocytes. Western blot confirmed an Aβ$_{1–42}$-induced significant increase of NLRP3 protein levels at 3 h (**a**) and 6 h (**b**). Co-treatment with A1AT significantly attenuated this increase at 3 h (**a**) and 6 h (**b**) stimulation time. Addition of MCC950 did not alter NLRP3-protein levels in all treatment groups. Treatment with Aβ$_{1–42}$ significantly increased mRNA levels of NLRP3 in astrocytes at 3 h (**c**) and 6 h (**d**). Co-treatment with A1AT significantly blocked this increase in NLRP3 mRNA expression. MCC950-pretreatment had no effects on NLRP3 mRNA expression at 3 h and 6 h. Data of $n = 3$ in triplicate represent mean ± SD. */^{a}$p < 0.05$; **/^{aa}$p < 0.01$; ***/^{aaa}$p < 0.001$, ns not significant compared to untreated cell control (ctr)

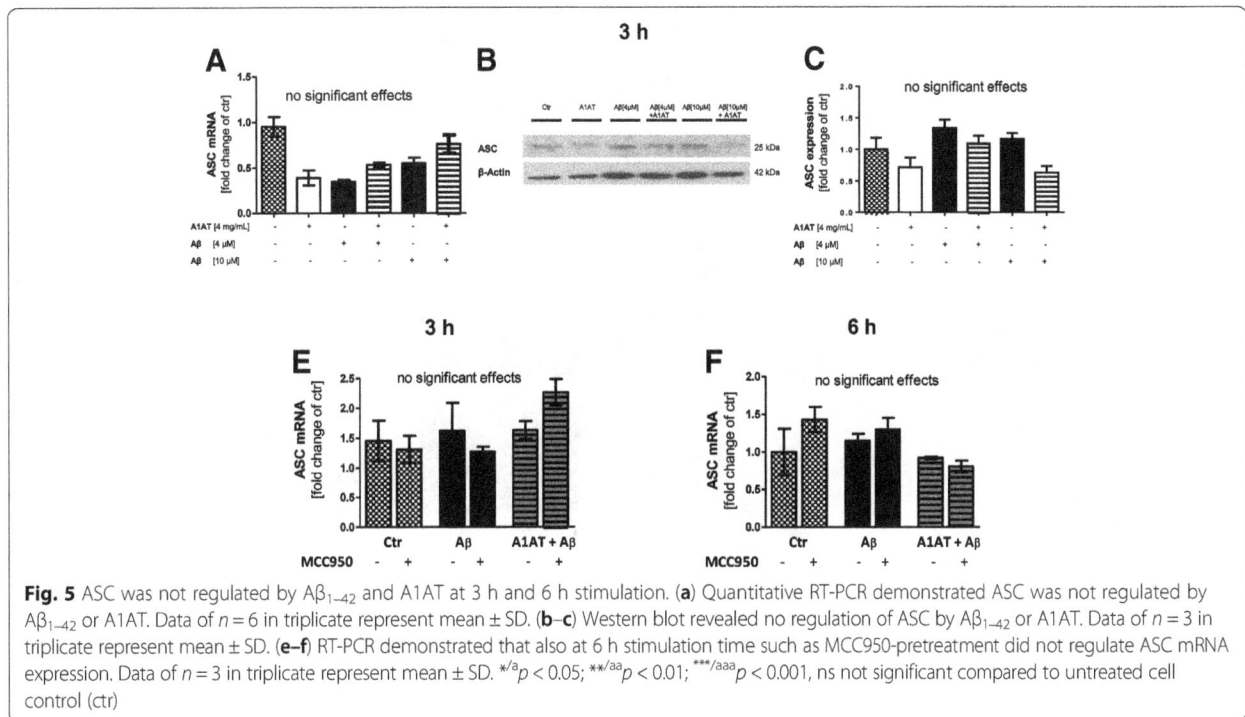

Fig. 5 ASC was not regulated by Aβ$_{1–42}$ and A1AT at 3 h and 6 h stimulation. (**a**) Quantitative RT-PCR demonstrated ASC was not regulated by Aβ$_{1–42}$ or A1AT. Data of $n = 6$ in triplicate represent mean ± SD. (**b–c**) Western blot revealed no regulation of ASC by Aβ$_{1–42}$ or A1AT. Data of $n = 3$ in triplicate represent mean ± SD. (**e–f**) RT-PCR demonstrated that also at 6 h stimulation time such as MCC950-pretreatment did not regulate ASC mRNA expression. Data of $n = 3$ in triplicate represent mean ± SD. */^{a}$p < 0.05$; **/^{aa}$p < 0.01$; ***/^{aaa}$p < 0.001$, ns not significant compared to untreated cell control (ctr)

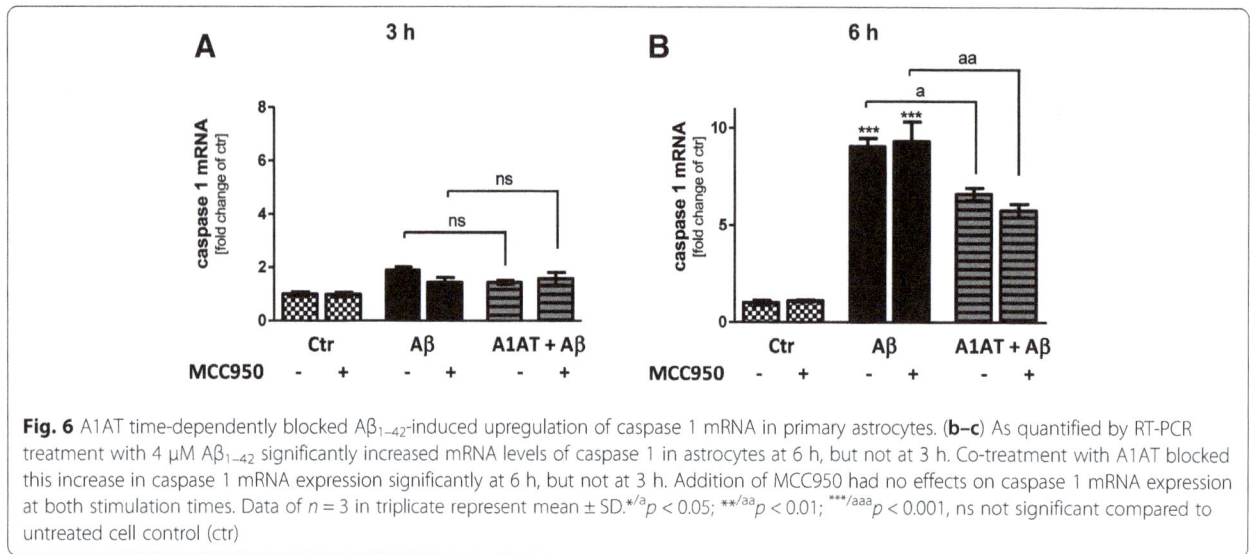

Fig. 6 A1AT time-dependently blocked Aβ$_{1-42}$-induced upregulation of caspase 1 mRNA in primary astrocytes. (**b–c**) As quantified by RT-PCR treatment with 4 μM Aβ$_{1-42}$ significantly increased mRNA levels of caspase 1 in astrocytes at 6 h, but not at 3 h. Co-treatment with A1AT blocked this increase in caspase 1 mRNA expression significantly at 6 h, but not at 3 h. Addition of MCC950 had no effects on caspase 1 mRNA expression at both stimulation times. Data of $n = 3$ in triplicate represent mean ± SD.$^{*/a}p < 0.05$; $^{**/aa}p < 0.01$; $^{***/aaa}p < 0.001$, ns not significant compared to untreated cell control (ctr)

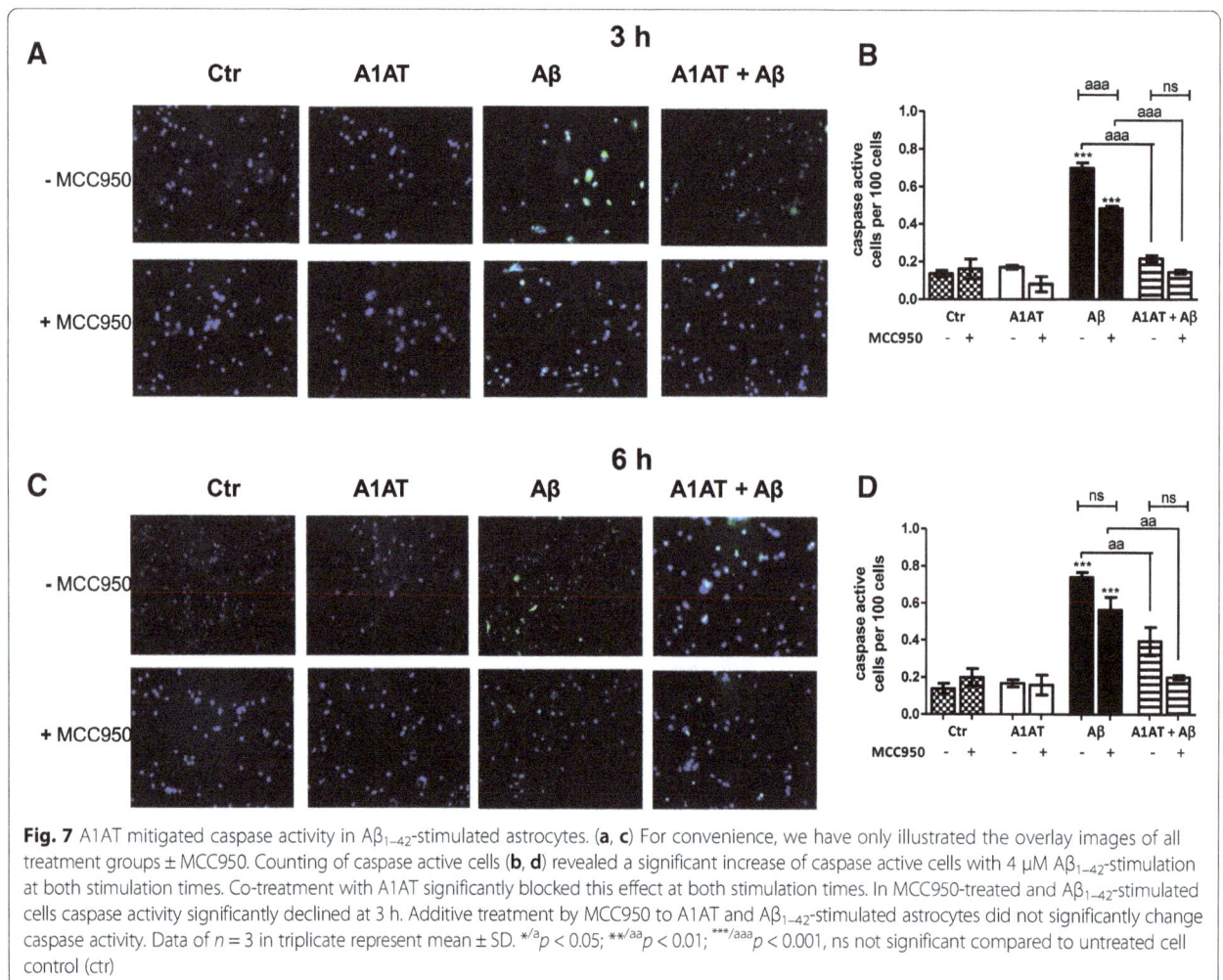

Fig. 7 A1AT mitigated caspase activity in Aβ$_{1-42}$-stimulated astrocytes. (**a**, **c**) For convenience, we have only illustrated the overlay images of all treatment groups ± MCC950. Counting of caspase active cells (**b**, **d**) revealed a significant increase of caspase active cells with 4 μM Aβ$_{1-42}$-stimulation at both stimulation times. Co-treatment with A1AT significantly blocked this effect at both stimulation times. In MCC950-treated and Aβ$_{1-42}$-stimulated cells caspase activity significantly declined at 3 h. Additive treatment by MCC950 to A1AT and Aβ$_{1-42}$-stimulated astrocytes did not significantly change caspase activity. Data of $n = 3$ in triplicate represent mean ± SD. $^{*/a}p < 0.05$; $^{**/aa}p < 0.01$; $^{***/aaa}p < 0.001$, ns not significant compared to untreated cell control (ctr)

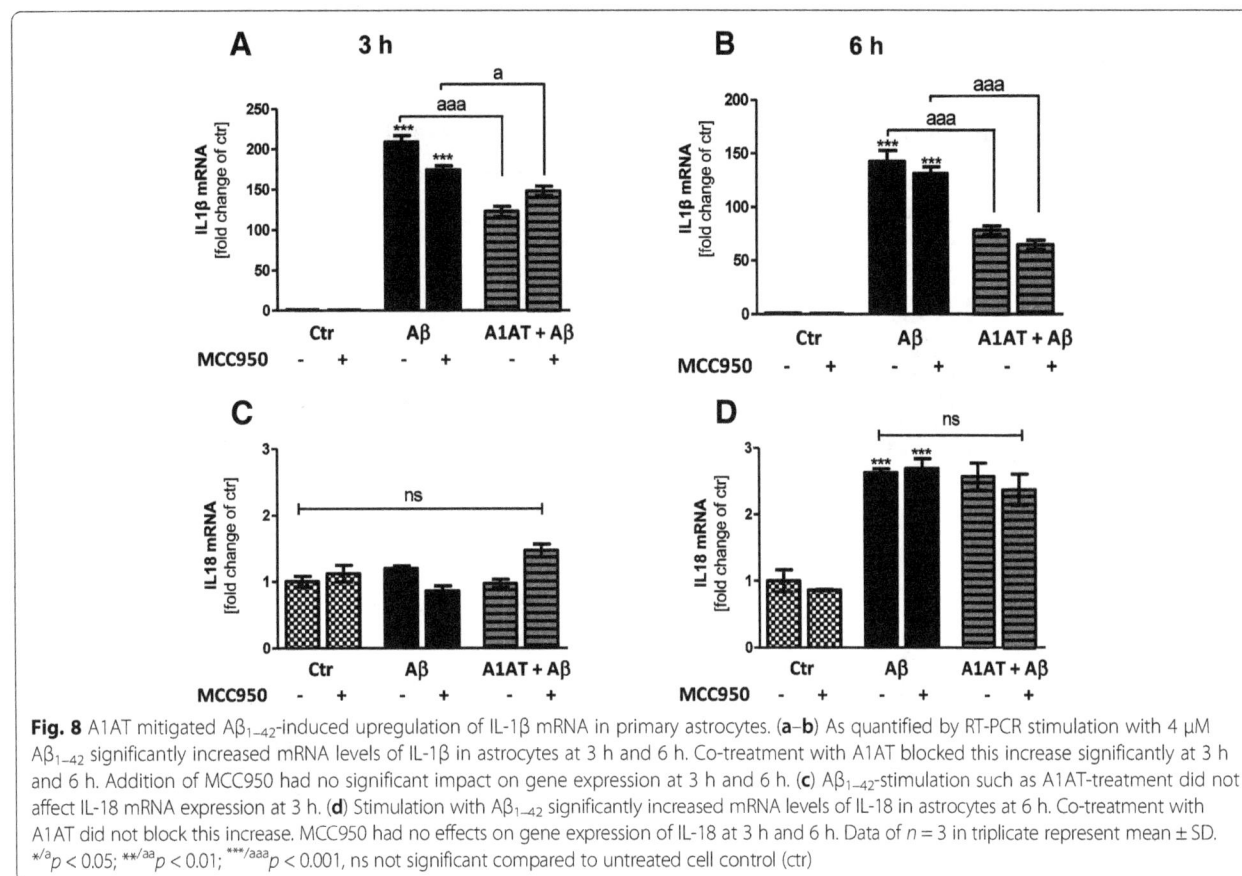

Fig. 8 A1AT mitigated Aβ$_{1-42}$-induced upregulation of IL-1β mRNA in primary astrocytes. (**a–b**) As quantified by RT-PCR stimulation with 4 μM Aβ$_{1-42}$ significantly increased mRNA levels of IL-1β in astrocytes at 3 h and 6 h. Co-treatment with A1AT blocked this increase significantly at 3 h and 6 h. Addition of MCC950 had no significant impact on gene expression at 3 h and 6 h. (**c**) Aβ$_{1-42}$-stimulation such as A1AT-treatment did not affect IL-18 mRNA expression at 3 h. (**d**) Stimulation with Aβ$_{1-42}$ significantly increased mRNA levels of IL-18 in astrocytes at 6 h. Co-treatment with A1AT did not block this increase. MCC950 had no effects on gene expression of IL-18 at 3 h and 6 h. Data of $n = 3$ in triplicate represent mean ± SD. $^{*/a}p < 0.05$; $^{**/aa}p < 0.01$; $^{***/aaa}p < 0.001$, ns not significant compared to untreated cell control (ctr)

though not significant (Fig. 9c, d). MCC950 did not affect Aβ-induced expression of IL-1β-precursor protein in western blot (Fig. 9a, b).

Co-treatment with A1AT and Aβ in the presence of MCC950 did not alter expression of NLRP3-inflammasome components

Examined by caspase 1 assay (Fig. 7), IL-1β western blot (Fig. 9a, b) and IL-1β-ELISA (Fig. 9c, d) co-treatment with A1AT and Aβ in the presence of MCC950 did not alter expression of inflammasome components compared to the same stimulation group in absence of MCC950. Therefore, we conclude that A1AT mitigated IL-1β mainly by inhibiting NLRP3-inflammasome.

Discussion

Activation of glia cells and overexpression of pro-inflammatory cytokines are regarded early events in Alzheimer's disease [56]. In recent years, astrocytes have come into focus in neurodegenerative disorders such as AD and are seen in a new way. Astrocytes express a plethora of receptors and modulate cells and their function in their surroundings [57]. In brief, they are involved in excitotoxic glutamate release, secretion of pro-inflammatory cytokines, growth factor production, stabilization, and organization of the blood-brain barrier

and Aβ$_{1-42}$ production [58]. In microglia cells, the activation of NLRP3 appears to be an essential step during AD. Following activation of NLRP3, inflammation is triggered by the activation of caspase 1 and generation of IL-1β. This hampers the phagocytic capability of microglia cells [39]. The NLRP3-inflammasome is important for the initiation and processing of neuroinflammatory processes, and especially in AD, NLRP3 is associated with age-related inflammation [59]. NLRP3 is known to be activated by Aβ$_{1-42}$-aggregates [14]. NLRP3 knock-out in transgenic animals carrying mutations associated with AD prevents AD pathology [24].

Our group has recently presented data in acute and chronic neurodegenerative disease models that different components of the NLRP3-inflammasome are allocated to astrocytes [60–64]. With respect to AD, Couturier and co-workers were able to show that astrocytes produce and release IL-1β following Aβ$_{1-42}$-stimulation [18]. In this animal model, the downregulation of NLRP3-inflammasome activation leads to decreased amyloid plaques and a better memory performance [35]. Our data now show that stimulation of primary astrocytes with Aβ$_{1-42}$ induces a dose-dependent upregulation of NLRP3. This in turn is known to stimulate the activation of caspase 1 and IL-1β [39]. Our work further demonstrates that such an effect

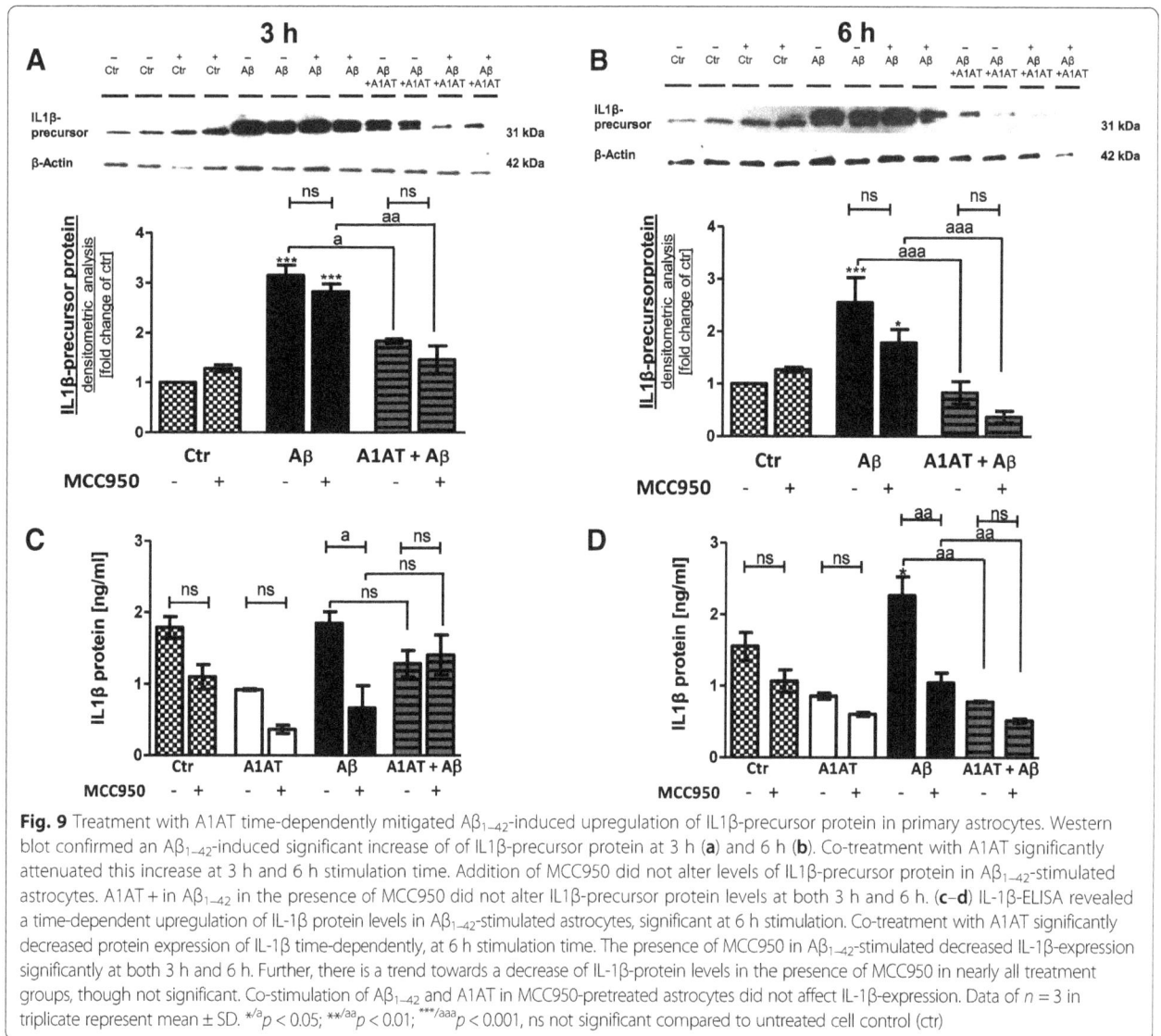

Fig. 9 Treatment with A1AT time-dependently mitigated Aβ₁₋₄₂-induced upregulation of IL1β-precursor protein in primary astrocytes. Western blot confirmed an Aβ₁₋₄₂-induced significant increase of of IL1β-precursor protein at 3 h (**a**) and 6 h (**b**). Co-treatment with A1AT significantly attenuated this increase at 3 h and 6 h stimulation time. Addition of MCC950 did not alter levels of IL1β-precursor protein in Aβ₁₋₄₂-stimulated astrocytes. A1AT + in Aβ₁₋₄₂ in the presence of MCC950 did not alter IL1β-precursor protein levels at both 3 h and 6 h. (**c–d**) IL-1β-ELISA revealed a time-dependent upregulation of IL-1β protein levels in Aβ₁₋₄₂-stimulated astrocytes, significant at 6 h stimulation. Co-treatment with A1AT significantly decreased protein expression of IL-1β time-dependently, at 6 h stimulation time. The presence of MCC950 in Aβ₁₋₄₂-stimulated decreased IL-1β-expression significantly at both 3 h and 6 h. Further, there is a trend towards a decrease of IL-1β-protein levels in the presence of MCC950 in nearly all treatment groups, though not significant. Co-stimulation of Aβ₁₋₄₂ and A1AT in MCC950-pretreated astrocytes did not affect IL-1β-expression. Data of $n = 3$ in triplicate represent mean ± SD. */ᵃ$p < 0.05$; **/ᵃᵃ$p < 0.01$; ***/ᵃᵃᵃ$p < 0.001$, ns not significant compared to untreated cell control (ctr)

also occurs after short-term stimulation with Aβ₁₋₄₂. In contrast, the co-treatment of astrocytes with Aβ₁₋₄₂ and A1AT blocks the induction of NLRP3. The regulation of NLRP3 is complex and usually requires a two-step activation process [22]. Currently, it is well accepted that the first step includes a priming signal, usually provided by NF-KB signaling or secretion of endogenous cytokines such as IL-1a [65]. NLRP3 is then activated by a variety of cellular signals, amongst them are misfolded proteins. The large variety of possible regulatory signals and pathways suggest that the activation is rather the consequence of a disturbance of cellular equilibrium [22]. In 2012, Lee and co-workers have identified calcium signaling as essential in NLRP3 activation [66]. In this study, increased intracellular calcium levels are associated with NLRP3 activation. In astrocytes, Aβ₁₋₄₂ potentiates calcium signaling which is triggered by mGlu, α7nAChR, and purinergic substances [57].

Yet, there is little evidence on the regulation of the NLRP3-inflammasome by A1AT. Toldo et al. 2011 stated that A1AT inhibits caspase-1 [67]. Aggarwal et al. 2016 found that—by the presence of polyunsaturated fatty acids—A1AT downregulates NLRP3 and caspase 1 [68]. For astrocytes, no data exist with respect to mechanisms of action of A1AT. In previous studies, we have presented data which show that A1AT reduces inflammation in microglia cells mainly by controlling calcium signaling pathways [15]. A1AT has no effect on classic signaling pathways such as MAPK p38, p44/42, JNK, and cAMP-coupled mechanisms [15]. Using a fluorescent calcium dye, we have shown that A1AT reduces intracellular calcium concentrations in a microglial cell line [15]. A1AT had no direct effect on Aβ₁₋₄₂-oligomerization [15]. We therefore hypothesize that A1AT effects on NLRP3 upregulation in primary astrocytes are mainly triggered by an inhibition of calcium and calpain. This hypothesis needs further evaluation, since other reports also demonstrate that A1AT is able to reduce glutamate-induced toxicity in murine primary neurons [45]. Since astrocytes release glutamate in response to $Aβ_{1-42}$-stimulation, this could represent another way how A1AT prevents deleterious $Aβ_{1-42}$-induced inflammatory cascades in microglia, neurons, and astrocytes. However, our current study does not include research on how A1AT could regulate the NLRP3-inflammasome complex. Further, it must be remarked that microglia might have partially contributed to the observed results due to the slight contamination of approximately 5%.

Our data demonstrate that NLRP3-inflammasome components are upregulated time-dependently following $Aβ_{1-42}$-stimulation. This can be blocked by A1AT application. NLRP3 is the sensor protein of the NLRP3-inflammasome complex, which explains its upregulation after $Aβ_{1-42}$-stimulation. ASC, in contrast, has the caspase activating and recruitment domain. In our experiments, ASC concentration on the mRNA and protein level was unchanged, indicating that $Aβ_{1-42}$ and A1AT mainly regulate NLRP3, but not ASC. We assume the total amount of ASC to be sufficient to lead to the NLRP3-ASC-complex formation and caspase 1 binding.

To further investigate the direct effect of A1AT on inflammasome-dependent IL-1β maturation, we used a specific NLRP3-inhibitor called MCC950. As previously shown by Coll et al., pre-treatment with MCC950 prevents complex formation of apoptosis-associated speck-like protein containing a CARD (ASC) and blocks the release of IL-1β in immunological active cells, without affecting priming of NLRP3 [46]. Furthermore, MCC950 stimulated Aβ phagocytosis in vitro, and it reduced Aβ accumulation in a mouse model of AD, which was associated with improved cognitive function [50]. In our studies, MCC950-pretreatment in cells co-treated with A1AT and Aβ did not further drop IL-1β protein expression. Thus, A1AT had no effect on protein expression, when NLRP3 was selectively blocked. We therefore conclude that A1AT reduces IL-1β by inhibiting NLRP3-inflammasome.

These observations not only clearly highlight the importance of astroglial-related pro-inflammatory processes in the brain and in particular during AD, but also point at A1AT as a potent antagonist in astrocyte-dependent inflammatory signaling.

Conclusion

We demonstrate that $Aβ_{1-42}$-stimulation results in an upregulation of NLRP3, caspase 1, and its cleavage products in astrocytes. A1AT time-dependently hampers $Aβ_{1-42}$-triggered neuroinflammation by attenuating NLRP3-inflammasome expression. This suggests that A1AT offers a therapeutic opportunity for AD treatment.

Additional files

Additional file 1: Figure S2. Cell counting revealed 95.2% astrocytes and 4.5% microglia. Approximately 0.4% of the cells remained undefined. $n = 12$. (PDF 336 kb)

Additional file 2: Figure S1. There are no oligodendrocytes contaminating the cell culture. Non-specific binding of Olig2 on astrocytes was observed. (PDF 316 kb)

Additional file 3: Figure S3. (A) Stimulation with $Aβ_{1-42}$ led to a concentration-dependent LDH-release. For further experiments, $Aβ_{1-42}$ (10 μM) was selected as the maximum concentration to not exceed 50% of cell death. (B) Ascending concentrations of A1AT did not affect cell viability. (C) Co-treatment with $Aβ_{1-42}$ and A1AT did not affect LDH-release, whereas LPS significantly increased LDH-release. Treatment with A1AT significantly reduced LDH-release in LPS-stimulated astrocytes. Data of $n = 6$ in triplicate represent mean ± SD. $*^{/a}p < 0.05$; $**^{/aa}p < 0.01$; $***^{/aaa}p < 0.001$, ns not significant compared control. (PDF 246 kb)

Additional file 4: Figure S4. No significant differences in cell metabolism were detected after increasing concentrations of $Aβ_{1-42}$ (A), A1AT (B) or co-treatment of A1AT, $Aβ_{1-42}$ and LPS (C). Data of $n = 6$ in triplicate represent mean ± SD, ns not significant compared to control. (PDF 260 kb)

Additional file 5: Figure S5. (A) Since there are no oligodendrocytes contaminating the cell culture, NLRP3-expression was not oligodendrocyte-induced. (B) NLRP3-expression was indeed induced by the few present microglia. But the majority of NLRP3-expression was not microglia-mediated. $n = 3$. (PDF 385 kb)

Additional file 6: Figure S6. (A) 10 μM $Aβ_{1-42}$ significantly increased caspase 1 mRNA. Co-treatment with A1AT blocked the increase of caspase 1 mRNA expression significantly. (B) Stimulation with $Aβ_{1-42}$ significantly increased IL-1β mRNA. Gene expression of IL-1β was significantly reduced with A1AT-co-treatment. (C) In contrast, $Aβ_{1-42}$-stimulation such as A1AT-treatment did not affect IL-18 mRNA expression. Data of $n = 6$ in triplicate represent mean ± SD. $*^{/a}p < 0.05$; $**^{/aa}p < 0.01$; $***^{/aaa}p < 0.001$ compared to control. (PDF 238 kb)

Abbreviations

A1AT: α1-antitrypsin; AD: Alzheimer's disease; ASC: Apoptosis-associated speck-like protein containing a CARD; Aβ: Amyloid β; CARD: Caspase activation and recruitment domain; Casp1: Caspase 1; CNS: Central nervous system; Ctr: Control; DMSO: Dimethylsulfoxid; GAPDH: Glycerinaldehyd-3-phosphate-dehydrogenase; GFAP: Glial fibrillary acidic protein; HPRT: Hypoxanthine phosphoribosyltransferase; Hsp90: Heat shock protein 90; Iba1: Ionized calcium binding adaptor molecule 1; ICC: Immunocytochemistry; IL-18: Interleukin-18; IL-1β: Interleukin-1β; LDH: Lactate dehydrogenase; LPS: Lipopolysaccharide; LRR: Leucine-rich repeat; NACHT: NAIP (NLP family apoptosis inhibitor protein), CIITA (class 2 transcription activator), HET-E (heterokaryon incompatibility), TEP1 (telomerase-associated protein 1); NLRP: NACHT, LRR, and PYD domains-containing; PCR: Polymerase chain reaction; Pos: Positive control; PYD: Pyrin domain; q-RT-PCR: Quantitative real-time PCR; RFU: Relative fluorescence units; sq-PCR: Semi-quantitative PCR

Funding

This work was supported by an internal grant from the Medical Clinic of the RWTH Aachen University (START grant, P. Habib). The funding body had no influence in the design of the study and was neither involved in collection, analysis, and interpretation of results nor in writing the manuscript.

Authors' contributions

JPB and PH conceived the conceptual idea, coordinated and designed the study, and corrected the manuscript. JPB and PH planned and supervised the experiments. TE conducted the experiments and drafted the manuscript. AS, PH, and TE performed the preparation of cells. MR assisted in the conduction of the experiments. TE, SNK, and AS carried out the western blots. AS and PH performed the statistical analysis. JPB, PH, and TE interpreted the results. CB, ARK, and JBS revised the manuscript and provided critical feedback. All authors read and approved the final manuscript.

Competing interests

All authors declare that they have no competing interests.

Author details

[1]Department of Neurology, RWTH Aachen University, Aachen, Germany.
[2]Institute of Neuroanatomy, RWTH Aachen University, Aachen, Germany.
[3]Department of Internal Medicine, Pulmonary and Critical Care Medicine, University Medical Center Giessen and Marburg, Marburg, Germany.
[4]JARA-Institute Molecular Neuroscience and Neuroimaging, Forschungszentrum Jülich GmbH and RWTH Aachen University, Aachen, Germany.

References

1. Prince M, Bryce R, Albanese E, Wimo A, Ribeiro W, Ferri CP. The global prevalence of dementia: a systematic review and metaanalysis. Alzheimers Dement. 2013;9(1):63–75.e62.
2. Brookmeyer R, Johnson E, Ziegler-Graham K, Arrighi HM. Forecasting the global burden of Alzheimer's disease. Alzheimers Dement. 2007;3(3):186–91.
3. Hirtz D, Thurman DJ, Gwinn-Hardy K, Mohamed M, Chaudhuri AR, Zalutsky R. How common are the "common" neurologic disorders? Neurology. 2007; 68(5):326–37.
4. Rosenberg PB, Lyketsos C. Mild cognitive impairment: searching for the prodrome of Alzheimer's disease. World Psychiatry. 2008;7(2):72–8.
5. Wilson RS, Leurgans SE, Boyle PA, Bennett DA. Cognitive decline in prodromal Alzheimer disease and mild cognitive impairment. Arch Neurol. 2011;68(3):351–6.
6. Ringman JM, Liang LJ, Zhou Y, Vangala S, Teng E, Kremen S, Wharton D, Goate A, Marcus DS, Farlow M, et al. Early behavioural changes in familial Alzheimer's disease in the dominantly inherited Alzheimer network. Brain. 2015;138(Pt 4):1036–45.
7. Bature F, Guinn BA, Pang D, Pappas Y. Signs and symptoms preceding the diagnosis of Alzheimer's disease: a systematic scoping review of literature from 1937 to 2016. BMJ Open. 2017;7(8):e015746.
8. Hsu D, Marshall GA. Primary and secondary prevention trials in Alzheimer disease: looking back, Moving Forward. Curr Alzheimer Res. 2017;14(4):426–40.
9. Karakaya T, Fusser F, Schroder J, Pantel J. Pharmacological treatment of mild cognitive impairment as a prodromal syndrome of Alzheimer's disease. Curr Neuropharmacol. 2013;11(1):102–8.
10. Dubois B, Zaim M, Touchon J, Vellas B, Robert P, Murphy MF, Pujadas-Navines F, Rainer M, Soininen H, Riordan HJ, et al. Effect of six months of treatment with V0191 in patients with suspected prodromal Alzheimer's disease. J Alzheimers Dis. 2012;29(3):527–35.
11. Caldwell CC, Yao J, Brinton RD. Targeting the prodromal stage of Alzheimer's disease: bioenergetic and mitochondrial opportunities. Neurotherapeutics. 2015;12(1):66–80.
12. Haass C, Selkoe DJ. Soluble protein oligomers in neurodegeneration: lessons from the Alzheimer's amyloid beta-peptide. Nat Rev Mol Cell Biol. 2007;8(2):101–12.
13. Baglioni S, Casamenti F, Bucciantini M, Luheshi LM, Taddei N, Chiti F, Dobson CM, Stefani M. Prefibrillar amyloid aggregates could be generic toxins in higher organisms. J Neurosci. 2006;26(31):8160–7.
14. Halle A, Hornung V, Petzold GC, Stewart CR, Monks BG, Reinheckel T, Fitzgerald KA, Latz E, Moore KJ, Golenbock DT. The NALP3 inflammasome is involved in the innate immune response to amyloid-beta. Nat Immunol. 2008;9(8):857–65.
15. Gold M, Dolga AM, Koepke J, Mengel D, Culmsee C, Dodel R, Koczulla AR, Bach JP. alpha1-antitrypsin modulates microglial-mediated neuroinflammation and protects microglial cells from amyloid-beta-induced toxicity. J Neuroinflammation. 2014;11:165.
16. Saresella M, La Rosa F, Piancone F, Zoppis M, Marventano I, Calabrese E, Rainone V, Nemni R, Mancuso R, Clerici M. The NLRP3 and NLRP1 inflammasomes are activated in Alzheimer's disease. Mol Neurodegen. 2016;11:23.
17. Glass CK, Saijo K, Winner B, Marchetto MC, Gage FH. Mechanisms underlying inflammation in neurodegeneration. Cell. 2010;140(6):918–34.
18. Kraft AD, Harry GJ. Features of microglia and neuroinflammation relevant to environmental exposure and neurotoxicity. Int J Environ Res Public Health. 2011;8(7):2980–3018.
19. Rama Rao KV, Kielian T. Neuron-astrocyte interactions in neurodegenerative diseases: role of neuroinflammation. Clin Exp Neuroimmunol. 2015;6(3):245–63.
20. Goedert M, Wischik CM, Crowther RA, Walker JE, Klug A. Cloning and sequencing of the cDNA encoding a core protein of the paired helical filament of Alzheimer disease: identification as the microtubule-associated protein tau. Proc Natl Acad Sci U S A. 1988;85(11):4051–5.
21. Goedert M, Spillantini MG, Jakes R, Rutherford D, Crowther RA. Multiple isoforms of human microtubule-associated protein tau: sequences and localization in neurofibrillary tangles of Alzheimer's disease. Neuron. 1989;3(4):519–26.
22. Song L, Pei L, Yao S, Wu Y, Shang Y. NLRP3 Inflammasome in neurological diseases, from functions to therapies. Front Cell Neurosci. 2017;11:63.
23. Agostini L, Martinon F, Burns K, McDermott MF, Hawkins PN, Tschopp J. NALP3 forms an IL-1beta-processing inflammasome with increased activity in Muckle-Wells autoinflammatory disorder. Immunity. 2004;20(3):319–25.
24. Heneka MT, Kummer MP, Stutz A, Delekate A, Schwartz S, Vieira-Saecker A, Griep A, Axt D, Remus A, Tzeng TC, et al. NLRP3 is activated in Alzheimer's disease and contributes to pathology in APP/PS1 mice. Nature. 2013; 493(7434):674–8.
25. Sutterwala FS, Haasken S, Cassel SL. Mechanism of NLRP3 inflammasome activation. Ann N Y Acad Sci. 2014;1319:82–95.
26. Martinon F. Detection of immune danger signals by NALP3. J Leukoc Biol. 2008;83(3):507–11.
27. Martinon F, Burns K, Tschopp J. The inflammasome: a molecular platform triggering activation of inflammatory caspases and processing of proIL-beta. Mol Cell. 2002;10(2):417–26.
28. Yatsiv I, Morganti-Kossmann MC, Perez D, Dinarello CA, Novick D, Rubinstein M, Otto VI, Rancan M, Kossmann T, Redaelli CA, et al. Elevated intracranial IL-18 in humans and mice after traumatic brain injury and evidence of neuroprotective effects of IL-18-binding protein after experimental closed head injury. J Cereb Blood Flow Metab. 2002;22(8):971–8.
29. Merrill JE, Benveniste EN. Cytokines in inflammatory brain lesions: helpful and harmful. Trends Neurosci. 1996;19(8):331–8.
30. Codolo G, Plotegher N, Pozzobon T, Brucale M, Tessari I, Bubacco L, de Bernard M. Triggering of inflammasome by aggregated alpha-synuclein, an inflammatory response in synucleinopathies. PLoS One. 2013;8(1):e55375.
31. Mao Z, Liu C, Ji S, Yang Q, Ye H, Han H, Xue Z. The NLRP3 Inflammasome is involved in the pathogenesis of Parkinson's disease in rats. Neurochem Res. 2017;42(4):1104–15.
32. Zhou Y, Lu M, Du RH, Qiao C, Jiang CY, Zhang KZ, Ding JH, Hu G. MicroRNA-7 targets nod-like receptor protein 3 inflammasome to modulate neuroinflammation in the pathogenesis of Parkinson's disease. Mol Neurodegener. 2016;11:28.
33. Zhang P, Shao XY, Qi GJ, Chen Q, Bu LL, Chen LJ, Shi J, Ming J, Tian B. Cdk5-dependent activation of neuronal Inflammasomes in Parkinson's disease. Mov Disord. 2016;31(3):366–76.
34. Yang F, Wang Z, Wei X, Han H, Meng X, Zhang Y, Shi W, Li F, Xin T, Pang Q, et al. NLRP3 deficiency ameliorates neurovascular damage in experimental ischemic stroke. J Cereb Blood Flow Metab. 2014;34(4):660–7.
35. Couturier J, Stancu IC, Schakman O, Pierrot N, Huaux F, Kienlen-Campard P, Dewachter I, Octave JN. Activation of phagocytic activity in astrocytes by reduced expression of the inflammasome component ASC and its implication in a mouse model of Alzheimer disease. J Neuroinflammation. 2016;13:20.
36. Dong Y, Benveniste EN. Immune function of astrocytes. Glia. 2001;36(2):180–90.
37. Akiyama H, Arai T, Kondo H, Tanno E, Haga C, Ikeda K. Cell mediators of inflammation in the Alzheimer disease brain. Alzheimer Dis Assoc Disord. 2000;14(Suppl 1):S47–53.
38. Salminen A, Ojala J, Suuronen T, Kaarniranta K, Kauppinen A. Amyloid-beta oligomers set fire to inflammasomes and induce Alzheimer's pathology. J Cell Mol Med. 2008;12(6A):2255–62.
39. Gold M, El Khoury J. beta-amyloid, microglia, and the inflammasome in Alzheimer's disease. Semin Immunopathol. 2015;37(6):607–11.
40. Freeman L, Guo H, David CN, Brickey WJ, Jha S, Ting JP. NLR members

NLRC4 and NLRP3 mediate sterile inflammasome activation in microglia and astrocytes. J Exp Med. 2017;214(5):1351–70.

41. Tumen J, Meyrick B, Berry L Jr, Brigham KL. Antiproteinases protect cultured lung endothelial cells from endotoxin injury. J Appl Physiol (1985). 1988; 65(2):835–43.

42. Libert C, Van Molle W, Brouckaert P, Fiers W. alpha1-Antitrypsin inhibits the lethal response to TNF in mice. J Immunol. 1996;157(11):5126–9.

43. Van Molle W, Libert C, Fiers W, Brouckaert P. Alpha 1-acid glycoprotein and alpha 1-antitrypsin inhibit TNF-induced but not anti-Fas-induced apoptosis of hepatocytes in mice. J Immunol. 1997;159(7):3555–64.

44. Janciauskiene S, Larsson S, Larsson P, Virtala R, Jansson L, Stevens T. Inhibition of lipopolysaccharide-mediated human monocyte activation, in vitro, by alpha1-antitrypsin. Biochem Biophys Res Commun. 2004;321(3):592–600.

45. Gold M, Koczulla AR, Mengel D, Koepke J, Dodel R, Dontcheva G, Habib P, Bach JP. Reduction of glutamate-induced excitotoxicity in murine primary neurons involving calpain inhibition. J Neurol Sci. 2015;359(1–2):356–62.

46. Coll RC, Robertson AA, Chae JJ, Higgins SC, Munoz-Planillo R, Inserra MC, Vetter I, Dungan LS, Monks BG, Stutz A, et al. A small-molecule inhibitor of the NLRP3 inflammasome for the treatment of inflammatory diseases. Nat Med. 2015;21(3):248–55.

47. Levy M, Thaiss CA, Elinav E. Taming the inflammasome. Nat Med. 2015;21(3):213–5.

48. Ismael S, Nasoohi S, Ishrat T. MCC950, the selective inhibitor of nucleotide oligomerization domain-like receptor Protein-3 inflammasome, protects mice against traumatic brain injury. J Neurotrauma. 2018;35(11):1294–303.

49. Perera AP, Fernando R, Shinde T, Gundamaraju R, Southam B, Sohal SS, Robertson AAB, Schroder K, Kunde D, Eri R. MCC950, a specific small molecule inhibitor of NLRP3 inflammasome attenuates colonic inflammation in spontaneous colitis mice. Sci Rep. 2018;8(1):8618.

50. Dempsey C, Rubio Araiz A, Bryson KJ, Finucane O, Larkin C, Mills EL, Robertson AAB, Cooper MA, O'Neill LAJ, Lynch MA. Inhibiting the NLRP3 inflammasome with MCC950 promotes non-phlogistic clearance of amyloid-beta and cognitive function in APP/PS1 mice. Brain Behav Immun. 2017;61:306–16.

51. Habib P, Dang J, Slowik A, Victor M, Beyer C. Hypoxia-induced gene expression of aquaporin-4, cyclooxygenase-2 and hypoxia-inducible factor 1alpha in rat cortical astroglia is inhibited by 17beta-estradiol and progesterone. Neuroendocrinology. 2014;99(3–4):156–67.

52. Kayed R, Head E, Thompson JL, McIntire TM, Milton SC, Cotman CW, Glabe CG. Common structure of soluble amyloid oligomers implies common mechanism of pathogenesis. Science. 2003;300(5618):486–9.

53. Habib P, Dreymueller D, Ludwig A, Beyer C, Dang J. Sex steroid hormone-mediated functional regulation of microglia-like BV-2 cells during hypoxia. J Steroid Biochem Mol Biol. 2013;138:195–205.

54. Dang J, Mitkari B, Kipp M, Beyer C. Gonadal steroids prevent cell damage and stimulate behavioral recovery after transient middle cerebral artery occlusion in male and female rats. Brain Behav Immun. 2011;25(4):715–26.

55. Johann S, Dahm M, Kipp M, Zahn U, Beyer C. Regulation of choline acetyltransferase expression by 17 beta-oestradiol in NSC-34 cells and in the spinal cord. J Neuroendocrinol. 2011;23(9):839–48.

56. Heneka MT, Golenbock DT, Latz E. Innate immunity in Alzheimer's disease. Nat Immunol. 2015;16(3):229–36.

57. Acosta C, Anderson HD, Anderson CM. Astrocyte dysfunction in Alzheimer disease. J Neurosci Res. 2017;95(12):2430–47.

58. Sofroniew MV. Molecular dissection of reactive astrogliosis and glial scar formation. Trends Neurosci. 2009;32(12):638–47.

59. Youm YH, Grant RW, McCabe LR, Albarado DC, Nguyen KY, Ravussin A, Pistell P, Newman S, Carter R, Laque A, et al. Canonical Nlrp3 inflammasome links systemic low-grade inflammation to functional decline in aging. Cell Metab. 2013;18(4):519–32.

60. Johann S, Heitzer M, Kanagaratnam M, Goswami A, Rizo T, Weis J, Troost D, Beyer C. NLRP3 inflammasome is expressed by astrocytes in the SOD1 mouse model of ALS and in human sporadic ALS patients. Glia. 2015;63(12):2260–73.

61. Heitzer M, Kaiser S, Kanagaratnam M, Zendedel A, Hartmann P, Beyer C, Johann S. Administration of 17beta-estradiol improves motoneuron survival and Down-regulates Inflammasome activation in male SOD1(G93A) ALS mice. Mol Neurobiol. 2017;54(10):8429–43.

62. Mortezaee K, Khanlarkhani N, Beyer C, Zendedel A. Inflammasome: its role in traumatic brain and spinal cord injury. J Cell Physiol. 2017;233(7):5160–9.

63. Zendedel A, Monnink F, Hassanzadeh G, Zaminy A, Ansar MM, Habib P, Slowik A, Kipp M, Beyer C. Estrogen attenuates local Inflammasome expression and activation after spinal cord injury. Mol Neurobiol. 2017;55(2):1364–75.

64. Debye B, Schmulling L, Zhou L, Rune G, Beyer C, Johann S. Neurodegeneration and NLRP3 inflammasome expression in the anterior thalamus of SOD1(G93A) ALS mice. Brain Pathol. 2016;28(1):14–27.

65. Bauernfeind FG, Horvath G, Stutz A, Alnemri ES, MacDonald K, Speert D, Fernandes-Alnemri T, Wu J, Monks BG, Fitzgerald KA, et al. Cutting edge: NF-kappaB activating pattern recognition and cytokine receptors license NLRP3 inflammasome activation by regulating NLRP3 expression. J Immunol. 2009;183(2):787–91.

66. Lee GS, Subramanian N, Kim AI, Aksentijevich I, Goldbach-Mansky R, Sacks DB, Germain RN, Kastner DL, Chae JJ. The calcium-sensing receptor regulates the NLRP3 inflammasome through Ca2+ and cAMP. Nature. 2012; 492(7427):123–7.

67. Toldo S, Seropian IM, Mezzaroma E, Van Tassell BW, Salloum FN, Lewis EC, Voelkel N, Dinarello CA, Abbate A. Alpha-1 antitrypsin inhibits caspase-1 and protects from acute myocardial ischemia-reperfusion injury. J Mol Cell Cardiol. 2011;51(2):244–51.

68. Aggarwal N, Korenbaum E, Mahadeva R, Immenschuh S, Grau V, Dinarello CA, Welte T, Janciauskiene S. alpha-Linoleic acid enhances the capacity of alpha-1 antitrypsin to inhibit lipopolysaccharide-induced IL-1beta in human blood neutrophils. Mol Med. 2016;22:680–93.

7

Ca^{2+}-dependent endoplasmic reticulum stress correlation with astrogliosis involves upregulation of KCa3.1 and inhibition of AKT/mTOR signaling

Zhihua Yu[1*], Fangfang Dou[3], Yanxia Wang[4], Lina Hou[1] and Hongzhuan Chen[1,2*]

Abstract

Background: The intermediate-conductance Ca^{2+}-activated K$^+$ channel KCa3.1 was recently shown to control the phenotype switch of reactive astrogliosis (RA) in Alzheimer's disease (AD).

Methods: KCa3.1 channels expression and cell localization in the brains of AD patients and APP/PS1 mice model were measured by immunoblotting and immunostaining. APP/PS1 mice and KCa3.1$^{-/-}$/APP/PS1 mice were subjected to Morris water maze test to evaluate the spatial memory deficits. Glia activation and neuron loss was measured by immunostaining. Fluo-4AM was used to measure cytosolic Ca^{2+} level in β-amyloid (Aβ) induced reactive astrocytes in vitro.

Results: KCa3.1 expression was markedly associated with endoplasmic reticulum (ER) stress and unfolded protein response (UPR) in both Aβ-stimulated primary astrocytes and brain lysates of AD patients and APP/PS1 AD mice. The KCa3.1 channel was shown to regulate store-operated Ca^{2+} entry (SOCE) through an interaction with the Ca^{2+} channel Orai1 in primary astrocytes. Gene deletion or pharmacological blockade of KCa3.1 protected against SOCE-induced Ca^{2+} overload and ER stress via the protein kinase B (AKT) signaling pathway in astrocytes. Importantly, gene deletion or blockade of KCa3.1 restored AKT/mechanistic target of rapamycin signaling both in vivo and in vitro. Consistent with these in vitro data, expression levels of the ER stress markers 78-kDa glucose-regulated protein and CCAAT/enhancer-binding protein homologous protein, as well as that of the RA marker glial fibrillary acidic protein were increased in APP/PS1 AD mouse model. Elimination of KCa3.1 in KCa3.1$^{-/-}$/APP/PS1 mice corrected these abnormal responses. Moreover, glial activation and neuroinflammation were attenuated in the hippocampi of KCa3.1$^{-/-}$/APP/PS1 mice, as compared with APP/PS1 mice. In addition, memory deficits and neuronal loss in APP/PS1 mice were reversed in KCa3.1$^{-/-}$/APP/PS1 mice.

Conclusions: Overall, these results suggest that KCa3.1 is involved in the regulation of Ca^{2+} homeostasis in astrocytes and attenuation of the UPR and ER stress, thus contributing to memory deficits and neuronal loss.

Keywords: Alzheimer's disease, Endoplasmic reticulum stress, Mouse model, Unfolded protein response, KCa3.1

* Correspondence: yuzhihua@shsmu.edu.cn; hongzhuan-chen@hotmail.com
[1]Department of Pharmacology and Chemical Biology, Shanghai Jiao Tong University School of Medicine, 280 South Chongqing Road, Shanghai 200025, China
Full list of author information is available at the end of the article

Introduction

Alzheimer's disease (AD) is a neurodegenerative disorder leading to a progressive decline in cognitive function that is characterized at the molecular level by β-amyloid (Aβ)-induced synaptic dysfunction, neuronal loss, tau pathology, and oxidative stress (Verkhratsky et al. 2010). Reactive gliosis, including microglia activation and astrocyte reactivation, plays a significant role in the pathogenesis of AD, both in transgenic rodent models and human patients [1, 2]. During the onset of AD, abnormal Aβ metabolism has a profound effect on the local community of neurons and glial cells in the central nervous system (CNS), while in the developmental stage of disease, the inflammatory response of reactive glial cells contributes to neuronal Ca^{2+} dysregulation.

In neurons, Aβ peptides induce neurotoxic effects that are mediated via deregulation of intracellular calcium ($[Ca^{2+}]_i$) homeostasis, which results in synaptic loss. However, little is known about the role of Aβ in the regulation of astrocytic Ca^{2+} homeostasis and subsequent pathological influences. Stimulation of Aβ in primary astrocytes triggers elevations in $[Ca^{2+}]_i$ and the formation of reactive oxygen species, which are associated with metabolic failure of astrocytes and may directly induce neuronal loss [3–5]. Notably, spontaneous $[Ca^{2+}]_i$ accumulation has been identified in astrocytes of amyloid precursor protein/presenilin 1 (APP/PS1) mice in vivo, independent of neuron hyperactivity [6].

The endoplasmic reticulum (ER) regulates $[Ca^{2+}]_i$ homeostasis and protein folding. Store-operated Ca^{2+} entry (SOCE) channels, which are complexes composed of stromal interaction molecule 1 (STIM1, an ER calcium sensor) and calcium release-activated calcium channel protein 1 (Orai1, a pore-forming protein), can be activated by the depletion of Ca^{2+} stores in the ER [7]. SOCE plays an essential role in the activation of non-excitable cells, including astrocytes and microglia, via triggering Ca^{2+} influx [8]. Disruption of protein folding in the ER triggers the unfolded protein response (UPR) via activation of three ER pathways: inositol-requiring enzyme 1 (IRE1), activating transcription factor 6 (ATF6), and PKR-like ER kinase (PERK) [9, 10]. The 78-kDa glucose-regulated protein (GRP78) dissociates from PERK, ATF6, and IRE1 during ER stress, and then initiates proapoptotic signaling via activation of the CCAAT/enhancer-binding protein homologous protein (CHOP). Accumulating evidence suggests that Ca^{2+}-dependent ER stress is correlated with reactive astrogliosis (RA) in both an AD mouse model and ischemic stroke [11, 12]. In addition, the intermediate-conductance Ca^{2+}-activated K^+ channel KCa3.1 is reported to be involved in cisplatin-initiated acute kidney injury [13] and the phenotypic switch of RA in ischemic stroke [12] via attenuation of ER stress.

KCa3.1 regulates K^+ efflux and subsequent Ca^{2+} entry via hyperpolarization of the membrane potential [14].

The KCa3.1 channel has been investigated as a therapeutic target in neurodegeneration diseases, vascular restenosis, and autoimmune diseases [15–17]. Our group recently reported that KCa3.1 inhibition significantly ameliorated neuronal loss, RA, microglial activation, and memory deficits in both APP/PS1 mice and senescence-accelerated mouse prone 8 (SAMP8) mice [15, 18]. KCa3.1 also plays a key role in mediating Aβ-induced RA, which includes activation of the mitogen-activated protein kinase/c-Jun N-terminal kinase (MAPK/JNK) signaling pathway and upregulation of reactive oxygen species (ROS) production. Blockade of KCa3.1 channels with triarylmethane-34 (TRAM-34) was shown to attenuate microglial-dependent indirect neurotoxicity in vivo, which emphasizes the role of Ca^{2+} in the process of neuroinflammation [19, 20]. Collectively, these data clearly demonstrate that KCa3.1 presents a potential therapeutic target in AD.

Therefore, the aim of present study was to elucidate the underlying mechanisms of Aβ-mediated ER stress in RA and to identify key molecules involved in the regulation of RA-induced neurotoxicity. We report that Ca^{2+} overload induces ER stress in primary astrocytes and ER stress is increased in AD patients and APP/PS1 AD mice. Blockade or gene deletion of KCa3.1 decreased SOCE-induced Ca^{2+} overload and attenuated ER stress via the protein kinase B/mechanistic target of rapamycin (AKT/mTOR) pathway in primary astrocytes, which is essential to protect neurons against RA-induced neurotoxicity. We also show that the absence of KCa3.1 channels attenuated ER stress, gliosis, neuroinflammation, memory deficits, and neuronal loss in KCa3.1$^{-/-}$/APP/PS1 mice. These results reveal an important correlation between KCa3.1 activation and cognitive deficits in APP/PS1 AD mice, suggesting that KCa3.1 may be an effective therapeutic target in AD.

Materials and methods
Brain autopsy material

Frozen tissues and paraffin-embedded brain slices from the hippocampi of postmortem human samples of control and AD patients were obtained from the Netherlands Brain Bank (Netherlands Institute for Neuroscience, Amsterdam, Netherlands). The Netherlands Brain Bank obtained written informed consent for brain autopsy specimens for research purposes after death. The Braak stage, neuropathological and clinical diagnoses, age and gender distributions, as well as diagnostic groupings are presented in Table 1. The frozen tissues were used to isolate proteins, and expression of proteins was evaluated by Western blotting as described below. Immunofluorescence was performed on 8-μm sections using antibodies against glial fibrillary acidic protein (GFAP), KCa3.1, Orai1, and GRP78 antibodies as described below.

Table 1 Demographic data of the cases studied

Diagnosis	Gender	Age	Braak stage	Amyloid	APOE	Analysis
Control-1	F	73	0	B	E3/E2	WB, IF
Control-2	M	99	2	C	–	WB, IF
Control-3	F	81	1	O	E3/E3	WB, IF
Control-4	F	89	2	B	–	WB, IF
Control-5	M	84	2	A	–	WB, IF
Control-6	F	64	0	A	E3/E2	WB, IF
AD-1	F	81	6	C	E4/E3	WB, IF
AD-2	F	62	6	C	E4/E3	WB, IF
AD-3	M	84	6	C	–	WB, IF
AD-4	F	72	6	C	E3/E2	WB, IF
AD-5	F	89	6	C	E4/E3	WB, IF
AD-6	M	96	6	C	–	WB, IF

Animals

Wild-type (WT) C57BL/6 mice (male, 25–30 g) were procured from the Shanghai Laboratory Animal Center (Shanghai, China). KCa3.1$^{-/-}$ mice were obtained from the Jackson Laboratory (Bar Harbor, ME, USA) and housed as described previously [18]. APP/PS1 transgenic mice (an AD model) were also purchased from the Jackson Laboratory (no. 003378) [15]. KCa3.1$^{-/-}$ mice were crossed with APP/PS1 mice and the offspring were intercrossed to generate mice with the KCa3.1$^{-/-}$/APP/PS1 genotype. Mouse cohorts of the four genotypes (WT, KCa3.1$^{-/-}$, KCa3.1$^{-/-}$/APP/PS1, and APP/PS1) were generated and used for behavioral analysis. The protocols of all animal experiments were approved by the Animal Experimentation Ethics Committee of Shanghai Jiao Tong University School of Medicine, Shanghai, China (ethics protocol number: A-2015-010).

Morris water maze test

The modified Morris water maze (MWM) test was performed as previously described [21]. Briefly, the test requires the mice to receive 5 consecutive training days (1 day with the visible platform and 4 days with the hidden platform) in a circular water tank (diameter = 80 cm; height = 50 cm) containing opaque water (22 °C, 25 cm deep). A spatial probe trial was performed on day 6 with no platform present. During the hidden platform training days, the mice were allowed to swim for 60 s to find the hidden platform (1 cm below the water surface). The platform was removed from the pool on day 6 of the spatial probe trial and the mice swam freely for 60 s. Performance of the MWM test was recorded using a video camera and analyzed using a video tracking system (Jiliang Software Technology Co., Ltd., Shanghai, China).

Immunostaining and data analysis

Confocal microscopy was performed as previously described [18]. Briefly, mice were anesthetized with chloral hydrate and perfused with 4% paraformaldehyde. Then, 10% goat serum in 0.01 M phosphate-buffered saline (PBS) was used to block 12-μm sections of the mice brain or 8-μm sections of the human brain for 1 h at room temperature. The brain sections were then incubated with the following primary antibodies: rabbit anti-GFAP (1:1000; Dako, Glostrup, Denmark), mouse anti-GFAP (1:200; Merck Millipore, Burlington, MA, USA), rabbit anti-NeuN (1:100; Merck Millipore, Burlington, MA, USA), rabbit anti-Iba1 (1:500; Wako Pure Chemical Industries, Ltd., Osaka, Japan), mouse anti-KCa3.1 (1:100; Alomone Labs, Ltd., Jerusalem, Israel), rabbit anti-GRP78 (1:100; Cell Signaling Technology, Inc., Beverly, MA, USA), mouse anti-NG2 (Sigma-Aldrich Corporation, St. Louis, MO, USA), and rabbit anti-Orai1 (1:100; Santa Cruz Biotechnology, Inc., Dallas, TX, USA). After incubation at 4 °C overnight, the brain sections were incubated with the respective Alexa Fluor® 488- or 568-conjugated secondary antibodies (1500; Invitrogen Corporation, Carlsbad, CA, USA). Images were collected using a TCS SP8 confocal laser scanning microscope (Leica Microsystems, Wetzlar, Germany) and processed with Leica LASAF Lite imaging software. The same reference position was used for each brain slice for quantification, i.e., between three and five random 0.01-mm^2 microscopic fields. Quantification was measured from six sections per brain (120-μm intervals) in a blinded manner.

Western blot analysis

Mice were anesthetized with chloral hydrate and perfused with saline. Mice or human brain tissues and cells were lysed on ice with radioimmunoprecipitation assay buffer (50 mM Tris (pH 7.4), 150 mM NaCl, 1% Triton X-100; 1% sodium deoxycholate, 0.1% sodium dodecyl sulfate, sodium orthovanadate, sodium fluoride, ethylenediaminetetraacetic acid, leupeptin) containing 1% phenylmethanesulfonyl fluoride. The supernatants were collected after centrifuging at 13,500 rpm for 5 min at 4 °C. Equal concentrations of proteins were separated by 10% (w/v) sodium dodecyl sulfate-polyacrylamide gel electrophoresis (SDS-PAGE) and then transferred to a polyvinylidene difluoride membrane, which was blocked for 1 h at room temperature (RT) in 5% milk in Tris-buffered saline with 0.05% Tween 20. The membrane was incubated with the following primary antibodies overnight at 4 °C: mouse anti-KCa3.1 (1:100; Alomone Labs, Ltd.), mouse anti-STIM1 (1:500; Santa Cruz Biotechnology, Inc.), rabbit anti-Orai1 (1:1000; Santa Cruz Biotechnology, Inc.), rabbit anti-GRP78, rabbit anti-mTOR, rabbit anti-phospho-mTOR (Ser2448), rabbit anti-phospho-PERK (Thr980), rabbit anti-phospho-eIF2α, rabbit anti-phospho-Akt (Thr308), rabbit anti-Akt, rabbit anti-phospho-4E-BP1, rabbit anti-phospho-p70 S6

Kinase, mouse anti-CHOP, rabbit anti-iNOS, rabbit anti-COX2 (1:1000; Cell Signaling Technology), and mouse anti-β-actin (1:1000; Beyotime Institute of Biotechnology, Haimen, China). The membranes were subsequently washed and incubated with anti-rabbit or anti-mouse HRP for 1 h at RT, and developed using BeyoECL solution (P0018A; Beyotime Institute of Biotechnology). Image Studio Lite Ver 5.2 software (LI-COR Biosciences, Lincoln, NE, USA) was used to analyze the proteins.

Enzyme-linked immunosorbent assay

ELISA was performed using the kit for TNF-α and IL-1β (Rapidbio Labs, Langka Trade Co. Ltd., Shanghai, China). The procedures were conducted according to manufacturer's protocols.

Preparation of oligomeric Aβ peptides

The oligomeric Aβ was prepared as described previously (Yi et al. 2016b). Briefly, monomeric peptide Aβ was dissolved in 1,1,1,3,3,3-hexafluoro 2-propanol (Sigma-Aldrich Corporation, St. Louis, MO, USA) at 1 mg/mL. The dried monomeric peptide Aβ was resolved in ddH$_2$O at a concentration of 100 mM and incubated at 4 °C for 24 h to induce aggregation.

Primary cultures

Primary cortical astrocyte cultures derived from newborn (P0–P2) WT or KCa3.1$^{-/-}$ C57BL/6 mouse brains were prepared from mixed glial cultures (10–14 days in vitro) as described previously [22]. Briefly, the cerebral cortices were dissociated into single cell suspensions. Dissociated single cells were grown in Dulbecco's modified Eagle's medium supplemented with 10% fetal bovine serum at 37 °C under an atmosphere of 5% CO$_2$. When the astrocytes grew to confluence (10–14 days later), the flasks were shaken overnight (200 rpm, 37 °C) to deplete microglia and oligodendrocytes. The purified astrocytes were then plated onto 6-well or 96-well plates in serum containing medium. Astrocytes were incubated with serum-free DMEM for 24 h after reaching confluence again, and then were treated with Aβ for different time periods before harvest. The culture medium (CM) was changed to neurobasal medium (NB) with B27 supplement (Invitrogen Corporation) after confluent astrocytes were serum-free for 24 h. The NB/B27-based WT and KCa3.1$^{-/-}$ astrocytes were then treated with 5 μM Aβ oligomer. The CM from the NB/B27-based cells was collected and used immediately. The primary cultured cortical neurons were isolated from neonatal (P0–P2) C57BL/6 mice and cultured as described previously (Yi et al. 2016b).

Neurite outgrowth assay

Cells were stained with primary antibody against microtubule-associated protein 2 (MAP2) and Alexa Fluor® 568-conjugated secondary antibody. A Cellomics Kinetic Scan reader (Thermo Fisher Scientific, Waltham, MA, USA) was used to scan the MAP2-positive cells. Extended Neurite Outgrowth software (Thermo Fisher Scientific) was used to analyze the data.

Calcium imaging

The purified astrocytes were plated in the wells of 96-well plates containing DMEM supplemented with 10% fetal bovine serum. After once again reaching confluence, the cells were incubated with the fluorescent calcium indicator Fluo-4AM (1.6 μM; Beyotime Institute of Biotechnology) for 25 min and then washed three times with 0.01 M PBS. Afterward, 2 μM ethylene glycol-bis (β-aminoethyl ether)-N,N,N',N'-tetraacetic acid was used to chelate the calcium in the DMEM and then 1 μM thapsigargin (Tg) was used to induce $[Ca^{2+}]_i$ release. After the $[Ca^{2+}]_i$ concentration was stable, 2 mM CaCl$_2$ solution was added to the DMEM to induce Ca^{2+} influx. Fluorescence signals were recorded and analyzed using a FlexStation 3 Multi-Mode Microplate Reader (Molecular Devices, Sunnyvale, CA, USA).

Statistical analysis

All data are presented as the mean ± standard error of the mean. Statistical analyses were performed using Prism software (GraphPad Software, Inc., La Jolla, CA, USA). Data were tested for Gaussian distribution with the Kolmogorov–Smirnov normality test and then analyzed by one-way analysis of variance (ANOVA) and the Dunnett's post-hoc test. Data were analyzed with an unpaired, two-tailed Student's t test when comparing between two groups or the non-parametric Mann–Whitney test was applied. Statistical significance was set at $p < 0.05$.

Results

Ca^{2+} overload induced ER stress in primary astrocytes and ER stress is increased in AD patients and APP/PS1 AD mice

ER stress induced by increased protein misfolding and upregulation of the UPR has been observed in AD patients and in an AD mouse model [23, 24]. Disruption of protein folding in the ER triggers the UPR via activation of three ER pathways: PERK, ATF6, and IRE1 [9, 10]. The GRP78 dissociates from PERK, ATF6, and IRE1 during ER stress, and then initiates proapoptotic signaling via activation of CHOP. GRP78 and CHOP protein levels were increased in both the brains of AD patients ($p < 0.05$, Fig. 1a, b) and the hippocampi of APP/PS1 mice ($p < 0.05$, Fig. 1c, d), as compared to control tissues.

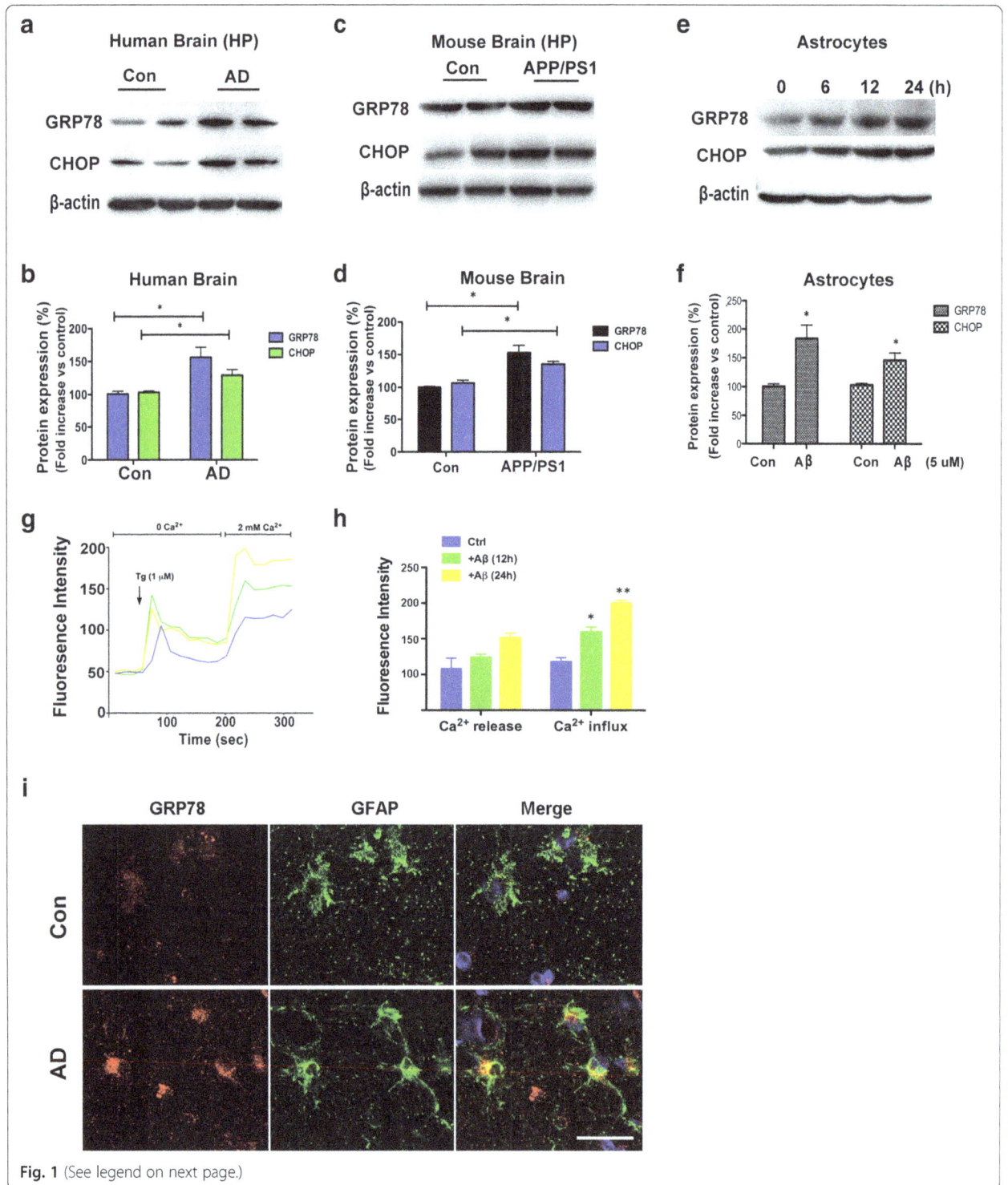

Fig. 1 (See legend on next page.)

(See figure on previous page.)
Fig. 1 Aβ induced intracellular Ca^{2+} overload by increasing SOCE, which resulted in ER stress. **a** Representative blots of GRP78 and CHOP from the hippocampi of postmortem human AD and age-matched controls. **b** Data are presented as the mean ± SEM ($n = 5$). The optical density (OD) values of GRP78 and CHOP were normalized to that of β-actin. *$p < 0.05$ vs. control brains (unpaired, two-tailed Student's t test). **c** Representative blots of GRP78 and CHOP from the hippocampi of APP/PS1 mice and age-matched controls. **d** Data are presented as the mean ± SEM ($n = 5$). The OD values of GRP78 and CHOP were normalized to that of β-actin. *$p < 0.05$ vs. control brains (unpaired, two-tailed Student's t test). **e** Primary astrocytes were treated with 5 μM Aβ for 6, 12, or 24 h. Then, the cell lysates were subjected to western blot analysis with β-actin as the loading control. **f** Data are presented as the mean ± SEM ($n = 3$). The OD values of GRP78 and CHOP were normalized to that of β-actin. *$p < 0.05$ vs. control cells (unpaired, two-tailed Student's t test). **g** Primary cultured astrocytes were treated with 5 μM Aβ for 12 or 24 h and then loaded with the Ca^{2+} sensitive dye Fluo-4AM at 37 °C for 30 min. Changes in $[Ca^{2+}]_i$ were monitored with a FlexStation 3 Multi-Mode Microplate Reader. Fluorescence intensities of $[Ca^{2+}]_i$ are shown. Fluorescence intensity was measured in the presence of 1 μM Tg with or without 2 mM Ca^{2+}. Tg thapsigargin. **h** Quantification (mean ± SEM) of fluorescence intensity. *$p < 0.05$, **$p < 0.01$ vs. control cells (one-way ANOVA followed by the Dunnett's multiple comparison test). **i** Upregulation of GRP78 in reactive astrocytes of AD patients. Double immunofluorescence staining of GRP78 with GFAP in brain sections of control and AD patients. Nuclei were stained blue with 4′,6-diamidino-2-phenylindole (DAPI). Scale bar: 25 μm

The Aβ oligomer was reported to disrupt Ca^{2+} homeostasis in the ER of astrocytes, which leads to ER stress-induced RA [25]. The addition of Aβ to primary cultured astrocytes significantly upregulated the protein levels of GRP78 and CHOP at 12 h, as compared with control cells, indicating that Aβ induces the activation of the UPR in astrocytes ($p < 0.05$, Fig. 1e, f). Overall, these data obtained from AD patients and APP/PS1 AD mouse models demonstrate a potential mechanism of ER stress activation in AD.

For evaluation of SOCE, Tg (1 μM), an ER Ca^{2+} ATPase pump blocker, was used to deplete ER Ca^{2+} stores. Without extracellular Ca^{2+} (0 Ca^{2+}), Tg-induced upregulation of $[Ca^{2+}]_i$ (first peak) showed no significant changes in response to treatment with 5 μM Aβ at 12 h, as compared to the control astrocytes ($p > 0.05$, Fig. 1g, h). However, SOCE, initiated by external Ca^{2+} (2 mM), was increased at 12 h ($p < 0.05$, Fig. 1g, h) and 24 h ($p < 0.01$, Fig. 1g, h) in response to treatment with 5 μM Aβ, as compared to control cells. Colocalization experiments were conducted using antibodies against the ER stress marker GRP78 and the RA marker GFAP. Double-labeled staining showed that GRP78 and GFAP colocalized in the AD brain tissues, but not the controls (Fig. 1i).

Aβ increases SOCE by upregulating KCa3.1 expression

The accumulation of Aβ oligomers and amyloid plaques in the brain is associated with neuroinflammation and abnormal gliosis, including reactive astrocytes [3, 26]. We previously reported that KCa3.1 gene deletion attenuated ER stress in RA via the c-Jun/JNK and MAPK/ERK signaling pathways in ischemic mice [12]. Given the key role of Aβ-induced astrocytes ER stress due to SOCE-induced Ca^{2+} overload, we then measured the expression levels of KCa3.1 and SOCE channels following stimulation by prolonged Aβ treatment. Although the exact SOCE molecular components in astrocytes are unknown, KCa3.1 and Orai1 have been reported as components of SOCE channels in some cell types [8, 27, 28]. Western blot analysis was performed to evaluate changes

in the expression profiles of KCa3.1, Orai1, and STIM1, which revealed upregulation of the KCa3.1 and Orai1 channels in response to stimulation with 5 μM Aβ for 24 h, as compared to the control group, whereas there was no obvious change in the expression of STIM1 (a regulator of KCa3.1 and Orai1) ($p > 0.05$, Fig. 2a, b). Colocalization experiments were conducted using specific KCa3.1 and Orai1 antibodies. Double-labeled staining showed that the colocalization of KCa3.1 and Orai1 was increased in primary astrocytes in response to stimulation with 5 μM Aβ for 24 h, as compared to the control cells (Fig. 2c).

We then further studied the potential relevance of KCa3.1 and Orai1 in the hippocampi of control and AD patients. The results showed that the expression levels of the KCa3.1 and Orai1 proteins, but not STIM1, were upregulated in the hippocampi of AD patients, as compared to the control tissues ($p < 0.05$, Fig. 2d, e). Colocalization experiments were conducted by immunostaining the brain tissues of AD patients and controls with specific KCa3.1 and Orai1 antibodies. Double-labeled staining showed that the colocalization of KCa3.1 and Orai1 was increased in the brain tissues of AD patients, as compared to the controls (Fig. 2f). In the present study, colocalization between KCa3.1 and astrocytes was detected in the brains of AD patients and 15-month-old APP/PS1 mice. Age-matched control humans and WT littermates were used as controls. In AD patients (Fig. 2g) and APP/PS1 mice (Fig. 2h), colocalization of KCa3.1 and GFAP+ astrocytes was increased, as compared to the controls.

Blockade or gene deletion of KCa3.1 decreased SOCE-induced Ca^{2+} overload and attenuated ER stress in primary astrocytes

The findings of the above experiments suggest that KCa3.1 plays a key role during the process of SOCE and in maintaining Ca^{2+} homeostasis in the ER. Pharmacological blockade of KCa3.1 was then conducted to further confirm the critical role of KCa3.1 in Ca^{2+}

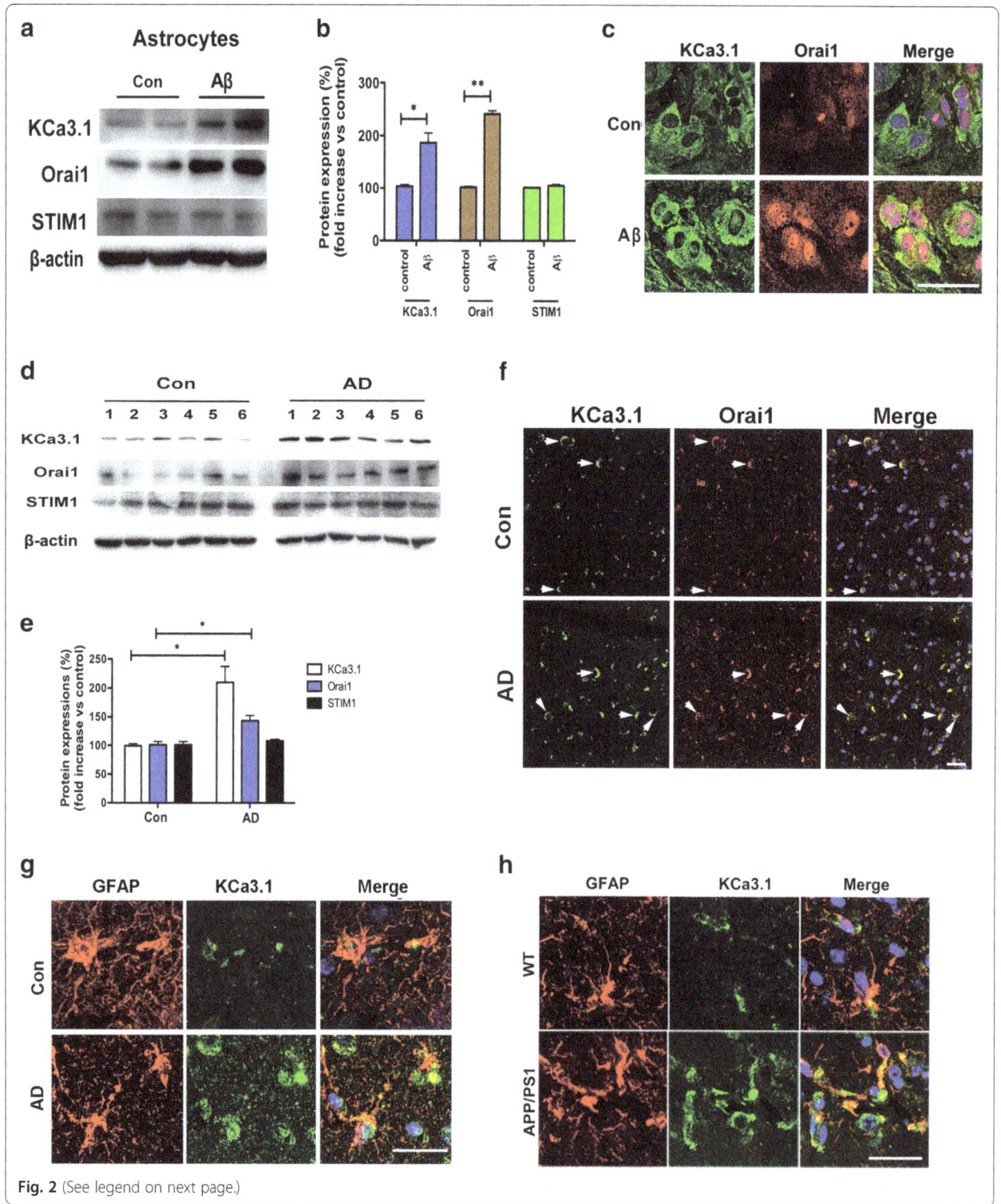

Fig. 2 (See legend on next page.)

homeostasis and stress in the ER. The results showed that blockade of KCa3.1 with 1 μM TRAM-34 attenuated Aβ-induced SOCE-induced Ca^{2+} overload, as compared with Aβ-treated cells ($p < 0.05$, Fig. 3a, b). Pharmacological blockade of KCa3.1 with 1 μM TRAM-34 decreased the upregulation of GRP78 and CHOP, which was induced by treatment with 5 μM Aβ for 24 h, indicating that blockade of KCa3.1 could inhibit prolonged UPR activation ($p < 0.05$, Fig. 3c, d). KCa3.1 gene deletion (KCa3.1$^{-/-}$) from astrocytes was stimulated with 5 μM Aβ or 1 μM Tg for 24 h, as compared to WT control cells. KCa3.1 gene deletion also decreased Aβ or Tg-induced upregulation of GRP78 ($p < 0.05$, Fig. 3e–h). As a critical transducer of the UPR, phosphorylation of PERK (p-PERK) was increased after stimulation with 5 μM Aβ or 1 μM Tg, but decreased in KCa3.1$^{-/-}$ astrocytes ($p < 0.05$, Fig. 3e–h). Similarly, prolonged UPR has been shown to activate eukaryotic initiation factor 2α (eIF2α), an important downstream signaling target, which was also increased in Aβ or Tg-treated WT astrocytes, but was restored to normal in KCa3.1$^{-/-}$ cells ($p < 0.05$, Fig. 3e–h).

WT and KCa3.1$^{-/-}$ astrocytes were used to test whether KCa3.1-mediated astrogliosis could induce dendritic damage. More dendritic damage was observed in the CM from 5 μM Aβ-stimulated WT astrocytes (WT/Aβ-CM) than in those treated with CM from WT astrocytes (WT/CM), as shown by immunofluorescent staining of the dendritic marker MAP2 (Fig. 3i). Incubation with WT/Aβ-CM decreased total neurite length ($p < 0.01$, Fig. 3j) and number of branch points ($p < 0.01$, Fig. 3k). Incubation with CM from 5 μM Aβ-stimulated KCa3.1$^{-/-}$ astrocytes (KCa3.1$^{-/-}$/Aβ-CM) attenuated the effect of WT/Aβ-CM by increasing total neurite length and the number of branch points ($p < 0.05$, Fig. 3j, k).

Levels of ER stress were decreased in the brains of APP/PS1 mice lacking KCa3.1

In the present study, APP/PS1 mice were crossed with KCa3.1$^{-/-}$ mice to study the role of KCa3.1 channels in RA-mediated neuronal toxicity. Offspring intercrossing generated mice with the WT, KCa3.1$^{-/-}$, APP/PS1, and KCa3.1$^{-/-}$/APP/PS1 genotypes.

Western blot analysis was conducted to identify changes in the expressions patterns of GRP78 and CHOP in the brains of 15-month-old APP/PS1 and KCa3.1$^{-/-}$/APP/PS1 mice, as compared with WT and KCa3.1$^{-/-}$ controls. Similar to previous results in AD patients (Fig. 1a, b), GRP78 and CHOP levels were significantly increased in APP/PS1 mice, as compared to WT and KCa3.1$^{-/-}$ mice ($p < 0.05$, Fig. 4a–c), while the expression levels of GRP78 and CHOP were significantly decreased in KCa3.1$^{-/-}$/APP/PS1 mice, as compared to APP/PS1 mice ($p < 0.05$, Fig. 4a–c).

It was reported that upregulation of GRP78 and phosphorylation of eIF2α in response to Aβ-induced ER stress contributed to RA in the AD mouse model and primary cultured astrocytes [25]. We then investigated whether KCa3.1 gene deletion could prevent changes in GRP78 expression levels in the astrocytes of APP/PS1 mice. To compare the response in astrocytes specifically, immunofluorescence was used to quantify GRP78 levels in GFAP$^+$ astrocytes in the hippocampi of WT, KCa3.1$^{-/-}$, APP/PS1, and KCa3.1$^{-/-}$/APP/PS1 mice. In the hippocampi of APP/PS1 mice, GRP78 expression was increased in GFAP$^+$ astrocytes, as compared to that of WT controls ($p < 0.01$, Fig. 4d, e). Meanwhile, hippocampal GRP78 immunoreactivity levels of KCa3.1$^{-/-}$/APP/PS1 mice were significantly decreased, as compared to that of APP/PS1 mice ($p < 0.01$, Fig. 4d, e).

Gene deletion of KCa3.1 activated the AKT/mTOR pathway

The foregoing data suggest that KCa3.1 gene deletion prevented activation of the UPR and attenuated astrocytic ER stress in an in vivo AD model. However, the signaling intermediates linking KCa3.1 and astrocytic ER stress in AD remain unknown. Given the reported relationship between the phosphatidylinositol 3-phosphate kinase/Akt pathway and ER stress [29], we tested whether the AKT pathway is involved in KCa3.1-mediated astrocytes ER stress.

Decreased phosphorylation of AKT (p-AKT) (Thr308) was observed in the brain tissues of AD patients ($p < 0.01$, Fig. 5a, b). In primary cultured astrocytes, Aβ treatment for 1 h significantly decreased p-AKT (Thr308) levels without inducing changes in

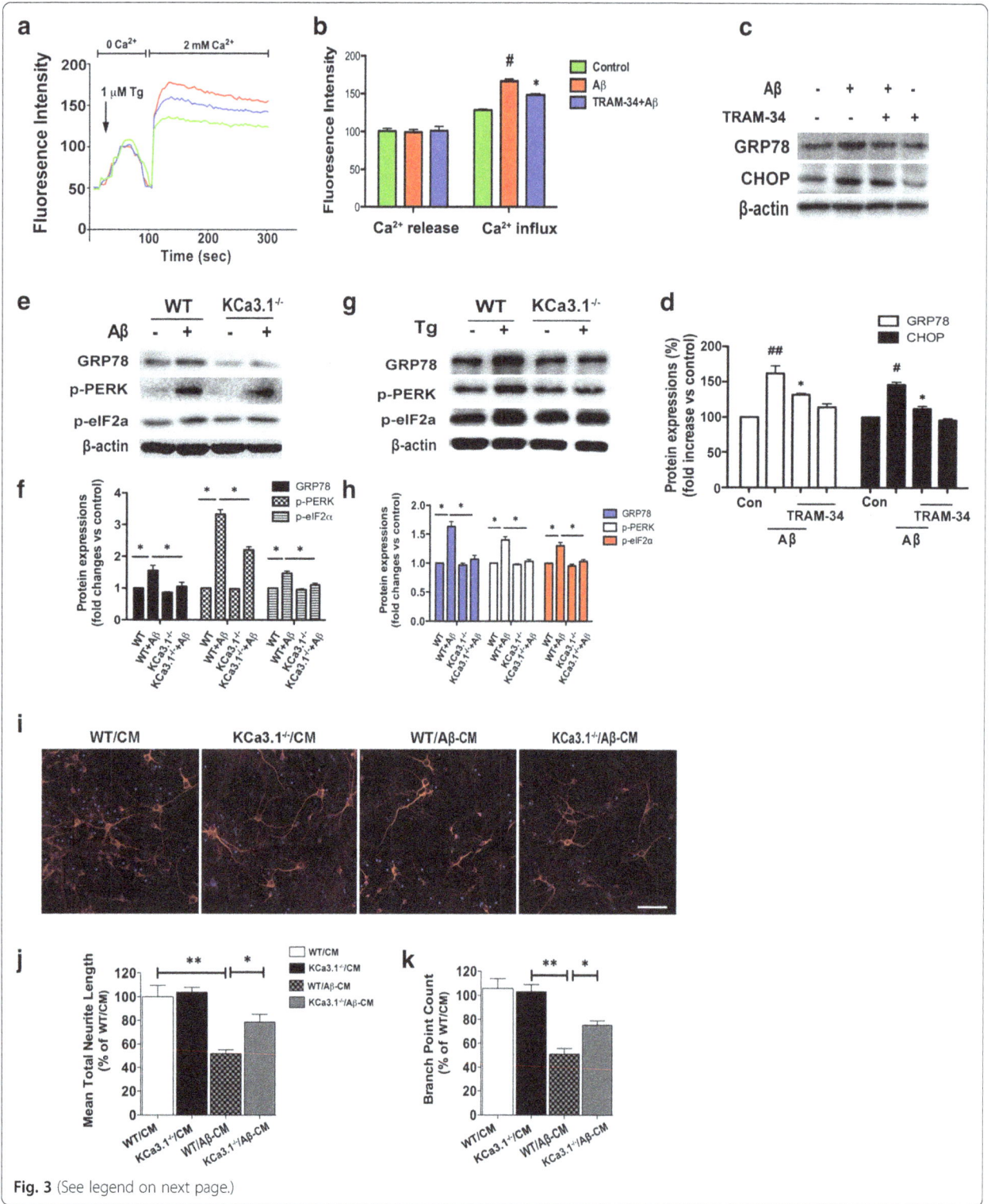

Fig. 3 (See legend on next page.)

(See figure on previous page.)

Fig. 3 KCa3.1 involved in astrocytes SOCE and ER stress. **a** Primary cultured astrocytes were treated with 5 μM Aβ for 12 h with or without pretreatment of the KCa3.1 blocker TRAM-34 (1 μM). Fluorescence intensities of [Ca^{2+}]$_i$ are shown. Fluorescence intensity was measured in the presence of 1 μM Tg with or without 2 mM Ca^{2+}. **b** Data are presented as the mean ± SEM ($n = 10$). #$p < 0.05$ vs. control, *$p < 0.05$ vs. Aβ-treated cells. **c** Astrocytes were treated with 5 μM Aβ for 24 h with or without 1 μM TRAM-34 pretreatment, and then subjected to western blot analysis with antibodies against GRP78 and CHOP. **d** Data are presented as the mean ± SEM ($n = 3$). #$p < 0.05$, ##$p < 0.01$ vs. controls, *$p < 0.05$ vs. Aβ-treated cells. One-way ANOVA followed by the Dunnett's multiple comparison test vs. control cells. **e, g** Representative images of GRP78, p-PERK, and phosphorylated eIF2α (p-eIF2α) in KCa3.1$^{-/-}$ astrocytes, responses to 5 μM Aβ (**e**) or 1 μM Tg (**g**) vs. WT cells. **f, h** Mean values of GRP78, p-PERK, and p-eIF2α relative to β-actin. Data are presented as the mean ± SEM ($n = 3$). *$p < 0.05$ (unpaired, two-tailed Student's t test). **i–k** Levels of the dendritic marker MAP2 were compared between neurons treated with CM from WT astrocytes (WT/CM), CM from KCa3.1$^{-/-}$ astrocytes (KCa3.1$^{-/-}$/CM), CM from 5 μM Aβ stimulated WT astrocytes (WT/Aβ-CM), or CM from 5 μM Aβ stimulated KCa3.1$^{-/-}$ astrocytes (KCa3.1$^{-/-}$/Aβ-CM). **i** Neuron dendrites were immunostained with MAP2 and nuclei were stained with DAPI (blue). Scale bars: 25 μm. Neurite length (**j**) and branch point counts (**k**) were analyzed by extended neurite outgrowth bioapplication software. Data represent mean ± SEM ($n = 3$). *$p < 0.05$, **$p < 0.001$ (one-way ANOVA followed by the Dunnett's multiple comparison test). *Tg* thapsigargin, *Con* control, *WT* wild-type

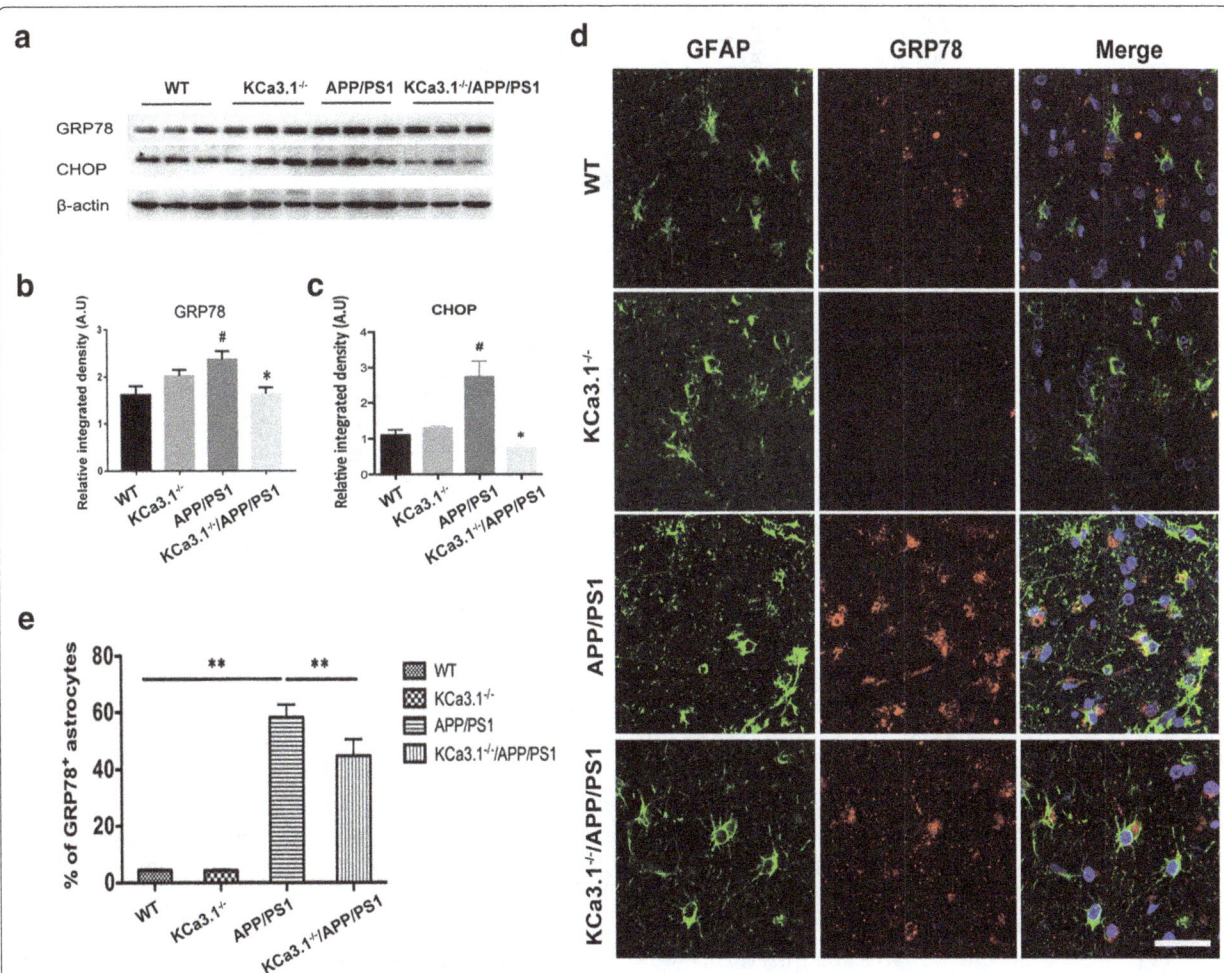

Fig. 4 KCa3.1 contributes to increased ER stress in APP/PS1 mice. **a** Western blot analysis of GRP78 and CHOP protein levels in hippocampal extracts of 15-month-old WT, KCa3.1$^{-/-}$, APP/PS1, and KCa3.1$^{-/-}$/APP/PS1 mice. **b, c** Data are presented as the mean ± SEM ($n = 3–5$). The OD values of GRP78 (**b**) and CHOP (**c**) were normalized to that of β-actin. #$p < 0.05$ vs. WT, *$p < 0.05$ vs. APP/PS1 (one-way ANOVA followed by the Dunnett's multiple comparison test). **d** Double immunofluorescence staining of GFAP with GRP78 in CA1 areas of the mouse hippocampus. DAPI (blue) was used to label nuclei. **e** Quantification of the percentage of GRP78$^+$ cells colabeled with GFAP. **$p < 0.01$ vs. control group (one-way ANOVA followed by the Dunnett's multiple comparison test) ($n = 4$). Scale bar: 25 μm. *WT* wild-type

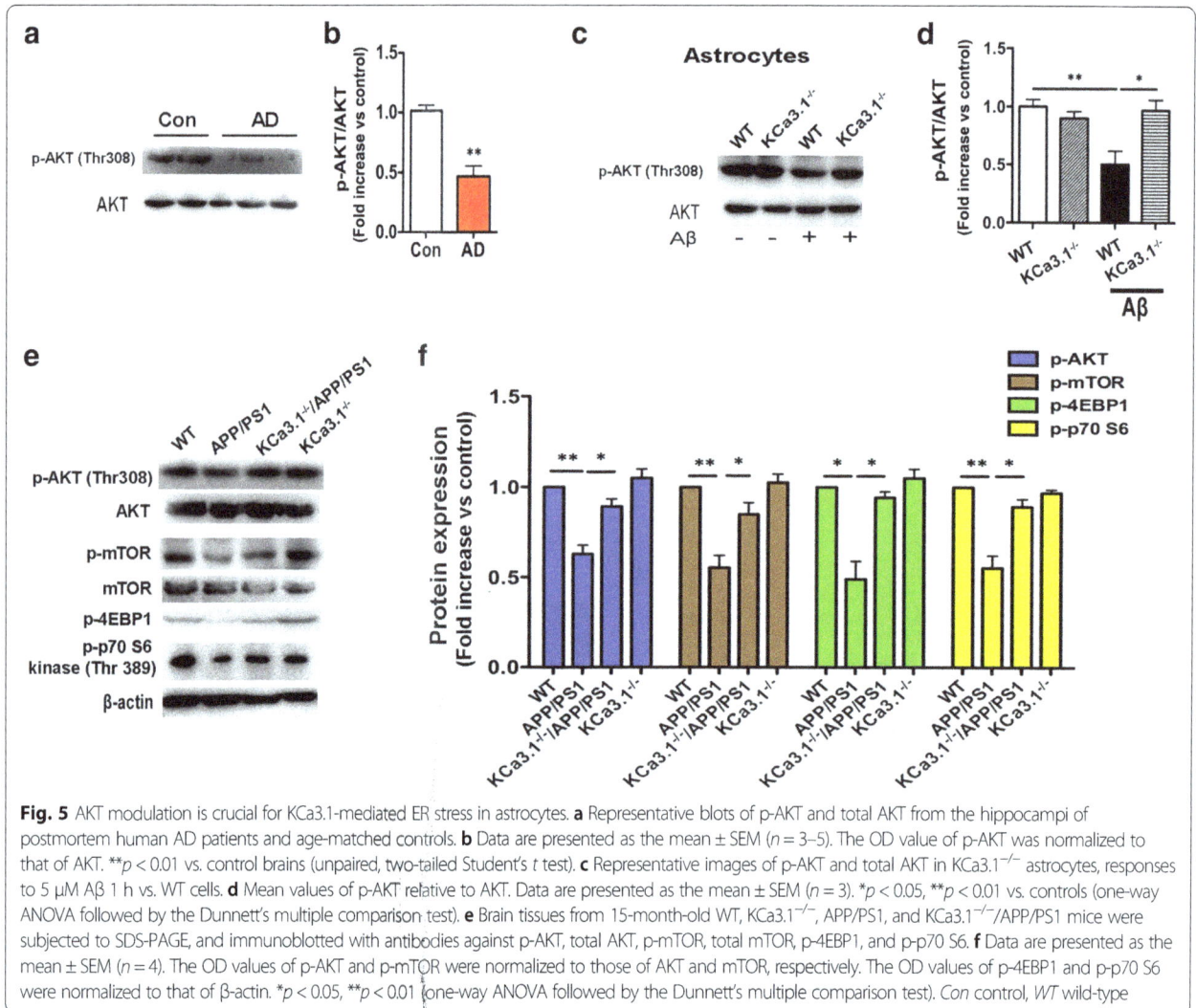

Fig. 5 AKT modulation is crucial for KCa3.1-mediated ER stress in astrocytes. **a** Representative blots of p-AKT and total AKT from the hippocampi of postmortem human AD patients and age-matched controls. **b** Data are presented as the mean ± SEM ($n = 3$–5). The OD value of p-AKT was normalized to that of AKT. **$p < 0.01$ vs. control brains (unpaired, two-tailed Student's t test). **c** Representative images of p-AKT and total AKT in KCa3.1$^{-/-}$ astrocytes, responses to 5 µM Aβ 1 h vs. WT cells. **d** Mean values of p-AKT relative to AKT. Data are presented as the mean ± SEM ($n = 3$). *$p < 0.05$, **$p < 0.01$ vs. controls (one-way ANOVA followed by the Dunnett's multiple comparison test). **e** Brain tissues from 15-month-old WT, KCa3.1$^{-/-}$, APP/PS1, and KCa3.1$^{-/-}$/APP/PS1 mice were subjected to SDS-PAGE, and immunoblotted with antibodies against p-AKT, total AKT, p-mTOR, total mTOR, p-4EBP1, and p-p70 S6. **f** Data are presented as the mean ± SEM ($n = 4$). The OD values of p-AKT and p-mTOR were normalized to those of AKT and mTOR, respectively. The OD values of p-4EBP1 and p-p70 S6 were normalized to that of β-actin. *$p < 0.05$, **$p < 0.01$ (one-way ANOVA followed by the Dunnett's multiple comparison test). *Con* control, *WT* wild-type

total AKT ($p < 0.01$, Fig. 5c, d), while KCa3.1 gene deletion (KCa3.1$^{-/-}$) inhibited the decrease in p-AKT (Thr308) after Aβ treatment ($p < 0.05$, Fig. 5c, d).

We then examined whether KCa3.1 gene deletion would activate the AKT/mTOR pathway in an in vivo AD model. Consistent with the in vitro results (Fig. 5c), p-AKT (Thr308) levels were decreased in the brain tissue of APP/PS1 mice ($p < 0.01$, Fig. 5e, f). KCa3.1 gene deletion in APP/PS1 mice (KCa3.1$^{-/-}$/APP/PS1) attenuated p-AKT (Thr308) suppression ($p < 0.05$, Fig. 5e, f). Importantly, the phosphorylation of mTOR, a kinase that regulates cell survival, was decreased in the brain tissue of APP/PS1 mice ($p < 0.01$, Fig. 5e, f). mTOR suppression, in turn, suppressed its downstream proteins, including phosphorylated 4EBP1 (p-4EBP1) and p70 S6 kinase (p-p70 S6 kinase) (Thr389), while KCa3.1 gene deletion in APP/PS1 mice (KCa3.1$^{-/-}$/APP/PS1) attenuated the suppression of mTOR phosphorylation ($p < 0.05$, Fig. 5e, f).

Attenuation of neuronal loss in APP/PS1 mice lacking KCa3.1

It was reported that blockade of KCa3.1 significantly reduced neuronal loss and memory deficits in both APP/PS1 mice and SAMP8 mice [11, 15]. Given that neuronal loss and decreased expression of synaptic proteins are likely correlated with the severity of AD [30], we compared expression levels of the neuron marker NeuN in the brain tissues of APP/PS1 mice with those of KCa3.1$^{-/-}$/APP/PS1 mutants. Immunostaining analysis revealed that NeuN-positive neuron levels were decreased in the CA1 areas of the hippocampi of APP/PS1 mice, as compared with that in the WT group, while KCa3.1 gene deletion in APP/PS1 mice (KCa3.1$^{-/-}$/APP/PS1) attenuated the decrease of NeuN staining ($p < 0.05$, Fig. 6a, b).

Decreased glial activation and neuroinflammation in APP/PS1 mice lacking KCa3.1

Both reactive astrocytes and microglial activation are predominant pathological features of AD [31]. Immunostaining

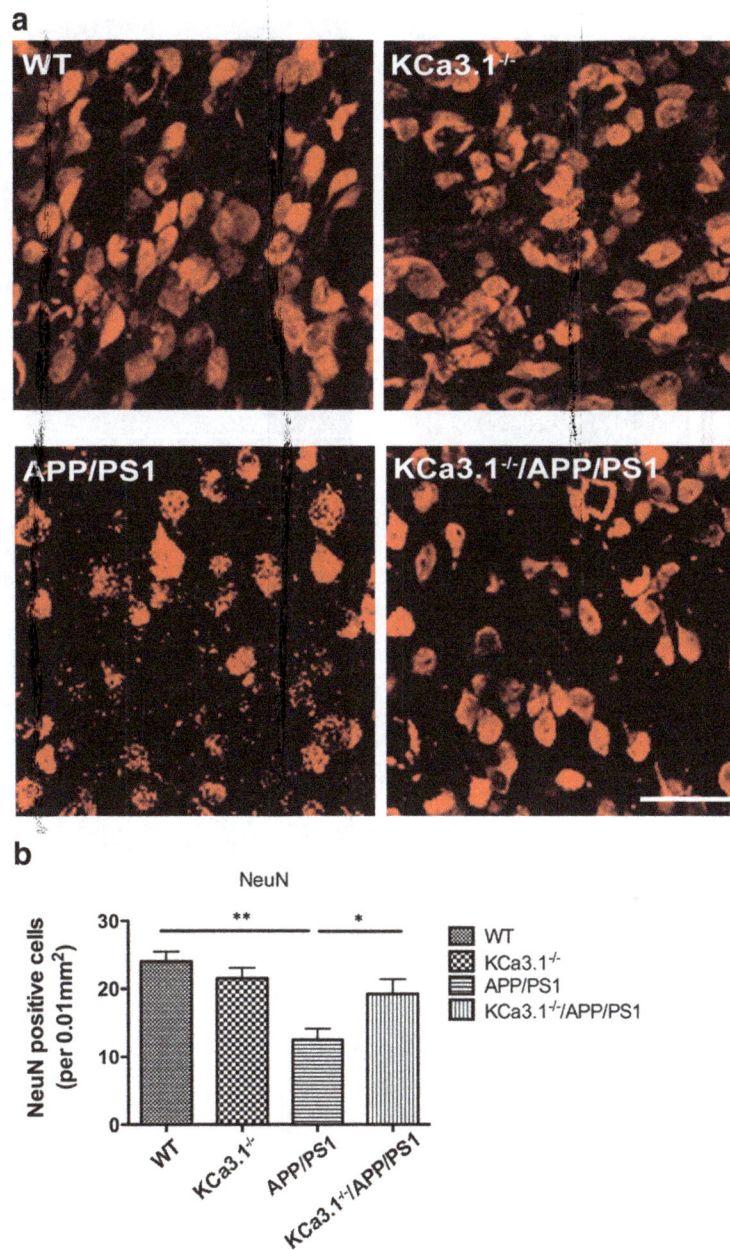

Fig. 6 Neuronal loss is rescued in brains of KCa3.1$^{-/-}$/APP/PS1 mice. **a** Immunofluorescence analysis of NeuN levels in the hippocampi of 15-month-old WT, KCa3.1$^{-/-}$, APP/PS1, and KCa3.1$^{-/-}$/APP/PS1 mice. **b** Quantification of neuron number/0.01 mm^2 in the hippocampus ($n = 6$). Data are presented as the mean ± SEM. *$p < 0.05$, **$p < 0.01$ (one-way ANOVA followed by Dunnett's post-hoc test). Scale bars: 25 μm

of the RA marker GFAP was measured to determine whether KCa3.1 gene deletion affects RA in APP/PS1 mice. Immunostaining of GFAP$^+$ astrocytes was increased in the brains of APP/PS1 mice, as compared with WT mice ($p < 0.05$, Fig. 7a, b), while KCa3.1 gene deletion in APP/PS1 mice (KCa3.1$^{-/-}$/APP/PS1) attenuated the increase in immunostaining of GFAP$^+$ astrocytes ($p < 0.05$, Fig. 7a, b).

We also investigated whether KCa3.1 gene deletion attenuates microglial activation in APP/PS1 mice by measuring expression levels of the microglia marker Iba1. Our data show that the content of Iba1$^+$ microglia was increased in the brains of APP/PS1 mice, as compared with that of WT mice ($p < 0.01$, Fig. 7c, d). KCa3.1 gene deletion in APP/PS1 mice (KCa3.1$^{-/-}$/APP/PS1) attenuated the increase of Iba1$^+$ microglia immunostaining ($p < 0.01$, Fig. 7c, d). Both the RA and microglia activation results suggest that, while brains of APP/PS1 mice show increased glial responses, these responses are attenuated in the brains of KCa3.1$^{-/-}$/APP/PS1 mice.

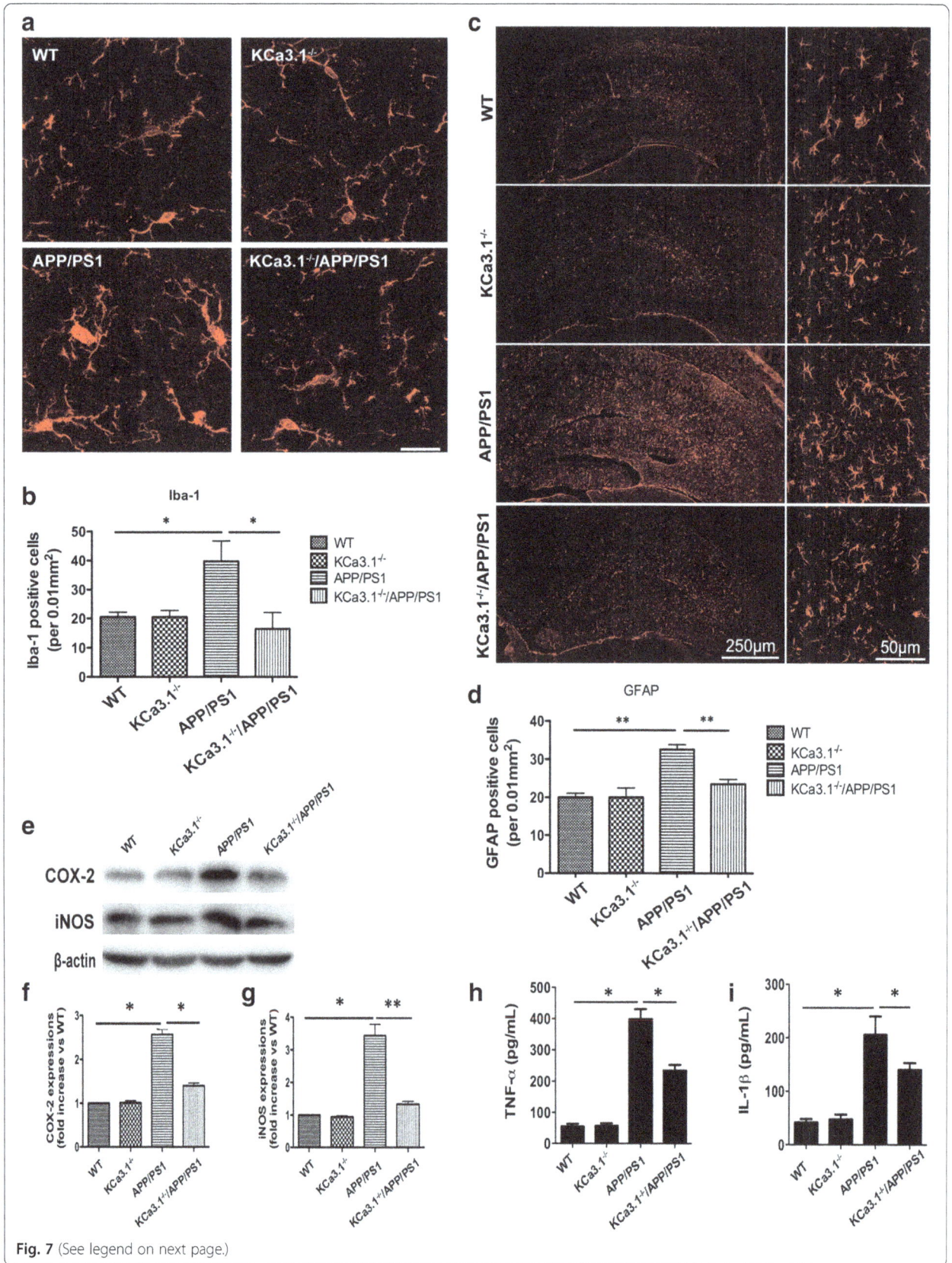

Fig. 7 (See legend on next page.)

(See figure on previous page.)

Fig. 7 Decreased neuroinflammation in brains of KCa3.1$^{-/-}$/APP/PS1 mice. **a** Levels of activated microglia in CA1 areas of the mouse hippocampus were analyzed by immunostaining of the microglia marker Iba1. **b** Quantification of activated microglia number/0.01 mm^2 in the hippocampus ($n = 3$). Data are presented as the mean ± SEM. *$p < 0.05$ (one-way ANOVA followed by Dunnett's post-hoc test). Scale bars: 25 μm. **c** Levels of reactive astrocytes in the CA1 area of the mouse hippocampus were analyzed by immunostaining of the astrocyte marker GFAP. **d** Quantification of reactive astrocytes number/0.01 mm^2 in the hippocampus ($n = 3$). Data are presented as the mean ± SEM. *$p < 0.05$ (one-way ANOVA followed by Dunnett's post-hoc test). Scale bars: 25 μm. **e–i** Gene deletion of KCa3.1 attenuated expression and release of inflammatory mediators in the brains of KCa3.1$^{-/-}$/APP/PS1 mice. **e–g** Western blots showing protein expressions of COX-2 (**e**, **f**) and iNOS (**e**, **g**) proteins. **f**, **g** Data are presented as the mean ± SEM ($n = 3$). *$p < 0.05$, **$p < 0.01$ (One-way ANOVA followed by the Dunnett's multiple comparison test). **h**, **i** Measurement of TNF-α (**h**) and IL-1β (**i**) released by ELISA in homogenated cortex of WT, KCa3.1$^{-/-}$, APP/PS1, and KCa3.1$^{-/-}$/APP/PS1 mice. Data represent mean ± SEM. *$p < 0.05$ (one-way ANOVA followed by the Dunnett's multiple comparison test)

KCa3.1 deficiency in KCa3.1$^{-/-}$/APP/PS1 mice attenuated the upregulation of COX-2 (Fig. 7e, f) and iNOS (Fig. 7e, g), compared with APP/PS1 mice. Levels of TNF-α and IL-1β in brain homogenates from WT, KCa3.1$^{-/-}$, APP/PS1, and KCa3.1$^{-/-}$/APP/PS1 group mice were measured by ELISA experiments (Fig. 7h, i). Levels of both TNF-α and IL-1β released were attenuated in the KCa3.1$^{-/-}$/APP/PS1 group compared with the APP/PS1 group. Together, these findings indicate that elimination of KCa3.1 ameliorated the pathological hallmarks of AD in KCa3.1$^{-/-}$/APP/PS1 mice, such as neuronal loss, microglial activation, RA, and neuroinflammation.

KCa3.1 elimination in APP/PS1 mice rescues spatial memory deficits

In this study, the MWM spatial memory test was used to determine whether loss of KCa3.1 had any effect on cognitive deficits in APP/PS1 mice. With the use of a hidden platform during the MWM test, 15-month-old APP/PS1 mice showed memory deficits, as compared with WT mice ($p < 0.01$, Fig. 8a). Furthermore, the KCa3.1$^{-/-}$/APP/PS1 mice showed improved spatial learning and memory, as compared with the APP/PS1 mice (Fig. 8a). In the spatial probe trial without an escape platform, significantly more KCa3.1$^{-/-}$/APP/PS1 mice were able to cross the target quadrant, as compared to APP/PS1 mice ($p < 0.05$, Fig. 8b), and spent more time and swam for greater distances in the target quadrant ($p < 0.05$, Fig. 8c, d). In conclusion, the MWM test results indicate that APP/PS1 mice present significant spatial memory deficits and that elimination of KCa3.1 channels ameliorates these deficits.

Discussion

The importance of KCa3.1 channels to CNS function is underscored by a series of studies implicating KCa3.1 in various diseases, including stroke/ischemia [32, 33], AD [11, 15], traumatic brain injury [34], and spinal cord injury [35]. These studies showed that upregulation of KCa3.1 activity can profoundly influence CNS pathology. Here, we report that KCa3.1 expression was markedly associated with ER stress and UPR in both Aβ-stimulated primary astrocytes and brain lysates of AD patients and APP/PS1

AD mice. Gene deletion or blockade of KCa3.1 attenuated SOCE-induced Ca^{2+} overload and ER stress, which regulates the AKT/mTOR pathway in RA to protect neurons from RA-induced neurotoxicity. Elimination of KCa3.1 can attenuate ER stress, neuronal loss, gliosis, neuroinflammation, and memory deficits observed in KCa3.1$^{-/-}$/APP/PS1 mice. These data suggest that KCa3.1 presents an effective therapeutic target in AD.

Astrocytes perform brain homeostatic maintenance within the CNS and communicate with neighboring neurons and glial cells via [Ca^{2+}]$_i$ signals triggering the gliotransmitters release [3, 36–40]. SOCE channels, composed of STIM1 and Orai1 (pore-forming proteins), can be activated by the depletion of Ca^{2+} stores in the ER [7]. SOCE, which is regulated by STIM1/2 and Orai1, plays an essential role in the activation of non-excitable cells, including astrocytes and microglia, via triggering Ca^{2+} influx [8]. STIM1/2 and Orai1 were identified as key molecules of SOCE in cortical and spinal astrocytes. SOCE plays an important role in the production of the cytokines tumor necrosis factor-α and interluekin-6 in spinal astrocytes in response to lipopolysaccharides [27].

Dysfunctional astrocytic Ca^{2+} signaling is involved in many pathological states, such as epilepsy and ischemia [41]. Vincent et al. reported that astrocytic Ca^{2+} homeostasis is disrupted in AD. Disruption of Ca^{2+} signaling of astrocytes was found both in the transgenic mouse models of AD in vivo and in Aβ-stimulated primary astrocytes in vitro [5, 6, 42, 43]. ER stress plays an important role in the pathophysiology of various neurodegenerative diseases, including AD [44, 45]. Much evidence indicates a relationship between ER stress and Aβ-induced cytotoxicity in the post-mortem brain tissue of AD patients and AD mouse models [45, 46]. Aβ severely disrupts ER function and induces ER stress in neurons and glial cells [25, 47]. Stimulation with Aβ oligomers deregulated ER Ca^{2+} homeostasis in neurons and astrocytes, which resulted in misfolding of proteins in the ER. Excessive and prolonged activation of ER stress may initiate apoptosis by regulation of several key proteins, including CHOP, caspase-12, and JNK, which can further aggravate Aβ cytotoxicity [48]. ER stress is reportedly linked with some inflammation signaling networks, suggesting that ER stress activation may be involved in the

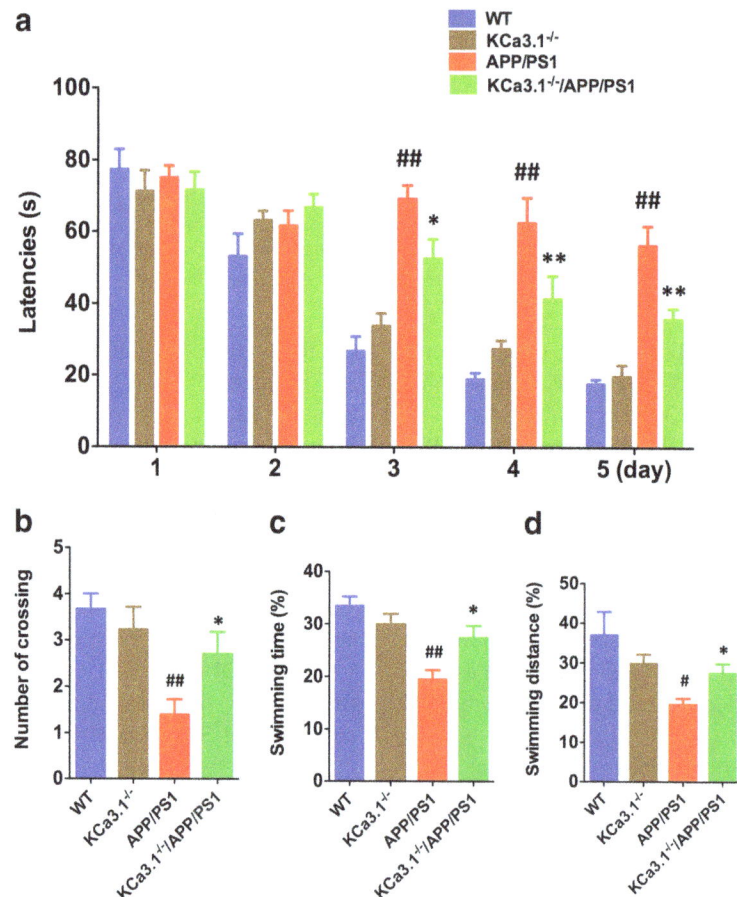

Fig. 8 Elimination of KCa3.1 in APP/PS1 mice rescues spatial memory deficits in the MWM test. MWM testing of 15-month-old WT, KCa3.1$^{-/-}$, APP/PS1, and KCa3.1$^{-/-}$/APP/PS1 mice was performed as described in the "Materials and methods" section. **a** Escape latency. **b** Number of crossing the target quadrant by each group during the probe trials (no platform). **c** Percentage of swimming time spent in the target quadrant by each group during the probe trials (no platform). **d** Percentage of swimming distance spent in the target quadrant by each group during the probe trials (no platform). Data are presented as the mean ± SEM ($n = 10–12$). #$p < 0.05$, ##$p < 0.01$ vs. WT mice. *$p < 0.05$, **$p < 0.01$ vs. APP/PS1 mice. *WT* wild-type

neuroinflammatory response [49]. In the present study, we demonstrated that Aβ induced ER stress in astrocytes in vitro and observed upregulation of CHOP and the ER-resident chaperone GRP78 [50, 51]. Gene deletion and pharmacological blockade of KCa3.1 were shown to attenuate the upregulation of UPR hallmarks.

APP/PS1 mice present the prodromal phase of AD, reflecting memory and spatial learning deficits, as assessed by performance in the MWM test [52]. Soluble and plaque-associated Aβ peptides, which are present starting at 6 months of age in APP/PS1 transgenic mice, induce ER stress and sequent phosphorylation of PERK and eIF2a, which are closely associated with the pathogenesis of AD [53]. The results of the present study also suggest that elimination of KCa3.1 ameliorated the pathological hallmarks of AD in KCa3.1$^{-/-}$/APP/PS1 mice, such as neuronal loss, microglial activation, and RA. Although the mechanisms underlying the attenuation of memory deficits by elimination of KCa3.1 are

not well known, they are likely associated with the decreased pathological markers noted in KCa3.1$^{-/-}$/APP/PS1 mice, as compared with APP/PS1 mice. Similar to AD patients, phosphorylation of GRP78 and eIF2α is upregulated in the brains of APP/PS1 mice [54]. APP/PS1 mice also showed decreased expression of NeuN and increased expression of Iba1 and GFAP, suggesting the presence of neuronal loss, microglial activation, and RA. Brain slices of KCa3.1$^{-/-}$/APP/PS1 mice showed significantly lower levels of these markers than those of APP/PS1 mice, indicating that KCa3.1 gene deletion might involve in ER stress and, thereby, attenuate neuronal loss and glia inflammation in AD mice.

Our data also demonstrated that KCa3.1 regulates ER stress via the downstream AKT/mTOR signaling pathway during RA in AD. We observed that Aβ decreased the activation of AKT by decreasing AKT phosphorylation in primary astrocytes. Interestingly, KCa3.1 elimination prevented Aβ-mediated loss of AKT activation via upregulation of AKT phosphorylation at Thr308. Growing evidence indicates that the mTOR signaling pathway plays a vital role during apoptosis and autophagy. Our results show that Aβ represses the phosphorylation of AKT, mTOR, p70 S6 kinase, and 4EBP1, and that a decrease in the phosphorylation of AKT led to UPR activation. The postmortem brain samples from patients with and without AD were also evaluated. The results indicate that KCa3.1 expression and activation of UPR-associated proteins are increased in the brains of AD patients.

Conclusions

Overall, these data indicate that KCa3.1 plays an important role in the process of Ca^{2+} homeostasis in the ER and that KCa3.1 upregulation involves in the activation of the UPR pathway, which subsequently leads to neurodegeneration in AD.

Abbreviations

ATF6: Activating transcription factor 6; CHOP: CCAAT enhancer-binding protein homologous protein; DAPI: 4′,6-Diamidino-2-phenylindole; EGTA: Ethylene glycol-bis(β-aminoethyl ether)-N,N,N′,N′-tetraacetic acid; GFAP: Glial fibrillary acidic protein; GRP78: 78 kDa glucose-regulated protein; IRE1: Inositol-requiring enzyme 1; KCa3.1: Intermediate-conductance calcium-activated potassium channel; PERK: PKR-like ER kinase; ROS: Reactive oxygen species; SAMP8: Senescence-accelerated mouse prone 8; SDS-PAGE: Sodium dodecyl sulfate-polyacrylamide gel electrophoresis; SOCE: Store-operated $Ca^2$$^+$ entry; TRAM-34: 1-((2-Chlorophenyl) (diphenyl) methyl)-1H–pyrazole; UPR: Unfolded protein response

Acknowledgments
We thank International Science Editing for editing the paper.

Funding
This work was supported by Science and Technology Commission of Shanghai Municipality grant 16ZR1418700, National Natural Science Foundation of China grant 81773699. The authors declare that the research was conducted in the absence of any commercial or financial relationships that could be construed as a potential conflict of interest.

Authors' contributions
ZY supervised the entire project, designed the research, and wrote the paper. HC conceived and designed the experiments, interpreted and analyzed the data, and supervised all the experimental procedure. FD and QL conceived and designed the experiments, performed the research interpreted, and analyzed the data. YW and LH performed the research and analyzed the data. All authors read and approved the final manuscript.

Competing interests
The authors declare that they have no competing interests.

Author details
[1]Department of Pharmacology and Chemical Biology, Shanghai Jiao Tong University School of Medicine, 280 South Chongqing Road, Shanghai 200025, China. [2]Shanghai University of Traditional Chinese Medicine, Shanghai 201203, China. [3]Basic Research Department, Shanghai Geriatric Institute of Chinese Medicine, Shanghai 200031, China. [4]Experimental Teaching Center of Basic Medicine, Shanghai Jiao Tong University School of Medicine, Shanghai 200025, China.

References
1. Mhatre SD, et al. Microglial malfunction: the third rail in the development of Alzheimer's disease. Trends Neurosci. 2015;38(10):621–36.
2. Zamanian JL, et al. Genomic analysis of reactive astrogliosis. J Neurosci. 2012;32(18):6391–410.
3. Verkhratsky A, et al. Astrocytes in Alzheimer's disease. Neurotherapeutics. 2010;7(4):399–412.
4. Abeti R, Abramov AY, Duchen MR. Beta-amyloid activates PARP causing astrocytic metabolic failure and neuronal death. Brain. 2011;134(Pt 6): 1658–72.
5. Abramov AY, Canevari L, Duchen MR. Changes in intracellular calcium and glutathione in astrocytes as the primary mechanism of amyloid neurotoxicity. J Neurosci. 2003;23(12):5088–95.
6. Kuchibhotla KV, et al. Synchronous hyperactivity and intercellular calcium waves in astrocytes in Alzheimer mice. Science. 2009;323(5918):1211–5.
7. Majewski L, Kuznicki J. SOCE in neurons: signaling or just refilling? Biochim Biophys Acta. 2015;1853(9):1940–52.
8. Michaelis M, et al. STIM1, STIM2, and Orai1 regulate store-operated calcium entry and purinergic activation of microglia. Glia. 2015;63(4):652–63.
9. Yang W, Paschen W. Unfolded protein response in brain ischemia: a timely update. J Cereb Blood Flow Metab. 2016;36(12):2044–50.
10. Gupta MK, et al. GRP78 interacting partner Bag5 responds to ER stress and protects cardiomyocytes from ER stress-induced apoptosis. J Cell Biochem. 2016;117(8):1813–21.
11. Yi M, et al. The potassium channel KCa3.1 constitutes a pharmacological target for astrogliosis associated with ischemia stroke. J Neuroinflammation. 2017;14(1):203.
12. Yu Z, et al. KCa3.1 inhibition switches the astrocyte phenotype during astrogliosis associated with ischemic stroke via endoplasmic reticulum stress and MAPK signaling pathways. Front Cell Neurosci. 2017;11:319.
13. Chen CL, et al. Blockade of KCa3.1 potassium channels protects against cisplatin-induced acute kidney injury. Arch Toxicol. 2016;90(9):2249–60.
14. Grossinger EM, et al. Ca(2+)-dependent regulation of NFATc1 via KCa3.1 in inflammatory Osteoclastogenesis. J Immunol. 2018;200(2):749–57.
15. Wei T, et al. The potassium channel KCa3.1 represents a valid pharmacological target for astrogliosis-induced neuronal impairment in a mouse model of Alzheimer's disease. Front Pharmacol. 2016;7:528.
16. Kahlfuss S, et al. Immunosuppression by N-methyl-D-aspartate receptor antagonists is mediated through inhibition of Kv1.3 and KCa3.1 channels in T cells. Mol Cell Biol. 2014;34(5):820–31.
17. Chiang EY, et al. Potassium channels Kv1.3 and KCa3.1 cooperatively and compensatorily regulate antigen-specific memory T cell functions. Nat Commun. 2017;8:14644.
18. Yi M, et al. KCa3.1 constitutes a pharmacological target for astrogliosis associated with Alzheimer's disease. Mol Cell Neurosci. 2016;76:21–32.
19. Maezawa I, et al. Microglial KCa3.1 channels as a potential therapeutic target for Alzheimer's disease. Int J Alzheimers Dis. 2012;2012:868972.
20. Kaushal V, et al. The Ca2+–activated K+ channel KCNN4/KCa3.1 contributes to microglia activation and nitric oxide-dependent neurodegeneration. J Neurosci. 2007;27(1):234–44.
21. Morris R. Developments of a water-maze procedure for studying spatial learning in the rat. J Neurosci Methods. 1984;11(1):47–60.
22. Yu Z, et al. Targeted inhibition of KCa3.1 attenuates TGF-beta-induced reactive astrogliosis through the Smad2/3 signaling pathway. J Neurochem. 2014;130(1):41–9.
23. Hoozemans JJ, et al. The unfolded protein response is activated in Alzheimer's disease. Acta Neuropathol. 2005;110(2):165–72.
24. Matus S, Glimcher LH, Hetz C. Protein folding stress in neurodegenerative diseases: a glimpse into the ER. Curr Opin Cell Biol. 2011;23(2):239–52.
25. Alberdi E, et al. Ca(2+) -dependent endoplasmic reticulum stress correlates

with astrogliosis in oligomeric amyloid beta-treated astrocytes and in a model of Alzheimer's disease. Aging Cell. 2013;12(2):292–302.

26. Sofroniew MV. Reactive astrocytes in neural repair and protection. Neuroscientist. 2005;11(5):400–7.

27. Gao X, et al. STIMs and Orai1 regulate cytokine production in spinal astrocytes. J Neuroinflammation. 2016;13(1):126.

28. Kraft R. STIM and ORAI proteins in the nervous system. Channels (Austin). 2015;9(5):245–52.

29. Selvaraj S, et al. Neurotoxin-induced ER stress in mouse dopaminergic neurons involves downregulation of TRPC1 and inhibition of AKT/mTOR signaling. J Clin Invest. 2012;122(4):1354–67.

30. Pozueta J, Lefort R, Shelanski ML. Synaptic changes in Alzheimer's disease and its models. Neuroscience. 2013;251:51–65.

31. Osborn LM, et al. Astrogliosis: an integral player in the pathogenesis of Alzheimer's disease. Prog Neurobiol. 2016;144:121–41.

32. Chen YJ, et al. The potassium channel KCa3.1 constitutes a pharmacological target for neuroinflammation associated with ischemia/reperfusion stroke. J Cereb Blood Flow Metab. 2016;36(12):2146–61.

33. Chen YJ, et al. Blood-brain barrier KCa3.1 channels: evidence for a role in brain Na uptake and edema in ischemic stroke. Stroke. 2015;46(1):237–44.

34. Yi M, et al. Activation of the KCa3.1 channel contributes to traumatic scratch injury-induced reactive astrogliosis through the JNK/c-Jun signaling pathway. Neurosci Lett. 2016;624:62–71.

35. Bouhy D, et al. Inhibition of the Ca(2)(+)-dependent K(+) channel, KCNN4/KCa3.1, improves tissue protection and locomotor recovery after spinal cord injury. J Neurosci. 2011;31(45):16298–308.

36. Bezzi P, et al. Prostaglandins stimulate calcium-dependent glutamate release in astrocytes. Nature. 1998;391(6664):281–5.

37. Bezzi P, et al. Astrocytes contain a vesicular compartment that is competent for regulated exocytosis of glutamate. Nat Neurosci. 2004;7(6):613–20.

38. Fellin T, et al. Neuronal synchrony mediated by astrocytic glutamate through activation of extrasynaptic NMDA receptors. Neuron. 2004;43(5):729–43.

39. Jourdain P, et al. Glutamate exocytosis from astrocytes controls synaptic strength. Nat Neurosci. 2007;10(3):331–9.

40. Volterra A, Meldolesi J. Astrocytes, from brain glue to communication elements: the revolution continues. Nat Rev Neurosci. 2005;6(8):626–40.

41. Nedergaard M, Rodriguez JJ, Verkhratsky A. Glial calcium and diseases of the nervous system. Cell Calcium. 2010;47(2):140–9.

42. Stix B, Reiser G. Beta-amyloid peptide 25-35 regulates basal and hormone-stimulated Ca2+ levels in cultured rat astrocytes. Neurosci Lett. 1998;243(1–3):121–4.

43. Chow SK, et al. Amyloid beta-peptide directly induces spontaneous calcium transients, delayed intercellular calcium waves and gliosis in rat cortical astrocytes. ASN Neuro. 2010;2(1):e00026.

44. Verkhratsky A. Physiology and pathophysiology of the calcium store in the endoplasmic reticulum of neurons. Physiol Rev. 2005;85(1):201–79.

45. Hoozemans JJ, et al. The unfolded protein response is activated in pretangle neurons in Alzheimer's disease hippocampus. Am J Pathol. 2009;174(4):1241–51.

46. Li HH, et al. Humic acid increases amyloid beta-induced cytotoxicity by induction of ER stress in human SK-N-MC neuronal cells. Int J Mol Sci. 2015;16(5):10426–42.

47. Umeda T, et al. Intraneuronal amyloid beta oligomers cause cell death via endoplasmic reticulum stress, endosomal/lysosomal leakage, and mitochondrial dysfunction in vivo. J Neurosci Res. 2011;89(7):1031–42.

48. Nakagawa T, et al. Caspase-12 mediates endoplasmic-reticulum-specific apoptosis and cytotoxicity by amyloid-beta. Nature. 2000;403(6765):98–103.

49. Lin JH, Walter P, Yen TS. Endoplasmic reticulum stress in disease pathogenesis. Annu Rev Pathol. 2008;3:399–425.

50. Ruiz A, Matute C, Alberdi E. Endoplasmic reticulum Ca(2+) release through ryanodine and IP(3) receptors contributes to neuronal excitotoxicity. Cell Calcium. 2009;46(4):273–81.

51. Ruiz A, Matute C, Alberdi E. Intracellular Ca2+ release through ryanodine receptors contributes to AMPA receptor-mediated mitochondrial dysfunction and ER stress in oligodendrocytes. Cell Death Dis. 2010;1:e54.

52. Webster SJ, et al. Using mice to model Alzheimer's dementia: an overview of the clinical disease and the preclinical behavioral changes in 10 mouse models. Front Genet. 2014;5:88.

53. Savonenko A, et al. Episodic-like memory deficits in the APPswe/PS1dE9 mouse model of Alzheimer's disease: relationships to beta-amyloid deposition and neurotransmitter abnormalities. Neurobiol Dis. 2005;18(3):602–17.

54. Hetz C, Mollereau B. Disturbance of endoplasmic reticulum proteostasis in neurodegenerative diseases. Nat Rev Neurosci. 2014;15(4):233–49.

8

HIV-1 Nef-induced lncRNA AK006025 regulates CXCL9/10/11 cluster gene expression in astrocytes through interaction with CBP/P300

Feng Zhou[1,2*†], Xiaomei Liu[2†], Dongjiao Zuo[2†], Min Xue[3†], Lin Gao[2], Ying Yang[2], Jing Wang[2], Liping Niu[2], Qianwen Cao[2], Xiangyang Li[2], Hui Hua[2], Bo Zhang[2], Minmin Hu[2], Dianshuai Gao[4], Kuiyang Zheng[2], Yoshihiro Izumiya[5] and Renxian Tang[2*] (iD)

Abstract

Background: HIV-associated neurocognitive disorder (HAND) is a neurodegenerative disease associated with persistent neuroinflammation and subsequent neuron damage. Pro-inflammatory factors and neurotoxins from activated astrocytes by HIV-1 itself and its encoded proteins, including the negative factor (Nef), are involved in the pathogenesis of HAND. This study was designed to find potential lncRNAs that regulate astrocyte functions and inflammation process.

Methods: We performed microarray analysis of lncRNAs from primary mouse astrocytes treated with Nef protein. Top ten lncRNAs were validated through real-time PCR analysis. Gene ontology (GO) and KEGG pathway analysis were applied to explore the potential functions of lncRNAs. RIP and ChIP assays were performed to demonstrate the mechanism of lncRNA regulating gene expression.

Results: There were 638 co-upregulated lncRNAs and 372 co-downregulated lncRNAs in primary astrocytes treated with Nef protein for both 6 h and 12 h. GO and KEGG pathway analysis showed that the biological functions of top differential-expressed mRNAs were associated with inflammatory cytokines and chemokine. Knockdown of lncRNA AK006025, not AK138360, inhibited significantly CXCL9, CXCL10 (IP-10), and CXCL11 expression in astrocytes treated with Nef protein. Mechanism study showed that AK006025 associated with CBP/P300 was enriched in the promoter of CXCL9, CXCL10, and CXCL11 genes.

Conclusions: Our findings uncovered the expression profiles of lncRNAs and mRNAs in vitro, which might help to understand the pathways that regulate astrocyte activation during the process of HAND.

Keywords: HIV-associated neurocognitive disorder, HIV-1, lncRNAs, Astrocytes, Nef, CBP/P300

* Correspondence: zhoufeng-xzmc@163.com; tangrenxian-t@163.com
†Feng Zhou, Xiaomei Liu, Dongjiao Zuo and Min Xue contributed equally to this work.
[1]Jiangsu Key Laboratory of Brain Disease Bioinformation, Research Center for Biochemistry and Molecular Biology, Xuzhou Medical University, Xuzhou 221004, Jiangsu, People's Republic of China
[2]Jiangsu Key Laboratory of Immunity and Metabolism, Department of Pathogen Biology and Immunology and Laboratory of Infection and Immunity, Xuzhou Medical University, Xuzhou 221004, Jiangsu, People's Republic of China
Full list of author information is available at the end of the article

Background

Human immunodeficiency virus type 1 (HIV-1) infection has been demonstrated to be associated with HIV-associated neurocognitive disorders (HAND) that is characterized by degenerative loss of neurons and ultimately develops into HIV-associated dementia (HAD), the most severe form of HAND [1, 2]. Despite the use of highly active antiretroviral therapy (HAART) has successfully prevented many of the former end-stage complications of acquired immunodeficiency syndrome (AIDS), neuronal cell death remains a problem that is frequently found in the brains of HIV-1-infected patients. With prolonged survival of AIDS patients, the prevalence of minor cognitive motor disorder appears to be rising among AIDS patients. Furthermore, HAD is still prevalent in treated AIDS patients.

HAND pathogenesis is associated with the direct and indirect effects of HIV-1 infection on the neuron damage and loss [3]. The direct effects from HIV-1 infection in the central nervous system (CNS) are from the neurotoxicity of HIV-1 itself [4–6] and HIV-1-encoded proteins including gp120 [7–10], transactivator of transcription (Tat) [3, 11–14], and negative factor (Nef) [15, 16], whereas the indirect toxicity is due to altered glutamate neurotransmission [5], as well as pro-inflammatory cytokines that are secreted by astrocytes or microglia infected with HIV-1 or stimulated with HIV-1 proteins [3, 17].

Astrocytes, the major glial cell type within the CNS [18], support neuron function through promoting formation and function of synapses and build the formation of the blood-brain barrier (BBB) [19]. Furthermore, astrocytes possess the capacity to interact with the peripheral immune system by recruiting leukocytes and monocytes into the CNS [20]. Reactive astrocytosis is an important feature in an inflammatory condition that occurs during HAND pathology [21]. Experimental data indicate that astrocyte activation is involved in the pathogenesis of HAND characterized by an increased expression of pro-inflammatory cytokines and chemokine [3, 17]. In response to HIV-1 and its encoded protein, Nef, in the CNS, astrocytes increase chemokine production to facilitate T cells and monocytes recruitment to the CNS [17]. However, the mechanisms by which astrocyte activation contribute to HAND by Nef remain still unknown.

Nef is a 27-kDa myristoylated protein released from HIV-infected cells in the exosome manner [22–24]. Nef interacts with a multitude of cellular factors and functions in trafficking, signal transduction, and gene expression. Nef leads to neural cell death directly and indirectly through the production of CXCL10 (IP-10) [25]. Functionally, Nef expressed in astrocytes results in impairing spatial and recognition memory in rats [26]. Clinical data display that Nef expresses in hippocampal neurons in HIV+ patients with HAD [27], consistent with this protein being involved in the memory impairment of those individuals. Of important, HIV-1 Nef induces CCL5 production in astrocytes to promote neuron death through p38-MAPK and PI3K/Akt pathway and utilization of transcription factors, such as NF-κB, C/EBP, and AP-1 [16]. These exciting results have prompted us to scan the expression profiles of inflammatory cytokines and chemokine in astrocytes induced by Nef and their roles in HAND pathogenesis.

Long non-coding RNAs (lncRNAs) have been defined as RNA transcripts more than 200 nucleotides in length that do not encode proteins. Based on the lncRNA-related position in the genome to the protein-coding genes, lncRNAs include five categories, which are sense, antisense, intronic, intergenic, and bidirectional [28]. Emerging evidence suggests that they play key roles in various biological and physiological processes including chromatin remodeling, epigenetic regulation, RNA splicing, and protein transport and directly relate to human diseases including neurodegenerative disorders [29–32]. One of the major functions of lncRNAs appears to be in the epigenetic regulation of gene transcription [32]. For example, lncRNAs have been shown to associate with a plethora of epigenetic modifier complexes including PRC2, PRC1, Cbx1, Cbx3, Tip60/P400, Setd8, ESET and Suv39h1, Jarid1b, Jarid1c, HDAC1, and YY1 [33, 34]. It has been reported that lncRNA H19 promotes neuroinflammation in ischemic stroke by driving HDAC1-dependent M1 microglial polarization [35]. In addition, lncRNAs activate NF-κB and MAP kinase pathway to regulate inflammation gene expression [36–39]. However, the roles of lncRNAs in the process of HAND are still unknown.

CREB-binding protein (CBP)/P300, histone acetyltransferase (HAT), is transcription co-activator that is cis-regulatory elements to control patterns of gene expression. By the enzymatic activity localized in HAT domain, CBP/P300 target both histones and numerous transcriptional factors (TFs), leading to elevated histone 3 lysine 27 acetylation (H3K27ac), p53, NF-κB, and RNA Pol II acetylation that forms a transcription network "hub" to promote gene expression [40–45]. Recent data show that CBP/P300 binds directly to enhancer RNAs (eRNAs) to stimulate histone acetylation and gene transcription [46]. Moreover, lncRNAs bind CBP/P300 activity to regulate gene expression [47].

In the present study, we analyzed the lncRNA and mRNA expression landscape of astrocytes treated by Nef protein in vitro. Our results suggest potential roles of lncRNAs in regulating inflammation in astrocytes during the process of HAND.

Methods

Animals

C57BL/6 mice were obtained from Nanjing University Laboratory Animal Center. Mice were housed at 25 ± 1 °

C with 55–65% humidity and maintained under specific pathogen-free conditions. All experimental procedures described in our study were performed according to the Provision and General Recommendation of the Chinese Laboratory Association. The protocol was approved by the Institutional Animal Care and Use Committee of Xuzhou Medical University.

Primary astrocyte culture

Primary mouse astrocytes from 0- to 1-day-old C57BL/6 mice were established as previously described [48]. In brief, the cerebral cortices freed of meninges were dissected, minced, and digested. After washed twice in DMEM/F12 medium containing 10% fetal bovine serum (FBS), the cells were filtrated, transferred to culture flasks pre-coated with 1 mg/ml poly-L-lysine (Sigma), and then cultured at 37 °C with 5% CO_2. Cells were passed for three passages and then glial fibrillary acidic protein (GFAP, astrocytic marker) expression was analyzed using immunofluorescence assays (IFA). Finally, at least 95% GAFP$^+$ cells were used to research.

Primary human astrocytes were obtained from ScienCell Research Laboratories with the help of Shanghai Zhong Qiao Xin Zhou Biotechnology Co., Ltd. in China. Human astrocytes were cultured in the Astrocyte Medium (AM, Cat. No. 1801) contained 2% FBS (Cat. No. 0010) and astrocyte growth supplement (AGS, Cat. No. 1852) at 37 °C with 5% CO_2. Cells were passed for three passages and performed to research.

RNA extraction

Total RNA was extracted from the primary astrocytes according to manufactures instructions. RNA quantity and quality was measured using NanoDrop ND-1000 spectrophotometer (Thermo Fisher Scientific).

Determination of lncRNA and mRNA profiles

The expression profiles of lncRNAs and mRNAs were detected as previously described [49]. Primary mouse astrocytes treated with 50 ng/ml Nef protein (Abcam, ab90462) were detected using Mouse LncRNA Microarray v2.0 (8 × 60 K, Arraystar) by Kangchen Bio-tech (Shanghai, China) that designed for the global profiling of mouse LncRNAs and protein-coding transcripts. Thirty-one thousand four hundred twenty-three LncRNAs and 25,376 coding transcripts can be detected by the second-generation LncRNA microarray. The LncRNAs are carefully collected from the most authoritative databases such as RefSeq, UCSC Known Genes, Ensembl, and many related literatures. Each transcript is represented by a specific exon or splice junction probe which can identify accurately individual transcript. Positive probes for housekeeping genes and negative probes are also printed onto the array as hybridization quality control.

According to previous experimental project, microarray assays had also been performed using pooled plasma, blood, liver, heart, or cell samples [50]. RNAs from mixed astrocytes treated with Nef protein three times were run microarray analysis. The acquired raw array images were processed by Agilent Feature Extraction software (version 11.0.1.1) and then normalized and analyzed by the Gene-Spring GX v12.0 software package (Agilent Technologies). Differentially expressed lncRNAs and mRNAs were then identified through fold change as well as P values calculated with t test. The threshold for up and downregulation was fold change > 2.0 and P value < 0.05. Afterwards, hierarchical clustering was performed to display the distinguishable lncRNA and mRNA expression patterns among the samples.

Real-time PCR assay

Real-time PCR (real-time PCR) assay was detected as previously described [49]. In brief, the total RNA from cultured astrocytes was extracted with TRIzol reagent (Invitrogen). First-strand cDNAs were generated using PrimeScriptTM RT reagent kit (TaKaRa, Japan), and SYBR Premix Ex TaqTM based on real-time PCR (TaKaRa) was performed to analyze the relative expression levels of lncRNAs and mRNAs. The relative gene expression was calculated using the $2^{-\Delta\Delta CT}$ method. The primers are listed in Additional file 1: Table S1.

Functional group analysis of mRNAs

Gene ontology (GO) and KEGG analysis were applied to determine the functions of differentially expressed mRNAs in biological pathways using the standard enrichment computation method [49]. The P value (hypergeometric P value) denotes the significance of the pathway correlated to the conditions. The recommend P value cut-off is 0.05.

ELISA

The levels of Cxcl9, Cxcl10, and Cxcl11 in the supernatants of cultured astrocytes were detected using Mouse ELISA kits (Abcam) according to the manufacturer's instructions.

RNA immunoprecipitation (RIP) assay

RIP assay was performed as previously described [51].In brief, after treated with Nef protein, 2×10^7 primary mouse astrocytes were treated with 0.3% formaldehyde in DMEM/F12 medium for 10 min at 37 °C. Glycine dissolved in PBS (1.25 M) was added to the final concentration of 0.125 M for 5 min at room temperature (RT). Cells were then washed twice in cold PBS and pelleted. The pellets were resuspended in RIPA buffer and incubated on ice with frequent vortex for 30 min, and the lysate was centrifugated at 13,000 RPM for 10 min.

Antibodies (5 μg) were added and incubated for 4 h at 4 °C. Samples were washed twice in RIPA buffer, four times in 1 M RIPA buffer, and then twice in RIPA in spin columns. The beads were resuspended in RIPA buffer and treated with proteinase K at 45 °C for 45 min. RNA samples were extracted with Trizol. Co-precipitated RNAs were purified with the RNeasy Mini Kit (QIAGEN) and detected by real-time PCR. The data of retrieved RNAs is calculated from the subtraction of RT/input ratio and non-RT/input ratio. The primer sequence was listed in Additional file 1: Table S1.

Chromatin immunoprecipitation (ChIP) assay

ChIP assays were performed as described previously [52]. Briefly, primary mouse astrocytes were treated with or without Nef protein for 3 h. Cells were cross-linked with 1% formaldehyde (final concentration) for 10 min at RT and then stopped by 1.25 mM of glycine (final concentration). 1×10^7 cells were used for each ChIP-enrichment. Chromatin was sheared to the fragment size of 200–500 bp using a Bioruptor (Diagenode). The antibodies used in the ChIP experiments were anti-NF-κB p65 antibody (Cell Signaling Technologies), anti-H3K27ac antibody (Abcam), anti-RNA Pol II antibody (Active Motif),

anti-CBP/P300 antibody (Cell Signaling Technologies), normal mouse IgG (Santa Cruz). All immunoprecipitated chromatin DNA was analyzed by real-time PCR. The primer sequences were listed in Additional file 1: Table S1.

Knockdown of lncRNAs

To silence the mouse lncRNA AK006025 and AK138360, siRNA sequences against AK006025 and AK138360 were designed. siRNA sequences were as follows: si-Ctrl, 5′-UUC UCC GAA CGU GUC ACG UTT-3′; si-AK006025, 5′-GCT GGG AAC CCA CAC ATA A-3′ and si-AK138360, 5′-GCA CCG GGC AAT GTT TAA T-3′.

Statistical analysis

SPSS version 18.0 was used for the statistical analysis of experimental data. Data presented as mean ± standard error of mean (SEM), calculated for all points from at least three independent experiments in triplicates. Statistical significance was determined using the two-tailed Student's t test or by one-way analysis of variance (ANOVA) when more than two groups were compared. $P < 0.05$ was considered significant.

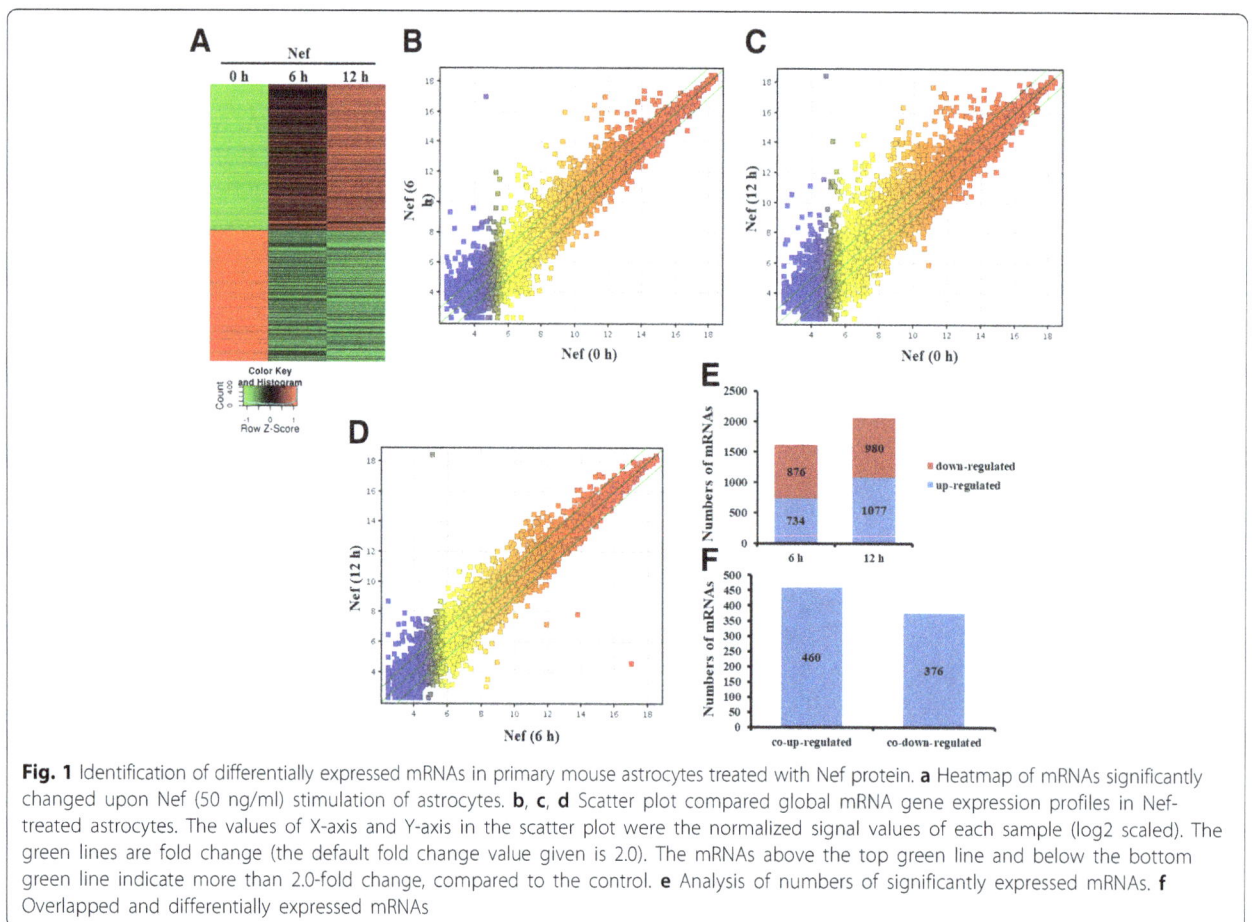

Fig. 1 Identification of differentially expressed mRNAs in primary mouse astrocytes treated with Nef protein. **a** Heatmap of mRNAs significantly changed upon Nef (50 ng/ml) stimulation of astrocytes. **b**, **c**, **d** Scatter plot compared global mRNA gene expression profiles in Nef-treated astrocytes. The values of X-axis and Y-axis in the scatter plot were the normalized signal values of each sample (log2 scaled). The green lines are fold change (the default fold change value given is 2.0). The mRNAs above the top green line and below the bottom green line indicate more than 2.0-fold change, compared to the control. **e** Analysis of numbers of significantly expressed mRNAs. **f** Overlapped and differentially expressed mRNAs

Results

Differentially expressed mRNA in the primary mouse astrocytes treated with Nef protein

To detect differentially expressed mRNAs in the activated mouse primary astrocytes, we performed a genome-wide analysis of mRNA expression profiles in the astrocytes stimulated with Nef protein (50 ng/ml) at the different time point (Fig. 1a). Firstly, a graphical overview of the expression signatures of mRNAs was performed by scatter plot analyses. The result displayed that a great number of mRNAs were differentially expressed in the astrocytes with Nef protein at 0 h, 6 h, and 12 h (Fig. 1b, c). Meanwhile, many mRNAs were differentially co-expressed in the astrocytes with Nef protein at 6 h and 12 h (Fig. 1d).

We then analyzed altered expression of mRNAs with fold change > 2, the criteria P value < 0.05 in the astrocytes stimulated by Nef protein at 6 h and 12 h compared with 0 h, respectively. Results showed that 734 mRNAs were upregulated, and 876 mRNAs were downregulated in the astrocytes stimulated by Nef protein for 6 h (Fig. 1e) and that 1077 upregulated and 980 downregulated mRNAs for 12 h (Fig. 1e). Notably, there were 460 co-upregulated and 376 co-downregulated mRNAs for between 6 h and 12 h (Fig. 1f). Importantly, there were many inflammatory cytokines and chemokine,

Table 1 Top 20 overlapped and upregulated mRNAs in mouse astrocytes treated with Nef protein (50 ng/ml) for 6 h and 12 h

Gene symbol	Upregulated folds	
	6 h/0 h	12 h/0 h
Cxcl11	105.05796	473.09506
Cxcl9	43.443104	213.93571
Ifnb1	112.73581	154.63144
Il1b	54.497185	153.78612
Gm4841	52.749744	149.3729
Cxcl2	98.37795	131.17091
Irg1	69.53818	101.9587
Ccl5	39.71899	94.32046
Il6	21.031158	74.925606
Ccl7	27.82146	74.49636
Fam26f	11.689228	64.880646
Cd69	30.492313	53.828453
Cxcl10	37.51984	45.796886
Cxcl1	20.680431	45.20861
Il1a	13.884002	49.921574
Cxcl3	38.239742	43.34039
Tnfsf10	4.3851957	24.53629
Tnf	30.36271	24.412766
Ccl3	11.2570715	15.065439
Ccl2	9.46433	10.722074

especially highly expressed *Cxcl11*, *Cxcl10* (IP-10), *Cxcl9*, *Cxcl3*, *Cxcl2*, *Cxcl1*, *Ccl5*, *Il-1β*, *Il-6*, and *Tnf*, among the co-upregulated mRNAs (Table 1).

To confirm the role of Nef protein in chemokine expression in human astrocytes, human primary astrocytes were treated with Nef protein for 6 h, *CXCL9*, *CXCL10*, and *CXCL11* mRNA levels were determined by real-time PCR assay. The results showed that mRNA levels of *CXCL9*, *CXCL10*, and *CXCL11* were significantly increased in human astrocytes treated with Nef at 6 h and 12 h (Fig. 2a), which was inconsistent with mouse astrocytes. To further determine upregulated mouse *Cxcl9*, *Cxcl10*, and *Cxcl11* by soluble recombinant Nef protein rather than by other factors like lipopolysaccharide (LPS), mouse primary astrocytes were immunoeluted with Nef (iNef) protein through using anti-Nef antibody (Abcam, ab42355) pretreatment prior to Nef stimulation for 6 h. Real-time PCR assay indicated that iNef did not induce mRNA levels of *Cxcl9*, *Cxcl10*, and *Cxcl11* (Fig. 2b). These results suggest that Nef itself enhances CXCL11, CXCL10, and CXCL9 expression in human and mouse astrocytes.

Go and KEGG pathway analysis of the molecular function of differentially expressed genes

To further explore potential molecular mechanism in HAND pathogenesis, GO and KEGG pathway analysis was performed for differentially expressed genes in astrocytes treated with Nef protein. GO analysis showed that the molecular function (MF) of differentially co-upregulated expressed transcripts was associated with cytokine and chemokine activity as well as their receptor binding in astrocytes treated with Nef protein (Fig. 3a). Furthermore, differentially co-downregulated genes were mainly related with protein binding in astrocytes treated with Nef protein (Fig. 3b).

KEGG pathway analysis indicated that 40 pathways were significantly involved in differentially expressed genes. Upregulated genes were enriched in cytokine and its receptor interaction, chemokine signaling pathway, NF-κB signaling pathway, and so on (Fig. 3c). Downregulated genes were involved in metabolism, lysosome, CoA biosynthesis, insulin signaling pathway, etc. (Fig. 3d). The above data represent that HAND is associated with the mRNA changes of inflammatory factors in the astrocytes.

Differentially expressed lncRNA in the primary mouse astrocytes treated with Nef protein

We further determined differentially expressed lncRNAs in the astrocytes treated with Nef protein at the different time point (Fig. 4a). Scatter plot analyses were firstly used to scan the expression signatures of lncRNAs. The result showed that a large number of lncRNAs were differentially expressed in the astrocytes with Nef protein at 0 h, 6 h, and 12 h (Fig. 4b, c). Meanwhile, lots of

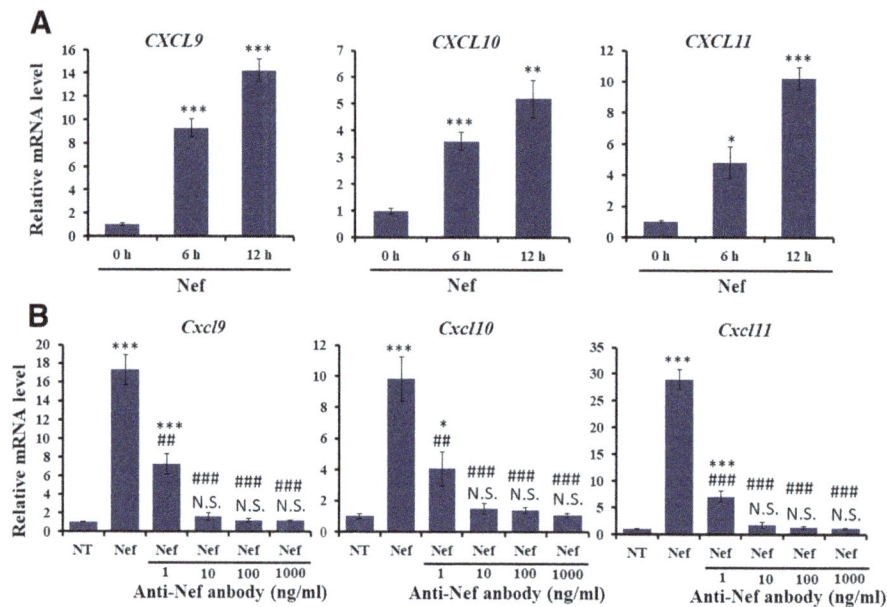

Fig. 2 Determination of effects of Nef protein on CXCL9/10/11 gene expression. **a** Primary human astrocytes were treated with soluble Nef protein (50 ng/ml) for 6 h and 12 h. Human *CXCL9*, *CXCL10*, and *CXCL11* mRNA levels were determined by real-time PCR assay (n = 3). Error bars represent means ± SEM. *P < 0.05, **P < 0.01, ***P < 0.001, vs 0 h. **b** Primary mouse astrocytes were pre-treated with different concentration of anti-Nef antibody followed by soluble Nef protein (50 ng/ml) for 6 h. Mouse *Cxcl9*, *Cxcl10*, and *Cxcl11* mRNA levels were determined by real-time PCR assay (n = 3). Error bars represent means ± SEM. *P < 0.05, ***P < 0.001, vs NT. ##P < 0.01, ###P < 0.001, vs Nef

lncRNAs were differentially expressed in the astrocytes with Nef protein at 12 h, compared to 6 h (Fig. 4d).

We then analyzed the differential expression of lncRNAs in the astrocytes stimulated by Nef protein at 6 h and 12 h compared with 0 h, respectively. Results showed that 1358 lncRNAs were upregulated, and 670

lncRNAs were downregulated in the astrocytes stimulated by Nef protein for 6 h (Fig. 4e) and that 1534 up-regulated and 1271 downregulated lncRNAs for 12 h (Fig. 4e). Notably, there were 638 co-upregulated and 372 co-downregulated lncRNAs for both 6 h and 12 h (Fig. 4f). The list of the top 20 differentially expressed

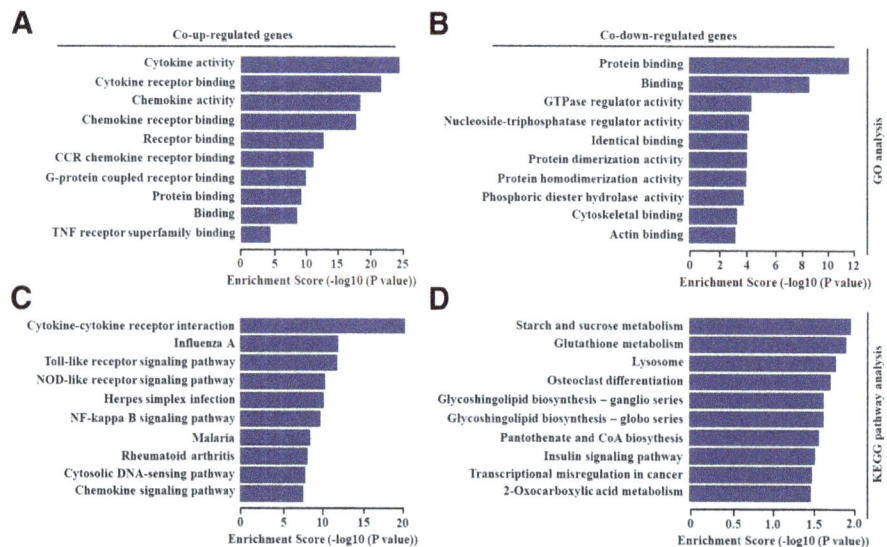

Fig. 3 Biological function of differentially overlapped genes with fold changes more than 2.0. **a, b** GO analysis of significant molecular function of co-upregulated and co-downregulated genes were shown in primary mouse astrocytes treated by Nef protein (50 ng/ml) with 6 h and 12 h. **c, d** KEGG pathway analysis of significant pathways for co-upregulated and co-downregulated genes were shown in primary mouse astrocytes treated by Nef protein with 6 h and 12 h

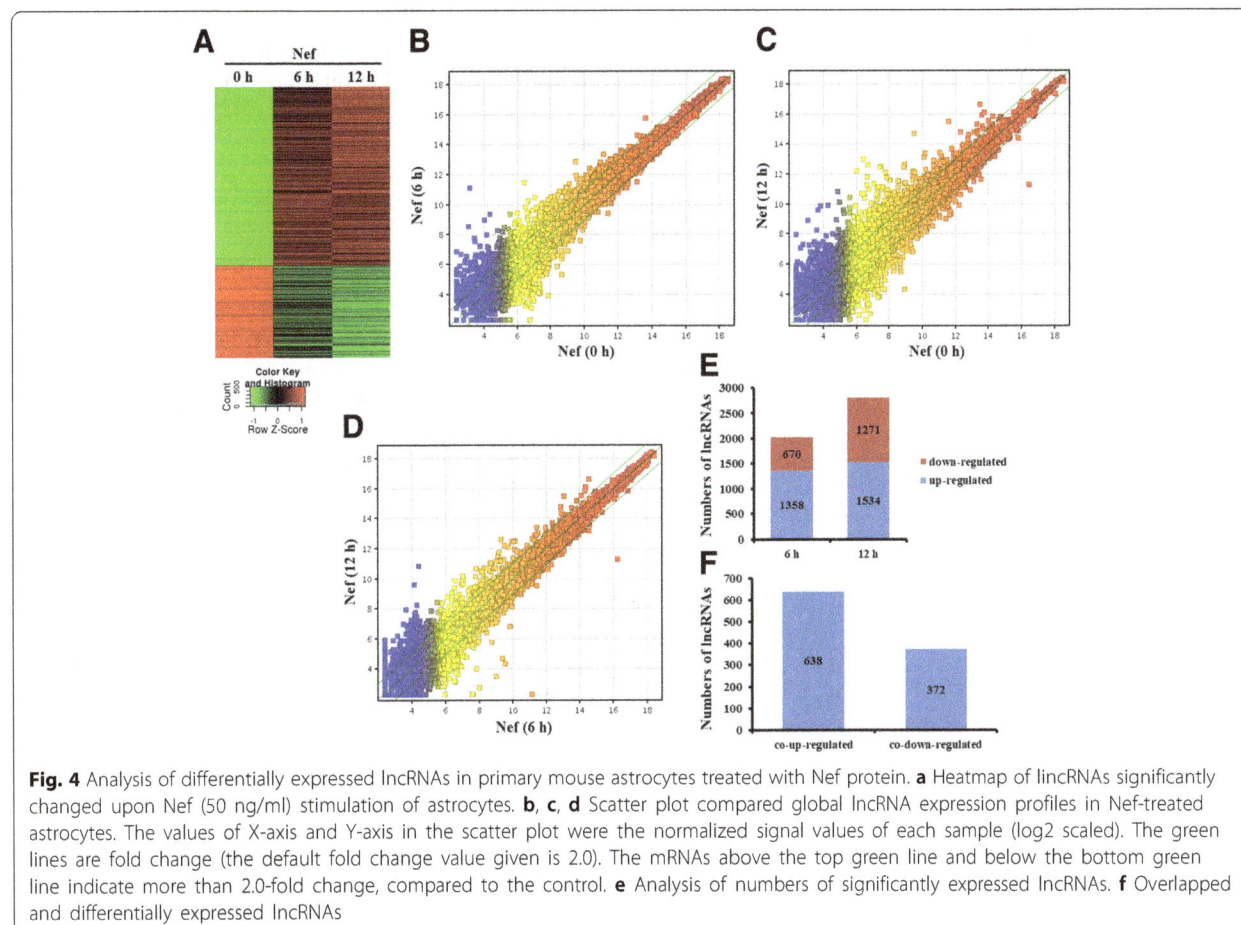

Fig. 4 Analysis of differentially expressed lncRNAs in primary mouse astrocytes treated with Nef protein. **a** Heatmap of lincRNAs significantly changed upon Nef (50 ng/ml) stimulation of astrocytes. **b**, **c**, **d** Scatter plot compared global lncRNA expression profiles in Nef-treated astrocytes. The values of X-axis and Y-axis in the scatter plot were the normalized signal values of each sample (log2 scaled). The green lines are fold change (the default fold change value given is 2.0). The mRNAs above the top green line and below the bottom green line indicate more than 2.0-fold change, compared to the control. **e** Analysis of numbers of significantly expressed lncRNAs. **f** Overlapped and differentially expressed lncRNAs

lncRNAs for both 6 h and 12 h identified by microarray analysis was shown in Additional file 1: Table S2 and Table 2.

Validation of the microarray data using real-time PCR

To further verify the accuracy of microarray data, we randomly assigned 10 lncRNAs from the differentially expressed lncRNAs, including 5 co-upregulated (Gm16685, Gm12250, AK151815, AK139352, and Gm8773) and 5 co-downregulated (AK038606, Gm12326, AK039511, Gm13484, and AK043126) and tested their expression through real-time PCR assay. As shown in Fig. 5, Gm16685, Gm12250, AK151815, AK139352, and Gm8773 expression were significantly increased, whereas AK038606, Gm12326, AK039511, Gm13484, and AK043126 expression were obviously decreased in the astrocytes stimulated by Nef protein for 6 h and 12 h, compared with 0 h. Overall, these data confirmed the accuracy of microarray data.

Analysis of upregulated lncRNAs on the chromosome 5 in the primary mouse astrocytes treated with Nef protein

Then, we analyze differentially co-upregulated lncRNAs on chromosome 5 in the primary mouse astrocytes treated with Nef protein for 6 h and 12 h. As shown in

Table 2, ten lncRNAs were selected as targeted ones. All of them were located at two terminals of Cxcl3/2/1 gene cluster and Cxcl/10/11 gene cluster (Additional file 1: Table S2). Among them, Uc008xxt.1 and AK138360 were close to 5′ terminal of Cxcl3/2/1 gene cluster while AK148399 and AK006025 were nearby the 3′ terminal of the Cxcl9/10/11 gene cluster (Fig. 6a). The class distribution of AK138360 and AK006025 were intergenic, Uc008xxt.1 was sense-overlap, and AK148399 was bidirectional (Additional file 1: Table S3).

We further measured above lncRNAs expression by real-time PCR in primary astrocytes stimulated with Nef protein. Results of real-time PCR showed that Uc008xxt.1, AK138360, AK148399, and AK006025 were significantly regulated (Fig. 6b), which was in accordance with the microarray data.

Knockdown of lncRNA AK006025 repressed Cxcl9/10/11 cluster gene expression

Intergenic lncRNA, as an in *cis*-regulatory element, regulates gene expression. To determine the role of intergenic lncRNAs in regulating Cxcl9/10/11 cluster gene expression, siRNA of AK138360 or AK006025 was transfected into primary mouse astrocytes for 48 h,

Table 2 Top 20 overlapped and upregulated lncRNAs in mouse astrocytes stimulated with Nef protein (50 ng/ml) for 6 h and 12 h

lncRNA seqname	Length	Upregulated folds	
		6 h/0 h	12 h/0 h
Gm16685	1592	33.808704	98.312874
Gm5970	1216	11.263321	75.315765
Gm12250	1274	6.2884264	61.74965
AK085771	1165	6.540899	66.45514
uc008roq.1	3961	45.042114	58.77
Gm4955	913	6.5966477	50.151352
A530040E14Rik	1262	10.544557	50.162678
Gm12407	720	6.1827254	33.648342
Gm13309	324	6.142315	30.465094
Mx2	2428	12.378684	37.599354
AK151815	1592	7.3327208	26.562384
MM9LINCRNAEXON11240-	1100	10.792236	20.239393
uc008smk.1	701	6.23503	32.482025
ENSMUST00000160565	1414	3.362174	22.119934
AK139352	4337	6.970084	36.466106
AK145170	2791	9.817351	20.934488
ENSMUST00000135659	1443	14.289103	18.727198
NR_003507	1848	3.7799745	14.091469
Gm8773	1268	5.3409157	10.783084
uc008zif.1	704	2.7248611	12.014651

followed by Nef protein treatment for 6 h and 12 h, respectively. We detected Cxcl9/10/11 expression using ELISA and real-time PCR. As seen from Fig. 7a, siRNA of AK138360 or AK006025 inhibited their expression. All of Cxcl9, Cxcl10, and Cxcl11 expression were significantly decreased in mouse astrocytes treated with Nef protein after knockdown of AK006025, not AK138360 (Fig. 7b).

AK006025 associated with CBP/P300 regulates Nef-induced Cxcl9/10/11 cluster gene expression

To further uncover the potential mechanism how lncRNA AK006025 regulated Cxcl9/10/11 cluster gene expression, RIP assay was used for detecting lncRNA AK006025 and NF-κB p65 and/or CBP/P300 interaction. RIP results showed that AK006025 was significantly associated with NF-κB p65 and CBP/P300 in mouse astrocytes treated with Nef protein for 3 h (Fig. 8a). Furthermore, ChIP assay indicated that NF-κB p65, CBP/P300, RNA Pol II, and H3K27ac were differentially enriched in in the promoter Cxcl9/10/11 gene cluster in mouse astrocytes treated with Nef protein for 3 h (Fig. 8b). Of importance, siRNA of AK006025 repressed dramatically NF-κB p65 and CBP/P300 enrichment in

the promoter Cxcl9/10/11 gene cluster in mouse astrocytes treated with Nef protein for 3 h (Fig. 8c). The data suggest that the interaction of AK006025 and CBP/P300 may regulate epigenetically Cxcl9/10/11 cluster gene transcription.

Discussion

HAND is a degenerative disease of the central nervous system with chronic inflammation, synapse dysfunction, and neuron loss. Many studies have determined that the blockade of pro-inflammatory cytokine and chemokine production in astrocytes could protect the neuron damage of HAND pathogenesis [13, 16, 17].

Nef, a myristoylated protein encoded by HIV-1, functions in the multifaceted biological process including trafficking, signal transduction, and gene expression in a paracrine manner. Nef is released from infected cells into the plasma of HIV-infected individuals [53]. The detectable concentration of soluble Nef in the serum ranges from 1 to 10 ng/ml [54, 55]. The soluble Nef can be taken up by several types of cells to regulate cellular function, such as B cells, primary effusion lymphoma (PEL) cells, pulmonary arterial endothelial cells as well as primary human umbilical vein endothelial cells (HUVECs) [56–59]. Although HIV-1 built latency in astrocytes in the brain, the expression of HIV-1 genes are low, for example, HIV p24 in HIV-1 [+] postmortem brain astrocytes is rarely detected [60]. Therefore, we used soluble Nef protein as an exogenous factor to explore its role in inducing the expression of lncRNAs and mRNAs. Here, our data showed that the exogenous Nef protein enhanced CCL5 and IP-10 expression in astrocytes, consistent with previous data of endogenous Nef expression [16, 25].

Over the past decades, the molecular mechanisms underlying HAND have been extensively explored. However, the understanding of the pathophysiological process of HAND is still limited. In recent years, a large number of evidence shows that lncRNAs have been associated with human diseases, such as cancer, neurological disorders, and so on [30, 31, 52, 61]. LncRNAs are found as important regulators of neuro-development and brain function [31]. However, there is no knowledge that lncRNAs are associated with a particular molecular or cellular function in HAND pathogenesis. To date, the functional characterization of lncRNAs during the HAND/HAD process and astrocyte activation has not been uncovered. Our recent study demonstrated the expression profiles of lncRNAs in Nef-treated astrocytes, analyzed the co-expression of lncRNAs in vivo and in vitro, and explored their characteristics and possible relations with protein-coding genes.

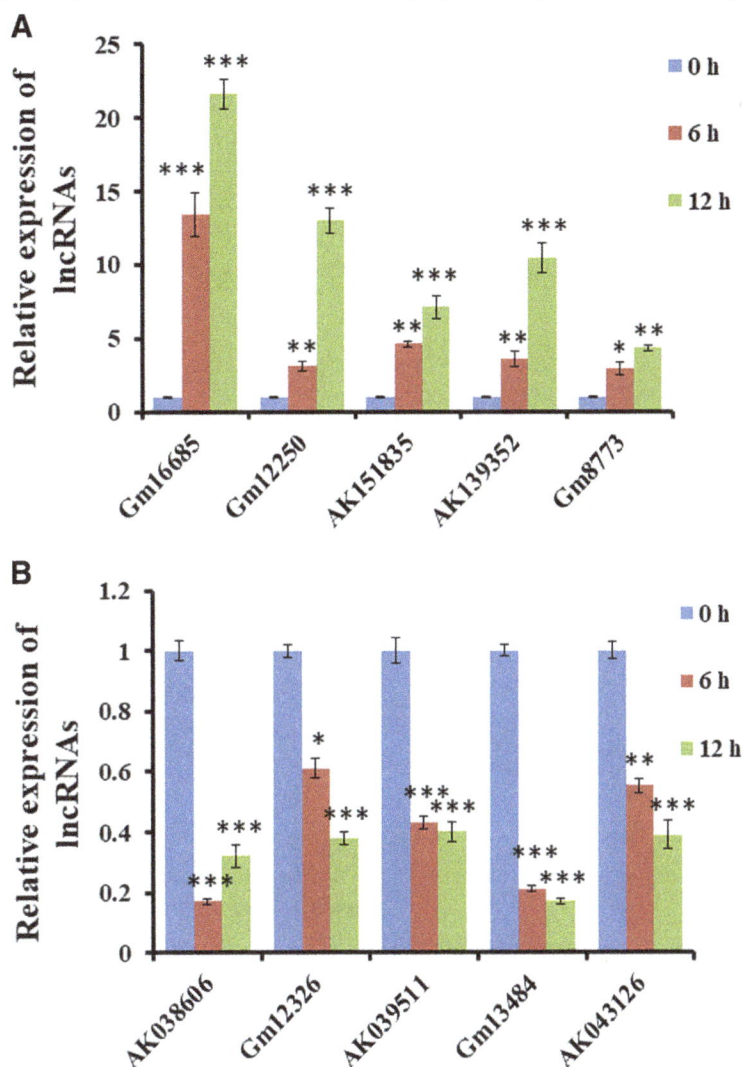

Fig. 5 Real-time PCR verification of differentially co-expressed lncRNAs in astrocytes stimulated with Nef. Ten lncRNAs were randomly chosen for real-time PCR validation. **a** The expressions of lncRNA Gm16685, Gm12250, AK151815, AK139352, and Gm8773 were significantly increased in astrocytes stimulated with Nef protein (50 ng/ml) with 0 h, 6 h, and 12 h. **b** The expressions of lncRNA AK038606, Gm12326, AK039511, Gm13484, and AK043126 were markedly downregulated in astrocytes. *$P < 0.05$, **$P < 0.01$, ***$P < 0.001$, vs 0 h. Error bars represent means $\pm$ SEM. These data are from three independent experiments

In our study, we found that there were 1385 upregulated lncRNAs and 734 upregulated mRNAs in the astrocytes stimulated by Nef protein for 6 h; meanwhile, 670 lncRNAs and 876 mRNAs were downregulated. Furthermore, 1534 lncRNAs and 1077 mRNAs were upregulated, and 1271 lncRNAs and 982 mRNAs were downregulated in the astrocytes stimulated by Nef for 6 h. Of importance, there were 638 lncRNAs and 460 mRNAs that differentially co-upregulated, and 372 lncRNAs and 376 mRNAs that differentially co-downregulated in the astrocytes treated with Nef for both 6 h and 12 h. Moreover, real-time PCR assay was performed to confirm parts of differentially expressed lncRNAs and mRNAs, which was consistent with the results of lncRNAs microarray.

Interestingly, the differentially-expressed lncRNAs appear to have a relationship with the levels of inflammatory cytokines and chemokine secreted by astrocytes, suggesting that these lncRNAs might uncover novel insight into the molecular basis of HAND pathogenesis.

In our studies, a large number of inflammatory genes were significantly co-upregulated in the astrocytes treated with Nef for both 6 h and 12 h, especially *Cxcl11*, *Cxcl10*, *Cxcl9*, *Cxcl3*, *Cxcl2*, *Cxcl1*, *Ccl5*, *Il-1β*, *Il-6*, and *Tnf*. Furthermore, some mRNAs including *Ifnb1*, *Irg1*, *Tnfsf10*, and *CD69* were also screened out and dramatically increased (Table 1), whose functions are associated with immune response, interferon (IFN) signal as well as apoptosis. Therefore, further studies

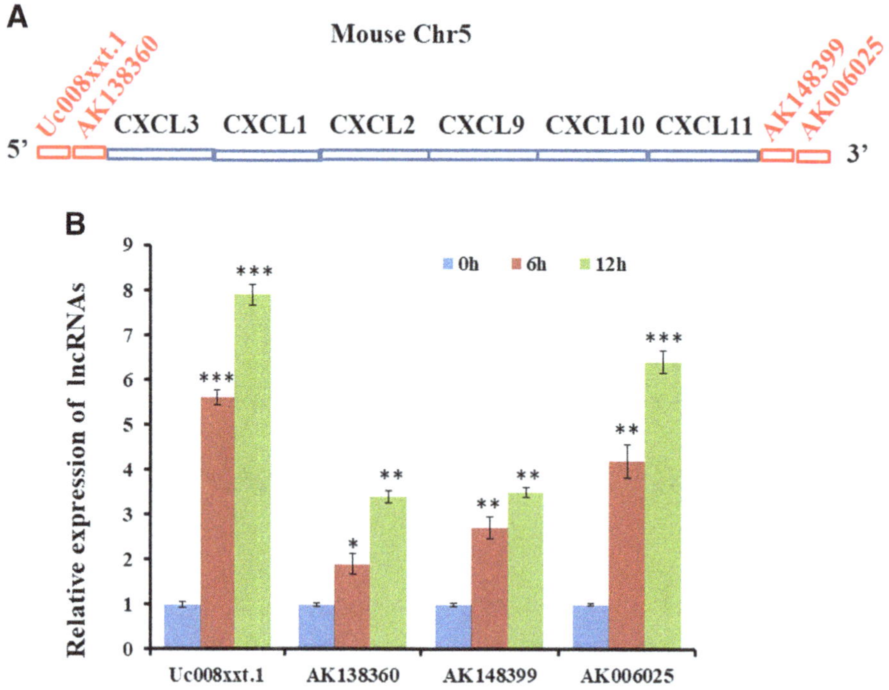

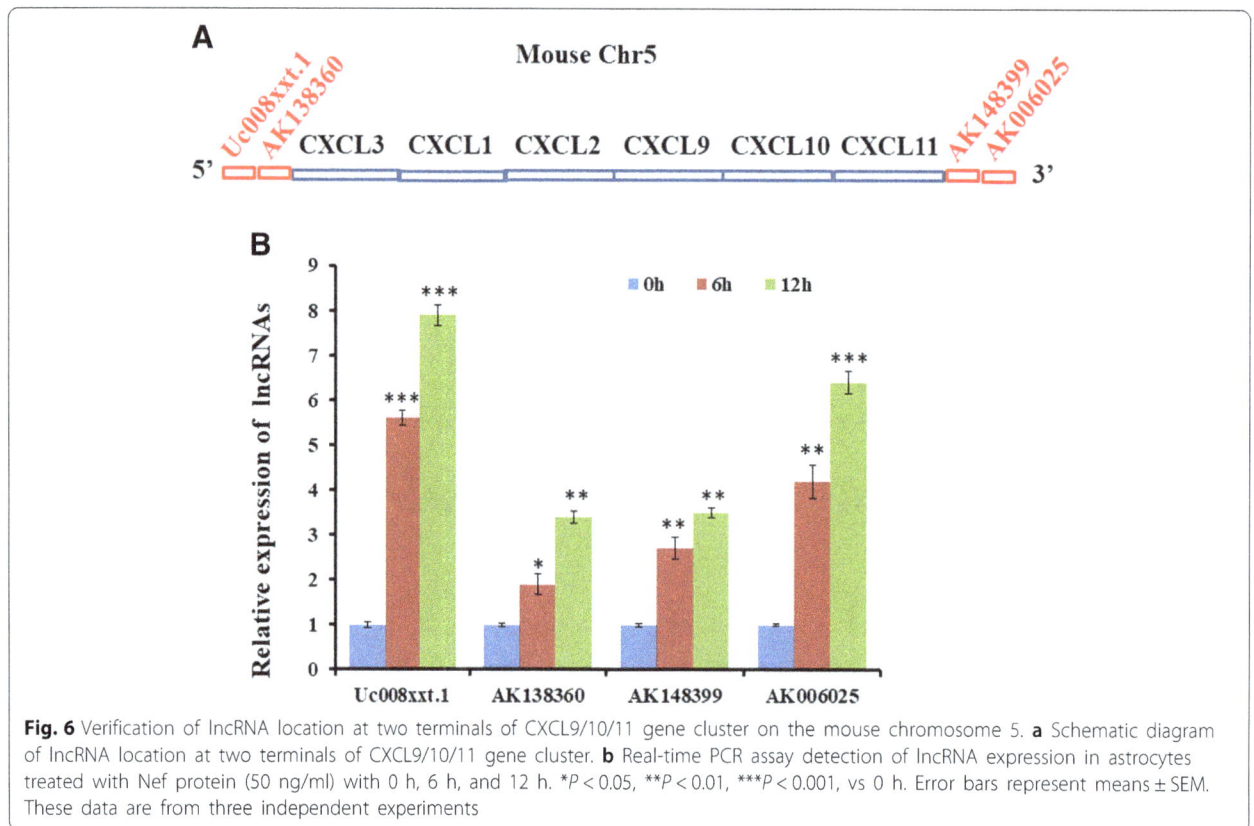

Fig. 6 Verification of lncRNA location at two terminals of CXCL9/10/11 gene cluster on the mouse chromosome 5. **a** Schematic diagram of lncRNA location at two terminals of CXCL9/10/11 gene cluster. **b** Real-time PCR assay detection of lncRNA expression in astrocytes treated with Nef protein (50 ng/ml) with 0 h, 6 h, and 12 h. *$P < 0.05$, **$P < 0.01$, ***$P < 0.001$, vs 0 h. Error bars represent means ± SEM. These data are from three independent experiments

are needed to demonstrate whether they are involved in HAND process.

CXC chemokine, structurally recognizable by the position of four conserved cysteine residues, are prominent mediators of chemotaxis. The Cxcl9/10/11 genes locate on the mouse chromosome 5 in cluster manner and are induced by IFN [62]. Previous data showed that Nef increased IP-10 expression in astrocytes [25]. Here, we scanned the chemokine expression profile in primary mouse astrocytes treated with Nef protein. The result showed that Cxcl9, Cxcl10, and Cxcl11 were all top differentially expressed; of importance, Nef increased CXCL9, CXCL10, and CXCL11, mRNA levels in human astrocytes, which suggests an important role in HAND pathogenesis.

Emerging data show that lncRNAs are involved in regulating NF-κB signaling, anti-viral response, and inflammatory response [36–39, 47]. In the present study, based on the GO term enrichment and pathway maps of mRNAs, we found that markedly enriched molecular functions and biological processes of upregulated genes in astrocytes were mainly associated with cytokine and chemokine activity as well as their receptor binding in astrocytes treated with Nef protein. These findings are consistent with previous data showing that the infiltration of immune cells and inflammation play a vital role in the pathogenesis of HAND [17].

It has been established that lncRNAs have been shown to link a number of epigenetic modified complexes with transcriptional factors including NF-κB, resulting in regulating gene expression [33, 34, 36]. In addition, lncRNAs bind CBP/P300 activity to regulate gene expression [47]. Here, we analyzed four lncRNAs located on 5′ terminal and 3′ terminal of Cxcl3/2/1 gene cluster and Cxcl9/10/11 gene cluster. Among them, AK138360 and AK006025 siRNA located on 3′ terminal of the Cxcl9/10/11 gene cluster. Unexpectedly, all of Cxcl9, Cxcl10, and Cxcl11 expression were dramatically decreased in mouse astrocytes treated with Nef protein after knockdown of AK006025, not AK138360. Furthermore, RIP and ChIP assay showed that AK006025 associated with NF-κB p65 and CBP/P300 was enriched in the promoter of Cxcl9, Cxcl10, and Cxcl11. These data suggest that interaction of AK006025 and CBP/P300 might regulate epigenetically Cxcl9/10/11 cluster gene transcription in HAND pathogenesis.

So far, our findings still have several limitations. First of all, these studies only were performed to scan lncRNA profiles in primary mouse astrocytes, which is possibly different from that of human astrocytes, particularly for ncRNAs that are heterogeneous expressions in mouse cells. Secondly, we only determined the role of a single acute exposure to Nef protein, which may differ from the effects of chronic exposure in HAND pathogenesis.

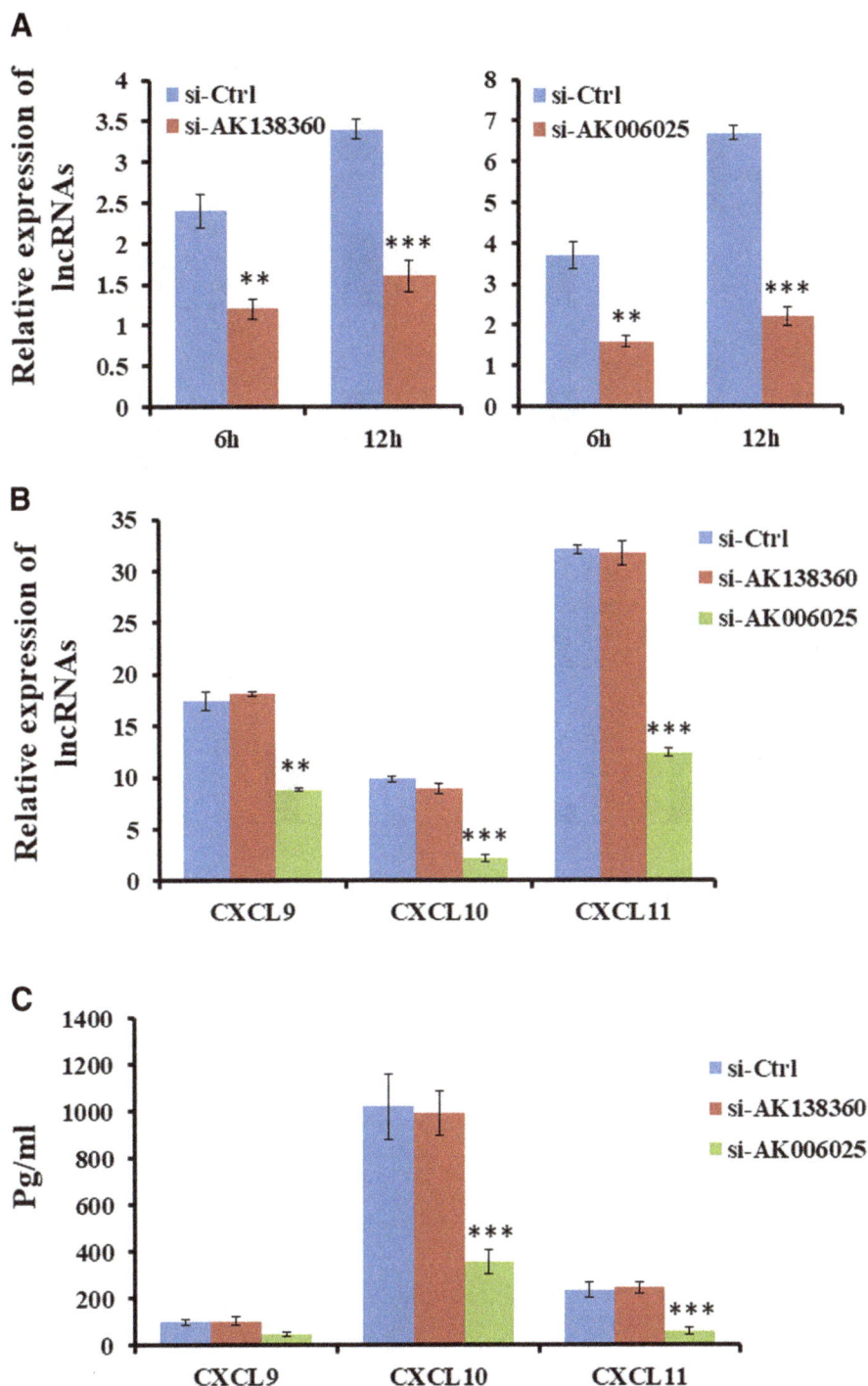

Fig. 7 Knockdown of lncRNA AK006025 reduced CXCL9/10/11 cluster gene expression in astrocytes treated with Nef. **a** Real-time PCR assay detection of lncRNA expression in astrocytes transfected siRNAs for 48 h, followed by treatment with Nef protein for 6 h and 12 h. **b** Real-time PCR assay analysis of CXCL9, CXCL10, and CXCL11 mRNA transcriptional level in astrocytes transfected siRNAs for 48 h, followed by treatment with Nef protein for 12 h. **c** ELISA analysis of CXCL9, CXCL10, and CXCL11 secretion in astrocytes transfected siRNAs for 48 h, followed by treatment with Nef protein for 24 h. $*P < 0.05$, $**P < 0.01$, $***P < 0.001$, vs 0 h. Error bars represent means $\pm$ SEM. These data are from three independent experiments

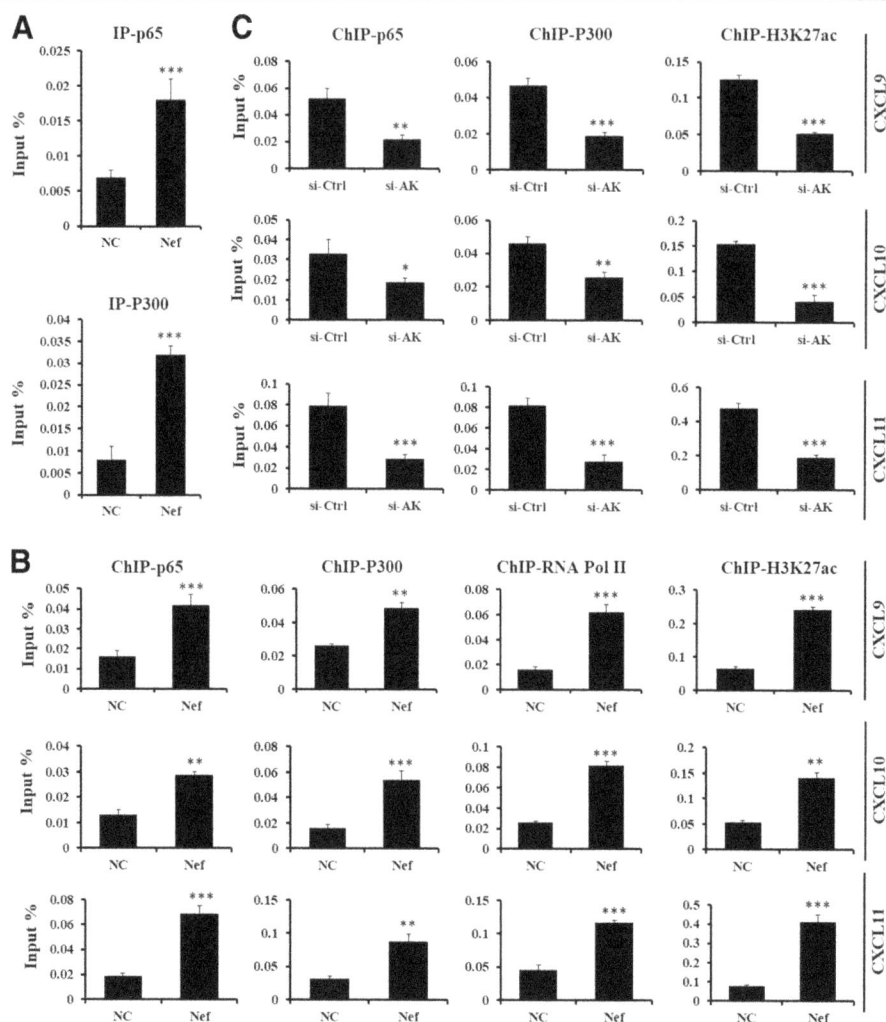

Fig. 8 Analysis of lncRNA AK006025 interaction with CBP/P300 to regulate CXCL9/10/11 cluster gene expression in astrocytes treated with Nef. **a** RIP assay analysis of the interaction of AK006025 with NF-κB p65 and CBP/P300 in astrocytes treatment with Nef protein for 3 h. NC: natural control. ***$P < 0.001$, vs NC. These data are from three independent experiments. **b** ChIP assay analysis of NF-κB p65, CBP/P300, RNA Pol II, and H3K27ac enrichment on the promoter of CXCL9/10/11 gene cluster in astrocytes treatment with Nef protein for 3 h. **$P < 0.01$, ***$P < 0.001$, vs NC. Error bars represent means ± SEM. These data are from three independent experiments. **c** ChIP assay analysis of NF-κB p65, CBP/P300, and H3K27ac enrichment on the promoter of CXCL9/10/11 gene cluster in astrocytes transfected siRNAs for 48 h, followed by treatment with Nef protein for 3 h. si-AK: si-AK006025. *$P < 0.05$, **$P < 0.01$, ***$P < 0.001$, vs his-Ctrl. Error bars represent means ± SEM. These data are from three independent experiments

Therefore, it is important to demonstrate how Nef influences lncRNAs expression in human astrocytes in HAND.

Conclusion

In summary, our results revealed that Nef induced thousands of differentially expressed lncRNAs in astrocytes. LincRNA AK006025 was involved in regulating Nef-induced CXCL9, CXCL10, and CXCL11 expression through interaction with NF-κB p65 and CBP/P300, which may play key roles in neuroinflammation and pathogenesis of HAND.

Abbreviations
AIDS: Acquired immunodeficiency syndrome; BBB: Blood-brain barrier; CBP/P300: CREB-binding protein; ChIP: Chromatin immunoprecipitation; CNS: Central nervous system; GFAP: Glial fibrillary acidic protein; GO: Gene ontology; HAART: Highly active antiretroviral therapy; HAD: HIV-associated dementia; HAND: HIV-associated neurocognitive disorder; HDAC1: Histone

deacetylase 1; HIV-1: Human immunodeficiency virus type 1; IL-1β: Interleukin-1 betta; IP-10: Interferon-gamma-inducible 10-Kd protein; lncRNAs: Long non-coding RNAs; MF: Molecular function; Nef: Negative factor; NF-κB: Nuclear factor-kappa B; RIP: RNA immunoprecipitation; Tat: Transactivator of transcription; TNF: Tumor necrosis factor

Acknowledgements
We thank that his work was supported by the Qing Lan Project.

Funding
This work was supported by Jiangsu Provincial Natural Science Foundation of China (BK20141136 to Zhou and BK20151168 to Liu), Jiangsu Key Laboratory of Brain Disease Bioinformation to Zhou (jsbl1205), the National Natural Science Foundation of China (81500914 to Xue; 81372598 and 81772688 to Gao and 81700794 to Hu), Dean Special Foundation of Xuzhou Medical University (2012KJZ09 to Xue), the Graduate Innovation Program in Science and Technology of Jiangsu Province (KYLX18_2169 to Cao), and the Priority Academic Program Development of Jiangsu Higher Education Institutions (2014 PAPD).

Authors' contributions
FZ, XmL, DZ, LG, JW, YY, and MX performed the analysis of lncRNA and mRNA profiles and real-time PCR assay. FZ, DZ, and LG performed the RIP and ChIP assay. XyL, DZ, QC, LN, and MX performed the real-time PCR verification. JW, XyL, MH, BZ, HH, and LN performed the ELISA assay and siRNA transfection. FZ, XmL, DG, KZ, YI, and RT conceived the design of experiments, collected and analyzed the data, and wrote the manuscript. All authors read and approved the final manuscript.

Competing interests
The authors declare that they have no competing interests.

Author details
[1]Jiangsu Key Laboratory of Brain Disease Bioinformation, Research Center for Biochemistry and Molecular Biology, Xuzhou Medical University, Xuzhou 221004, Jiangsu, People's Republic of China. [2]Jiangsu Key Laboratory of Immunity and Metabolism, Department of Pathogen Biology and Immunology and Laboratory of Infection and Immunity, Xuzhou Medical University, Xuzhou 221004, Jiangsu, People's Republic of China. [3]Department of Physiology, Xuzhou Medical University, Xuzhou 221004, Jiangsu, People's Republic of China. [4]Department of Neurobiology and Anatomy, Xuzhou Medical University, Xuzhou 221004, Jiangsu, People's Republic of China. [5]Department of Dermatology, University of California Davis (UC Davis) School of Medicine, Sacramento, CA, USA.

References
1. Clifford DB, Ances BM. HIV-associated neurocognitive disorder. Lancet Infect Dis. 2013;13(11):976–86.
2. Ghafouri M, Amini S, Khalili K, Sawaya BE. HIV-1 associated dementia: symptoms and causes. Retrovirology. 2006;3:28.
3. Gaskill PJ, Miller DR, Gamble-George J, Yano H, Khoshbouei H. HIV, Tat and dopamine transmission. Neurobiol Dis. 2017;105:51–73.
4. Gonzalez E, Rovin BH, Sen L, Cooke G, Dhanda R, Mummidi S, Kulkarni H, Bamshad MJ, Telles V, Anderson SA, et al. HIV-1 infection and AIDS dementia are influenced by a mutant MCP-1 allele linked to increased monocyte infiltration of tissues and MCP-1 levels. Proc Natl Acad Sci U S A. 2002;99(21):13795–800.
5. Huang Y, Zhao L, Jia B, Wu L, Li Y, Curthoys N, Zheng JC. Glutaminase dysregulation in HIV-1-infected human microglia mediates neurotoxicity: relevant to HIV-1-associated neurocognitive disorders. J Neurosci. 2011; 31(42):15195–204.
6. Spudich S. HIV and neurocognitive dysfunction. Curr HIV/AIDS Rep. 2013; 10(3):235–43.
7. Silverstein PS, Shah A, Weemhoff J, Kumar S, Singh DP, Kumar A. HIV-1 gp120 and drugs of abuse: interactions in the central nervous system. Curr HIV Res. 2012;10(5):369–83.
8. Xu C, Liu J, Chen L, Liang S, Fujii N, Tamamura H, Xiong H. HIV-1 gp120 enhances outward potassium current via CXCR4 and cAMP-dependent protein kinase a signaling in cultured rat microglia. Glia. 2011;59(6): 997–1007.
9. Shah A, Kumar A. HIV-1 gp120-mediated increases in IL-8 production in astrocytes are mediated through the NF-kappaB pathway and can be silenced by gp120-specific siRNA. J Neuroinflammation. 2010;7:96.
10. Wyss-Coray T, Masliah E, Toggas SM, Rockenstein EM, Brooker MJ, Lee HS, Mucke L. Dysregulation of signal transduction pathways as a potential mechanism of nervous system alterations in HIV-1 gp120 transgenic mice and humans with HIV-1 encephalitis. J Clin Invest. 1996;97(3):789–98.
11. Green MV, Thayer SA. NMDARs adapt to neurotoxic HIV protein Tat downstream of a GluN2A-ubiquitin ligase signaling pathway. J Neurosci. 2016;36(50):12640–9.
12. Bruce-Keller AJ, Chauhan A, Dimayuga FO, Gee J, Keller JN, Nath A. Synaptic transport of human immunodeficiency virus-tat protein causes neurotoxicity and gliosis in rat brain. J Neurosci. 2003;23(23):8417–22.
13. D'Aversa TG, Yu KO, Berman JW. Expression of chemokine by human fetal microglia after treatment with the human immunodeficiency virus type 1 protein Tat. J Neuro-Oncol. 2004;10(2):86–97.
14. Kim BO, Liu Y, Ruan Y, Xu ZC, Schantz L, He JJ. Neuropathologies in transgenic mice expressing human immunodeficiency virus type 1 Tat protein under the regulation of the astrocyte-specific glial fibrillary acidic protein promoter and doxycycline. Am J Pathol. 2003;162(5):1693–707.
15. Bergonzini V, Calistri A, Salata C, Del Vecchio C, Sartori E, Parolin C, Palu G. Nef and cell signaling transduction: a possible involvement in the pathogenesis of human immunodeficiency virus-associated dementia. J Neuro-Oncol. 2009; 15(3):238–48.
16. Liu X, Shah A, Gangwani MR, Silverstein PS, Fu M, Kumar A. HIV-1 Nef induces CCL5 production in astrocytes through p38-MAPK and PI3K/Akt pathway and utilizes NF-kB, CEBP and AP-1 transcription factors. Sci Rep. 2014;4:4450.
17. Hong S, Banks WA. Role of the immune system in HIV-associated neuroinflammation and neurocognitive implications. Brain Behav Immun. 2015;45:1–12.
18. Allen NJ, Barres BA. Neuroscience: glia - more than just brain glue. Nature. 2009;457(7230):675–7.
19. Barres BA. The mystery and magic of glia: a perspective on their roles in health and disease. Neuron. 2008;60(3):430–40.
20. Wilson EH, Weninger W, Hunter CA. Trafficking of immune cells in the central nervous system. J Clin Invest. 2010;120(5):1368–79.
21. Budka H, Wiley CA, Kleihues P, Artigas J, Asbury AK, Cho ES, Cornblath DR, Dal Canto MC, DeGirolami U, Dickson D, et al. HIV-associated disease of the nervous system: review of nomenclature and proposal for neuropathology-based terminology. Brain Pathol. 1991;1(3):143–52.
22. Kestler HW 3rd, Ringler DJ, Mori K, Panicali DL, Sehgal PK, Daniel MD, Desrosiers RC. Importance of the nef gene for maintenance of high virus loads and for development of AIDS. Cell. 1991;65(4):651–62.
23. Puzar Dominkus P, Ferdin J, Plemenitas A, Peterlin BM, Lenassi M. Nef is secreted in exosomes from Nef.GFP-expressing and HIV-1-infected human astrocytes. J Neuro-Oncol. 2017;23(5):713–24.
24. Khan MB, Lang MJ, Huang MB, Raymond A, Bond VC, Shiramizu B, Powell MD. Nef exosomes isolated from the plasma of individuals with HIV-associated dementia (HAD) can induce Abeta(1-42) secretion in SH-SY5Y neural cells. J Neuro-Oncol. 2016;22(2):179–90.
25. van Marle G, Henry S, Todoruk T, Sullivan A, Silva C, Rourke SB, Holden J, McArthur JC, Gill MJ, Power C. Human immunodeficiency virus type 1 Nef protein mediates neural cell death: a neurotoxic role for IP-10. Virology. 2004;329(2):302–18.

26. Chompre G, Cruz E, Maldonado L, Rivera-Amill V, Porter JT, Noel RJ, Jr. Astrocytic expression of HIV-1 Nef impairs spatial and recognition memory. Neurobiol Dis 2013; 49:128–136.

27. Torres-Munoz J, Stockton P, Tacoronte N, Roberts B, Maronpot RR, Petito CK. Detection of HIV-1 gene sequences in hippocampal neurons isolated from postmortem AIDS brains by laser capture microdissection. J Neuropathol Exp Neurol. 2001;60(9):885–92.

28. Mercer TR, Dinger ME, Mattick JS. Long non-coding RNAs: insights into functions. Nat Rev Genet. 2009;10(3):155–9.

29. Qureshi IA, Mehler MF. Emerging roles of non-coding RNAs in brain evolution, development, plasticity and disease. Nat Rev Neurosci. 2012; 13(8):528–41.

30. Johnson R. Long non-coding RNAs in Huntington's disease neurodegeneration. Neurobiol Dis. 2012;46(2):245–54.

31. Roberts TC, Morris KV, Wood MJ. The role of long non-coding RNAs in neurodevelopment, brain function and neurological disease. Philos Trans R Soc Lond Ser B Biol Sci. 2014;369(1652).

32. Gibb EA, Vucic EA, Enfield KS, Stewart GL, Lonergan KM, Kennett JY, Becker-Santos DD, MacAulay CE, Lam S, Brown CJ, Lam WL. Human cancer long non-coding RNA transcriptomes. PLoS One. 2011;6(10):e25915.

33. Khalil AM, Guttman M, Huarte M, Garber M, Raj A, Rivea Morales D, Thomas K, Presser A, Bernstein BE, van Oudenaarden A, et al. Many human large intergenic noncoding RNAs associate with chromatin-modifying complexes and affect gene expression. Proc Natl Acad Sci U S A. 2009; 106(28):11667–72.

34. Guttman M, Donaghey J, Carey BW, Garber M, Grenier JK, Munson G, Young G, Lucas AB, Ach R, Bruhn L, et al. lincRNAs act in the circuitry controlling pluripotency and differentiation. Nature. 2011;477(7364):295–300.

35. Wang J, Zhao H, Fan Z, Li G, Ma Q, Tao Z, Wang R, Feng J, Luo Y, Long Noncoding RNA. H19 promotes neuroinflammation in ischemic stroke by driving histone deacetylase 1-dependent M1 microglial polarization. Stroke. 2017;48(8):2211–21.

36. NE II, Heward JA, Roux B, Tsitsiou E, Fenwick PS, Lenzi L, Goodhead I, Hertz-Fowler C, Heger A, Hall N, et al. Long non-coding RNAs and enhancer RNAs regulate the lipopolysaccharide-induced inflammatory response in human monocytes. Nat Commun. 2014;5:3979.

37. Zhou X, Han X, Wittfeldt A, Sun J, Liu C, Wang X, Gan LM, Cao H, Liang Z. Long non-coding RNA ANRIL regulates inflammatory responses as a novel component of NF-kappaB pathway. RNA Biol. 2016;13(1):98–108.

38. Zhao G, Su Z, Song D, Mao Y, Mao X. The long noncoding RNA MALAT1 regulates the lipopolysaccharide-induced inflammatory response through its interaction with NF-kappaB. FEBS Lett. 2016;590(17):2884–95.

39. Zhang F, Wu L, Qian J, Qu B, Xia S, La T, Wu Y, Ma J, Zeng J, Guo Q, et al. Identification of the long noncoding RNA NEAT1 as a novel inflammatory regulator acting through MAPK pathway in human lupus. J Autoimmun. 2016;75:96–104.

40. Barlev NA, Liu L, Chehab NH, Mansfield K, Harris KG, Halazonetis TD, Berger SL. Acetylation of p53 activates transcription through recruitment of coactivators/histone acetyltransferases. Mol Cell. 2001; 8(6):1243–54.

41. Schroder S, Herker E, Itzen F, He D, Thomas S, Gilchrist DA, Kaehlcke K, Cho S, Pollard KS, Capra JA, et al. Acetylation of RNA polymerase II regulates growth-factor-induced gene transcription in mammalian cells. Mol Cell. 2013;52(3):314–24.

42. Tie F, Banerjee R, Stratton CA, Prasad-Sinha J, Stepanik V, Zlobin A, Diaz MO, Scacheri PC, Harte PJ. CBP-mediated acetylation of histone H3 lysine 27 antagonizes Drosophila Polycomb silencing. Development. 2009;136(18): 3131–41.

43. Wang F, Marshall CB, Ikura M. Transcriptional/epigenetic regulator CBP/p300 in tumorigenesis: structural and functional versatility in target recognition. Cell Mol Life Sci. 2013;70(21):3989–4008.

44. Bedford DC, Kasper LH, Fukuyama T, Brindle PK. Target gene context influences the transcriptional requirement for the KAT3 family of CBP and p300 histone acetyltransferases. Epigenetics. 2010;5(1):9–15.

45. Jin Q, Yu LR, Wang L, Zhang Z, Kasper LH, Lee JE, Wang C, Brindle PK, Dent SY, Ge K. Distinct roles of GCN5/PCAF-mediated H3K9ac and CBP/p300-mediated H3K18/27ac in nuclear receptor transactivation. EMBO J. 2011; 30(2):249–62.

46. Bose DA, Donahue G, Reinberg D, Shiekhattar R, Bonasio R, Berger SL. RNA binding to CBP stimulates histone acetylation and transcription. Cell. 2017; 168(1–2):135–49 e22.

47. Cui W, Yoneda R, Ueda N, Kurokawa R. Arginine methylation of translocated in liposarcoma (TLS) inhibits its binding to long noncoding RNA, abrogating TLS-mediated repression of CBP/p300 activity. J Biol Chem. 2018;293(28): 10937–48.

48. Liu XM, He FX, Pang RR, Zhao D, Qiu W, Shan K, Zhang J, Lu YL, Li Y, Wang YW. Interleukin-17 (IL-17)-induced microRNA 873 (miR-873) contributes to the pathogenesis of experimental autoimmune encephalomyelitis by targeting A20 ubiquitin-editing enzyme. J Biol Chem. 2014;289(42): 28971–86.

49. Liu X, Zhang Q, Wang W, Zuo D, Wang J, Zhou F, Niu L, Li X, Qin S, Kou Y, et al. Analysis of long noncoding RNA and mRNA expression profiles in IL-9-activated astrocytes and EAE mice. Cell Physiol Biochem. 2018;45(5): 1986–98.

50. Kang Z, Altuntas CZ, Gulen MF, Liu C, Giltiay N, Qin H, Liu L, Qian W, Ransohoff RM, Bergmann C, et al. Astrocyte-restricted ablation of interleukin-17-mediated signaling ameliorates autoimmune encephalomyelitis. Immunity. 2010;32(3):414–25.

51. Tsai MC, Manor O, Wan Y, Mosammaparast N, Wang JK, Lan F, Shi Y, Segal E, Chang HY. Long noncoding RNA as modular scaffold of histone modification complexes. Science. 2010;329(5992):689–93.

52. Zhou F, Shimoda M, Olney L, Lyu Y, Tran K, Jiang G, Nakano K, Davis RR, Tepper CG, Maverakis E, et al. Oncolytic reactivation of KSHV as a therapeutic approach for primary effusion lymphoma. Mol Cancer Ther. 2017;16(11): 2627–38.

53. Raymond AD, Campbell-Sims TC, Khan M, Lang M, Huang MB, Bond VC, Powell MD. HIV type 1 Nef is released from infected cells in CD45(+) microvesicles and is present in the plasma of HIV-infected individuals. AIDS Res Hum Retrovir. 2011;27(2):167–78.

54. Cullen BR. HIV-1 auxiliary proteins: making connections in a dying cell. Cell. 1998;93(5):685–92.

55. Fujii Y, Otake K, Tashiro M, Adachi A. Soluble Nef antigen of HIV-1 is cytotoxic for human CD4+ T cells. FEBS Lett. 1996;393(1):93–6.

56. Qiao X, He B, Chiu A, Knowles DM, Chadburn A, Cerutti A. Human immunodeficiency virus 1 Nef suppresses CD40-dependent immunoglobulin class switching in bystander B cells. Nat Immunol. 2006;7(3):302–10.

57. Yan Q, Ma X, Shen C, Cao X, Feng N, Qin D, Zeng Y, Zhu J, Gao SJ, Lu C. Inhibition of Kaposi's sarcoma-associated herpesvirus lytic replication by HIV-1 Nef and cellular microRNA hsa-miR-1258. J Virol. 2014;88(9): 4987–5000.

58. Marecki JC, Cool CD, Parr JE, Beckey VE, Luciw PA, Tarantal AF, Carville A, Shannon RP, Cota-Gomez A, Tuder RM, et al. HIV-1 Nef is associated with complex pulmonary vascular lesions in SHIV-nef-infected macaques. Am J Respir Crit Care Med. 2006;174(4):437–45.

59. Xue M, Yao S, Hu M, Li W, Hao T, Zhou F, Zhu X, Lu H, Qin D, Yan Q, et al. HIV-1 Nef and KSHV oncogene K1 synergistically promote angiogenesis by inducing cellular miR-718 to regulate the PTEN/AKT/mTOR signaling pathway. Nucleic Acids Res. 2014;42(15):9862–79.

60. Narasipura SD, Kim S, Al-Harthi L. Epigenetic regulation of HIV-1 latency in astrocytes. J Virol. 2014;88(5):3031–8.

61. Prensner JR, Iyer MK, Sahu A, Asangani IA, Cao Q, Patel L, Vergara IA, Davicioni E, Erho N, Ghadessi M, et al. The long noncoding RNA SChLAP1 promotes aggressive prostate cancer and antagonizes the SWI/SNF complex. Nat Genet. 2013;45(11):1392–8.

62. Ogawa N, Ping L, Zhenjun L, Takada Y, Sugai S. Involvement of the interferon-gamma-induced T cell-attracting chemokine, interferon-gamma-inducible 10-kd protein (CXCL10) and monokine induced by interferon-gamma (CXCL9), in the salivary gland lesions of patients with Sjogren's syndrome. Arthritis Rheum. 2002;46(10):2730–41.

9

Human neural stem cell-derived neuron/astrocyte co-cultures respond to La Crosse virus infection with proinflammatory cytokines and chemokines

Brian E. Dawes[1], Junling Gao[2], Colm Atkins[3], Jacob T. Nelson[3], Kendra Johnson[1], Ping Wu[2] and Alexander N. Freiberg[3,4,5]* (iD)

Abstract

Background: La Crosse virus (LACV) causes pediatric encephalitis in the USA. LACV induces severe inflammation in the central nervous system, but the recruitment of inflammatory cells is poorly understood. A deeper understanding of LACV-induced neural pathology is needed in order to develop treatment options. However, there is a severe limitation of relevant human neuronal cell models of LACV infection.

Methods: We utilized human neural stem cell (hNSC)-derived neuron/astrocyte co-cultures to study LACV infection in disease-relevant primary cells. hNSCs were differentiated into neurons and astrocytes and infected with LACV. To characterize susceptibility and responses to infection, we measured viral titers and levels of viral RNA, performed immunofluorescence analysis to determine the cell types infected, performed apoptosis and cytotoxicity assays, and evaluated cellular responses to infection using qRT-PCR and Bioplex assays.

Results: hNSC-derived neuron/astrocyte co-cultures were susceptible to LACV infection and displayed apoptotic responses as reported in previous in vitro and in vivo studies. Neurons and astrocytes are both targets of LACV infection, with neurons becoming the predominant target later in infection possibly due to astrocytic responses to IFN. Additionally, neuron/astrocyte co-cultures responded to LACV infection with strong proinflammatory cytokine, chemokine, as well as MMP-2, MMP-7, and TIMP-1 responses.

Conclusions: hNSC-derived neuron/astrocyte co-cultures reproduce key aspects of LACV infection in humans and mice and are useful models to study encephalitic viruses. Specifically, we show astrocytes to be susceptible to LACV infection and that neurons and astrocytes are important drivers of the inflammatory responses seen in LACV infection through the production of proinflammatory cytokines and chemokines.

Keywords: La Crosse virus, Neural stem cells, Neurons, Astrocytes, Inflammation, Encephalitis, Central nervous system

* Correspondence: anfreibe@utmb.edu
[3]Department of Pathology, University of Texas Medical Branch, 301 University Boulevard, Galveston 77555-0609, USA
[4]Center for Biodefense and Emerging Infectious Diseases, University of Texas Medical Branch, Galveston, USA
Full list of author information is available at the end of the article

Background

La Crosse virus (LACV), family *Peribunyaviridae* (genus *Orthobunyavirus*), is a leading cause of pediatric arboviral encephalitis in the USA [1]. The primary vector of LACV is the eastern tree-hole mosquito (*Ochlerotatus triseriatus*). LACV was responsible for 665 confirmed cases of encephalitis from 2003 to 2012, although the true incidence of disease is thought to be underestimated [2]. Endemic areas of infection include the Midwest and Appalachian regions, with county-level incidence of 0.2–228 cases per 100,000 children under the age of 15, but LACV is also becoming an important emerging pathogen of the Southern and Western United States [3]. Despite the threats posed, there are currently no approved therapeutics or vaccines available against LACV.

LACV encephalitis is almost exclusively found in children under 15 years of age [4]. Like other arboviruses, the majority of cases present as mild febrile illness, but in a minority of cases, LACV causes severe neuroinvasive disease including encephalitis, meningitis, and meningoencephalitis [5]. Neuroinvasive LACV typically presents with fever, headache, lethargy, and vomiting, and nearly half of patients experience seizures [4, 5]. While the disease is rarely (< 1%) fatal, neurological deficits such as epilepsy (in 10–28% of cases), reduced IQ, and attention-deficit-hyperactivity disorder (ADHD) are not uncommon [4–6].

LACV replicates peripherally and likely invades the central nervous system (CNS) via the olfactory bulb in the mouse model of LACV encephalitis after the compromise of the blood-brain barrier (BBB) [7]. In human infection, cortical and basal ganglia neurons appear to be the primary target of infection in the CNS leading to foci of neuronal necrosis [8]. Additionally, inflammatory lesions with largely monocytic infiltration and lymphocytic perivascular cuffing are noted [8]. The understanding of LACV neuropathogenesis has been advanced by studies using the suckling mouse model which closely resembles human disease including age-related susceptibility [9, 10]. Infection of adult mice and rhesus macaques result in asymptomatic infections and antibody responses [9, 10]. Most studies agree that neurons comprise the main target cell in the CNS [9, 11]. Infected neurons appear to undergo apoptosis via mitochondrial antiviral-signaling protein (MAVS)-induced oxidative stress [12]. However, some groups report low levels of astrocyte infection in vitro and in vivo [1, 11]. Especially interesting is the finding that when NSs, a LACV encoded interferon (IFN) antagonist, is deleted, astrocytes significantly increase production of IFN, suggesting that IFN production in astrocytes is antagonized by LACV [11]. Regarding the inflammatory component of the disease, a recent study showed that lymphocytes play a protective role during LACV infection of adult mice

and do not contribute to the pathogenesis of weanling mice [13]. The majority of inflammatory cells noted in human and mouse brains during LACV infection are monocytes and macrophages. Recent work has demonstrated that in the mouse model, CCL2 is important for inflammatory monocytic migration within the brain and that astrocytes are a source of CCL2 in the brain [8, 14]. Importantly, it is becoming increasingly clear that CNS parenchymal cells play a major role in the development of innate immune responses during LACV infection [15–17]. Additionally, cytokine responses can also negatively impact BBB integrity and lead to worsened neuroinvasion [18, 19]. While our knowledge on the pathogenesis and molecular mechanisms of LACV-induced disease using animal models is increasing, there is still a need to verify many of these results with a human-based system.

Primary human neurons are terminally differentiated, post-mitotic, and difficult to obtain. Most studies of encephalitic viruses rely on primary rat or mouse neuronal cells or human neuroblastoma cell lines. While these models are strong tools for understanding pathogenesis, species differences and the genetic and signaling abnormalities found in these models require validation using human cells without genetic modification. Furthermore, most studies rely on the use of a single cell type, although it has been shown that neuronal cells behave differently in co-culture compared to monoculture [20, 21]. In recent years, human neural stem cells (hNSC), embryonic stem cells (hESCs), and induced pluripotent cells (iPCs) have become important tools in studying neurologic diseases, including encephalitic viruses. Varicella zoster virus (VZV) has been extensively studied using such systems, which has provided accurate models for VZV productive infection, latency, and reactivation. [22–26].

In this study, we use a well-validated hNSC-derived neuron/astrocyte co-culture system which has previously been used in the study of neurodegenerative diseases [27–29]. Importantly, this primary human neural cell system was recently used to assess Zika virus-induced changes in hNSC differentiation, although this study mainly focused on the direct infection of hNSCs rather than differentiated neuronal cells [30]. We have reported susceptibility of neuron/astrocyte co-cultures to infection with henipaviruses, but an in-depth characterization of the cellular responses to infection has not been reported yet [31]. In the present study, we infected hNSC-derived neuron/astrocyte co-cultures with LACV. Our results indicate that both neurons and astrocytes are highly susceptible to LACV, and that LACV infection induces strong proinflammatory responses, which likely play a major role in the observed neuroinflammation and breakdown in the BBB.

Methods

Cells and viruses

Vero CCL81 cells were acquired from American Type Culture Collection (ATCC, Manassas, VA). Vero cells were propagated using MEM (Corning) supplemented with 10%FBS. K048 hNSCs were originally obtained from the cortex of a 9-week-old male fetus and were propagated as described previously [27]. Briefly, hNSCs were cultured as nonadherent neurospheres in DMEM/F12 (Corning) media supplemented with epidermal growth factor (EGF) (20 ng/mL) (R&D Systems), fibroblast growth factor (FGF) (20 ng/mL) (R&D Systems), leukocyte inhibitory factor (LIF) (10 ng/mL) (Chemicon), heparin (5 μg/mL) (Sigma-Aldrich), and insulin (25 μg/mL) (Sigma-Aldrich). Cells were passaged every 10 days and maintained at 37 °C and 8.5% CO_2.

hNSCs were plated onto wells coated with 0.01% poly-D-Lysine (Sigma-Aldrich) and 1 μg/cm^2 laminin. Cells were primed for 4 days with a priming media containing EGF (20 ng/mL), LIF (10 ng/mL), and laminin (1 μg/mL) (GIBCO). K048 hNSCs were primed and differentiated into neurons and astrocytes in a roughly 1:1 ratio. The neurons in this system have previously been characterized as being both GABAergic and glutamatergic, and the overall composition is similar to that found in the cerebral cortex [32]. Cells were then differentiated for 9 days in a differentiation media containing N2 basal media supplemented with glutathione (1 μg/mL) (Sigma-Aldrich), biotin (0.1 μg/mL) (Sigma-Aldrich), superoxide dismutase (2.5 μg/mL) (Sigma-Aldrich), DL-α-tocopherol (1 μg/mL) (Sigma-Aldrich), DL-α-tocopherol acetate (1 μg/mL) (Sigma-Aldrich), and catalase (2.5 μg/mL) (Sigma-Aldrich).

LACV was obtained from the World Reference Center for Emerging Viruses and Arboviruses at the University of Texas Medical Branch (kindly provided by R. Tesh). The strain used was isolated from a human brain in Wisconsin in 1964. This strain had undergone nine passages in suckling mice and was amplified in our lab in one passage in Vero cells.

Growth curves

Neuron/astrocyte co-cultures were infected with 0.1, 1, or 10 multiplicity of infection (MOI) of LACV for 1 h at 37 °C and 8.5% CO_2. Virus inoculum was removed, cells gently washed with PBS, and fresh culture medium re-added. Cells only underwent one PBS wash due to the fragility of the neurons to avoid their detachment. Supernatant aliquots were then collected at various time points after infection. Samples were titrated via standard plaque assay. Cell culture supernatant aliquots were serially diluted in MEM supplemented with 2% FBS and used to infect Vero CCL81 cells for 1 h. Cells were washed with PBS and given a media overlay of MEM with 0.8% tragacanth (Sigma-Aldrich). At 4 days post-infection, the overlay was removed, cells were fixed in 10% formalin (Thermo Fisher) and stained using crystal violet (Thermo Fisher), and plaques were counted.

Immunofluorescence

Neuron/astrocyte co-cultures on glass coverslips were infected with 0.1, 1, or 10 MOI of LACV as described above. Infected cells were fixed in formalin at various times post-infection. Cells were stained with primary antibodies and fluorophore-conjugated secondary antibodies along with DAPI (Sigma Aldrich) as previously described [20]. Antibodies used were rabbit-anti-microtubule associated protein 2 (MAP2) polyclonal (Millipore, AB5622) used at 1:500, rabbit-anti-glial fibrillary acidic protein (GFAP) polyclonal (Millipore, AB5804) used at 1:2,000, and mouse-anti-LACV Gc monoclonal (ThermoFisher, MA1–10801) used at 1:1,000. Secondary antibodies were Alexa Fluor goat-anti-rabbit 594 and goat-anti-mouse 488 used at 1:500 (ThermoFisher). Images were acquired on an Olympus IX71 fluorescent microscope and cells were quantified visually using six random fields per condition with an average of over 200 cells/field.

Cytotoxicity and apoptosis assays

Neuron/astrocyte co-cultures were grown in 96-well plates and infected with 1 MOI of LACV as in other experiments along with media only controls and 10 μM staurosporine (Abcam) treatment. Cells were then assayed using the ApoTox-Glo triplex assay (Promega) according to the manufacturer's protocols. Plates were assayed on a BioTek Synergy HT plate reader at 485nm$_{Ex}$/505nm$_{Em}$ for cytotoxicity (extracellular protease activity) and luminescence for apoptosis (caspase 3/7 activity).

TUNEL assay

Neuron/astrocyte co-cultures were infected with 1 MOI LACV as described previously and fixed at 96 HPI. Additionally, staurosporine-treated cells were fixed at 12 h post-treatment. Formalin-fixed monolayers were prepared for immunofluorescence staining as previously described. Terminal deoxynucleotidyl transferase dUTP nick end labeling (TUNEL) staining (TACS 2 TdT-Fluor In Situ Apoptosis Detection Kit, R&D systems) was performed as per manufacturer instructions. Briefly, following DAPI stain, cells were incubated in labeling buffer, followed by labeling reaction mix. Strep-FITC was added for 20 min before final washes. Slides were briefly rinsed in ddH$_2$O to remove residual salt and inverted onto Fluoromount G (Southern Biotech) and allowed to cure overnight at 4 °C in the dark. Samples were imaged on an Olympus BX61 microscope.

BioPlex assays

Co-cultures were infected as in previous experiments with 0.1, 1, or 10 MOI of LACV or treated with heat-inactivated LACV (60 °C for 30 min) (1 MOI) or 10 μM polyinosinic:polycytidylic acid (poly I:C) (Sigma Aldrich). Supernatant samples were collected at various time points post-infection and γ-irradiated with a dose of 5 Mrad to inactivate the infectious virus. Cells treated with Poly I:C or heat-inactivated virus were collected at 48 h post-infection (HPI) only. Samples were then used for BioPlex assay analysis (Bio-Plex Pro Human Cytokine, Group 1, 27-Plex, Bio-Plex) according to manufacturer's protocols. Standard curves were developed using fresh standards provided in each kit. The assays were run on a Bio-Plex 200 system (Bio-Rad), and data was analyzed using Bio-Plex Manager (Bio-Rad).

qRT-PCR

Co-cultures were grown and infected with 0.1, 1, 10 MOI or treated with heat-inactivated virus or poly I:C. Cells were lysed and collected in TRIzol (Thermo Fisher) reagent, and RNA was isolated using Direct-zol RNA Miniprep kits (Zymo Research). cDNA was obtained using High Capacity RNA-to-cDNA kit (Thermo-Fisher). cDNA was then amplified using SYBR green mix (Bio-Rad) on a Bio-Rad CFX384 instrument. Data was analyzed using CFX Manager (Bio-Rad), and mRNA expression differences were determined via change in threshold cycle (ΔCT) and normalized to 18S RNA ($\Delta\Delta$CT). PrimeTime qPCR primers (IDT) were used to target MMP7, MMP2, and TIMP2. PrimePCR PCR primers (Bio-Rad) were used to target IL-6, IL-8, CXCL10, CCL2, CCL4, CCL5, and TNF-α. Additional primers (IDT) were used to target 18S (For-GTAA CCCGTTGAACCCCATT, Rev-CCATCCAATCGGTA GTAGCG), IFN-α (For-GACTCCATCTTGGCTGTGA, Rev-TGATTTCTGCTCTGACAACCT), IFN-β (For-TCTG GCACAGGTAGTAGGC, Rev-GAGAAGCACAACAG GAGAGCAA) and LACV (For-ATTCTACCCGCTGA CCATTG, Rev-GTGAGAGTGCCATAGCGTTG).

MMP activity assay

Supernatants of LACV-infected neuron/astrocyte co-cultures were assayed for the activities of matrix metalloproteinases (MMPs) using MMP Activity Assay Kit (Fluorometric-Green) (Abcam, #ab112146) as per manufacturer's instructions. Briefly, pro-MMPs in solution are activated by incubating with APMA, immediately prior to enzyme reaction. Samples were read on a Bio-Tek Synergy multimode plate reader at 490/525 nm at 60 min incubation. Substrate and culture media controls were used to reduce background in analyzed values. All conditions were performed in singlicate from biological triplet samples.

Statistical analysis

All experiments were performed in biological triplicate. All statistical analysis and figure preparation was performed with Prism (GraphPad Software). Cytotoxicity and apoptosis assays were subjected to two-way ANOVA with Bonferroni's multiple comparisons test. BioPlex control experiments were subjected to one-way ANOVA with Tukey's multiple comparisons test. The qRT-PCR and BioPlex experiments of the stimulated controls were subjected to one-way ANOVA with Dunnett's multiple comparisons test. The qRT-PCR, BioPlex, MMP activity assays, and immunofluorescence experiments of virus-infected samples were subjected to two-way ANOVA with Tukey's multiple comparisons test. TUNEL assays were subjected to one-way ANOVA with Tukey's (percent of cells TUNEL positive) or Sidak's (percent of TUNEL positive cells expressing GFAP or MAP2) multiple comparisons tests.

Results

hNSC-derived neuron/astrocyte co-cultures are susceptible to LACV infection

We first set out to demonstrate that hNSC-derived neuron/astrocyte co-cultures are susceptible to LACV infection and accurately replicate key aspects of LACV infection seen in other models including the susceptibility of neurons and apoptosis [9, 12, 33, 34]. Differentiated co-cultures were infected with 0.1, 1, or 10 MOI of LACV and images taken at 24, 48, and 72 HPI. At 48 HPI, the lytic nature of LACV infection could be observed, which is consistent with human and animal pathology (Fig. 1a) [8, 9, 33]. Cytopathic effect (CPE) was correlated with initial MOI, with 10 MOI infections resulting in maximum cell rounding and cell death as opposed to 0.1 MOI (not shown), which had only minimal observable CPE.

Supernatant aliquots were collected and titrated via plaque assay (Fig. 1b). High initial titers are due to the fragility of the co-culture system, and the limited ability to wash cells after the initial infection period. Regardless, a sharp increase in viral titers was observed within the first 24 HPI. The 10, 1, and 0.1 MOI infections reached peak titers by 24, 48, and 72 HPI, respectively. Peak titers were approximately 10^6–10^7 PFU/ml and remained within that range for the duration of the study. Additionally, we confirmed viral replication via qRT-PCR (Fig. 1c). An increase in viral RNA within the first 24 HPI was also noted; however, there was a decline at 48 HPI. By 72 HPI, viral RNA had once again increased. Our results indicate that the hNSC-derived neuron/astrocyte co-culture system is susceptible to LACV infection and supports replication and that viral infection leads to noticeable cytopathic effect.

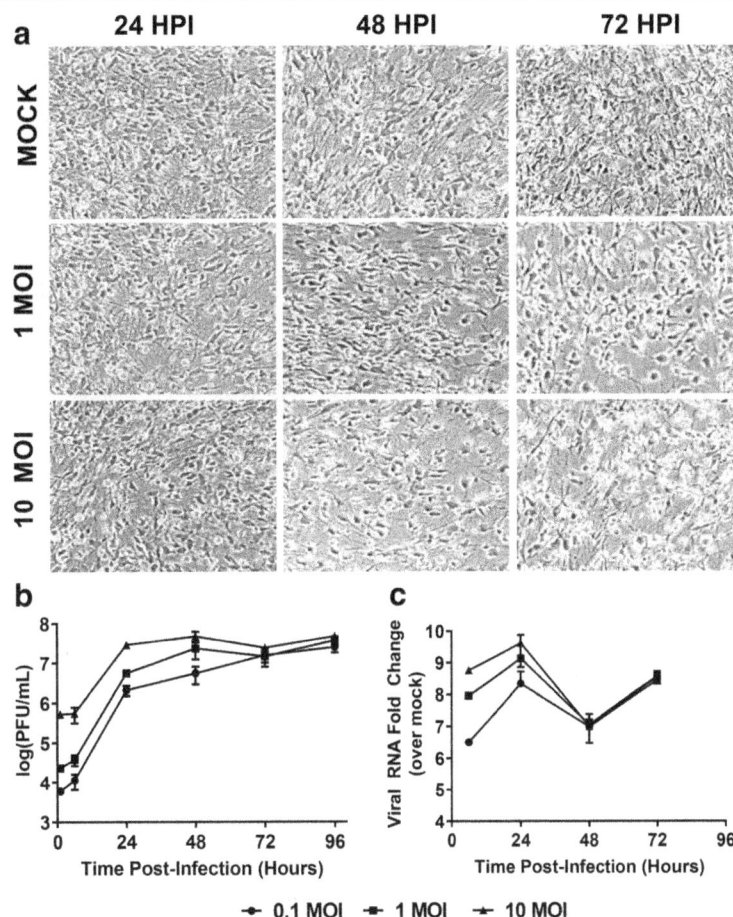

Fig. 1 Susceptibility and replication kinetics in differentiated hNSC neuron/astrocyte co-cultures. hNSCs were primed and differentiated into mature neuron/astrocyte co-cultures for 9 days prior to infection with mock, 0.1, 1, or 10 MOI of LACV. **a** Co-cultures were imaged at various times post-infection via phase contrast microscopy. **b** Supernatant was collected at various times post-infection and titrated via plaque assay. **c** Cells were lysed and RNA was collected and qRT-PCR was used to determine viral replication. Anti-LACV N gene primers were used, and levels were determined as fold change relative to the mock-infected background

Neurons and astrocytes both support LACV replication

We next determined the cell types infected with LACV in the neuron/astrocyte co-cultures. We stained infected cells against LACV glycoprotein and either an astrocytic marker (GFAP) or a neuronal marker (MAP2) with a DAPI counterstain (Fig. 2a). These experiments demonstrated that both neurons and astrocytes were infected. Interestingly, different distribution patterns were noted, particularly at 96 HPI. Neurons either had small punctuate patterns or cell-wide distribution of viral antigen, while in astrocytes antigen was much more apparent in a larger cluster. To further quantify the cell types infected, fields with evident infection were counted and ratios of neuron to astrocyte (Additional file 1: Figure S1), the percentage of neurons or astrocytes infected (Fig. 2b), and the ratio of neurons to astrocytes infected (Fig. 2c) determined. The data indicate that, as previously reported, there is an approximate 1:1 ratio of neurons to astrocytes present in the co-cultures (Additional file 1:

Figure S1) [27, 30]. As early as 12 HPI, the virus was detectable in both cell types, and the percentage of cells infected increases in a time and dose-dependent manner (Fig. 2b). By 96 HPI, about 60% of neurons are infected, and 30% of astrocytes are infected. At early time points, neurons and astrocytes appear to be infected at an approximate 1:1 ratio with a trend towards greater neuronal infection (Fig. 2c). However, by 72 HPI, neurons became the more prevalent infected cell type. By 96 HPI, the ratio of neurons to astrocytes infected was approximately 2:1. At higher MOIs, this trend was weaker, with approximately equal percentages of neurons and astrocytes infected (Additional file 2: Figure S2a), but neurons become the predominant cell type infected later in infection (Additional file 2: Figure S2b). Taken together, these data indicate that in the hNSC-derived neuron/astrocyte co-culture system neurons and astrocytes are both susceptible to LACV infection, but neuronal infection is enriched later during the course of infection.

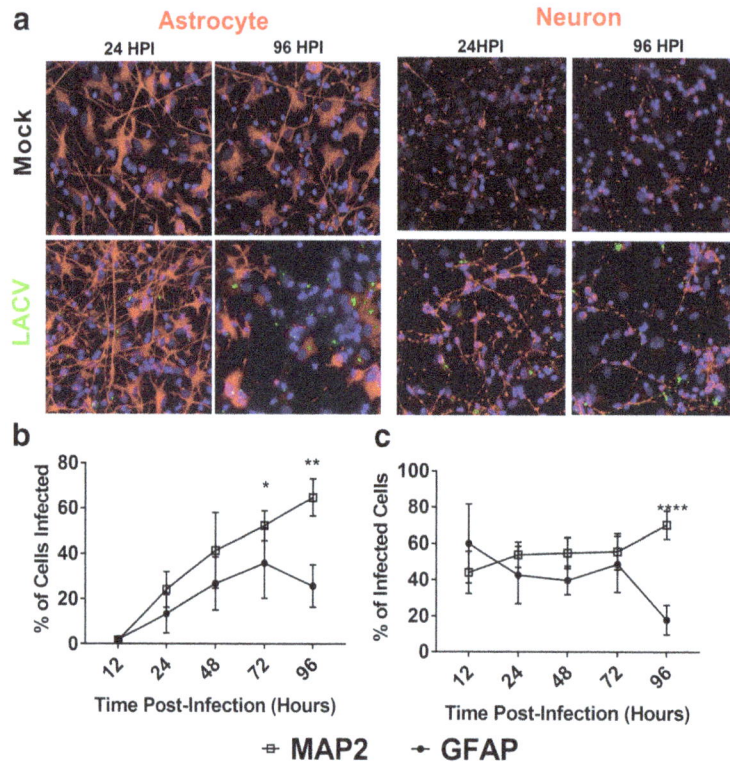

Fig. 2 Identification of LACV target cells in neuron/astrocyte co-cultures. Neuron/astrocyte co-cultures were infected with 0.1, 1, and 10 MOI of LACV and formalin fixed at various times post-infection. **a** Cells were then stained for DAPI, LACV Gc protein, and either neuronal marker MAP2 or astrocytic marker GFAP. Representative images from the mock-infected and 1 MOI LACV-infected group are shown. **b** The percentage of neurons and astrocytes infected was determined over the course of infection for the 0.1 MOI group. The 1 and 10 MOI are available in Additional file 2: Figure S2a. **c** The percentage of infected cells expressing either MAP2 or GFAP was quantified for the set of cells infected with 0.1 MOI. The 1 and 10 MOI have similar trends and are available in Additional file 2: Figure S2b. $*P < 0.05$, $**P < 0.01$, $****P < 0.0001$

LACV induces apoptosis in hNSC-derived neuron/astrocyte co-cultures

Previous studies have demonstrated that neurons in vivo and in vitro undergo apoptosis in response to LACV infection [9, 12, 33]. To further validate this system, we performed necrosis and apoptosis assays to confirm apoptotic cell death. Neuron/astrocyte co-cultures were either mock-infected, infected with LACV, or treated with staurosporine. A single dose (1 MOI) was selected because at this MOI CPE is apparent, titers are comparable to 10 MOI infections, and cells remain viable for longer which allowed us to assay later time points. A cytotoxicity assay (Fig. 3a) assessed supernatant for cell-impermeable proteases via fluorescence, and an apoptosis assay (Fig. 3b) detected caspase 3/7 activity via luminescence. As expected, mock-infected controls displayed low levels of cytotoxicity and caspase activation throughout the course of the experiment. Staurosporine controls were only measured for the first 24 h but demonstrated significant cytotoxicity and caspase 3/7 activation at that time point indicating an apoptotic response. LACV-infected co-cultures began displaying significant cytotoxicity at 48 HPI (Fig. 3a) consistent with CPE

observed in Fig. 1a. Additionally, at 48 HPI, significant increases in caspase 3/7 activity were measured in LACV-infected neuron/astrocyte co-cultures (Fig. 3b). Taken together, these results indicate that apoptosis is a primary mediator of cytotoxicity in LACV-infected neuron/astrocyte co-cultures.

To determine which cells were dying as a result of apoptosis, we performed TUNEL staining on LACV-infected neuron/astrocyte co-cultures at 96 HPI. Around 20% of cells at 96 HPI were apoptotic in the absence of LACV infection, and staurosporine treatment led to roughly 50% of cells undergoing apoptosis (Fig. 3c). LACV infection resulted in similar levels of apoptosis to staurosporine treatment (Fig. 3c). To determine which cells were undergoing apoptosis, cells were double stained with TUNEL staining and either GFAP or MAP2 (Fig. 3d). Apoptotic cells in mock-infected co-cultures were both MAP2 and GFAP positive, but neurons appeared to be more susceptible. Staurosporine induced apoptosis in both neurons and astrocytes equally. LACV induced apoptosis in both neurons and astrocytes. However, apoptotic cells were nearly twice as likely to be neurons. These data indicate that LACV infection

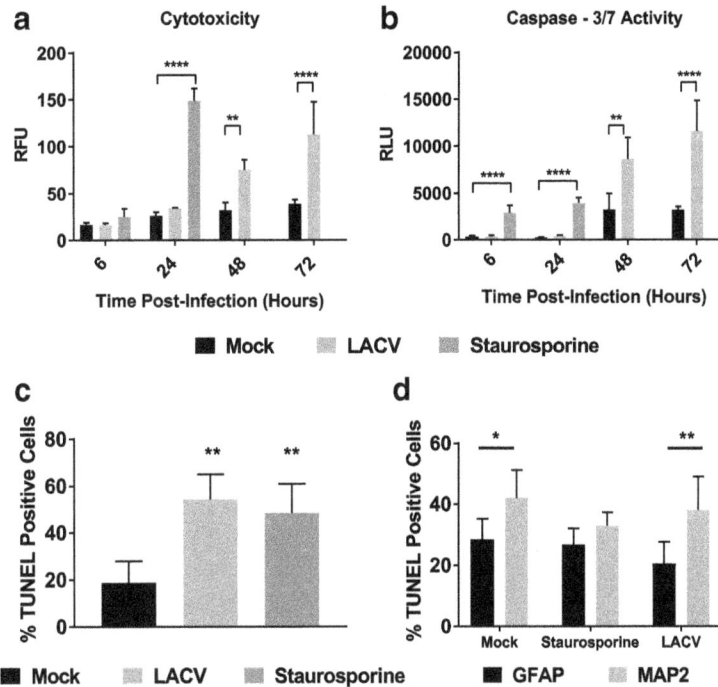

Fig. 3 Apoptosis of LACV-infected neuron/astrocyte co-cultures. Neuron/astrocyte co-cultures were infected with 1 MOI of LACV and assayed for **a** cytotoxicity or **b** apoptosis at various time points. Staurosporine treatment was included up to 24 HPI as a positive control for apoptosis. Cytotoxicity was measured via fluorescence activity of a non-permeable protease substrate, and apoptosis was measured via luminescence from a caspase 3/7 substrate. **c** TUNEL staining was performed at 96 HPI to determine the percentage of apoptotic cells. **d** Double staining with TUNEL and cell markers was performed. Results reported are the percentages of TUNEL positive cells expressing either GFAP or MAP2. *$P < 0.05$ **$P < 0.01$ ****$P < 0.0001$

induces apoptosis in both neurons and astrocytes, but neurons appear to be more susceptible to apoptosis.

hNSC-derived neuron/astrocyte co-cultures are responsive to proinflammatory stimuli

After demonstrating that the hNSC-derived neuron/astrocyte co-culture system reproduced the basic pathology seen in LACV, we next confirmed the innate immune responses of these primary human cells to inflammatory stimuli [8, 9, 33]. For these studies, neuron/astrocyte co-cultures were either mock-treated or treated with heat-inactivated LACV or Poly I:C (Additional file 3: Figure S3). No significant increases were noted with inactivated LACV for any of the tested analytes at the transcriptional level (Additional file 3: Figure S3a). In contrast, the majority of analytes were significantly upregulated after Poly I:C exposure including IFN-β, proinflammatory cytokines IL-6 and TNF-α, and proinflammatory chemokines IL-8, CCL2, CCL4, CCL5, and CXCL10. IFN-α was not significantly upregulated in response to Poly I:C similar to previous studies [35, 36]. Translational changes were confirmed using BioPlex assays (Additional file 3: Figure S3b). Among the upregulated proteins were the proinflammatory cytokines IFN-γ, IL-6, and TNF-α and the proinflammatory chemokines IL-8,

CCL4, CCL5, and CXCL10 (Fig. 4b). Surprisingly, no significant increase in CCL2 protein expression was detected in comparison to mock- and heat-inactivated LACV-treated cells. These data indicate that neuron/astrocyte co-cultures have the ability to respond to proinflammatory stimuli in a physiologically relevant manner with the production of interferons, cytokines, and chemokines.

hNSC-derived neuron/astrocyte co-cultures respond to LACV infection with proinflammatory chemokine and cytokine responses

After demonstrating that hNSC derived neuron/astrocyte co-cultures are capable of responding to insult with the production of cytokines and chemokines, we measured the co-cultures' responses to LACV infection. To accomplish this, co-cultures were infected with 0.1, 1, or 10 MOI of LACV and responses measured over time. RNA was collected and analyzed via qRT-PCR. IFN-α responses were detected as early as 6 HPI and continued until 48 HPI before decreasing to near baseline levels at 72 HPI (Additional file 4: Figure S4a). IFN-β responses were detected later (24 HPI through 48 HPI) but were much stronger (Fig. 4a). The other cytokines and chemokines investigated (IL-6, TNF-α, IL-8, CCL2, CCL4, CCL5, and CXCL10) displayed significant increases with

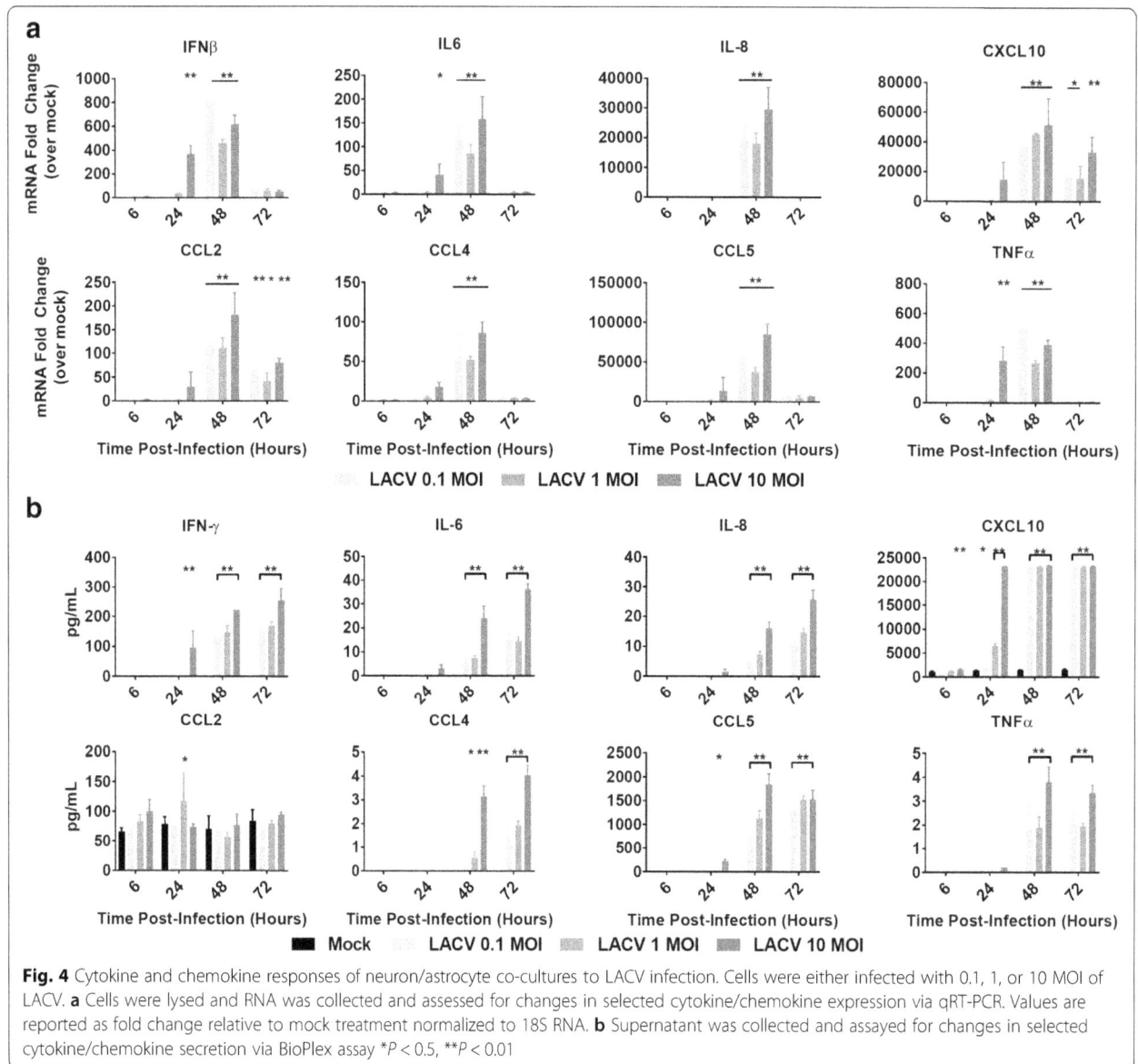

Fig. 4 Cytokine and chemokine responses of neuron/astrocyte co-cultures to LACV infection. Cells were either infected with 0.1, 1, or 10 MOI of LACV. **a** Cells were lysed and RNA was collected and assessed for changes in selected cytokine/chemokine expression via qRT-PCR. Values are reported as fold change relative to mock treatment normalized to 18S RNA. **b** Supernatant was collected and assayed for changes in selected cytokine/chemokine secretion via BioPlex assay *P < 0.5, **P < 0.01

the peak mRNA induction at 48 HPI (Fig. 4a). In general, these responses were stronger in the 10 MOI group than in the 0.1 and 1 MOI groups. Additionally, responses in the 10 MOI group had a tendency to show significant upregulation earlier (24 HPI), which correlated with the viral growth kinetics (Fig. 1b, c).

Protein secretion patterns closely mirrored mRNA responses. Most measured analytes had significant upregulation at 48 and 72 HPI, with some analytes such as IFN-γ, CXCL10, and CCL5 responding at 24 HPI (Fig. 4b). In general, the responses were stronger in the 10 MOI group. Interestingly, again, we noted no significant differences in CCL2 secretion opposed to large mRNA increases. PDGF, IL-1Rα, IL-4, IL-7, IL-9, Eotaxin, FGF, G-CSF, VEGF, MIP-1α, and GM-CSF also displayed upregulation at 48 and 72 HPI, IL-12,

IL-10, and IL-13 displayed mild increases over mock, and IL-1β, IL-2, IL-5, IL-15, and IL-17 did not display significant increases (Additional file 4: Figure S4b). These data demonstrate that neuron/astrocyte co-culture responded to LACV infection with a strong pro-inflammatory cytokine profile, with particularly large increases in monocytic and lymphocytic chemokines.

hNSC-derived neuron/astrocyte co-cultures alter MMP and TIMP expression in response to LACV infection

In addition to cytokine and chemokine responses, we also determined expression levels of matrix metalloproteinases (MMPs) or tissue inhibitor of metalloproteinases (TIMPs), which can influence the permeability of the BBB [37–39]. To determine the changes in MMP and TIMP expression in the neuron/astrocyte co-culture system, cells were treated as in previous experiments and RNA analyzed by qRT-PCR. Here, we assayed MMP2, MMP7, MMP9, TIMP1, and TIMP2, which have previously been described to be differentially expressed after infection of the CNS [19, 40–42]. No responses were measured for MMP9 (data not shown). Low but significant increases were detected for MMP2, although interestingly, Poly I:C failed to induce a significant change (Fig. 5a). Of note, the increase at 48 HPI, while statistically significant, was very similar to that of inactive virus controls, and may constitute a measurement artifact. MMP7 had the largest induction with significant upregulation for all three MOIs at 48 and 72 HPI (Fig. 5a). TIMP-1 was also significantly upregulated in response to viral infection and Poly I:C at 48 and 72 HPI. Lastly, upregulation was not noted for TIMP2. We instead measured significant downregulation of TIMP2 mRNA for co-cultures infected with 10 MOI at 72 HPI (Fig. 5a). Additionally, while not significant, Poly I:C treatment trended to similar levels of downregulation. Taken together, these data suggest that later responses in neurons and/or astrocytes significantly upregulate MMP7 and TIMP1 while potentially downregulating TIMP2.

As both MMPs and TIMPs were upregulated, we assessed the overall MMP activity during LACV infection via a MMP activity assay. Supernatant from LACV infected, inactivated LACV infected, or Poly I:C treated co-cultures was assessed for MMP substrate cleavage activity throughout the course of infection (Fig. 5b). Poly I:C and inactive virus was only assayed at 48 HPI. Poly I:C and inactive virus significantly increased MMP substrate cleavage activity at 48 HPI. LACV failed to induce any changes in MMP activity until 72 HPI, and only at the highest MOI. These results suggest that while LACV does increase MMP expression, these changes do not result in a functional change until very late during the course of infection.

Discussion

CNS infections continue to be an important facet of emerging viral disease. Despite this threat, in vitro models of CNS infection remain limited. Clinical samples are rarely obtained outside of autopsy due to the challenging nature of CNS biopsy. Animal models, both in vivo and ex vivo studies with primary cells, have been the primary models and provided many important insights [43, 44]. However, animal models often do not accurately model all aspects of clinical disease described in patients. Many studies have now demonstrated profound differences between murine and human cellular responses [45, 46]. Differences also exist in the structure and function of human and murine parenchymal cells. For example, astrocytes are much larger and perform

more complex signaling in humans than in mice [47]. Human primary CNS cells are relevant models, but they are difficult to obtain and introduce donor variability. Immortalized cell lines offer a useful alternative for in vitro studies, but the interpretation of results is limited by alterations in specific pathways and differences among different cell lines. Here, we report the use of a primary hNSC-derived neuron/astrocyte cell co-culture system as a more accurate and reproducible in vitro model to study encephalitic viruses. In addition to allowing for the repeated study of human primary cells without donor variability, co-culturing neurons and astrocytes allows for a more physiologically relevant model than neuronal monoculture. While the lack of donor variability is useful for the identification of pathogenic mechanisms, it may also obscure different aspects of disease as seen in other studies where different hNSC strains responded differently to infection [30]. Astrocytes play a key role in the physiologic support of neuronal health and function such as synaptic development, protection from glutamate toxicity and oxidative stress, and metabolic support [48]. Astrocytes also are increasingly recognized as major contributors to inflammatory responses during CNS infection. In addition to pathogenesis studies, neuron/astrocyte co-cultures may provide a relevant in vitro system for the evaluation of antiviral therapies against neurotropic viruses.

Neuron/astrocyte co-cultures were susceptible to LACV infection (Fig. 1) and high viral titers were reached regardless of initial viral inoculum (Fig. 1b). However, there was a drop in viral RNA measured at 48 HPI (Fig. 1c), for which the reasons are unknown, but the timing coincides with the peak IFN-β response suggesting that cells may become less susceptible to infection during this period (Fig. 4a). Future studies should evaluate the role of IFNs and the viral IFN antagonist NSs during LACV neuron/astrocyte infection. CPE was also observed at later time points consisting of cell rounding in detachment (Fig. 1a). Indeed, cytotoxicity and apoptosis assays indicate increased numbers of apoptotic cells beginning at 48 HPI (Fig. 3). Additionally, it seems that neurons are more susceptible to apoptosis than astrocytes in response to LACV infection (Fig. 3d). These data mirror those seen in previous work using murine models and the human NT2N cell line [9, 12, 33, 34]. Of note, while cytotoxicity and apoptosis were noted, large amounts of viable cells remain as late as 96 HPI. This contrasts reports of LACV as a highly cytopathic virus in mouse primary neurons and human NT2N cells and are likely due to intact IFN responses and the protective effects of astrocytic co-culture resulting in a more physiologic response and greater resilience to infection [12, 33].

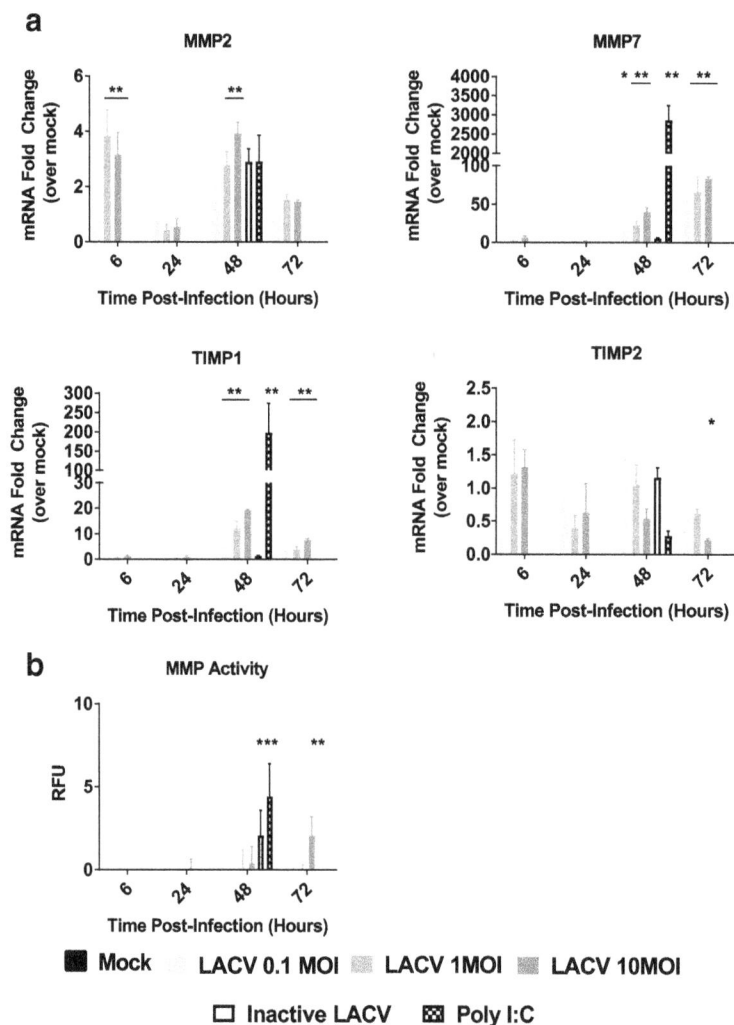

Fig. 5 MMP and TIMP responses of LACV infected neuron/astrocyte co-cultures. Neuron/astrocyte co-cultures were either mock infected, treated with inactivated LACV, treated with Poly I:C, or infected with 0.1, 1, 10 MOI of LACV. **a** RNA was collected and analyzed via qRT-PCR against selected MMPs and TIMPs. Values are reported as fold change relative to mock treatment normalized to 18S RNA. **b** MMP activity assays were performed to determine MMP cleavage activity. *$P < 0.5$, **$P < 0.01$

The overall percentage of cells infected during this study was lower than expected, reaching maximums of 64% neuronal infection and 50% astrocytic infection (Fig. 2b). Again, this is likely due to intact antiviral sensing pathways and IFN responses. Multiple studies have indicated that both neurons and astrocytes are important producers of type I IFN during LACV infection, but astrocytes appear to be responsible for greater responses [11, 15]. Therefore, astrocytic IFN production may be responsible for limiting the magnitude of infection. The current study also demonstrates neurons as astrocytes are both highly susceptible to LACV infection. Neurons have long been recognized as a target of infection, but astrocytic infection has been largely ignored [8, 9, 11, 15]. One study demonstrated that in the weanling mouse model of LACV encephalitis, less than 1% of infected

cells were astrocytes [11]. However, in the same study, deleting the LACV NSs gene (an IFN antagonist) resulted in large increases of astrocytic IFN-β production suggesting nonproductive infections or infections below the detection limit of utilized assays may be higher than previously thought [11]. Another group has proposed in a review that astrocytic infections are common and that the rapid death of infected astrocytes leads to a lack of detection in vivo [1]. Here, we have shown that human astrocytes are indeed highly susceptible to LACV infection in vitro (Fig. 2). At early time points, neurons and astrocytes are infected at a nearly 1:1 ratio, and at an MOI of 10, the infection in astrocytes is significantly higher than in neurons at 12 HPI (Additional file 2: Figure S2c). However, by 72 HPI, neurons became the predominant cell type infected in the 0.01 MOI infections.

Despite the shifting tropism of viral infection, no changes were detected in the overall ratio of neurons to astrocytes, and astrocytes seemed to be less susceptible to apoptosis compared to neurons (Additional file 1: Figure S1, Fig. 3d). This suggests that rapid astrocytic death is not a major driver in the shift in tropism in vitro. This shift may be due to the type I IFN response which begins at 48 HPI. Astrocytes may be more sensitive to type I IFN signaling and induce strong antiviral states, protecting this cell type while leaving neurons more vulnerable. This shift is less prominent at higher MOIs, likely because too many cells are infected early to adequately demonstrate changes in tropism and/or IFN responses were mounted too late to counter the heavy infection. However, when comparing only infected cells, neurons still tend to dominate at later timepoints even at late MOIs (Additional file 2: Figure S2b). Future studies will attempt to determine the relative roles of IFN on neurons and astrocytes during viral infection.

Neurons and astrocytes are increasingly recognized as important components of CNS immune responses. We tested the responsiveness of hNSC-derived neuron/astrocyte co-cultures by stimulating with the inactivated virus and a dsRNA analogue, Poly I:C (Additional file 3: Figure S3). The co-cultures are highly responsive to Poly I:C, responding with large increases in IFNs and proinflammatory cytokines and chemokines at both the RNA and protein level. It is reasonable to conclude that these cells have intact antiviral sensing pathways and are capable of initiating inflammatory responses. No responses to inactivated LACV were detected, suggesting that viral replication is necessary for such cellular responses. Alternatively, these results may indicate that viral entry is necessary as heat inactivation may denature attachment and entry glycoproteins. Another interesting finding was that while CCL2 mRNA is induced following Poly I:C treatment, the levels of CCL2 secretion remain unchanged. This suggests additional levels of regulation of CCL2 at the translational level.

LACV infection generated similar, but more limited, proinflammatory responses in these neuron/astrocyte co-cultures with mRNA levels peaking around 48 HPI and protein levels closely mirroring (Fig. 4 and Additional file 4: Figure S4). Interestingly, LACV, but not Poly I:C induced an increase in IFN-α mRNA similar to previous studies [35, 36]. At the same time, unlike Poly I:C, LACV failed to induce IL-1β, IL-2, IL-5, IL-15, and IL-17. Additionally, LACV only resulted in modest increases in IL-10, IL-12, IL-9, and IL-13 only at late time points with high MOIs. This may be explained as either viral inhibition of select responses, lower levels of stimulation relative to Poly I:C, or differences in signaling pathways used to detect Poly I:C versus LACV. Indeed, Poly I:C was added to the supernatant without transfection, which typically stimulates

TLR3 while LACV infection likely stimulates a larger range of endosomal and cytosolic RNA sensing receptors. These results clearly show that neurons and astrocytes are likely important factors in shaping the immune response to LACV encephalitis. This has been demonstrated for the type I IFN responses, but not yet the proinflammatory chemokines [11, 15].

Human pathology reports and animal models note inflammation primarily composed of macrophages and lymphocytes [8, 9, 14]. A recent study by Winkler et al. revealed that lymphocytes do not appear to be important in the development of neuropathology [13]. The same group has also shown inflammatory monocytes to be the primary infiltrating cell type, although their role in immune-mediated neuropathology was not addressed [14]. In the same study, it was noted that CCR2 was necessary for monocytes to migrate to lesions in the CNS, but not for recruitment to the CNS. Interestingly, while changes in mRNA expression for CCL2 were noted, protein expression in the cell culture supernatant was unchanged. Neurons and astrocytes constitutively express low levels of CCL2 in the healthy brain, as seen in our results, but some studies have noted a microglial requirement for upregulation after infection [17, 49]. Microglia are missing from this system and should be further evaluated for their effect on responses after LACV infection. Their response is potentially via bystander effects, as preliminary experiments infecting primary human microglia did not yield productive infection or chemokine responses (data not shown). Future studies should address the role of inflammatory monocytes during LACV encephalitis.

The strongest responses in our study were in the monocytic and lymphocytic chemokines, CCL5 and CXCL10. These chemokines have been associated with a wide range of viral CNS infections and are important for lymphocyte recruitment [50]. As previously mentioned, lymphocytes do not appear to play a role in immunopathology, but it is likely that during human infection their role is critical in the recovery from LACV encephalitis [13]. The receptors for these CCL5 and CXCL10 (CCR5 and CXCR3, respectively) have been shown to be critical for T cell recruitment for several encephalitic viruses such as West Nile virus (WNV), murine hepatitis virus (MHV), and herpes simplex virus (HSV) [51–53]. CCR5 has also been shown to be important for the control of WNV [54]. Our data therefore suggest that neurons and/or astrocytes are important for the recruitment of T cells to the CNS during LACV encephalitis, although in vivo studies will be required to confirm this hypothesis. Additionally, we show strong IFN-γ responses which have been shown to be critical for the control of several viral CNS infections such as HSV, Sindbis virus, measles virus, and Theiler's murine encephalomyelitis virus [55–58].

One limitation of the current study is the difficulty in determining which cell types are responsible for signaling. Predictions can be made using other models, but as cells behave differently in co-culture, simple assessment of primary astrocytes and neurons may not be accurate. Both cell types appear to be important for cytokine responses in WNV infection, with astrocytes producing CXCL10, CCL2, and CCL5, but not IL-1β or IL-6 [59]. Neuronal cells were then shown to produce IL-1β, IL-6, IL-8, and TNF-α [60]. Both neurons and astrocytes appear to be important producers of CXCL10 during viral infection [59, 61]. However, these differences are often virus-specific, with H7N9 influenza inducing IL-6 and IL-8 in both neuronal and astrocytic cells [62]. Another layer of complexity is that host species differences are known to exist in cytokine expression and IFN responses [63]. These conflicting data highlight the need for species-specific models for viral infection. However, immunofluorescent or immunohistochemical staining for cytokines and chemokines is often problematic due to low intercellular levels of protein, and separation via FACS is difficult due to the fragility of the cells. Future effort needs to focus on better understanding cell-specific responses.

The neuron/astrocyte co-cultures in this system also demonstrated a potential to disrupt the BBB. While initial LACV neuroinvasion is thought to occur via hematogenous spread through capillaries in the olfactory bulb, further disruption of the BBB after neuroinvasion may contribute to greater viral neuroinvasion or increased inflammatory responses leading to greater damage [7]. Rift Valley fever virus, a related bunyavirus, is likely to also use the olfactory bulb for CNS entry, but generally maintains BBB integrity during infection in contrast to LACV [64, 65]. TNF-α, IL-6, and VEGF had modest upregulation in this study and have long been associated with increased BBB permeability (Fig. 5 and Additional file 4: Figure S4) [18, 19]. We additionally assessed MMPs and TIMPs (Fig. 5). MMP9 and MMP2 are typically the primary MMPs associated with BBB disruption [19]. Initial BioPlex screens and RT-PCR did not detect MMP9 after virus infection (data not shown). We did however observe modest increases in MMP2 at 6 HPI and large increases in MMP7. MMP7 has not been commonly studied in the context of viral encephalitis and its relevance is unknown. However, MMP7 is important for leukocyte infiltration during experimental autoimmune encephalomyelitis and is found in the CSF during AIDS dementia [40, 41]. TIMP-2 is constitutively expressed in the brain while TIMP-1 is inducible [42]. The current study demonstrates that TIMP-1 is induced following LACV infection and that TIMP-2 appears to be downregulated (Fig. 5a). As both MMPs and TIMPs are upregulated, the functional status of MMP activity

required further study. An MMP substrate cleavage assay revealed that high MOI LACV infection could induce an increased MMP response at 96 HPI. However, this is very late in infection, and the MMP activity was not high (Fig. 5b). This suggests that TIMP upregulation may be limiting BBB breakdown by MMP upregulation during LACV infection, but the functional activity of these enzymes on the BBB during LACV infection in vivo remains to be assessed.

Conclusion

Our results demonstrate the feasibility, accuracy, and usefulness of hNSC-derived neuron/astrocyte co-cultures to study encephalitic viruses. In the current study, many aspects of LACV encephalitis such as neurotropism and apoptosis were replicated. In addition, we noted the susceptibility of astrocytes early in infection with a shifting tropism later during the course of infection. This may explain why while low levels of astrocyte infection have been noted in experimental models, they do not appear to be prevalent in vivo. We also demonstrate intact viral sensing pathways and proinflammatory cytokine and chemokine responses. These neuron/astrocyte responses may drive the observed monocytic and lymphocytic infiltration observed during LACV encephalitis as well as prolonged disruption of the BBB.

Additional files

Additional file 1: Figure S1. Neurons and astrocytes are present in a 1:1 ratio, which is not altered during LACV infection. Neuron/astrocyte co-cultures were either mock infected or infected with 0.1, 1, or 10 MOI of LACV. Cells were formalin fixed and stained for MAP2 or GFAP with DAPI counterstain. Percentages of GFAP or MAP2 positive cells were calculated across 6 fields of at least 200 cells. (PDF 187 kb)

Additional file 2: Figure S2. Neurons and astrocytes are both targets of LACV infection across various MOIs. Neuron/astrocyte co-cultures were either mock infected or infected with 0.1 or 10 MOI of LACV. Cells were formalin fixed and stained for MAP2 or GFAP, LACV antigen and with DAPI counterstain. (a) Percentages of neurons and astrocytes infected with LACV were calculated (b) Percentages of infected cells positive for GFAP and MAP2 were calculated. *P < 0.05, **P < 0.01 (PDF 38 kb)

Additional file 3: Figure S3. Innate immune responses to inflammatory stimuli in neuron/astrocyte co-cultures. RT-PCR and BioPlex assays were performed to determine the cytokine and chemokine responses of neuron/astrocyte co-cultures. (a) Co-cultures were treated with either mock, Poly I:C, or heat inactivated LACV and at 48 HPI assessed for changes in gene expression for selected cytokines/chemokines via qRT-PCR. Values are reported as fold change relative to mock treatment normalized to 18S RNA. (b) Supernatant was collected and assayed for changes in selected cytokine/chemokine secretion via BioPlex assay. * P < 0.5, **P < 0.01, ***P < 0.001, ****P < 0.0001. (PDF 207 kb)

Additional file 4: Figure S4. Full cytokine and chemokine responses of neuron/astrocyte co-cultures to LACV infection. Cells were either infected with 0.1, 1, or 10 MOI of LACV. (a) Cells were lysed and RNA was collected and assessed for changes in selected cytokine/chemokine expression via qRT-PCR. Values are reported as fold change relative to mock treatment normalized to 18S. (b) Supernatant was collected and assayed for changes in selected cytokine/chemokine secretion via BioPlex assay *P < 0.5, **P < 0.01. (PDF 461 kb)

Abbreviations

ADHD: Attention-deficit-hyperactivity disorder; BBB: Blood-brain barrier; CNS: Central nervous system; CPE: Cytopathic effect; EGF: Epidermal growth factor; FGF: Fibroblast growth factor; GFAP: Glial fibrillary acidic protein; hESCs: Embryonic stem cells; hNSC: Human neural stem cells; HPI: Hours post-infection; HSV: Herpes simplex virus; IFN: Interferon; iPCs: Induced pluripotent cells; LACV: La Crosse virus; LIF: Leukocyte inhibitory factor; MAPS 2: Microtubule associated protein 2; MAVS: Mitochondrial antiviral-signaling protein; MHV: Murine hepatitis virus; MMPs: Metalloproteinases; MOI: Multiplicity of infection; PFU: Plaque forming units; Poly I:C: Polyinosinic:polycytidylic acid; TIMPs: Tissue inhibitor of metalloproteinases; TUNEL: Terminal deoxynucleotidyl transferase dUTP nick end labeling; VZV: Varicella zoster virus; WNV: West Nile virus

Acknowledgements

The authors would like to thank Dr. Robert Tesh for providing the LACV used in this study.

Funding

BED was supported by a UTMB Jeane B. Kempner Scholar pre-doctoral fellowship and a NIAID T32 Emerging and Tropical Infectious Diseases Training program fellowship (2T32AI007526). This project was supported through a pilot project of the Institute of Human Infections and Immunity at UTMB (PW and ANF).

Authors' contributions

BED and JG cultured and differentiated hNSCs. BED and JTN performed cytotoxicity and apoptosis assays. BED performed all growth curves, immunofluorescence, qRT-PCR, and BioPlex assays and analyzed all data. CA and KJ performed all TUNEL staining. BED, PW, and ANF designed the experiments. BED and AF wrote the manuscript. All authors read and approved the final manuscript.

Competing interests

The authors declare that they have no competing interests.

Author details

[1]Department of Microbiology and Immunology, University of Texas Medical Branch, Galveston, USA. [2]Department of Neuroscience, Cell Biology and Anatomy, University of Texas Medical Branch, Galveston, USA. [3]Department of Pathology, University of Texas Medical Branch, 301 University Boulevard, Galveston 77555-0609, USA. [4]Center for Biodefense and Emerging Infectious Diseases, University of Texas Medical Branch, Galveston, USA. [5]Sealy Institute for Vaccine Sciences, University of Texas Medical Branch, Galveston, USA.

References

1. Soldan SS, González-Scarano F. The Bunyaviridae. Handb Clin Neurol. 2014; 123:449–63.
2. Gaensbauer JT, Lindsey NP, Messacar K, Staples JE, Fischer M. Neuroinvasive arboviral disease in the United States: 2003 to 2012. Pediatrics. 2014;134: e642–50 Available from: http://pediatrics.aappublications.org/content/early/2014/08/06/peds.2014-0498.abstract.
3. Haddow AD, Odoi A. The incidence risk, clustering, and clinical presentation of La Crosse virus infections in the Eastern United States, 2003-2007. PLoS One. 2009;4:2003–7.
4. McJunkin JE, de los Reyes EC, Irazuzta JE, Caceres MJ, Khan RR, Minnich LL, et al. La Crosse encephalitis in children. N Engl J Med. 2001;344:801–7 Available from: http://www.nejm.org/doi/abs/10.1056/NEJM200103153441103.
5. Rust RS, Thompson WH, Matthews CG, Beaty BJ, Chun RWM. Topical review: La Crosse and other forms of California encephalitis. J Child Neurol. 1999;14: 1–14 Available from: http://jcn.sagepub.com/cgi/doi/10.1177/088307389901400101.
6. Balfour HH, Siem A, Quie G, Ph D. CALIFORNIA I . Clinical ARBOVIRUS (LA CROSSE) findings with meningoencephalitis. 1973;52.
7. Winkler CW, Race B, Phillips K, Peterson KE. Capillaries in the olfactory bulb but not the cortex are highly susceptible to virus-induced vascular leak and promote viral neuroinvasion. Acta Neuropathol. Springer Berlin Heidelberg. 2015;130:233–45.
8. Kalfayan B. Pathology of La Crosse virus infection in humans. Prog Clin Biol Res. United States. 1983;123:179–86.
9. Bennett RS, Cress CM, Ward JM, Firestone CY, Murphy BR, Whitehead SS. La Crosse virus infectivity, pathogenesis, and immunogenicity in mice and monkeys. Virol J. 2008;5:1–15.
10. Johnson RT. Pathogenesis of La Crosse virus in mice. Prog Clin Biol Res United States. 1983;123:139–44.
11. Kallfass C, Ackerman A, Lienenklaus S, Weiss S, Heimrich B, Staeheli P. Visualizing production of beta interferon by astrocytes and microglia in brain of La Crosse virus-infected mice. J Virol. 2012;86:11223–30 Available from: http://jvi.asm.org/cgi/doi/10.1128/JVI.01093-12.
12. Mukherjee P, Woods TA, Moore RA, Peterson KE. Activation of the innate signaling molecule MAVS by bunyavirus infection upregulates the adaptor protein SARM1, leading to neuronal death. Immunity; 2013;38:705–716. Elsevier Inc. Available from: https://doi.org/10.1016/j.immuni.2013.02.013
13. Winkler CW, Myers LM, Woods TA, Carmody AB, Taylor KG, Peterson KE. Lymphocytes have a role in protection, but not in pathogenesis, during La Crosse virus infection in mice. J Neuroinflammation. 2017;14:1–14.
14. Winkler CW, Woods TA, Robertson SJ, McNally KL, Carmody AB, Best SM, et al. Cutting edge: CCR2 is not required for Ly6C [hi] monocyte egress from the bone marrow but is necessary for migration within the brain in La Crosse virus encephalitis. J Immunol. 2018;200:471–6 Available from: http://www.jimmunol.org/lookup/doi/10.4049/jimmunol.1701230.
15. Delhaye S, Paul S, Blakqori G, Minet M, Weber F, Staeheli P, et al. Neurons produce type I interferon during viral encephalitis. Proc Natl Acad Sci. 2006;103:7835–40 Available from: http://www.pnas.org/cgi/doi/10.1073/pnas.0602460103.
16. Schultz KLW, Vernon PS, Griffin DE. Differentiation of neurons restricts arbovirus replication and increases expression of the alpha isoform of IRF-7. J Virol. 2015;89:48–60 Available from: http://jvi.asm.org/lookup/doi/10.1128/JVI.02394-14.
17. Hou Y-J, Banerjee R, Thomas B, Nathan C, Garcia-Sastre A, Ding A, et al. SARM is required for neuronal injury and cytokine production in response to central nervous system viral infection. J Immunol. 2013;191: 875–83 Available from: http://www.jimmunol.org/cgi/doi/10.4049/jimmunol.1300374.
18. Daniels BP, Holman DW, Cruz-Orengo L, Jujjavarapu H, Durrant DM, Klein RS. Viral pathogen-associated molecular patterns regulate blood-brain barrier integrity via competing innate cytokine signals. MBio. 2014;5:1–13.
19. Chang C-Y, Li J-R, Chen W-Y, Ou Y-C, Lai C-Y, Hu Y-H, et al. Disruption of in vitro endothelial barrier integrity by Japanese encephalitis virus-infected astrocytes: Glia; 2015. United States. https://doi.org/10.1002/glia.22857.
20. Jordan PM, Cain LD, Wu P. Astrocytes enhance long-term survival of cholinergic neurons differentiated from human fetal neural stem cells. J Neurosci Res. 2008;86:35–47 United States.
21. Faissner S, Ambrosius B, Schanzmann K, Grewe B, Potthoff A, Münch J, et al. Cytoplasmic HIV-RNA in monocytes determines microglial activation and neuronal cell death in HIV-associated neurodegeneration. Exp Neurol. 2014;261:685–697. Elsevier Inc.;Available from: https://doi.org/10.1016/j.expneurol.2014.08.011
22. Grigoryan S, Kinchington PR, Yang IH, Selariu A, Zhu H, Yee M, et al. Retrograde axonal transport of VZV: kinetic studies in hESC-derived neurons. J Neuro-Oncol. 2012;18:462–70.
23. Markus A, Grigoryan S, Sloutskin A, Yee MB, Zhu H, Yang IH, et al. Varicella-zoster virus (vzv) infection of neurons derived from human embryonic stem

cells: direct demonstration of axonal infection, transport of VZV, and productive neuronal infection. J Virol. 2011;85:6220–33 Available from: http://jvi.asm.org/cgi/doi/10.1128/JVI.02396-10.

24. Pugazhenthi S, Nair S, Velmurugan K, Liang Q, Mahalingam R, Cohrs RJ, et al. Varicella-zoster virus infection of differentiated human neural stem cells. J Virol. 2011;85:6678–86 Available from: http://jvi.asm.org/cgi/doi/10.1128/JVI.00445-11.

25. Markus A, Lebenthal-Loinger I, Yang IH, Kinchington PR, Goldstein RS. An in vitro model of latency and reactivation of Varicella zoster virus in human stem cell-derived neurons. PLoS Pathog. 2015;11:1–22.

26. Lee KS, Zhou W, Scott-McKean JJ, Emmerling KL, Cai GY, Krah DL, et al. Human sensory neurons derived from induced pluripotent stem cells support Varicella-zoster virus infection. PLoS One. 2012;7:e53010.

27. Wu P, Tarasenko YI, Gu Y, Huang L-YM, Coggeshall RE, Yu Y. Region-specific generation of cholinergic neurons from fetal human neural stem cells grafted in adult rat. Nat Neurosci. 2002;5:1271–8 Available from: http://www.nature.com/articles/nn974.

28. Cai Y, Wu P, Ozen M, Yu Y, Wang J, Ittmann M, et al. Gene expression profiling and analysis of signaling pathways involved in priming and differentiation of human neural stem cells. Neuroscience. 2006;138: 133–48.

29. Tarasenko YI, Yu Y, Jordan PM, Bottenstein J, Wu P. Effect of growth factors on proliferation and phenotypic differentiation of human fetal neural stem cells. J Neurosci Res. 2004;78:625–36.

30. McGrath EL, Rossi SL, Gao J, Widen SG, Grant AC, Dunn TJ, et al. Differential responses of human fetal brain neural stem cells to Zika virus infection. Stem Cell Reports. 2017;8:715–27.

31. Yun T, Park A, Hill TE, Pernet O, Beaty SM, Juelich TL, et al. Efficient reverse genetics reveals genetic determinants of budding and fusogenic differences between Nipah and Hendra viruses and enables real-time monitoring of viral spread in small animal models of Henipavirus infection. J Virol. 2015; 89(2):1242-1253. Available from: http://jvi.asm.org/lookup/doi/10.1128/JVI.02583-14 .

32. Herculano-Houzel S. The glia/neuron ratio: how it varies uniformly across brain structures and species and what that means for brain physiology and evolution. Glia. 2014;62:1377–91 United States.

33. Pekosz A, Phillips J, Pleasure D, Merry D, Gonzalez-Scarano F. Induction of apoptosis by La Crosse virus infection and role of neuronal differentiation and human bcl-2 expression in its prevention. J Virol. 1996;70:5329–35 Available from: http://www.pubmedcentral.nih.gov/articlerender.fcgi?artid= 190490&tool=pmcentrez&rendertype=abstract.

34. Soldan SS, Hollidge BS, Wagner V, Weber F, González-Scarano F. La Crosse virus (LACV) Gc fusion peptide mutants have impaired growth and fusion phenotypes, but remain neurotoxic. Virology. 2010;404:139–47 Academic Press; [cited 17 Feb 2018]; Available from: https://www.sciencedirect.com/science/article/pii/S0042682210002473?via%3Dihub.

35. Costello DA, Lynch MA. Toll-like receptor 3 activation modulates hippocampal network excitability, via glial production of interferon-?? Hippocampus. 2013;23:696–707.

36. Gesuete R, Packard AEB, Vartanian KB, Conrad VK, Stevens SL, Bahjat FR, et al. Poly-ICLC preconditioning protects the blood-brain barrier against ischemic injury in vitro through type i interferon signaling. J Neurochem. 2012;123:75–85.

37. Savarin C, Bergmann CC, Hinton DR, Stohlman SA. MMP-independent role of TIMP-1 at the blood brain barrier during viral encephalomyelitis. ASN Neuro. United States. 2013;5:e00127.

38. Groters S, Alldinger S, Baumgartner W. Up-regulation of mRNA for matrix metalloproteinases-9 and -14 in advanced lesions of demyelinating canine distemper leukoencephalitis. Acta Neuropathol. Germany. 2005;110:369–82.

39. Toft-Hansen H, Buist R, Sun X-J, Schellenberg A, Peeling J, Owens T. Metalloproteinases control brain inflammation induced by pertussis toxin in mice overexpressing the chemokine CCL2 in the central nervous system. J Immunol. United States. 2006;177:7242–9.

40. Buhler LA, Samara R, Guzman E, Wilson CL, Krizanac-Bengez L, Janigro D, et al. Matrix metalloproteinase-7 facilitates immune access to the CNS in experimental autoimmune encephalomyelitis. BMC Neurosci. England. 2009;10:17.

41. Conant K, McArthur JC, Griffin DE, Sjulson L, Wahl LM, Irani DN. Cerebrospinal fluid levels of MMP-2, 7, and 9 are elevated in association with human immunodeficiency virus dementia. Ann Neurol. United States. 1999;46:391–8.

42. Gardner J, Ghorpade A. Tissue inhibitor of metalloproteinase (TIMP)-1: the TIMPed balance of matrix metalloproteinases in the central nervous system. J Neurosci Res. United States. 2003;74:801–6.

43. Morrey JD, Siddharthan V, Wang H. Neurological approaches for investigating West Nile virus disease and its treatment in rodents. Antiviral Res. 2013;100:535–545. Elsevier B.V.; Available from: https://doi.org/10.1016/j.antiviral.2013.09.010

44. Salimi H, Cain MD, Klein RS. Encephalitic arboviruses: emergence, clinical presentation, and neuropathogenesis. Neurotherapeutics. 2016;13:514–34 Available from: https://doi.org/10.1007/s13311-016-0443-5.

45. Seok J, Warren HS, Cuenca AG, Mindrinos MN, Baker HV, Xu W, et al. Genomic responses in mouse models poorly mimic human inflammatory diseases. Proc Natl Acad Sci. 2013;110:3507–12 Available from: http://www.pnas.org/lookup/doi/10.1073/pnas.1222878110.

46. Mestas J, Hughes CCW. Of mice and not men: differences between mouse and human immunology. J Immunol. 2004;172:2731–8 Available from: http://www.jimmunol.org/cgi/doi/10.4049/jimmunol.172.5.2731.

47. Oberheim NA, Takano T, Han X, He W, Lin JHC, Wang F, et al. Uniquely hominid features of adult human astrocytes. J Neurosci. 2009;29:3276–87 Available from: http://www.jneurosci.org/cgi/doi/10.1523/JNEUROSCI.4707-08.2009.

48. Hill E, Nagel D, Parri R, Coleman M. Stem cell-derived astrocytes: are they physiologically credible? J Physiol. 2016;594:6595–606.

49. Banisadr G, Gosselin R-D, Mechighel P, Kitabgi P, Rostene W, Parsadaniantz SM. Highly regionalized neuronal expression of monocyte chemoattractant protein-1 (MCP-1/CCL2) in rat brain: evidence for its colocalization with neurotransmitters and neuropeptides. J Comp Neurol. United States. 2005; 489:275–92.

50. Metcalf TU, Baxter VK, Nilaratanakul V, Griffin DE. Recruitment and retention of B cells in the central nervous system in response to alphavirus encephalomyelitis. J Virol. 2013;87:2420–9 Available from: http://jvi.asm.org/cgi/doi/10.1128/JVI.01769-12.

51. Michlmayr D, McKimmie CS, Pingen M, Haxton B, Mansfield K, Johnson N, et al. Defining the chemokine basis for leukocyte recruitment during viral encephalitis. J Virol. 2014;88:9553–67 Available from: http://jvi.asm.org/cgi/doi/10.1128/JVI.03421-13.

52. Liu MT, Chen BP, Oertel P, Buchmeier MJ, Armstrong D, Hamilton TA, et al. Cutting edge: the T cell chemoattractant IFN-inducible. Protein 10 is essential in host defense against viral-induced neurologic disease. J Immunol. 2000;165:2327–30 Available from: http://www.jimmunol.org/cgi/doi/10.4049/jimmunol.165.5.2327.

53. Wuest TR, Carr DJJ. Dysregulation of CXCR3 signaling due to CXCL10 deficiency impairs the antiviral response to herpes simplex virus 1 infection. J Immunol. 2008;181:7985–93 Available from: http://www.jimmunol.org/cgi/doi/10.4049/jimmunol.181.11.7985.

54. Glass WG, McDermott DH, Lim JK, Lekhong S, Yu SF, Frank WA, et al. CCR5 deficiency increases risk of symptomatic West Nile virus infection. J Exp Med. 2006;203:35 LP–40 Available from: http://jem.rupress.org/content/203/1/35.abstract.

55. Patterson CE, Lawrence DMP, Echols LA, Rall GF. Immune-mediated protection from measles virus-induced central nervous system disease is noncytolytic and gamma interferon dependent. J Virol. 2002;76:4497–506 Available from: http://www.pubmedcentral.nih.gov/articlerender.fcgi?artid= 155105&tool=pmcentrez&rendertype=abstract.

56. Smith PM, Wolcott RM, Chervenak R, Jennings SR. Control of acute cutaneous herpes simplex virus infection: T cell-mediated viral clearance is dependent upon interferon-gamma (IFN-gamma). Virology. United States. 1994;202:76–88.

57. Rodriguez M, Zoecklein LJ, Howe CL, Pavelko KD, Gamez JD, Nakane S, et al. Gamma interferon is critical for neuronal viral clearance and protection in a susceptible mouse strain following early intracranial Theiler's murine encephalomyelitis virus infection. J Virol. United States. 2003;77:12252–65.

58. Burdeinick-Kerr R, Griffin DE. Gamma interferon-dependent, noncytolytic clearance of sindbis virus infection from neurons in vitro. J Virol United States. 2005;79:5374–85.

59. Cheeran MC-J, Hu S, Sheng WS, Rashid A, Peterson PK, Lokensgard JR. Differential responses of human brain cells to West Nile virus infection. J Neurovirol. 2005;11:512–24 Available from: http://link.springer.com/10.1080/13550280500384982.

60. Kumar M, Verma S, Nerurkar VR. Pro-inflammatory cytokines derived from West Nile virus (WNV)-infected SK-N-SH cells mediate neuroinflammatory

markers and neuronal death. J Neuroinflammation. 2010;7:73 BioMed Central Ltd;. Available from: http://www.jneuroinflammation.com/content/7/1/73.

61. Mathieu C, Guillaume V, Sabine A, Ong KC, Wong KT, Legras-Lachuer C, et al. Lethal Nipah virus infection induces rapid overexpression of cxcl10. PLoS One. 2012;7:e32157.

62. Ng YP, Yip TF, Peiris JSM, Ip NY, Lee SMY. Avian influenza A H7N9 virus infects human astrocytes and neuronal cells and induces inflammatory immune responses. J Neurovirol. 2018;1. https://doi.org/10.1007/s13365-018-0659-8.

63. Lin CC, Wu YJ, Heimrich B, Schwemmle M. Absence of a robust innate immune response in rat neurons facilitates persistent infection of Borna disease virus in neuronal tissue. Cell Mol Life Sci. 2013;70:4399–410.

64. Reed C, Lin K, Wilhelmsen C, Friedrich B, Nalca A, Keeney A, et al. Aerosol exposure to Rift Valley fever virus causes earlier and more severe neuropathology in the murine model, which has important implications for therapeutic development. PLoS Negl Trop Dis. 2013;7:e2156.

65. Dodd KA, McElroy AK, Jones TL, Zaki SR, Nichol ST, Spiropoulou CF. Rift Valley fever virus encephalitis is associated with an ineffective systemic immune response and activated T cell infiltration into the CNS in an immunocompetent mouse model. PLoS Negl Trop Dis. 2014;8:e2874.

10

Distinct contributions of hyperglycemia and high-fat feeding in metabolic syndrome-induced neuroinflammation

Brooke J. Wanrooy[1], Kathryn Prame Kumar[1], Shu Wen Wen[1], Cheng Xue Qin[2], Rebecca H. Ritchie[2,3] and Connie H. Y. Wong[1*]

Abstract

Background: High-fat feeding and hyperglycemia, key risk factors for the development of metabolic syndrome (MetS), are emerging to associate with increased risk of developing dementia and cognitive decline. Despite this, clinical and experimental studies have yet to elucidate the specific contributions of either high-fat feeding or hyperglycemia to potential neuroinflammatory components. In this study, we delineate these individual components of MetS in the development of neuroinflammation.

Methods: Male C57Bl/6 J adult mice were treated with either citrate vehicle (CIT) or streptozotocin (STZ; 55 mg/kg) 3, 5 and 7 days before commencement of either a normal or high-fat diet for 9 or 18 weeks. By creating separate models of high-fat feeding, STZ-induced hyperglycemia, as well as in combination, we were able to delineate the specific effects of a high-fat diet and hyperglycemia on the brain. Throughout the feeding regime, we measured the animals' body weight and fasting blood glucose levels. At the experimental endpoint, we assessed plasma levels of insulin, glycated haemoglobin and performed glucose tolerance testing. In addition, we examined the effect of high fat-feeding and hyperglycemia on the levels of systemic inflammatory cytokines, gliosis in the hippocampus and immune infiltration in cerebral hemispheric tissue. Furthermore, we used intravital multiphoton microscopy to assess leukocyte-endothelial cell interactions in the cerebral vasculature of mice in vivo.

Results: We showed that acute hyperglycemia induces regional-specific effects on the brain by elevating microglial numbers and promotes astrocytosis in the hippocampus. In addition, we demonstrated that chronic hyperglycemia supported the recruitment of peripheral GR1[+] granulocytes to the cerebral microvasculature in vivo. Moreover, we provided evidence that these changes were independent of the systemic inflammation associated with high-fat feeding.

Conclusions: Hyperglycemia alone preferentially induces microglial numbers and astrocytosis in the hippocampus and is associated with the peripheral recruitment of leukocytes to the cerebrovasculature, but not systemic inflammation. High-fat feeding alone, and in combination with hyperglycemia, increases the systemic pro-inflammatory cytokine milieu but does not result in brain-specific immune gliosis. These results shed light on the specific contributions of high-fat feeding and hyperglycemia as key factors of MetS in the development of neuroinflammation.

Keywords: Neuroinflammation, High-fat feeding, Microglia, Astrocytes, Hippocampus, Streptozotocin, Hyperglycemia

* Correspondence: connie.wong@monash.edu
[1]Centre for Inflammatory Diseases, Department of Medicine, School of Clinical Sciences at Monash Health, Monash Medical Centre, Monash University, Clayton, VIC 3168, Australia
Full list of author information is available at the end of the article

Background

The prevalence of metabolic syndrome (MetS) in adults is increasing worldwide [1], largely due to several factors such as ageing of the population, increased life expectancy and chronic overnutrition and physical inactivity [2]. MetS refers to a cluster of inter-connected metabolic abnormalities involving glucose metabolism (diabetes milletus), lipid metabolism (hypercholesterolaemia and dyslipidaemia), elevated blood pressure and central obesity. In particular, obesity is emerging as a major health concern owing to its key role in MetS and being a well-recognised risk factor for the development of type 2 diabetes (T2D) and related cardiovascular diseases (CVDs) [3]. Recently, interdisciplinary research in neuroscience and immunology has linked overnutrition to neuroinflammation, particularly in the hypothalamus and hippocampus [4]. A growing body of evidence suggests that a complex interplay exists between accelerated adiposity, hyperglycemia and cognitive decline [5]. Indeed, clinical studies demonstrate that patients with T2D are more susceptible to symptoms of neurological impairment, but how T2D may induce neurological deficits remains undetermined.

The recently identified systemic and chronic inflammatory component of MetS is a primary candidate to confer the increased risk of cognitive decline in both obese and hyperglycemic individuals, perhaps by priming the specialised resident macrophage population (microglia) towards an inflammatory state to establish a form of low-grade neuroinflammation [6]. Chronic hyperglycemia in its own right is known to have deleterious effects on the brain. Meta-analyses of non-obese hyperglycemic type 1 diabetes patients show mild declines in mental speed and flexibility compared to non-diabetic individuals [7]. Moreover, increased blood-brain barrier permeability, oxidative damage and neuronal apoptosis are all associated with hyperglycemia in experimental animal models of hyperglycemia [8–10]. These conditions are seen similarly in conjunction with obesity, where negative relationships exist between body mass index (BMI) and neuronal viability, myelin integrity and grey matter volumes of the hippocampus in middle-aged adults [11, 12] However, both clinical and experimental studies have yet to elucidate the specific contributions of either obesity or hyperglycemia to its implicated neuroinflammatory component. Foundational animal studies have primarily investigated the contributions of obesity and hyperglycemia in mice deficient in either the leptin (*ob/ob*) or leptin receptor (*db/db*) as a result of genetic mutations. While beneficial, findings in these models have often proven difficult to translate to, and do not accurately reflect, the disease aetiology of obesity and diabetes in humans [13]. Furthermore, these models do not allow for the analysis of individual components of MetS in the development of neuroinflammation.

The present study was designed to dissect the specific contributions of high-fat feeding and hyperglycemia to neuroinflammation. We hypothesise that the systemic inflammatory component as a result of high-fat feeding is required to initially activate the brain's immune system, which may be worsened by progressive hyperglycemia. To test our hypothesis, we assessed changes to systemic inflammatory cytokines, microglia numbers and astrocytosis in the hippocampus, and immune cell infiltrate in the brains of high-fat diet (HFD)-fed and streptozotocin (STZ)-treated C57BL/6 mice over 9 and 18 weeks. We also used intravital multiphoton microscopy to assess leukocyte-endothelial cell interactions in the cerebral vasculature of these mice in vivo.

Methods

Mice

Five to 6-week-old adult male C57Bl/6 J mice were obtained from the Monash Animal Research Platform and were housed in specific pathogen-free (SPF) conditions with access to food and water ad libitum (Monash Medical Centre Animal Facility, Clayton, VIC, Australia). Mice were housed 2–5 per cage in temperature-controlled rooms (22 °C) under a standard 12 h light-dark cycle. Prior to the start of experiments, mice were acclimatised for a minimum of 7 days before use. Mice were monitored every 3–4 days for specific health monitoring parameters including body weight, alertness, activity, coat health, dehydration, and gait. All procedures were approved by the Monash University Animal Ethics Committee under regulations that comply with the National Institute of Health guidelines for the care and use of laboratory animals.

Induction of hyperglycemia and high-fat feeding

After acclimatisation, all mice were randomly assigned treatment groups. Mice for use in the control group underwent three intraperitoneal (IP) injections of citrate vehicle (CIT, 0.01 M, pH 4.5) 3, 5 and 7 days prior to commencement of control diet (CON; SF09-091, 16% kilojoules from lipids, Speciality Feeds, WA) for 9 or 18 weeks. These mice were designated with the group name "CIT + CON". To develop a high-fat feeding model, a separate group of mice was treated identically with citrate vehicle and were placed on a high-fat diet (HFD; SF16-104, 44% kilojoules from lipids, Specialty Feeds, WA) for 9 or 18 weeks and designated "CIT + HFD". To develop a mild hyperglycemia-only model, mice were treated with three separate IP injections of low-dose streptozotocin within 5 min of preparation (STZ; 55 mg/kg in 0.01 M CIT) 3, 5 and 7 days prior to the commencement of control diet for 9 or 18 weeks. These mice were designated with the group name "STZ + CON". To develop a combination model of both hyperglycemia and high-fat feeding, mice were treated with three separate IP injections of STZ (55 mg/kg in 0.01 M CIT) 3, 5 and 7 days prior to the commencement of a HFD for 9 or 18 weeks. These mice were designated the group name "STZ + HFD". Low-dose streptozotocin (STZ) treatment was selected as it causes the targeted destruction of the insulin-producing β cells of the pancreas to produce mild hyperglycemia [14].

Glucose and insulin measurements

Fasting blood glucose was monitored fortnightly in all mice as a health monitoring parameter using a hand-held glucometer (Accu-Chek Performa, Roche) from whole blood collected via saphenous tail vein bleeds. Mice were fasted for 3 h prior to blood collection. Two weeks before end-point, a glucose tolerance test was performed. Baseline fasting blood glucose levels were obtained and mice were then injected IP with 0.8 g/kg glucose solution. Further measurements were taken at 15, 30, 45, 60, 90 and 120 min post-injection via tail vein bleeds. In addition, glycated haemoglobin (HbA1c) was assessed at the experimental endpoint. Mice were anaesthetised with isofluorane prior to transcardiac puncture with a heparinised 26G needle (100 I.U/mL). A small aliquot of whole blood (20 μL) was used for HbA1c analysis, via the Cobas B 101 (Roche Diagnostics). Plasma was collected from the remaining blood and stored at – 80 °C until required. Insulin levels were evaluated from plasma using a mouse ultrasensitive insulin ELISA kit (Alpco, Beijing, China) in single replicates according to the manufacturer's instructions.

Flow cytometry of brain immune cell isolates

The left cerebral hemisphere was cut into small pieces and digested in 500 μL collagenase digestion buffer at 37 °C for 30 min (collagenase XI (125 U/mL), hyaluronidase (60 U/mL) and collagenase type I-S (450 U/mL) in DPBS (Ca^{2+}/Mg^{2+} supplemented)). Samples were kept on ice and passed through a 70 μm nylon cell strainer. Single-cell suspensions were subjected to 30% isotonic Percoll, underlaid with 70% Percoll and centrifuged for 20 min at $600g$ at room temperature. The interphase containing the mononuclear cells was collected, washed and stained with eFluor 506-conjugated anti-mouse CD45 (30-F11, eBioscience), FITC-conjugated anti-mouse CD3 (145-2CC, eBioscience), eFluor 450-conjugated anti-mouse B220 (RA3-6B2, eBioscience), PE-Cy7-conjugated anti-mouse CD11b (M1/70, eBioscience) and PE-conjugated anti-mouse CD68 (FA/11, eBioscience) with Fc-receptor blocker (1:100, 2.4G2, BD Pharmingen) for 15 min on ice in the dark. After staining, the cells were washed, resuspended with counting bead mixture (50 / μL) and 7AAD live-dead viability stain (1:50, 420404, Biolegend) in FACS buffer. Samples were run using a flow cytometer (BD FACSCanto II) and analysed using FlowJo (v10.3.0). Cell numbers were normalised to the left cerebral hemisphere weight of each mouse.

Immunofluorescence

Mice were deeply anaesthetised with a cocktail of ketamine (150 mg/kg) and xylazine (10 mg/kg) prior to cardiac perfusion. An 18G needle was inserted into the left ventricle to perfuse ice-cold PBS and subsequent 4% paraformaldehyde (PFA; in PBS, pH 7.4). After perfusion, the brain was left to fix in PFA for 1 h and cryoprotected in 20% sucrose overnight. Brains were frozen in isopentane for cutting using a cryostat. Tissue anterior to the hippocampus was discarded until the defining bowtie-like structures of Cornu Ammonis (CA1) could be visually identified. Sections were cut at 10 μm and left at room temperature for 30 min prior to storage at – 80 °C until required. Upon use, sections were acclimatised to room temperature prior to rehydration with Tris-buffered saline containing 0.1% Tween 20 (TBST, pH 7.6), thrice, for 5 min. Sections were encircled with hydrophobic ink to maintain a staining well. Sections were permeabilised in 0.5% Triton X-100 (in 1x TBST, pH 7.6) at room temperature for 15 min in a humidifying chamber. Sections were then incubated for 48 h at 4 °C with either APC-conjugated anti-mouse Iba1 (1:1000, NCNP24, Wako Chemicals) to label microglia, anti-mouse GFAP (1:250, 1B4, BD Pharmingen) to label only activated astrocytes or PE-conjugated anti-mouse CD45 (1:200, 30F11, eBioscience) in TBST to label general immune cells. After incubation, excess stain was removed and sections were washed thrice with TBST for 10 min at room temperature, followed by a deionised water wash for 5 min. Sections were cover-slipped using DAPI ProLong Diamond Antifade Mountant (Invitrogen) to stain all nuclei and were left to cure for a minimum of 1 h at 4 °C in the dark. The 18-week cohort was stained with primary mouse anti-Iba1 (1:200, NCNP24, Wako Chemicals) and secondary anti-rabbit IgG (1:200, AlexaFluor-568, A-11011, Life Technologies) according to the manufacturer's recommended instructions. To perform neuronal counts, the sections were stained with guinea pig anti-mouse NeuN (1:1000, MAB3777, Merck Millipore) and donkey anti-guinea pig IgG (1:400, AlexaFluor-647, Jackson Immunoresearch).

Quantification of neurons and immune cells

Imaging of Immunofluorescence sections was performed on a Nikon C1 confocal laser-scanning microscope (Hamamatsu, Japan) at × 20 magnification with 405 nm (DAPI), 568 nm (PE) and 637 nm (APC) lasers. All microscope settings and laser powers were kept identical between each batch of sections imaged. Cell counts were performed manually, under blinded conditions, selected by appropriate cell body co-localisation of DAPI+ and either CD45+, IBA1+, or NeuN cells using FIJI (v1.51, NIH). Adjustments to brightness and contrast were made to individual files to allow optimal visualisation of

CD45$^+$, Iba1$^+$ and NeuN$^+$ cells only. Quantification of GFAP$^+$ activated astrocytes per area stained was performed using identical threshold settings for all samples within each cohort using FIJI.

Cytometric bead array

Plasma cytokine levels were measured by cytometric bead array (CBA) using the BD CBA Mouse Th1/Th2/Th17 Cytokine Kit (BD Biosciences, San Jose, CA, USA). The kit was used for parallel detection of mouse interleukin-2 (IL-2), interleukin-4 (IL-4), interleukin-6 (IL-6), interferon-γ (IFNγ), tumour necrosis factor (TNF), interleukin-17A (IL-17A) and interleukin-10 (IL-10). Standards were reconstituted with 2 mL of assay diluent to a maximum concentration of 5000 pg/mL and serially diluted to a concentration of 2.5 pg/mL. Capture bead mix was prepared by adding 60% of total capture beads to 40% assay diluent as per the kit instructions. Thereafter, 25 μL of bead mix, 25 μL of plasma and 15 μL phycoerythrin (PE) detection reagent were added consecutively to each well and incubated at room temperature for 2 h in the dark. Samples were washed and resuspended in wash buffer. Assay diluent was used as an internal control in place of sample plasma and returned negative values for all cytokines. Samples were measured using the Navios flow cytometer (Beckman Coulter Inc) and analysed using FlowJo (v 10.3.0). Standard curves and interpolations were constructed using GraphPad Prism 7.0 software.

Real-time in vivo imaging of cerebral vasculature

To examine the leukocyte-endothelial cell interactions in the brain at experimental endpoints, intravital multiphoton microscopy of the brain was performed. Mice were anaesthetised by IP injection of an anaesthetic cocktail consisting of 150 mg/kg ketamine hydrochloride and 10 mg/kg xylazine and the tail vein was cannulised to administer fluorescently labelled antibodies and/or additional anaesthetic, if required. Body temperature was maintained using a heat pad. Mice were immobilised in a stereotactic frame, whereby the skin overlying the skull was swabbed with ethanol and a 1 cm vertical incision was made to expose the skull. The skin was retracted, and a 5 mm × 5 mm cranial window was shaved to a thin membrane using a dental drill. PE-conjugated anti-mouse CD31 (390, 1 mg/25 g mouse, eBioscience) and PacBlue-conjugated anti-mouse GR1 (RB6-8C5, 1 mg/25 g mouse, eBioscience,) were injected through the intravenous cannula to label the cerebral brain vasculature and neutrophils/monocytes, respectively. At least three post-capillary venules of approximately 20–40 μm in diameter were chosen per mouse. Images and videos were acquired using a multiphoton microscope (Leica SP5), equipped with a × 20 water-dipping objective (NA 1.0) and a MaiTai pulsed

infrared laser (SpectraPhysics) set to an excitation wavelength of 810 nm. A 512 × 512 pixel image was acquired every 1.5 s for 9 min. Adjustments to brightness and contrast were made to individual files to allow optimal visualisation and measurements of blood vessels and cells. Multiple measurements of the width of blood vessels were taken and averaged, while the length of the vessel was measured along its centre, both using the segmented line tool. The number of adherent, intravascular cells was normalised to the vessel surface area and time of recording. Cells were considered adherent if they interacted with the vessel wall for 30 s or more. The measurements from all fields of view from one mouse were averaged with the final data representing neutrophil/monocyte numbers from one mouse.

Statistical analysis

All statistical analyses were performed using GraphPad Prism Software (La Jolla, CA, USA). The normality of all data were first assessed using a Shapiro-Wilk normality test and analysed using a one-way analysis of variance (ANOVA) or Kruskal-Wallis posthoc test if appropriate. Each group was compared to the CIT + CON group. Some data were excluded due to outliers, determined using Grubbs' test (Prism 7) at $P \leq 0.05$. All values are mean ± SEM. A value of $P \leq 0.05$ was considered statistically significant.

Results

Establishment of high-fat feeding and hyperglycemia experimental models at 9-week time point

To investigate the effect of high-fat feeding on neuroinflammation, we first established a mouse model with high-fat feeding. We show that mice on a HFD (CIT + HFD) exhibited significant weight gain compared to mice fed on a control diet (CIT + CON) as confirmed by the area under the curve (AUC) (Fig. 1a, b). In contrast, STZ-treated mice (STZ + CON) had retarded weight gain compared to CIT-treated mice (CIT + CON) on the same diet (Fig. 1b). Despite this, all STZ-treated mice developed hyperglycemia, regardless of diet, as determined by the increase in percentage glycated haemoglobin at the 9-week endpoint (Fig. 1c). However, high-fat feeding alone did not alter the percentage of glycated haemoglobin at the 9-week endpoint (Fig. 1c), likely attributable to significantly elevated plasma insulin in this group of mice (Fig. 1d).

Next, we performed a glucose tolerance test to assess glucose absorption from the bloodstream in our experimental groups. At the 9-week experimental endpoint, a 20% glucose solution was injected into fasting mice and blood glucose levels were assessed at various time points thereafter. As shown in the CIT + CON group, the metabolism of glucose is normally cleared from the bloodstream

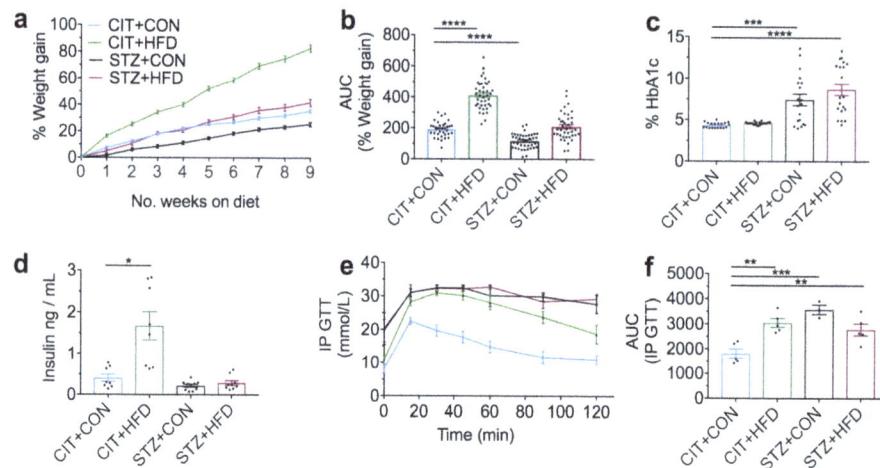

Fig. 1 Diet-induced weight gain and STZ-induced hyperglycemia after 9 weeks. Male C57BL/6 J mice (5–6-week-old) were treated IP with either citrate vehicle (CIT) or streptozotocin (STZ; 55 mg/kg) 3, 5 and 7 days prior to commencement of a control diet (CON; 16% kilojoules from lipids) or high-fat diet (HFD; 44% kilojoules from lipids) for 9 weeks. **a** Mice were weighed every 3–4 days, and percentage change in body mass compared to baseline following the high-fat diet (HFD), control diet (CON) and STZ treatment was calculated at the end of each week. **b** Corresponding percentage weight gain as the area under the curve (AUC). **c** Percentage of glycated haemoglobin (HbA1c) from heparanised whole blood was measured as an indicator of hyperglycemia at the endpoint. **d** Plasma levels of insulin at the endpoint. **e** Following a 3 h fast, blood glucose measurements of the vehicle and STZ-induced mice were assessed via tail tip vein collection (time zero) and then administered 0.8 mg/g glucose solution for IP glucose tolerance test (GTT). Blood samples were collected from the tail tip vein at 15, 30, 45, 60, 90 and 120 min after glucose challenge. **f** Corresponding AUC of the IP GTT. Data are shown as mean ± S.E.M. of **a** and **b**, $n = 39$–40; **c**, $n = 19$–20; **d**, $n = 8$–10; **e** and **f**, $n = 3$–5 per group. Data in **c** and **d** analysed by Kruskal-Wallis test followed by Dunn's, **b** and **f** by one-way ANOVA with Dunnett's. *$P < 0.05$, **$P < 0.01$, ***$P < 0.001$, ****$P < 0.0001$ vs CIT + CON control group

at 90 min post-injection (Fig. 1e). On the contrary, all of the other three experimental groups demonstrated marked delay in the absorption of circulating glucose, failing to return to baseline levels after 120 min (Fig. 1e). As confirmed by AUC, all three experimental groups demonstrated significant impairment in glucose tolerance when compared to mice in the CIT + CON group at the 9-week experimental endpoint (Fig. 1f). Taken together, we have established a high-fat feeding only group (CIT + HFD) whereby the mice are significantly overweight and demonstrate impairment in glucose tolerance. The mice in the STZ + CON group exhibit elevated blood glucose, increased percentage of glycated haemoglobin and inefficient glucose metabolism, forming the hyperglycemia-only group.

High-fat feeding and hyperglycemia modify immune populations in the brain

To assess the effect of high-fat feeding, hyperglycemia, or a combination of both, on the immune changes in the brain at the 9-week experimental time point, we used flow cytometry to quantify innate and adaptive immune cells present in the cerebral tissue. Using CD45 as a pan-leukocyte marker, we identified approximately 3×10^6 cells per gram of hemispheric tissue in the CIT + CON control group (Fig. 2a). Interestingly, mice treated with STZ on a high-fat diet exhibited significantly less CD45+ cells compared to the CIT + CON control group

(Fig. 2a). Moreover, the majority of these CD45+ live cells were CD11b+ and were significantly decreased in STZ + HFD mice (Fig. 2b). Despite lower CD45+CD11b+ numbers, the number of CD11b+CD68+ cells was significantly increased in STZ + HFD mice despite reduced CD45+ leukocyte numbers (Fig. 2c). Using B220 and CD3 as general B and T cell markers respectively, we observed that mice in the hyperglycemia-only group (STZ + CON) showed a significant increase in the number of B cells (Fig. 2d), whilst those on high-fat diet (STZ + HFD) exhibited a significant decrease in the numbers of T cells compared to control (Fig. 2e). Collectively, these data indicate more robust changes in the cerebral immune population were seen in STZ-treated mice, particularly in the presence of a high-fat diet after 9 weeks.

Hyperglycemia increases microglia numbers and activates astrocytes

The hippocampus is a region of the brain responsible for consolidating short and long-term memory and has been shown to be particularly prone to inflammation and damage during metabolic disease [15]. Therefore, we next examined whether there is evidence of neuroinflammation localised to CA1b of the hippocampus in our models of MetS. Using immunofluorescence, we quantified the numbers of Iba1+ microglia and assessed the area of astrocytosis as denoted with GFAP+ staining. At the 9-week experimental endpoint, mice in the STZ

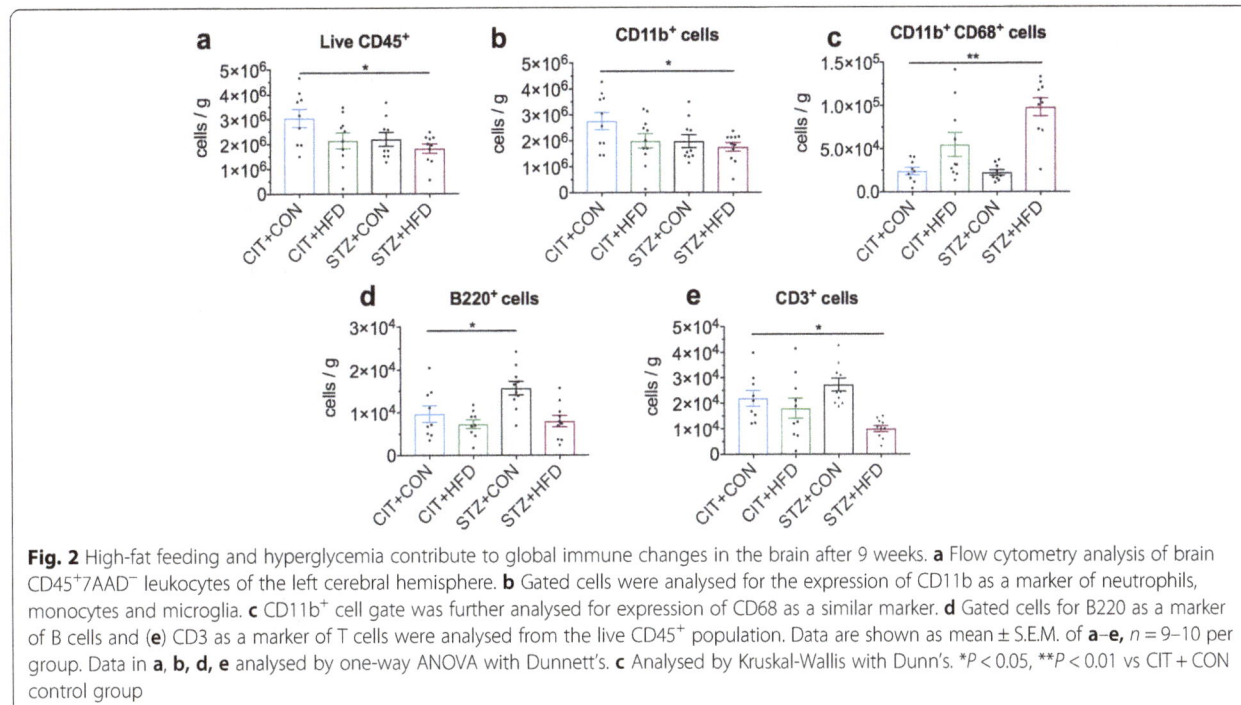

Fig. 2 High-fat feeding and hyperglycemia contribute to global immune changes in the brain after 9 weeks. **a** Flow cytometry analysis of brain CD45$^+$7AAD$^-$ leukocytes of the left cerebral hemisphere. **b** Gated cells were analysed for the expression of CD11b as a marker of neutrophils, monocytes and microglia. **c** CD11b$^+$ cell gate was further analysed for expression of CD68 as a similar marker. **d** Gated cells for B220 as a marker of B cells and (**e**) CD3 as a marker of T cells were analysed from the live CD45$^+$ population. Data are shown as mean ± S.E.M. of **a–e**, $n = 9$–10 per group. Data in **a, b, d, e** analysed by one-way ANOVA with Dunnett's. **c** Analysed by Kruskal-Wallis with Dunn's. *$P < 0.05$, **$P < 0.01$ vs CIT + CON control group

+ CON group showed significantly increased numbers of microglia (Fig. 3a–c). In addition, the degree of astrocytosis in CA1b of the hippocampus was more pronounced in the STZ + CON group compared to CIT + CON control (Fig. 3d–f). Interestingly, no significant increases in microglia number were observed in any of the experimental groups in sections of the cortex (Additional file 1: Figure S1), suggesting a regional-specific

effect. Intriguingly, the enhanced microglial numbers and astrocytosis were not observed in the CIT + HFD or STZ + HFD group (Additional file 1: Figure S2), suggesting that increased microglial numbers and astrocytosis as indicators of inflammation after hyperglycemia may be mitigated by the effects of a high-fat diet. To assess whether the hyperglycemia-induced gliosis was associated with neurodegeneration or neuronal loss, we

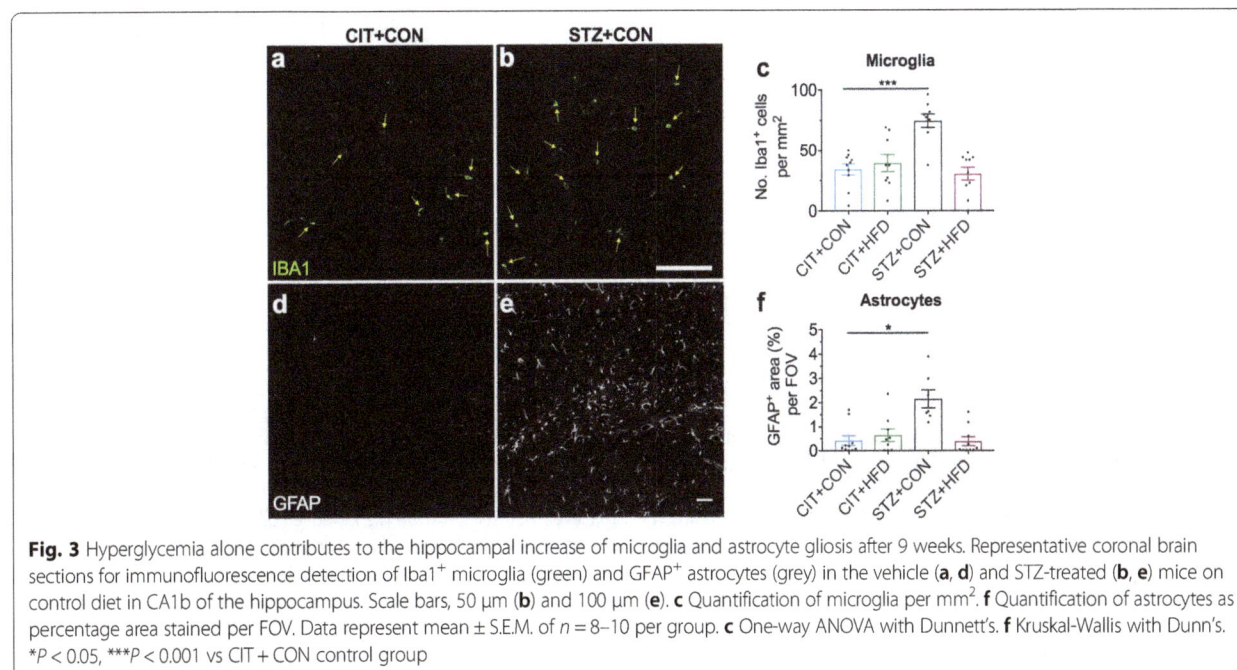

Fig. 3 Hyperglycemia alone contributes to the hippocampal increase of microglia and astrocyte gliosis after 9 weeks. Representative coronal brain sections for immunofluorescence detection of Iba1$^+$ microglia (green) and GFAP$^+$ astrocytes (grey) in the vehicle (**a, d**) and STZ-treated (**b, e**) mice on control diet in CA1b of the hippocampus. Scale bars, 50 μm (**b**) and 100 μm (**e**). **c** Quantification of microglia per mm^2. **f** Quantification of astrocytes as percentage area stained per FOV. Data represent mean ± S.E.M. of $n = 8$–10 per group. **c** One-way ANOVA with Dunnett's. **f** Kruskal-Wallis with Dunn's. *$P < 0.05$, ***$P < 0.001$ vs CIT + CON control group

quantified the number of NeuN⁺ cells in the pyramidal layer of CA1, its thickness and general NeuN⁺ cells in CA1 (Additional file 1: Figure S3), but noted no significant change.

Establishment of chronic high-fat diet and hyperglycemia experimental models at 18-week time point

To examine whether the brain immune population changes and inflammatory state worsened with a longer period of a high-fat feeding and/or hyperglycemia, we assessed a separate cohort of animals on these experimental parameters after 18 weeks. Both CIT- and STZ-treated mice fed a HFD exhibited significant weight gain over 18 weeks compared to CIT + CON group, gaining up to 110% and 50% of their original body weight respectively (Fig. 4a, b). Similar to the findings of the 9-week model, all STZ-treated mice developed hyperglycemia as determined by the increase in percentage of glycated haemoglobin at the 18-week endpoint (Fig. 4c). However, high-fat feeding on its own (CIT + HFD)

did not elevate the percentage of glycated haemoglobin at the 18-week endpoint (Fig. 4c). Again, this may be attributable to the substantially elevated plasma insulin in this group of mice (Fig. 4d).

In addition, we performed glucose tolerance testing to assess any impairment in glucose absorption from the bloodstream that could suggest the presence of insulin resistance in the experimental groups after 18 weeks. As shown in our CIT + CON group, the metabolism of glucose is normally cleared from the bloodstream at 90 min post-injection (Fig. 4e). In contrast to the findings of the 9 weeks experimental endpoint, only STZ-treated mice on high-fat diet (STZ + HFD) demonstrated a significant impairment in glucose tolerance compared to CIT + CON controls at 18 weeks after the onset of the model. This was confirmed by the quantification of the AUC (Fig. 4f). Furthermore, as both chronic high-fat feeding and hyperglycemia are associated with systemic inflammation both clinically and experimentally, we assessed systemic levels of pro-inflammatory IL-6 in our

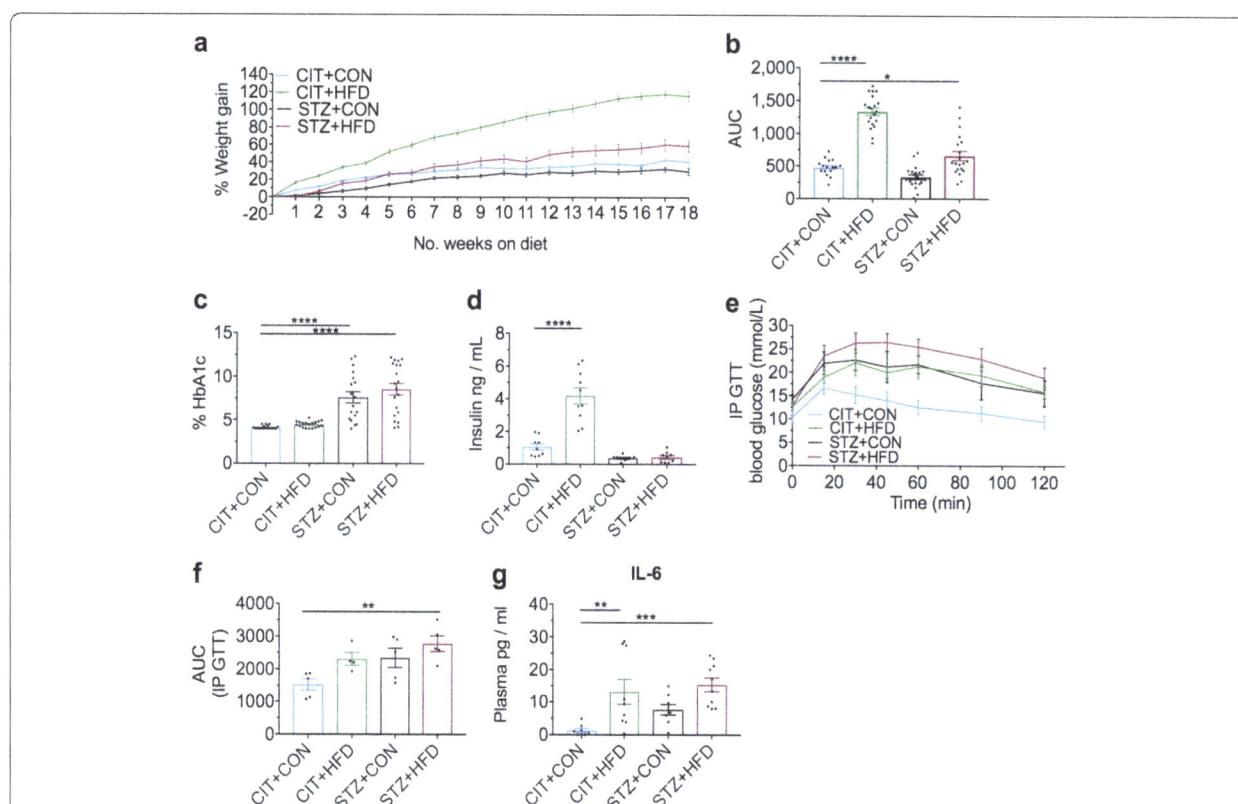

Fig. 4 Diet-induced weight gain and STZ-induced hyperglycemia after 18 weeks. a Mice were weighed every 3–4 days and percentage gain in body mass compared to baseline following the high-fat diet (HFD), control diet (CON) and STZ treatment was calculated at the end of each week. b Corresponding percentage weight gain as the area under the curve (AUC). c Percentage of glycated haemoglobin or HbA1c from heparanised whole blood was measured as an indicator of hyperglycemia at the endpoint. d Plasma levels of insulin from whole blood. e Following a 3 h fast, blood glucose measurements of the vehicle and STZ-induced mice were assessed via tail tip vein collection (time zero) and then administered 0.8 mg/g glucose solution for IP glucose tolerance test (GTT). Blood samples were collected from the tail tip vein at 15, 30, 45, 60, 90 and 120 min after glucose challenge. f Corresponding AUC of the IP GTT. g Proinflammatory cytokine interleukin-6 was measured from plasma using cytometric bead array. Data are shown as mean ± S.E.M. of a–c, n = 18–20; d, n = 9–10; e and f, n = 4–5; g, n = 8–10 per group. b, d and f analysed by ordinary one-way ANOVA with Dunn's. c and g analysed by Kruskal-Wallis with Dunnett's. *P < 0.05, **P < 0.01, ***P < 0.001, ****P < 0.0001 vs CIT + CON control group

respective models. Both CIT- and STZ-treated mice on a HFD exhibited significantly greater levels of circulating IL-6 compared to CIT + CON controls. (Fig. 4g). No detectable levels of cytokines were found in the 9-week cohort (data not shown).

The effect of chronic high-fat feeding and hyperglycemia on the brain

We provided support for the presence of neuroinflammation (altered immune populations, increased number of hippocampal microglia and astrocytosis) mostly in the STZ + CON group at the 9-week time point. We next assessed these parameters in the long-term model after 18 weeks of treatment. We hypothesised that the elevated systemic inflammation evident at the 18-week time point would elicit more pronounced neuroinflammation in the brain compared to 9 weeks of high-fat feeding and hyperglycemia. Interestingly, we found no significant differences in the numbers of total leukocytes, CD11b$^+$ and phagocyte-like cells (Fig. 5a–c), or in the number of B (Fig. 5d) and T cells (Fig. 5e) in the brains of any of

the experimental groups compared to the CIT + CON control counterparts. However, it is important to note that the number of the various immune populations reported here in the chronic model was distinctly different to the findings of the 9-week time point. In fact, the total number of leukocytes per gram of brain tissue was approximately 50% less in the 18-week experimental groups compared to 9-week, and this was consistent for both innate and adaptive immune populations. Similarly, despite the lack of significant changes in the number of microglia (Fig. 5f) or degree of astrocytosis (Fig. 5g) in the hippocampus of any of the experimental groups compared to the CIT + CON controls at the 18-week time point, the number of Iba1$^+$ microglia and the degree of activated astrocytes denoted by GFAP$^+$ staining were elevated in an age-dependent manner. Indeed, there was a ~ 5-fold and 2.5-fold increase in Iba1$^+$ cells and GFAP$^+$ staining in CIT + CON mice at 18 weeks compared to the 9-week cohort (Fig. 5h, i), suggesting ageing supersedes high-fat or hyperglycemia-induced inflammation on the brain.

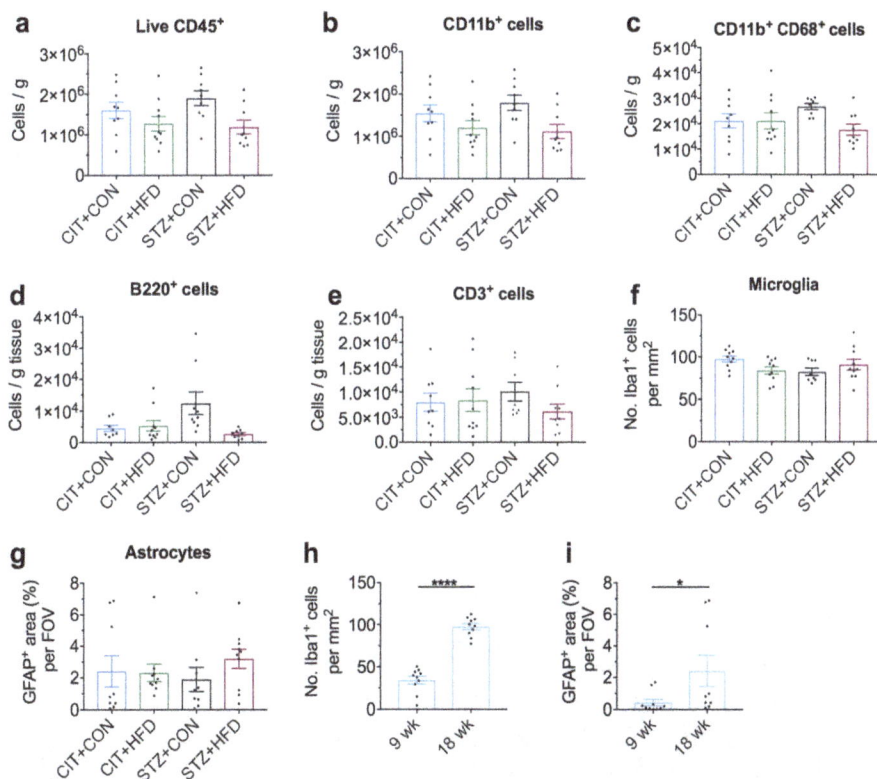

Fig. 5 Global brain immune changes return to baseline after 18 weeks of high-fat feeding and/or hyperglycemia. **a** Flow cytometry analysis of brain CD45$^+$7AAD$^-$ leukocytes of the left cerebral hemisphere. **b** Gated cells were analysed for the expression of CD11b as a marker of neutrophils, monocytes and microglia. **c** CD11b$^+$ cell gate was further analysed for expression of CD68 as a phagocytic marker. **d** Gated cells for B220 as a marker of B cells and (**e**) CD3 as a marker of T cells were analysed. **f** Number of Iba1$^+$ microglia and (**g**) GFAP$^+$ astrocytes in CA1 of the hippocampus were quantified at 20 weeks, and (**h**) microglial and (**i**) astrocyte numbers were compared between time points in CIT + CON mice. Data are shown as mean ± S.E.M. of **a**–**e**, n = 8–10 per group. Data in **a**–**c** analysed by one-way ANOVA with Dunnett's. **d** and **e** analysed by Kruskal-Wallis with Dunn's. **h** and **i** by Student's t test. *P < 0.05, ****P < 0.0001 vs CIT + CON control group

Chronic hyperglycemia promotes cerebral leukocyte-endothelial cell interactions

To assess whether the regional-specific neuroinflammation observed in the hyperglycemic mice at 9 weeks or systemic inflammation evident in the mice on 18 weeks of HFD was associated with recruitment of peripheral immune cells to the brain, we used intravital multiphoton microscopy to assess cerebral leukocyte-endothelial interactions. We delivered fluorescently conjugated anti-GR1 antibody into mice intravenously to study the interaction of monocytes and/or neutrophils with the cerebral vasculature in vivo. We did not observe any cerebral leukocyte-endothelial cell interactions in all groups at the 9-week time point (data not shown). However, after 18 weeks following induction of hyperglycemia, there was a significant increase in the number of GR1$^+$ leukocytes adherent to the post-capillary venules in the brain of mice from the STZ + CON group (Fig. 6a–c). No cerebral leukocyte-endothelial cell interactions were detected in any other experimental groups. In addition, to examine if chronic hyperglycemia induces the recruitment of blood-derived leukocytes into the brain, we used immunofluorescence to quantify the numbers of CD45$^+$ cells in the cortex of a separate cohort of mice. We found a significantly increased number of CD45$^+$ cells in the cortex of STZ + CON mice compared to control (Fig. 6d).

Discussion

In this study, we dissect the specific contributions of high-fat feeding and hyperglycemia to neuroinflammation in experimental mouse models of MetS. We demonstrate that acute hyperglycemia induces regional-specific effects on the brain by elevating microglial numbers and promotes astrocytosis in the hippocampus. In addition, we demonstrate that chronic hyperglycemia supports the recruitment of peripheral leukocytes, particularly GR1$^+$ granulocytes, to the cerebral microvasculature. Moreover, we provide evidence that these changes are independent of the systemic inflammation associated with high-fat feeding. Taken together, our findings suggest that hyperglycemia rather than high-fat feeding contributes to the development of regional neuroinflammation in animal models of MetS.

MetS in humans is associated with a wide-array of phenotypes. Therefore, the need for clinically relevant and highly reproducible animal models is paramount. Research has primarily centered on using monogenetic deletions or mutations that indirectly induce severe obesity, yet in the case of T2D, obesity is usually second only to environmental influences, not manifestations of genetic mutations [16]. Thus, the clinical relevance of these models to obesity in MetS and T2D in humans remains controversial. In this study, we used a high-fat diet as a method of inducing weight gain and low-dose STZ-treatment in producing a form of mild hyperglycemia. While a definitive diagnosis of hyperglycemia in T2D can vary depending on the weight, gender and race of an individual, clinical benchmarks constitute mild hyperglycemia as > 7–9% glycosylated haemoglobin [17]. Our findings indicate that the STZ treatment regime induced a clinically comparable mild hyperglycemia (8–9%), which was sustained over both 9-week and 18-week time points. To induce weight gain, high-fat feeding was selected to reflect the macronutrient composition of the westernised diet, strongly implicated in the development of obesity and insulin resistance in MetS [18]. We found that high-fat feeding (ad libitum) significantly induced weight gain. Similarly, high-fat feeding was associated with significant impairments to glucose metabolism and hyperinsulinaemia, but not hyperglycemia. Previous studies of HFD in C57Bl/6 J mice note percentage weight gain and insulin resistance consistent with our findings, yet contrastingly, with induced hyperglycemia, which may in part be due to the composition of lipids in our diet (22% fat), compared to these studies (60% fat) [19]. Our attempt of a combination model (STZ + HFD) resulted in weight gain at 18 weeks, but not

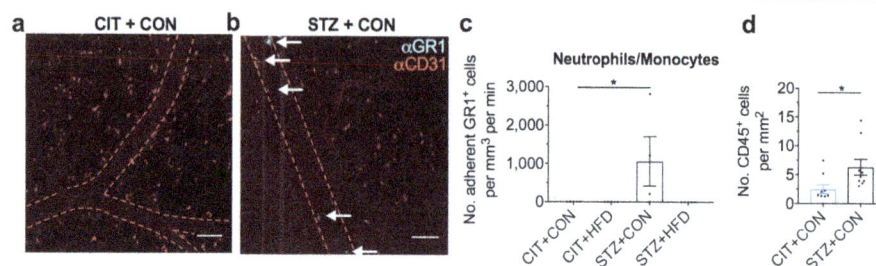

Fig. 6 Hyperglycemia drives peripheral recruitment of neutrophils and monocytes to the brain after 18 weeks. **a** Intravital multiphoton microscopy of the cerebral vasculature of vehicle-treated mice on control diet. **b** Intravital multiphoton microscopy of the cerebral vasculature of STZ-treated mice on control diet. Monocytes/neutrophils are visualised in blue, labelled with anti-GR1 mAb (clone RB6-8C5). Endothelium is visualised in red, labelled with anti-CD31 mAb and outlined with the red dotted line. Scale bars, 50 μm. **c** Quantification of GR1+ neutrophils/monocytes. Each data point represents the average of three fields of view per mouse. **d** Immunofluorescence of CD45$^+$ leukocytes in the cortex. Data represent mean ± S.E.M. of n = 4–5 per group. Kruskal-Wallis with Dunn's. *P < 0.05 vs CIT + CON control group

9 weeks. The delayed progression of weight gain in the mice of STZ + HFD group may be attributed to preferential lipid metabolism following impairment of glucose uptake. While only observational, these are critically important findings. Our use of high-fat feeding and STZ-treatment seemingly echo a sounder model of weight gain and hyperglycemia after 18 weeks, reflecting similar conditions and levels relevant to those seen in clinical MetS, without the need of gene deletions or mutations to induce these conditions. Although beyond the scope of this study, it would be important to validate whether our models demonstrate the diverse comorbidities of MetS, such as cardiovascular disease, nephropathy and atherosclerosis. The presence of these complications that arise from MetS patients would lend credence to our models in more accurately representing the more complex physiology and clinical presentation of MetS patients.

Administration of STZ alone to male C57BL/6 mice is commonly associated with retarded weight gain, as we and others routinely observe [20]. Similar retarded weight gain is also evident in rats subjected to STZ alone [21], as well as other mouse models where there is also hyperglycemia in the absence of high-fat diet [22, 23]. This retarded weight gain is a direct result of the degree of hyperglycemia, as it is not evident at a milder hyperglycemia [21], and is preventable by insulin replacement [23]. Rather than proposing that high glucose protects against the weight-gaining effect of a HFD, we would hence propose that a HFD protects against the retarded weight gain effect of hyperglycemia in rodent models. This protective effect of HFD on retarded weight gain as a result of impaired insulin availability may reflect a specific rodent phenomenon rather than a potential means of preventing obesity in diabetic humans. Interestingly, however, patients diagnosed with type 1 diabetes (insulin deficiency) exhibit a more severe hyperglycemia than patients diagnosed with type 2 diabetes (insulin resistance), yet it is the latter that are more commonly associated with obesity [24]. Clinical and experimental evidence has established that chronic hyperglycemia and weight gain in MetS are associated with both localised and systemic inflammation, yet studies struggle to delineate this from the effects of hyperglycemia alone. Our current study is able to shed light on this. By giving a HFD to both CIT- and STZ-treated mice, we examined whether systemic inflammation was driven solely by high-fat feeding, or in conjunction with hyperglycemia. Our findings show that mice in the CIT + HFD and STZ + HFD groups had increased levels of systemic pro-inflammatory IL-6 after 18 weeks, but not STZ + CON mice, suggesting that high-fat feeding is more likely to contribute to systemic inflammation over hyperglycemia. Previous experimental studies of high-fat feeding in C57Bl/6 J mice note significant increases in IL-6 and other pro-inflammatory cytokines after only

8 weeks [25], while studies involving the use of STZ-treatment in mice vary, noting the presence of IL-1β and TNFα in pancreatic tissue [26] and IFNγ and TNFα systemically [27]. In accordance with these studies, our results demonstrate that chronic weight gain induced by 18 weeks of high-fat feeding impacts significantly on systemic inflammation.

Inflammation is recognised as a key mechanism of diabetes progression and its multifactorial complications; its likely contribution to diabetes-induced neuropathy is now also clearly emerging [28]. Indeed, diabetes is regarded as a low-grade, chronic inflammatory disorder [29, 30]. Systemic inflammation is unmistakably present in diabetic patients [31, 32] and is considered a contributing mechanism to peripheral disease progression [33]. CD68 is a protein highly expressed by monocytes and macrophages, as well as microglia. Our observation that a combination of hyperglycemia and high-fat feeding leads to elevated CD11b$^+$CD68$^+$ cells is consistent with a diabetes-driven phenotype of increased circulating monocytes and tissue microglia, and suggests that inflammatory signalling is also likely to be implicated in both the systemic and central complications of diabetes, analogous to the known contribution of inflammation to other neurological disorders [28].

Under steady-state conditions, the number and function of microglia are tightly regulated, comprising the immune-dominant cell type in the brain. In response to an acute immune stimulus, microglia proliferate, increase phagocytosis, and clear the pathogenic insult—a process referred to as priming [34]. Generally, microglia will undergo apoptosis upon resolving inflammation, but in response to a chronic stimulus, microglia may become notoriously long-lived, contributing to—and thus enhancing—neuro-destructive effects. In our study, mice in the STZ + CON group demonstrated marked increases in the number of hippocampal Iba1$^+$ microglia after 9 weeks of treatment. This finding is consistent with a previous study that reported hippocampal-specific elevations in Iba1$^+$ microglia in STZ-treated rats [35]. Moreover, mice in the STZ + CON group demonstrated a significant increase in activated astrocytes, as indicated by elevated GFAP staining. Intriguingly, these changes were seemingly ameliorated at the 18 weeks endpoint, with no difference found amongst the experimental groups. As neuroinflammatory responses are concomitant with the correct homeostasis functioning of the CNS and are capable of resolving over time, our findings suggest that the STZ-induced changes in microglial numbers and astrocytosis are representative of an acute insult, in this case, hyperglycemia. Chronic hyperglycemia has been associated with cerebral endothelial cell dysfunction and apoptosis, which may provide an entry-point for circulating inflammatory cytokines [36]. We propose that with more severe weight gain (i.e. obesity) and hyperglycemia, beyond the endpoints examined here, the effects of systemic inflammation and peripheral leukocyte recruitment could establish a form of chronic, non-resolving neuroinflammation in the brain. This would reflect the reasoning by which systemic cytokine increases in obese T2D patients are thought to become evident later in life and support the concept that neurological impairments are primarily seen in aged individuals [37]. While only conjecture, the notion that hyperglycemia could act as the primary insult in priming microglia prior to the systemic inflammation formed by the secondary insult (obesity and/or ageing) is an interesting prospect that remains to be fully examined.

Having established the presence of systemic inflammation in HFD-fed mice, we characterised whether this was associated with the presence of adherent leukocytes to the cerebral vasculature. The extravasation of leukocytes from the peripheral vasculature into the brain parenchyma is a critical component in both acute and chronic neuroinflammatory disorders. This phenomenon has been predominantly explored in rodent models of multiple sclerosis (MS) and ischaemic stroke in vivo [38, 39], yet the influences by which this occurs are not fully understood. Here, we observed adherent GR1$^+$ granulocytes (neutrophils/monocytes) in the surface cerebrovasculature of STZ + CON mice after 18, but not 9 weeks. Interestingly, this adherence was not associated with any increases of IL-6 or other cytokines measured, suggesting that the recruitment of these cells is independent of systemic inflammation and high-fat feeding. Hyperglycemic conditions have been shown to induce endothelial cell dysfunction and promote low-grade inflammation [40]. Indeed, previous in vitro studies of human brain endothelial cell cultures reveal a high degree of apoptosis under hyperglycemic conditions [41]. To our knowledge, this is the first study of its kind to demonstrate in vivo granulocyte trafficking along the cerebrovasculature of hyperglycemic mice. Moreover, immunofluorescence of the cortex of STZ + CON mice after 18 weeks demonstrated an increase in the presence of CD45$^+$ blood-derived leukocytes. Given the lack of changes in inflammatory cells and markers measured using flow cytometry at the level of hemispheric tissue, it is possible that the GR1$^+$ granulocytes detected with intravital microscopy eventually transmigrated into the brain parenchyma and presented as this CD45$^+$ population.

Although not specifically examined in this study, the notion of whether high-fat feeding under hyperglycemic conditions seemingly protected against the gliosis we observed at 9 weeks is an interesting prospect. High-fat feeding or the "ketogenic diet" has recently been shown to provide disease-modifying activity in a broad range of neurodegenerative disorders including Alzheimer's disease [42]. These observations are supported by studies in animal models and isolated cells that showed ketone bodies, especially β-hydroxybutyrate, to confer neuroprotection against diverse types of cellular injury [43]. A recent study in young mice highlights that ketogenic diet intervention in mice induces significant increases in cerebral blood flow and P-glycoprotein transports on the blood-brain barrier to facilitate clearance of amyloid-β, a hallmark of Alzheimer's disease [44]. Therefore, the absence of hyperglycemia-associated elevation of microglia and astrocytosis in the STZ + HFD group may further suggest a neuroprotective role of high-fat feeding.

Despite the overwhelming evidence linking ageing to a wide array of systemic and neuroinflammatory disorders [45], it is important to note that the mice used in these experiments were not considered aged. It would be pertinent, therefore, to repeat this investigation in aged mice to examine whether age-associated risk factors could provide the necessary threshold to drive chronic neuroinflammation. In support of this, we observed that both microglial numbers and the degree of astrocytosis in control mice hippocampus increased significantly by four and fivefold, respectively, between 9 and 18 weeks of treatment. Previous studies in aged mice also note increases in CA1-specific gliosis [46] and that both microglia and astrocytes are more susceptible to inflammatory stimuli [47]. However, impairments to microglial function have also been observed in aged mice with regard to phagocytosis and motility [48, 49], which may suggest that this increase in microglial numbers may be a mechanism of compensation for otherwise dysfunctional microglia. Indeed, this age-associated increase in key immune populations of the hippocampus may explain the increased vulnerability to cognitive functions of psychomotor speed and working memory in MetS patients [50].

Conclusions

In summary, the findings of this study indicate that the hyperglycemic component of metabolic syndrome confers a more inflammatory role in the brain than high-fat feeding. Hyperglycemia alone promotes microglial numbers and astrocytosis in the hippocampus and is associated with the peripheral recruitment of leukocytes to the cerebrovasculature. On the contrary, chronic high-fat feeding is sufficient to induce a systemic inflammation, which may have other consequences on the brain over time. Further studies in older (12–18 months) mice will more accurately address the contributions of these components to the development of neuroinflammation and cognitive decline or dementia. Nevertheless, our results shed light on the specific contributions of high-fat feeding and hyperglycemia in the development of neuroinflammation.

Additional file

Additional file 1: Figure S1. Microglial numbers in cortex was unchanged after 9 weeks. Cell counts of Iba1$^+$ microglia in the cortex. Data represent mean ± S.E.M. of $n = 8$–10 per group. **Figure S2.**

Representative coronal brain sections for immunofluorescence detection of Iba1$^+$ microglia (green, denoted by yellow arrow) in the hippocampus of (a) CIT+HFD and (b) STZ+HFD mice. Scale bar, 100 μm. **Figure S3.** Neuronal numbers of CA1 hippocampus unchanged after 9-weeks of treatment. (a) Schematic diagram of the designated quantification area for neuronal counts. (b) Number of neurons in the pyramidal layer of CA1. (c) Area of pyramidal layer of CA1 (d) Number of neurons within CA1. Data represent mean ± S.E.M. of $n = 8$–10 per group. (DOCX 1055 kb)

Abbreviations

AUC: Area under the curve; BMI: Body mass index; CA1: Cornu Ammonis 1; CD: Cluster of differentiation; CIT: Citrate vehicle; CON: Control diet; CVD: Cardiovascular disease; ELISA: Enzyme-linked immunosorbent assay; GFAP: Glial fibrillary acidic protein; GR1: Granulocytic marker 1; HFD: High-fat diet; IBA1: Ionised calcium-binding adapter molecule 1; IL-6: Interleukin 6; MetS: Metabolic syndrome; PFA: Paraformaldehyde; STZ: Streptozotocin; T2D: Type 2 diabetes; TNFα: Tumour necrosis factor alpha

Acknowledgements

We thank Angela Vais from the Monash Histology Platform for her assistance with immunofluorescence and cryostat sectioning and Monash Medical Centre Animal Facility staff for the care of animals. We also thank the staff at Monash Medical Imaging and the Monash FlowCore facility.

Funding

This work was supported by the Future Leaders Fellowship to C.H.Y.W. from the National Heart Foundation (NHF, Australia; 100863). R.H.R is supported by a senior research fellowship from the National Health and Medical Research Council of Australia (CID; 1059960). The funding bodies had no role in the design of the study or collection, analysis, interpretation of data, or in writing the manuscript.

Authors' contributions

CHYW conceived of, designed, obtained ethics approval, supervised the project and performed in vivo experiments. BJW performed animal monitoring, conducted experiments, analysed the data and wrote the manuscript draft. KPK assisted with all animal monitoring and all endpoint collections. SW and BJW performed flow cytometry and data analysis. RHR and CHQ provided the use of and expertise in the STZ-treated combination model, use of equipment, provided input into the study design and participated in manuscript preparation and discussion. All authors read and approved the final manuscript.

Competing interests

The authors declare that they have no competing interests.

Author details

[1]Centre for Inflammatory Diseases, Department of Medicine, School of Clinical Sciences at Monash Health, Monash Medical Centre, Monash University, Clayton, VIC 3168, Australia. [2]Baker Heart and Diabetes Institute, Melbourne, Australia. [3]Department of Diabetes, Monash University, Melbourne, Australia.

References

1. Information on the IDF concensus worldwide definiton of the metabolic sydrome. http://www.idf.org/component/attachments/attachments.html?id=705&task=download. Accessed 1 June 2018.
2. James AM, Collins Y, Logan A, Murphy MP. Mitochondrial oxidative stress and the metabolic syndrome. Trends Endocrinol Metab. 2012;23:429–34.
3. Lavie CJ, Milani RV, Ventura HO. Obesity and cardiovascular disease: risk factor, paradox, and impact of weight loss. J Am Coll Cardiol. 2009;53:1925–32.
4. Cai D. Neuroinflammation and neurodegeneration in overnutrition-induced diseases. Trends Endocrinol Metab. 2013;24:40–7.
5. Moreno-Navarrete JM, Blasco G, Puig J, Biarnes C, Rivero M, Gich J, Fernandez-Aranda F, Garre-Olmo J, Ramio-Torrenta L, Alberich-Bayarri A, et al. Neuroinflammation in obesity: circulating lipopolysaccharide-binding protein associates with brain structure and cognitive performance. Int J Obes. 2017;41:1627–35.
6. Drake C, Boutin H, Jones MS, Denes A, McColl BW, Selvarajah JR, Hulme S, Georgiou RF, Hinz R, Gerhard A, et al. Brain inflammation is induced by co-morbidities and risk factors for stroke. Brain Behav Immun. 2011;25:1113–22.
7. Brands AMA, Biessels GJ, de Haan EHF, Kappelle LJ, Kessels RPC. The effects of type 1 diabetes on cognitive performance. Diabetes Care. 2005;28:726.
8. Hawkins BT, Lundeen TF, Norwood KM, Brooks HL, Egleton RD. Increased blood-brain barrier permeability and altered tight junctions in experimental diabetes in the rat: contribution of hyperglycaemia and matrix metalloproteinases. Diabetologia. 2007;50:202–11.
9. Sharma R, Buras E, Terashima T, Serrano F, Massaad CA, Hu L, Bitner B, Inoue T, Chan L, Pautler RG. Hyperglycemia induces oxidative stress and impairs axonal transport rates in mice. PLoS One. 2010;5:e13463.
10. Russell JW, Sullivan KA, Windebank AJ, Herrmann DN, Feldman EL. Neurons undergo apoptosis in animal and cell culture models of diabetes. Neurobiol Dis. 1999;6:347–63.
11. Gazdzinski S, Kornak J, Weiner MW, Meyerhoff DJ. Body mass index and magnetic resonance markers of brain integrity in adults. Ann Neurol. 2008; 63:652–7.
12. Taki Y, Kinomura S, Sato K, Inoue K, Goto R, Okada K, Uchida S, Kawashima R, Fukuda H. Relationship between body mass index and gray matter volume in 1,428 healthy individuals. Obesity (Silver Spring). 2008;16:119–24.
13. Wang B, Chandrasekera PC, Pippin JJ. Leptin- and leptin receptor-deficient rodent models: relevance for human type 2 diabetes. Curr Diabetes Rev. 2014;10:131–45.
14. Wu J, Yan L-J. Streptozotocin-induced type 1 diabetes in rodents as a model for studying mitochondrial mechanisms of diabetic β cell glucotoxicity. Diabetes Metab Syndr Obes. 2015;8:181–8.
15. Wu W, Brickman AM, Luchsinger J, Ferrazzano P, Pichiule P, Yoshita M, Brown T, DeCarli C, Barnes CA, Mayeux R, et al. The brain in the age of old: the hippocampal formation is targeted differentially by diseases of late life. Ann Neurol. 2008;64:698–706.
16. King AJ. The use of animal models in diabetes research. Br J Pharmacol. 2012;166:877–94.
17. Kilpatrick ES, Bloomgarden ZT, Zimmet PZ. International Expert Committee report on the role of the A1C assay in the diagnosis of diabetes: response to the International Expert Committee. Diabetes Care. 2009;32:e159 author reply e160.
18. Kothari V, Luo Y, Tornabene T, O'Neill AM, Greene MW, Geetha T, Babu JR. High fat diet induces brain insulin resistance and cognitive impairment in mice. Biochim Biophys Acta. 2017;1863:499–508.
19. Gallou-Kabani C, Vige A, Gross MS, Rabes JP, Boileau C, Larue-Achagiotis C, Tome D, Jais JP, Junien C. C57BL/6J and A/J mice fed a high-fat diet delineate components of metabolic syndrome. Obesity (Silver Spring). 2007; 15:1996–2005.
20. Deeds MC, Anderson JM, Armstrong AS, Gastineau DA, Hiddinga HJ, Jahangir A, Eberhardt NL, Kudva YC. Single dose streptozotocin-induced diabetes: considerations for study design in islet transplantation models. Lab Anim. 2011;45:131–40.
21. Kahlberg N, Qin CX, Anthonisz J, Jap E, Ng HH, Jelinic M, Parry LJ, Kemp-Harper BK, Ritchie RH, Leo CH. Adverse vascular remodelling is more sensitive than endothelial dysfunction to hyperglycaemia in diabetic rat mesenteric arteries. Pharmacol Res. 2016;111:325–35.

22. Sharma A, Rizky L, Stefanovic N, Tate M, Ritchie RH, Ward KW, de Haan JB. The nuclear factor (erythroid-derived 2)-like 2 (Nrf2) activator dh404 protects against diabetes-induced endothelial dysfunction. Cardiovasc Diabetol. 2017;16:33.

23. Tate M, Deo M, Cao AH, Hood SG, Huynh K, Kiriazis H, Du XJ, Julius TL, Figtree GA, Dusting GJ, et al. Insulin replacement limits progression of diabetic cardiomyopathy in the low-dose streptozotocin-induced diabetic rat. Diab Vasc Dis Res. 2017;14:423–33.

24. Abbasi A, Juszczyk D, van Jaarsveld CHM, Gulliford MC. Body mass index and incident type 1 and type 2 diabetes in children and young adults: a retrospective cohort study. J Endocr Soc. 2017;1:524–37.

25. Kim KA, Gu W, Lee IA, Joh EH, Kim DH. High fat diet-induced gut microbiota exacerbates inflammation and obesity in mice via the TLR4 signaling pathway. PLoS One. 2012;7:e47713.

26. Han X, Tao YL, Deng YP, Yu JW, Cai J, Ren GF, Sun YN, Jiang GJ. Metformin ameliorates insulitis in STZ-induced diabetic mice. PeerJ. 2017;5:e3155.

27. Lee YS, Eun HS, Kim SY, Jeong JM, Seo W, Byun JS, Jeong WI, Yi HS. Hepatic immunophenotyping for streptozotocin-induced hyperglycemia in mice. Sci Rep. 2016;6:30656.

28. Wong CHY, Wanrooy BJ, Bruce DG. Chapter 10 - Neuroinflammation, type 2 diabetes, and dementia. In: Srikanth V, Arvanitakis Z, editors. Type 2 diabetes and dementia. New York: Academic Press, Elsevier; 2018. p. 195–209.

29. Devaraj S, Dasu MR, Jialal I. Diabetes is a proinflammatory state: a translational perspective. Expert Rev Endocrinol Metab. 2010;5:19–28.

30. Huynh K, Bernardo BC, McMullen JR, Ritchie RH. Diabetic cardiomyopathy: mechanisms and new treatment strategies targeting antioxidant signaling pathways. Pharmacol Ther. 2014;142:375–415.

31. Hanley AJG, Festa A, D'Agostino RB, Wagenknecht LE, Savage PJ, Tracy RP, Saad MF, Haffner SM. Metabolic and inflammation variable clusters and prediction of type 2 diabetes. Diabetes. 2004;53:1773.

32. Schalkwijk CG, Poland DCW, van Dijk W, Kok A, Emeis JJ, Dräger AM, Doni A, van Hinsbergh VWM, Stehouwer CDA. Plasma concentration of C-reactive protein is increased in type I diabetic patients without clinical macroangiopathy and correlates with markers of endothelial dysfunction: evidence for chronic inflammation. Diabetologia. 1999;42:351–7.

33. Donath MY, Shoelson SE. Type 2 diabetes as an inflammatory disease. Nat Rev Immunol. 2011;11:98.

34. Perry VH, Holmes C. Microglial priming in neurodegenerative disease. Nat Rev Neurol. 2014;10:217–24.

35. Nagayach A, Patro N, Patro I. Astrocytic and microglial response in experimentally induced diabetic rat brain. Metab Brain Dis. 2014;29:747–61.

36. Schalkwijk CG, Stehouwer CD. Vascular complications in diabetes mellitus: the role of endothelial dysfunction. Clin Sci (Lond). 2005;109:143–59.

37. Umegaki H. Type 2 diabetes as a risk factor for cognitive impairment: current insights. Clin Interv Aging. 2014;9:1011–9.

38. Schmitt C, Strazielle N, Ghersi-Egea JF. Brain leukocyte infiltration initiated by peripheral inflammation or experimental autoimmune encephalomyelitis occurs through pathways connected to the CSF-filled compartments of the forebrain and midbrain. J Neuroinflammation. 2012;9:187.

39. Jickling GC, Liu D, Ander BP, Stamova B, Zhan X, Sharp FR. Targeting neutrophils in ischemic stroke: translational insights from experimental studies. J Cereb Blood Flow Metab. 2015;35:888–901.

40. Sena CM, Pereira AM, Seica R. Endothelial dysfunction - a major mediator of diabetic vascular disease. Biochim Biophys Acta. 2013;1832:2216–31.

41. Shao B, Bayraktutan U. Hyperglycaemia promotes human brain microvascular endothelial cell apoptosis via induction of protein kinase C-ssl and prooxidant enzyme NADPH oxidase. Redox Biol. 2014;2:694–701.

42. Reger MA, Henderson ST, Hale C, Cholerton B, Baker LD, Watson GS, Hyde K, Chapman D, Craft S. Effects of beta-hydroxybutyrate on cognition in memory-impaired adults. Neurobiol Aging. 2004;25:311–4.

43. Gasior M, Rogawski MA, Hartman AL. Neuroprotective and disease-modifying effects of the ketogenic diet. Behav Pharmacol. 2006;17:431–9.

44. Ma D, Wang AC, Parikh I, Green SJ, Hoffman JD, Chlipala G, Murphy MP, Sokola BS, Bauer B, Hartz AMS, Lin AL. Ketogenic diet enhances neurovascular function with altered gut microbiome in young healthy mice. Sci Rep. 2018;8:6670.

45. Franceschi C, Campisi J. Chronic inflammation (inflammaging) and its potential contribution to age-associated diseases. J Gerontol A Biol Sci Med Sci. 2014;69(Suppl 1):S4–9.

46. Hayakawa N, Kato H, Araki T. Age-related changes of astrocytes, oligodendrocytes and microglia in the mouse hippocampal CA1 sector. Mech Ageing Dev. 2007;128:311–6.

47. Godbout JP, Chen J, Abraham J, Richwine AF, Berg BM, Kelley KW, Johnson RW. Exaggerated neuroinflammation and sickness behavior in aged mice following activation of the peripheral innate immune system. FASEB J. 2005; 19:1329–31.

48. Hefendehl JK, Neher JJ, Suhs RB, Kohsaka S, Skodras A, Jucker M. Homeostatic and injury-induced microglia behavior in the aging brain. Aging Cell. 2014;13:60–9.

49. Floden AM, Combs CK. Microglia demonstrate age-dependent interaction with amyloid-beta fibrils. J Alzheimers Dis. 2011;25:279–93.

50. Yates KF, Sweat V, Yau PL, Turchiano MM, Convit A. Impact of metabolic syndrome on cognition and brain: a selected review of the literature. Arterioscler Thromb Vasc Biol. 2012;32:2060–7.

11

Interaction of systemic oxidative stress and mesial temporal network degeneration in Parkinson's disease with and without cognitive impairment

Pi-Ling Chiang[1], Hsiu-Ling Chen[1], Cheng-Hsien Lu[2], Yueh-Sheng Chen[1], Kun-Hsien Chou[3], Tun-Wei Hsu[4], Meng-Hsiang Chen[1], Nai-Wen Tsai[2], Shau-Hsuan Li[5] and Wei-Che Lin[1*]

Abstract

Background: To identify the vulnerable areas associated with systemic oxidative stress and further disruption of these vulnerable areas by measuring the associated morphology and functional network alterations in Parkinson's disease (PD) patients with and without cognitive impairment.

Methods: This prospective study was approved by the institutional review board of KCGMH, and written informed consent was obtained. Between December 2010 and May 2015, 41 PD patients with different levels of cognitive functions and 29 healthy volunteers underwent peripheral blood sampling to quantify systemic oxidative stress, as well as T1W volumetric and resting state functional MRI (rs-fMRI) scans. Rs-fMRI was used to derive the healthy intrinsic connectivity patterns seeded by the vulnerable areas associated with any of the significant oxidative stress markers. The two groups were compared in terms of the functional connectivity correlation coefficient (fc-CC) and gray matter volume (GMV) of the network seeded by the vulnerable areas.

Results: The levels of oxidative stress markers, including leukocyte apoptosis and adhesion molecules, were significantly higher in the PD group. Using whole-brain VBM-based correlation analysis, the bilateral mesial temporal lobes (MTLs) were identified as the most vulnerable areas associated with lymphocyte apoptosis ($P < 0.005$). We found that the MTL network of healthy subjects resembled the PD-associated atrophy pattern. Furthermore, reduced fc-CC and GMV were further associated with the aggravated cognitive impairment.

Conclusion: The MTLs are the vulnerable areas associated with peripheral lymphocyte infiltration, and disruptions of the MTL functional network in both architecture and functional connectivity might result in cognitive impairments in Parkinson's disease.

Keywords: Parkinson's disease, Systemic oxidative stress, Lymphocyte apoptosis, Mesial temporal network, Gray matter volume, Functional connectivity, Cognitive impairment

* Correspondence: u64lin@yahoo.com.tw
[1]Department of Diagnostic Radiology, Kaohsiung Chang Gung Memorial Hospital, Chang Gung University College of Medicine, 123 Ta-Pei Road, Niao-Sung, Kaohsiung 83305, Taiwan
Full list of author information is available at the end of the article

Background

Parkinson's disease (PD) is the second most common neurodegenerative movement disorder among the elderly and also presents as a spectrum of cognitive dysfunction, ranging from PD with normal cognition (PDN) to PD with mild cognitive impairment (PDMCI) to PD with dementia (PDD) [1]. PDMCI is an early form of neurodegeneration that carries a risk of further degeneration into dementia. It is now known that early cognitive deficits constitute an important issue for diagnostic, therapeutic, and prognostic factors in PD [1]. In previous studies, dementia in PD has been demonstrated to be associated with widespread gray matter (GM) atrophy [2], especially in the mesial temporal lobe (MTL) [3]. Although the brain is less affected in cases of PDMCI than dementia, the initial atrophy patterns seen in PDMCI can be used for dementia prediction [3, 4].

In addition to structural changes, alterations of both dopaminergic and non-dopaminergic transmitter systems in the PD brain have also been found to modify several distinct functional networks underlying the different cognitive impairments [3]. The functional network disruptions assessed with "resting state" or intrinsic connectivity fMRI has shown distinct patterns of global network disruption or disruption within specific networks in PD in recent studies. Different network connectivity changes affect different types of cognitive impairment in PD Different network connectivity changes result in different types of cognitive impairment in PD [5–8]. Progressive cognitive decline in PD is associated with altered resting status functional connectivity in multiple brain regions, including the MTL [9]. Several studies have also discussed dopamine-dependent functional connectivity disruptions and other network alternations in PD [10]. Furthermore, a previous review study has shown worsening memory storage deficits associated with worsening MTL atrophy and further damage to the MTL network with the progression from PD to PDD. Another network implicated in memory is the basal nucleus of Meynert (BNM) cholinergic network. The volume of the BNM cholinergic network degenerates significantly in PDD, which correlates with progressive electrocortical depression in magnetoencephalography [3].

In the large-scale study of human brain networks by Seeley et al., it was reported that spatial disease atrophy patterns reflect the healthy brain's intrinsic functional network architecture. These findings support the network neurodegeneration hypothesis of Seeley et al. [11] and suggest that human neural networks can be defined by synchronous baseline activity and selective vulnerability to neurodegenerative illness. However, while these functional networks are associated with cognitive dysfunctions, the specific factors that affect the vulnerable areas, and their locations and contributions to the

degeneration from mild cognitive impairment to dementia in PD are still undetermined.

Systemic oxidative stress is an important etiology of the neuroinflammation seen in PD and is associated with further progression of the disease via various pathways, such as blood-brain barrier (BBB) dysfunction and the infiltration of peripheral immune cells and circulating cytokines [12, 13]. The infiltration of peripheral immune cells, especially lymphocytes and monocytes, which can mediate apoptosis [14], is one of the interactive pathways of systemic oxidative stress and neuroinflammation. The migration of lymphocytes to the central nervous system (CNS) through the BBB is dependent on lymphocyte function-associated antigen 1 (LFA-1) [15]. This association has been further been demonstrated by the increased peripheral leukocyte apoptosis with striatal dopamine neuron loss [16] and white matter alteration observed through the use of diffusion tensor imaging [17]. In addition, increased oxidative stress has been found to be associated with cognitive function status even in the early stage of the disease in young PD patients [18]. The accumulating evidence has shown an association between inflammation and cognitive impairment not only in PD [19] but also in other neurodegenerative diseases such as AD [20] and even in changes due to normal aging [21]. Peripheral immune cells, which reflect the level of systemic oxidative stress, might play important roles both in disease progression and cognitive function deterioration in PD.

The main focus with respect to peripheral immune cells was on their role in dopamine neuron loss in the substantia nigra (SN) or striatum in previous studies. Although the peripheral immune cells are associated with the initial pathogenesis of PD [22], it is still not known whether this association is widely spread in a non-specific manner to all brain tissues or if it is only focused on particular regions, i.e., the so-called vulnerable areas. Some recent studies have demonstrated the correlational relationships between structural alterations of various areas and different peripheral oxidative stress markers [17, 18, 23]. Moreover, two mediation studies by our team revealed the interactions between altered brain structures and elevated serum oxidative stress [24, 25]. A related important question that has yet to be clearly answered by existing research is whether peripheral inflammation affects these vulnerable areas and, if so, whether it disrupts cognition-related networks, thus causing subsequent downstream degradation and functional impairment. In any case, the identification of any highly sensitive areas might be helpful in the early detection of cognitive deficits, in treatment monitoring, and in dementia progression prevention.

In the present study, we used voxel-based morphometry (VBM) and resting state functional MRI (rs-fMRI) to evaluate the effects of systemic oxidative stress on brain morphology and functional network alterations, respectively, in PD patients with different cognitive statuses. More specifically, the study's aims were (1) to evaluate the differences in systemic oxidative stress and GM volume changes in PD patients and healthy controls, (2) to investigate the vulnerable areas and associated functional networks in the brain that are highly sensitive to systemic oxidative parameters, and (3) to evaluate the relationships between cognitive impairment and the structural and functional integrity of the networks of the vulnerable areas.

Methods

This prospective study enrolled 41 patients who were diagnosed with idiopathic PD from December 2010 to May 2015 according to the United Kingdom Brain Bank criteria [26] by an experienced neurologist from our hospital. For comparison, 29 sex- and age-matched healthy volunteers were recruited as a normal control (NC) group. All the participants in both groups had no other history of neurologic or psychiatric illness. All the evaluations for the PD patients, including the evaluations of clinical disease status, the MRI studies, and the neuropsychological tests, were initially assessed in the OFF-medication state achieved by the withdrawal of dopaminergic medications 12 to 18 h before testing. The Chang Gung Memorial Hospital Ethics Committee approved the study, and all of the participants provided written informed consent.

Each patient's disease severity and cognitive functional status were evaluated using the Unified Parkinson's Disease Rating Scale (UPDRS), the modified Hoehn and Yahr Staging Scale, the Schwab and England Activities of Daily Living Scale, and the MiniMental State Examination (MMSE). Neuropsychological evaluations of five cognitive domains (i.e., attention and working memory, executive, language, memory, and visuospatial) were conducted using subtests from the Cognitive Ability Screening Instrument [27] and the Wechsler Adult Intelligence Scale-III [28].

All the patients were classified as having PDN, PDMCI, or PDD. PDMCI was defined according to the Movement Disorder Society Task Force Guidelines [1]. Cognitive impairment was defined as a score 1.5 SD below the normative mean in each of the domains [29]. PDN was defined as less than two domains of cognitive impairment. PDMCI was defined as one score at -1.5 SD in each of two or more domains but without dementia. PDD was defined as impairment in more than one cognitive domain with an MMSE score of less than 26 [30]. The analyses of the five cognitive function domains were used with the average Z-score of all the subtest scores in each domain.

Blood samples were drawn by venipuncture on the same day as the MRI study and neuropsychological testing were conducted. Systemic inflammation was evaluated in terms of the percentage of apoptotic peripheral leukocytes and the levels of cellular adhesion molecules. The level of leukocyte apoptosis was assessed using APO 2.7-phycoerythrin (PE). The quantities of cellular adhesion molecules were expressed as the mean fluorescence intensity of anti-LFA-1 or anti-macrophage-1 antigen (Mac-1) antibody-positive leukocytes. All the leukocytes and their subtypes were analyzed by flow cytometry. The statistical analyses were performed using the Statistical Package for Social Sciences (SPSS, version 22, SPSS Inc. Chicago, IL, USA). The group differences were compared by analysis of covariance (ANCOVA), with age and sex controlled for as potential confounding variables. Statistical significance was set at Bonferroni corrected $P < 0.05$.

For each subject, an MRI scan was performed using a 3.0 Tesla whole-body GE Signa MRI system equipped with an eight-channel head coil. A 3D high-resolution T1-weighted anatomical image was acquired using an inversion recovery fast spoiled gradient-recalled echo pulse sequence (TR/TE/inversion time = 9.5/3.9/450 ms; flip angle = 20°; FOV = 256 mm; matrix size = 512 × 512). A resting state functional image was also acquired using 300 contiguous echo planar imaging whole-brain functional scans (TR = 2 s, TE = 30 ms, FOV = 240 mm, flip angle 80°, matrix size 64 × 64, thickness = 4 mm). During the resting experiment, the scanner room was darkened and the participants were instructed to relax, with their eyes closed, without falling asleep. All patients were in the OFF-dopaminergic-medication state during the MRI scans.

T1-weighted structural MRI data were analyzed using VBM and the Statistical Parametric Mapping software program (SPM12, Wellcome Institute of Neurology, University College London, UK, http://www.fil.ion.ucl.a-c.uk/spm/) with default settings. All native space T1-weighted structural MRI scans were segmented into GM, white matter (WM), and cerebrospinal fluid (CSF) components. During normalization, the GM and WM images were affine-registered to the tissue probability maps in the Montreal Neurological Institute standard space. The resulting GM tissue segment images were transformed by the DARTEL registration procedure and were smoothed with a Gaussian kernel of full width at half maximum of 8 mm. The final GM images were analyzed within the framework of a full factorial design, whereas ANCOVA was performed with age, sex, and total intracranial volume (TIV) as covariates to investigate the gray matter volume (GMV) differences between the PD and control groups. The resulting statistical inferences were considered significant if the cluster-level family-wise error corrected P value was < 0.05. For the correlation analyses, whole-brain voxel-based multiple regression analysis with age and gender controlled for was used to identify the GM vulnerable areas associated with significant oxidative stress markers in PD.

The rs-fMRI data were preprocessed using the SPM software program and the Data Processing Assistant for Resting-State fMRI software program. After normalization and smoothing by SPM, the waveform of each voxel was finally used for removal of the linear trends of time courses and for temporal band-pass filtering (0.01 to 0.08 Hz) [31]. For network construction of the vulnerable areas associated with oxidative stress, the GM regions previously identified as vulnerable to any significant levels of oxidative stress markers were set as seeds. The voxel-wise FC analyses of the four groups were performed by computing the temporal correlations between the mean time series of each seed and the time series of each voxel within the whole brain. The correlation coefficients of each voxel were normalized to z-scores with Fisher's r-to-z transformation. A head movement parameter, the mean frame-wise displacement (FD), which indexes the volume-to-volume changes in head position, was also assessed for each participant. There was no significant difference between the NC and PD groups or among the PD subgroups.

To test whether the changes in FC patterns were associated with the underlying structural atrophy, the GMV values of the four groups were calculated under the intrinsic connectivity networks of the healthy controls connecting to the vulnerable areas. ANCOVAs with age, sex, and TIV (only for GMV) as the covariates were then used to compare the groups in terms of the mean GMV and functional connectivity correlation coefficient (fc-CC) values of the network area. The intergroup differences in the seed-based functional connectivity to the vulnerable areas were tested using the voxel-wise two-sample t test embedded in SPM. Analyses of the correlations between the fc-CC and GMV of the network and the correlations among the fc-CC, disease severity, and cognitive impairment were also performed, with the former analyses controlling for TIV and the latter analyses controlling for age and sex. The cluster size was determined over 1000 Monte Carlo simulations using the AlphaSim program distributed with the REST software tool (http://resting-fmri.sourceforge.net/). A corrected significance level of $P = 0.01$ was obtained by a combined threshold of $P = 0.01$ for each voxel and an extent threshold of 43 voxels (cluster size > 1161 mm^3). The threshold for statistical significance was set at $P < 0.05$.

Results

Clinical characteristics and oxidative parameters among groups

The demographic characteristics and oxidative parameters of the 41 PD patients and 29 healthy volunteers are shown in Table 1. There were no significant differences in age, sex, and years of education between the NC group and overall PD group. However, the PDD subgroup had, on average, significantly fewer years of education, higher MMSE and UPDRS I scores, and higher medication doses. Meanwhile, the apoptosis percentage and the LFA-1 levels of monocytes and lymphocytes were significantly higher in the PDN subgroup than in the controls (Bonferroni corrected $P < 0.05$) (Table 1 and Additional file 1: Figure S1). The apoptosis percentage of monocytes and especially lymphocytes were still significantly higher in the PDN subgroup after removal of outliers (Additional file 2: Table S1).

Changes of gray matter volume in PD subgroups

Compared with the NC group, the PDD subgroup showed significantly diffuse GMV loss throughout the whole brain; the PDMCI and PDN subgroups showed significantly smaller GMV values (Additional file 3: Figure S2). There was no brain region in which the PD subgroups had significantly greater GMV than the NC group.

Vulnerable areas associated with oxidative parameters in PD group

Using whole-brain voxel-based correlation analysis for the PD group, the bilateral MTLs (MNI space[x,y,z]: [−32,− 6,− 29] and [18,− 2,− 35]) were identified as the vulnerable areas associated with lymphocyte apoptosis ($P < 0.005$, cluster > 288) (Fig. 1). This meant that the GMV of the MTL vulnerable areas was correlated with the lymphocyte apoptosis marker in the PD group. No vulnerable areas associated with other oxidative parameters in the PD brains were identified.

Analysis of intrinsic connectivity networks connected to the vulnerable areas

The intrinsic connectivity network of the vulnerable area was constructed by using the bilateral MTLs as seed regions. We found that the functional connectivity with the bilateral MTL vulnerable areas became limited and disrupted in the PD patients (Fig. 2). The MTL functional network profile derived from the healthy subjects resembled the PD-associated GM atrophy pattern (Fig. 2 and Additional file 3: Figure S2). However, there were no significant fc-CC value differences of the bilateral MTL functional network among the PD subgroups.

By using the MTL functional network of the healthy controls as a mask, we found that the GMVs underlying the MTL functional network were significantly smaller in the PDD subgroup than in the NC group and other PD subgroups ($P < 0.001$) (Fig. 3a).

Finally, the two-sample t test conducted to compare all the PD patients and the NC group showed significant

Table 1 Demographic characteristics of the PD patients and normal controls

	Normal group (n = 29)	Patients with PD (n = 41)			F†	P† value
		PDN (n = 16)	PDMCI (n = 13)	PDD (n = 12)		
Sex (male/female)	13/16	8/8	7/6	6/6		0.954
Age	62.17 ± 4.82	61.44 ± 7.33	61.54 ± 7.52	64.50 ± 5.65	0.690	0.561
Education	9.93 ± 4.05	11.94 ± 4.17 #	9.08 ± 3.62	5.67 ± 4.01 #	5.169	0.003†
Disease duration		2.33 ± 1.38 #	2.44 ± 2.19	5.65 ± 5.32 #	4.340	0.020†
Medicine dose		261.38 ± 151.91 #	413.25 ± 283.20	512.75 ± 317.41 #	3.739	0.034†
MMSE		26.69 ± 3.59 #	27.31 ± 1.55 §	19.75 ± 3.60 #§	21.416	0.000†
UPDRS I		2.69 ± 2.24 #	3.00 ± 2.61	5.08 ± 3.34 #	3.722	0.034†
UPDRS II		9.00 ± 6.36	10.54 ± 9.00	13.33 ± 9.38	0.843	0.439
UPDRS III		18.06 ± 13.24	26.00 ± 17.92	31.50 ± 19.94	2.042	0.145
UPDRS total		29.75 ± 20.49	39.54 ± 28.60	49.92 ± 31.25	1.832	0.175
H&Y score		1.94 ± 1.24	2.27 ± 1.07	2.54 ± 1.01	0.710	0.499
S&E score		83.75 ± 18.93	83.08 ± 21.36	77.50 ± 18.65	0.300	0.743
Oxidation parameters						
Monocyte LFA-1	13.21 ± 4.34 ¤*	17.83 ± 5.58 ¤	17.67 ± 6.20	18.69 ± 6.02*	4.562	0.006†
Lymphocyte LFA-1	12.31 ± 3.10 ¤	15.37 ± 4.00 ¤	14.72 ± 1.78	14.43 ± 3.17	4.250	0.008†
Granulocyte LFA-1	5.42 ± 1.34	6.11 ± 1.17	6.15 ± 0.72	6.29 ± 1.69	1.841	0.149
Monocyte Mac-1	40.26 ± 30.28	49.69 ± 19.87	63.75 ± 53.22	52.90 ± 28.68	1.575	0.204
Lymphocyte Mac-1	9.91 ± 1.89	10.03 ± 2.66	10.94 ± 5.24	10.58 ± 2.37	0.477	0.699
Granulocyte Mac-1	41.42 ± 15.35	49.66 ± 20.81	56.41 ± 25.01	50.71 ± 27.27	1.921	0.135
Monocyte APO2.7 (%)	2.28 ± 1.30 ¤	8.00 ± 9.82 ¤	4.13 ± 3.44	4.83 ± 4.52	4.361	0.007†
Lymphocyte APO2.7 (%)	0.48 ± 0.38 ¤	1.04 ± 0.71 ¤	0.56 ± 0.38	0.62 ± 0.41	5.305	0.002†
Granulocyte APO2.7 (%)	0.82 ± 0.58	1.03 ± 0.57	1.17 ± 1.19	1.11 ± 0.79	0.799	0.499

Data are presented as mean ± standard deviation. Sex data were compared by Pearson chi-square test. Age data were compared by independent t test. Education year, oxidation parameters, clinical severity score, medication, and cognitive function data were compared by analysis of covariance (ANCOVA) after controlling for age and sex. F† and P† represent the comparison amounts of the PDN, PDMCI, and PDD patients and the normal control group, controlling for age and sex, with Bonferroni correction

¤ Significant differences between NC and PDN; * Significant differences between NC and PDD; # Significant differences between PDN and PDD; § Significant differences between PDMCI and PDD; †Significant differences among groups

changes of the fc-CC values in the middle occipital lobe (MOL) and pons within the MTL functional network (Additional file 4: Figure S3). The MOL fc-CC value was significantly decreased in the PDD subgroup compared with the NC group and other PD subgroups. Otherwise, the fc-CC value of the pons was significantly increased in the PDN and PDD subgroups compared with the NC group (Fig. 3b, c).

Relationship between functional connectivity and gray matter volume of MTL functional network

Within the MTL functional network, we found that the reduced GMV was associated with decreased fc-CC ($r = -0.332$, $P = 0.036$) values in the PD patients. Disruptions to the MTL network were seen in both its architecture and functional connectivity, and these architectural and functional disruptions were associated with each other.

Relationships among disease severity, cognitive function, and the MTL functional network

Correlation analyses were conducted to evaluate the relationships among the disease severity, cognitive function, and fc-CC values. In general, the aggregated disease severity and cognitive impairment were associated with lower functional connectivity in the PD patients. Due to the exploratory design of the study, we performed the correlation analyses with and without controlling clinical parameters, such as education year, disease duration, and medication.

With controlling age and gender only, the reduced fc-CC values of the MTL functional network were associated with greater disease severity, including in terms of the UPDRS part I ($r = -0.439$, $P = 0.006$) and III ($r = -0.454$, $P = 0.004$) and total scores ($r = -0.435$, $P = 0.006$) (Fig. 4a). In addition, the reduced fc-CC values between the MOL and MTL of the PD patients were also associated with greater disease severity as indicated by the

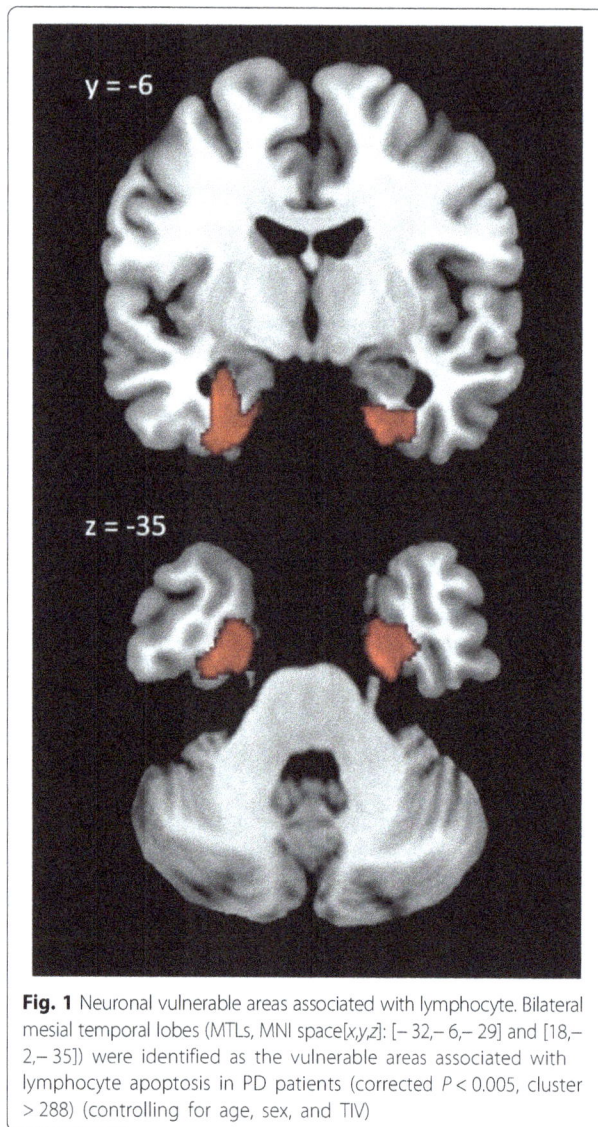

Fig. 1 Neuronal vulnerable areas associated with lymphocyte. Bilateral mesial temporal lobes (MTLs, MNI space[x,y,z]: [− 32,− 6,− 29] and [18,− 2,− 35]) were identified as the vulnerable areas associated with lymphocyte apoptosis in PD patients (corrected $P < 0.005$, cluster > 288) (controlling for age, sex, and TIV)

the MOL and disease severity as indicated by the UPDRS I ($r = − 0.320$, $P = 0.061$) and MMSE scores ($r = 0.411$, $P = 0.014$), as well as greater cognitive impairment in the attention ($r = 0.330$, $P = 0.053$) and memory ($r = 0.327$, $P = 0.055$) domains were weakened.

Discussion

In the comparison between the PD patients and healthy controls, the PD patients presented with higher levels of systemic oxidative stress, including increased apoptosis percentages and increased LFA-1 values. Compared with the NC group, the PD patients had significantly lower GMVs with diffuse atrophy patterns, especially the PDD patients. The MTL atrophy was used to identify the MTLs as the vulnerable areas associated with lymphocyte apoptosis, indicating their relationship with systemic oxidative stress. In addition, we also found deterioration of the structural and functional network integrity of the MTL network, a finding which further associated the network with the progression of disease severity and cognitive deficits. These associations may reflect the possible key role of lymphocyte apoptosis in the GMV atrophy and functional connectivity alterations seen in the development of PD.

Increased apoptosis of lymphocytes and monocytes and increased expression of LFA-1 might support the view that there is only one primary pathophysiology of PD: abnormal systemic oxidative stress and the acceleration of peripheral immune cell infiltration into the brain. Neurodegeneration in PD associated with systemic inflammation via various pathways has been thoroughly discussed [12, 13, 16–18, 24, 25]. Several previous studies showed that higher percentages of peripheral apoptotic lymphocytes [32] and the CNS infiltration of lymphocytes and monocytes contribute to neurodegeneration [22, 33, 34]. The activation of LFA-1 has been shown to mediate the recruitment of peripheral lymphocytes and monocytes into the PD brain [22]. Although researchers have faced some difficulty in verifying the direct interactions between systemic oxidative stress and neuroinflammation in PD subjects, the infiltration of peripheral immune cells into the SN of animal PD models [13] and the association between leukocyte apoptosis and striatal dopamine neuron loss [16] constitute indirect forms of evidence provided by previous studies. Current study may further provide an indirect evidence of peripheral inflammation communicating with the brain with immune cells in PD.

UPDRS I ($r = − 0.359$, $P = 0.027$) and MMSE scores ($r = 0.384$, $P = 0.017$), as well as with greater cognitive impairment in the attention ($r = 0.353$, $P = 0.03$) and memory ($r = 0.325$, $P = 0.046$) domains (Fig. 4b).

In further analyses with education year, disease duration and medication as covariates, the reduced fc-CC values of the MTL functional network were less significantly associated with greater disease severity, including in terms of the UPDRS part I ($r = − 0. 381$, $P = 0.024$) and III ($r = − 0.406$, $P = 0.016$) and total scores ($r = − 0.385$, $P = 0.022$). The associations of the increased pons fc-CC values with greater disease severity as indicated by the UPDRS I ($r = 0.404$, $P = 0.016$) and MMSE scores ($r = − 0.388$, $P = 0.021$), as well as with greater cognitive impairment in the attention ($r = − 0.466$, $P = 0.005$) and memory ($r = − 0.471$, $P = 0.004$) domains were emphasized. But the associations between the fc-CC values of

In terms of comparisons among the PD subgroups, our data revealed that the PDN group had a higher level oxidative stress than the other PD subgroups. At the same time, the trajectory of oxidative stress presented double peaks in the PDMCI and PDD subgroups (Table 1 and Additional file 1: Figure S1). To the best of our

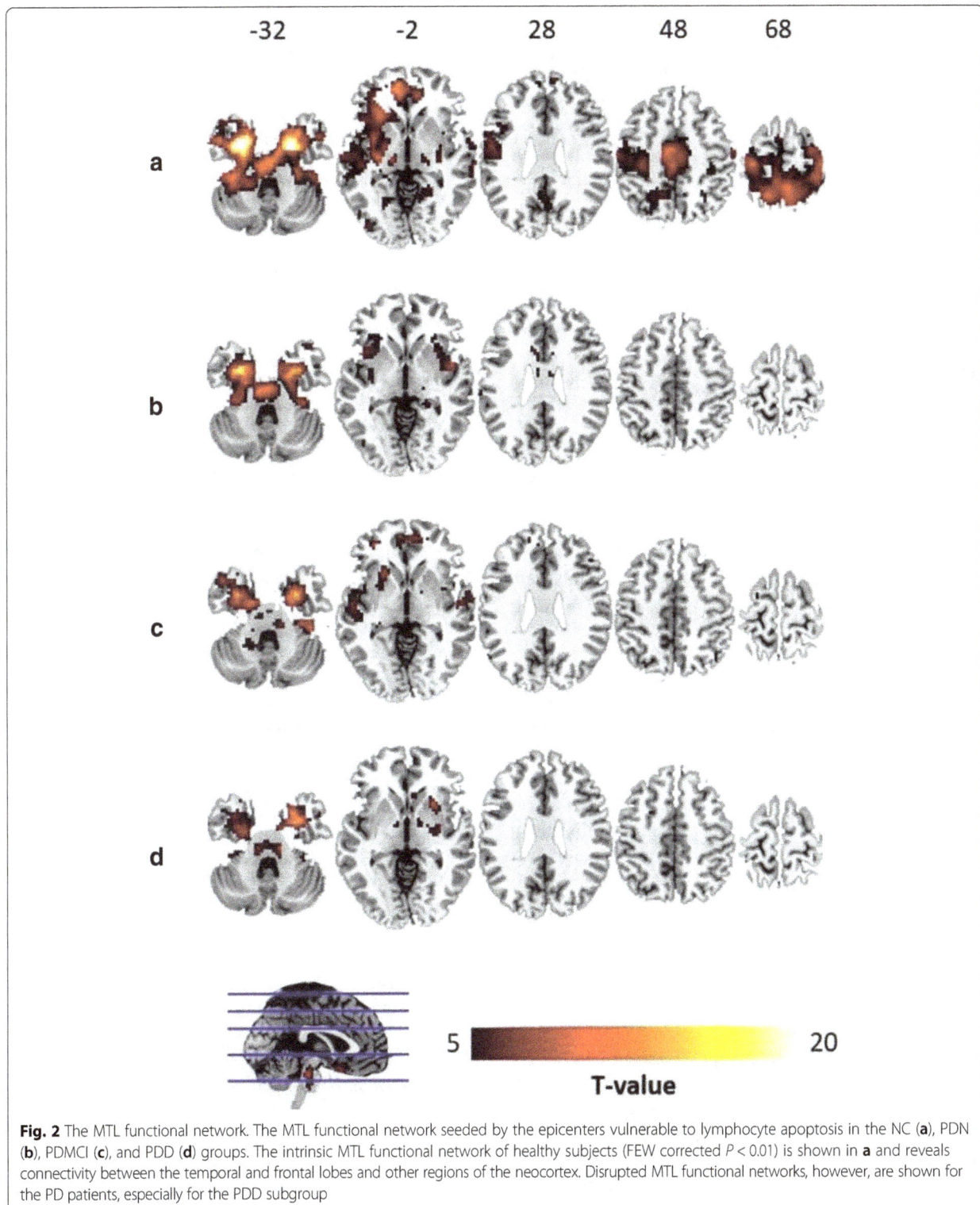

Fig. 2 The MTL functional network. The MTL functional network seeded by the epicenters vulnerable to lymphocyte apoptosis in the NC (**a**), PDN (**b**), PDMCI (**c**), and PDD (**d**) groups. The intrinsic MTL functional network of healthy subjects (FEW corrected *P* < 0.01) is shown in **a** and reveals connectivity between the temporal and frontal lobes and other regions of the neocortex. Disrupted MTL functional networks, however, are shown for the PD patients, especially for the PDD subgroup

knowledge, there have been no previous studies discussing the changes in oxidative stress in PD in terms of different cognitive functions. The trajectory of oxidative stress seen in the present study, however, was similar to that of the hypothetical model of a dual peak of microglial activation in Alzheimer's disease proposed by Fan et al. [35], wherein ramified microglia transform into anti-inflammatory and pro-inflammatory phenotypes. Dynamic changes to the peripheral immune system in mild (early) and severe (late) cognitive status might also

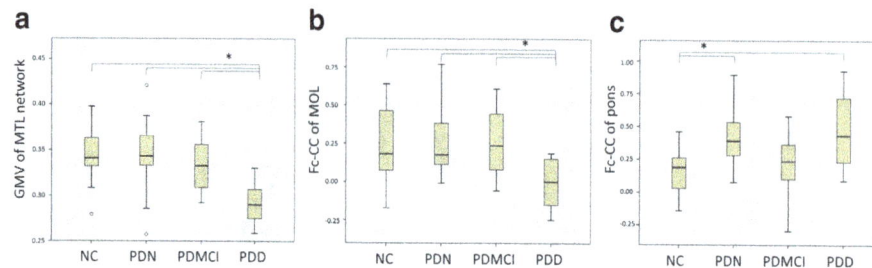

Fig. 3 The structural and functional alteration in the MTL network. (**a**) Comparison of GMVs under the intrinsic MTL functional network among the NC group and PD subgroups revealed significant atrophy in the PDD subgroup. (**b**) The functional connectivity between the MTL and middle occipital lobe (MOL) within the MTL functional network was significantly decreased in the PDD subgroup, (**c**) but the functional connectivity between the MTL and pons was significantly increased in the PDN and PDD subgroups

reflect the progression of neurodegeneration in a non-cell-autonomous fashion with respect to neurons [35]. Although we could not verify the phenotypes of leukocytes in the present study, the higher immune response seen in PD without dementia might suggest a stage with higher levels of CNS pro-inflammatory phenotypes, such as increased apoptosis percentage and LFA-1 values.

Although GMV was diffusely and significantly reduced in all the PD patients relative to the normal controls in the present study, only the GMV reductions in the bilateral MTLs were significantly associated with peripheral lymphocyte apoptosis accompanied with cognitive impairment. The high susceptibility of the MTL suggests its role as an important area in maintaining cognitive ability in PD. The cell-autonomous factors of neuron govern both for and against the influence of peripheral immune cells [36], might determine the different sensitivity over different brain regions. The MTL is known as a very sensitive area for chronic stress and hypoxia conditions [37–39] and is among the brain areas most easily affected in Alzheimer's disease [40]. The neurons in the MTL have large cell surfaces and high-energy requirements, which makes these neurons more prone to receiving multiple forms of oxidative stress [40]. Our whole-brain VBM-based correlation analysis with lower presumptions further highlights the reliability of the observed findings.

We found that the topographic distribution of the MTL functional network derived from the healthy subjects was partially overlaid with the key components of the cholinergic pathways from the BNM network to the frontal and temporal cortices [3]. The BNM network is responsible for maintaining fronto-executive and memory functions [41]. Relatedly, decreased cholinergic neurons in the frontal and temporal lobes are believed to be associated with the cognitive impairments seen in PDMCI and PDD [3]. Alterations of MTL intra-network functional connectivity between the MTL and MOL were also found. Meanwhile, attention and memory impairments were observed to be associated with decreased

functional connectivity between the MTL and MOL. Interestingly, the MTL-pons connectivity in the PDMCI subgroup was lower than that for the other PD subgroups. The cause of this presentation is still uncertain and requires further investigation and research.

We also found progressive underlying structural deficits of the MTL network in PDN, PDMCI, and PDD. Those temporo-spatial degradation results reflect the functional and anatomical proximity of the MTL network to presumed disease vulnerable areas, and highlight the value of systemic lymphocyte levels in the evaluation of the network degenerative mechanisms in PD. According to the network degeneration hypothesis [11], the different pathological molecules, such as misfolded proteins, target different specific brain vulnerable areas and their networks. These selective forms of neuronal vulnerability may be related to the weakening of synaptic convergence zones, the loss of retrograde growth factor supplement, the transsynaptic spread of mis-folded protein, and other factors related to network destabilization [11]. The concordance between disease-related atrophy and healthy intrinsic functional connectivity reflects the network-driven neuronal vulnerability. However, the accumulation of mis-folded alpha-synuclein in Lewy bodies and Lewy neurites, a major hallmark of PD [42], was not evaluated in the present study. Its effects and interactions with systemic inflammation in the MTL were thus not determined, and a further validation study should therefore be conducted.

This study has some limitations. First, it was a small-sized and cross-sectional study, which limits any interpretations that can be made from it regarding the trajectory of oxidative stress markers, the structural or functional alterations as the disease progresses, and any causal relationships among the above parameters. Second, multiple comparison correction was not applied for the correlational analyses due to the small sample sizes after subgrouping, the exploratory nature of the study, and the possibility of overcorrection owing to the high collinearity of the studied clinical and

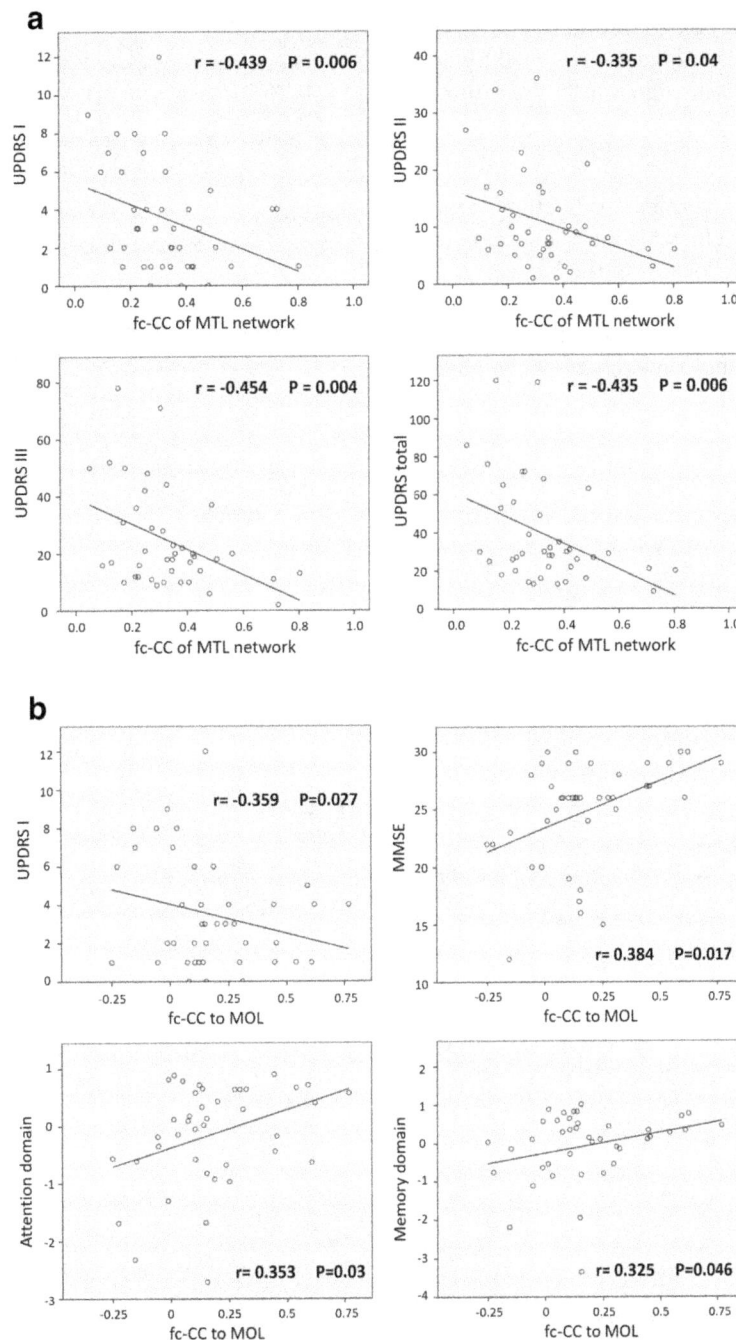

Fig. 4 a The correlation between disease severity and functional connectivity within the MTL functional network. The reduced fc-CC values of the MTL functional network were associated with worsening clinical symptoms, including UPDRS part I (mentation and mood) and part III (motor) and total scores (controlling for age and sex, Bonferroni corrected $P < 0.05$). **b** The correlation between cognition and functional connectivity within the MTL functional network. The reduced fc-CC values of the middle occipital lobe were associated with worsening cognitive impairment, including UPDRS part I (mentation and mood), MMSE, attention, and memory function scores (controlling for age and sex, Bonferroni corrected $P < 0.05$)

cognitive parameters. As such, the correlational analyses might be underpowered, and the significance of the associated results should be interpreted cautiously. Third, we did not verify the phenotypes of peripheral immune cells. As such, only successful therapeutic trials targeting those oxidative stress makers, their upstream causes, or their downstream effects will confirm that PD are indeed caused by processes related to immune cell infiltration. Manipulations of the systemic immune system and mis-folded proteins and evaluations of their effects in PD animal models might help to verify the role of the MTL in cognition in the future.

Conclusion

In terms of cognitive impairment, this study demonstrates that the neuronal vulnerable areas associated with lymphocyte infiltration are located in the bilateral MTLs, with such infiltration resulting in the disruption of both architectural and functional connectivity. Lymphocyte-associated MTL atrophy may thus represent the possible etiology of PD.

Additional files

Additional file 1: Figure S1. Systemic oxidative stress in PD. Systemic oxidative stress was significantly increased in the PD patients. Compared with the NC group, the LFA-1 levels of monocytes were significantly higher in the PDD subgroup. Furthermore, the apoptosis percentage and the LFA-1 levels of monocytes and lymphocytes were significantly higher in the PDN subgroup than in the controls. (MFI: mean fluorescence intensity) (*Bonferroni corrected $P < 0.05$). (DOCX 376 kb)

Additional file 2: Table S1. Oxidation parameters of the PD patients and normal controls after removal of outliers. (DOCX 18 kb)

Additional file 3: Figure S2. The alternation of gray matter volume in PD. Gray matter atrophy patterns in the PD subgroups compared with the NC group and with each other. The PDD subgroup showed significantly diffuse GMV loss compared with the PDMCI and PDN subgroups, as well as the NC group. The PDN and PDMCI subgroups showed only small areas of GMV loss compared with the NC group, and there was no significant difference between them. (Corrected $P < 0.005$, cluster> 350). (DOCX 210 kb)

Additional file 4: Figure S3. The alternation of functional connectivity within the MTL functional network in PD. The two-sample t test between all the PD patients and the NC group showed significant changes of the fc-CC values in the middle occipital lobe (MOL) and pons within the MTL functional network. (Corrected $P < 0.001$, cluster = 19). (DOCX 74 kb)

Abbreviations

ANCOVA: Analysis of covariance; BBB: Blood-brain barrier; BNM: Basal nucleus of Meynert; CNS: Central nervous system; CSF: Cerebrospinal fluid; fc-CC: Functional connectivity correlation coefficient; GM: Gray matter; GMV: Gray matter volume; LFA-1: Lymphocyte function-associated antigen 1; Mac-1: Macrophage-1 antigen; MMSE: MiniMental State Examination; MOL: Middle occipital lobe; MTLs: Mesial temporal lobes; NC: Normal control; PD: Parkinson's disease; PDD: PD with dementia; PDMCI: PD with mild cognitive impairment; PDN: PD with normal cognition; PE: Phycoerythrin; rs-fMRI: Resting state functional MRI; SN: Substantia nigra; SPM: Statistical Parametric Mapping software program; SPSS: Statistical Package for Social Sciences; TIV: Total intracranial volume; UPDRS: Unified Parkinson's Disease Rating Scale; VBM: Voxel-based morphometry; WM: White matter

Acknowledgements

The authors wish to thank the MRI Core Facility of Chang Gung Memorial Hospital, as well as Yi-Wen Chen, Ting-Yi Chen, and Yi-Fan Chiang, and all the subjects who participated in this study.

Funding

This work was supported by funds from the National Ministry of Science and Technology (MOST106-2314-B-182A-031-MY2 to W-C Lin).

Authors' contributions

PLC and HLC analyzed and interpreted the patient data regarding the systemic inflammation in Parkinson's disease, and PLC was a major contributor in writing the manuscript. PLC, YSC, KHC, and TWH analyzed and interpreted the MRI data. CHL, NWT, and SHL made contributions to acquisition of data. MHC and WCL made contributions to the conception and design of this study. All authors read and approved the final manuscript.

Competing interests

The authors declare that they have no competing interests.

Author details

[1]Department of Diagnostic Radiology, Kaohsiung Chang Gung Memorial Hospital, Chang Gung University College of Medicine, 123 Ta-Pei Road, Niao-Sung, Kaohsiung 83305, Taiwan. [2]Department of Neurology, Kaohsiung Chang Gung Memorial Hospital, Chang Gung University College of Medicine, Kaohsiung, Taiwan. [3]Brain Research Center, National Yang-Ming University, Taipei, Taiwan. [4]Department of Radiology, Taipei Veterans General Hospital, Taipei, Taiwan. [5]Department of Hematology and Oncology, Kaohsiung Chang Gung Memorial Hospital, Chang Gung University College of Medicine, Kaohsiung, Taiwan.

References

1. Litvan I, Goldman JG, Troster AI, Schmand BA, Weintraub D, Petersen RC, Mollenhauer B, Adler CH, Marder K, Williams-Gray CH, et al. Diagnostic criteria for mild cognitive impairment in Parkinson's disease: Movement Disorder Society task force guidelines. Mov Disord. 2012;27(3):349–56.
2. Melzer TR, Watts R, MacAskill MR, Pitcher TL, Livingston L, Keenan RJ, Dalrymple-Alford JC, Anderson TJ. Grey matter atrophy in cognitively impaired Parkinson's disease. J Neurol Neurosurg Psychiatry. 2012;83(2):188–94.
3. Gratwicke J, Jahanshahi M, Foltynie T. Parkinson's disease dementia: a neural networks perspective. Brain. 2015;138(Pt 6):1454–76.
4. Chen FX, Kang DZ, Chen FY, Liu Y, Wu G, Li X, Yu LH, Lin YX, Lin ZY. Gray matter atrophy associated with mild cognitive impairment in Parkinson's disease. Neurosci Lett. 2016;617:160–5.
5. Baggio HC, Segura B, Sala-Llonch R, Marti MJ, Valldeoriola F, Compta Y, Tolosa E, Junque C. Cognitive impairment and resting-state network connectivity in Parkinson's disease. Hum Brain Mapp. 2015;36(1):199–212.
6. Putcha D, Ross RS, Cronin-Golomb A, Janes AC, Stern CE. Altered intrinsic functional coupling between core neurocognitive networks in Parkinson's disease. Neuroimage Clin. 2015;7:449–55.
7. Hacker CD, Perlmutter JS, Criswell SR, Ances BM, Snyder AZ. Resting state functional connectivity of the striatum in Parkinson's disease. Brain. 2012;135(Pt 12):3699–711.
8. Pievani M, de Haan W, Wu T, Seeley WW, Frisoni GB. Functional network disruption in the degenerative dementias. Lancet. 2011;10(9):829–43.
9. Lopes R, Delmaire C, Defebvre L, Moonen AJ, Duits AA, Hofman P, Leentjens AF, Dujardin K. Cognitive phenotypes in parkinson's disease differ in terms of brain-network organization and connectivity. Hum Brain Mapp. 2017;38(3):1604–21.
10. Baggio HC, Segura B, Junque C. Resting-state functional brain networks in Parkinson's disease. CNS Neurosci Ther. 2015;21(10):793–801.
11. Seeley WW, Crawford RK, Zhou J, Miller BL, Greicius MD. Neurodegenerative diseases target large-scale human brain networks. Neuron. 2009;62(1):42–52.
12. Su X, Federoff HJ. Immune responses in Parkinson's disease: interplay between central and peripheral immune systems. Biomed Res Int. 2014;2014:275178.
13. Chung YC, Ko HW, Bok E, Park ES, Huh SH, Nam JH, Jin BK. The role of neuroinflammation on the pathogenesis of Parkinson's disease. BMB Rep. 2010;43(4):225–32.
14. Grozdanov V, Bliederhaeuser C, Ruf WP, Roth V, Fundel-Clemens K, Zondler L, Brenner D, Martin-Villalba A, Hengerer B, Kassubek J, et al. Inflammatory dysregulation of blood monocytes in Parkinson's disease patients. Acta Neuropathol. 2014;128(5):651–63.
15. Greenwood J, Wang Y, Calder VL. Lymphocyte adhesion and transendothelial migration in the central nervous system: the role of LFA-1, ICAM-1, VLA-4 and VCAM-1. Off. Immunology. 1995;86(3):408–15.

16. Lin WC, Tsai NW, Huang YC, Cheng KY, Chen HL, Li SH, Kung CT, Su YJ, Lin WM, Chen MH, et al. Peripheral leukocyte apoptosis in patients with parkinsonism: correlation with clinical characteristics and neuroimaging findings. Biomed Res Int. 2014;2014:635923.

17. Chiang PL, Chen HL, Lu CH, Chen PC, Chen MH, Yang IH, Tsai NW, Lin WC. White matter damage and systemic inflammation in Parkinson's disease. BMC Neurosci. 2017;18(1):48.

18. Chen YS, Chen MH, Lu CH, Chen PC, Chen HL, Yang IH, Tsai NW, Lin WC. Associations among cognitive functions, plasma DNA, and white matter integrity in patients with early-onset Parkinson's disease. Front Neurosci. 2017;11:9.

19. Lindqvist D, Hall S, Surova Y, Nielsen HM, Janelidze S, Brundin L, Hansson O. Cerebrospinal fluid inflammatory markers in Parkinson's disease--associations with depression, fatigue, and cognitive impairment. Brain Behav Immun. 2013;33:183–9.

20. Bettcher BM, Kramer JH. Longitudinal inflammation, cognitive decline, and Alzheimer's disease: a mini-review. Clin Pharmacol Ther. 2014;96(4):464–9.

21. Sartori AC, Vance DE, Slater LZ, Crowe M. The impact of inflammation on cognitive function in older adults: implications for healthcare practice and research. J Neurosci Nurs. 2012;44(4):206–17.

22. Brochard V, Combadiere B, Prigent A, Laouar Y, Perrin A, Beray-Berthat V, Bonduelle O, Alvarez-Fischer D, Callebert J, Launay JM, et al. Infiltration of CD4+ lymphocytes into the brain contributes to neurodegeneration in a mouse model of Parkinson disease. J Clin Invest. 2009;119(1):182–92.

23. Naduthota RM, Bharath RD, Jhunjhunwala K, Yadav R, Saini J, Christopher R, Pal PK. Imaging biomarker correlates with oxidative stress in Parkinson's disease. Neurol India. 2017;65(2):263–8.

24. Lin WC, Chou KH, Lee PL, Huang YC, Tsai NW, Chen HL, Cheng KY, Wang HC, Lin TK, Li SH, et al. Brain mediators of systemic oxidative stress on perceptual impairments in Parkinson's disease. J Transl Med. 2015;13:386.

25. Chen MH, Chen PC, Lu CH, Chen HL, Chao YP, Li SH, Chen YW, Lin WC. Plasma DNA mediate autonomic dysfunctions and white matter injuries in patients with Parkinson's disease. Oxidative Med Cell Longev. 2017; 2017:7371403.

26. Hughes AJ, Ben-Shlomo Y, Daniel SE, Lees AJ. What features improve the accuracy of clinical diagnosis in Parkinson's disease: a clinicopathologic study. Neurology. 1992;42(6):1142–6.

27. Teng EL, Hasegawa K, Homma A, Imai Y, Larson E, Graves A, Sugimoto K, Yamaguchi T, Sasaki H, Chiu D, et al. The cognitive abilities screening instrument (CASI): a practical test for cross-cultural epidemiological studies of dementia. Int Psychogeriatr. 1994;6(1):45–58 discussion 62.

28. D. W. Wechsler adult intelligence scale. New York: Psychological Cooperation; 1981.

29. Dalrymple-Alford JC, Livingston L, MacAskill MR, Graham C, Melzer TR, Porter RJ, Watts R, Anderson TJ. Characterizing mild cognitive impairment in Parkinson's disease. Mov Disord. 2011;26(4):629–36.

30. Emre M, Aarsland D, Brown R, Burn DJ, Duyckaerts C, Mizuno Y, Broe GA, Cummings J, Dickson DW, Gauthier S, et al. Clinical diagnostic criteria for dementia associated with Parkinson's disease. Mov Disord. 2007;22(12): 1689–707 quiz 1837.

31. Zhong Y, Wang H, Lu G, Zhang Z, Jiao Q, Liu Y. Detecting functional connectivity in fMRI using PCA and regression analysis. Brain Topogr. 2009; 22(2):134–44.

32. Battisti C, Formichi P, Radi E, Federico A. Oxidative-stress-induced apoptosis in PBLs of two patients with Parkinson disease secondary to alpha-synuclein mutation. J Neurol Sci. 2008;267(1–2):120–4.

33. London A, Cohen M, Schwartz M. Microglia and monocyte-derived macrophages: functionally distinct populations that act in concert in CNS plasticity and repair. Front Cell Neurosci. 2013;7:34.

34. Theriault P, ElAli A, Rivest S. The dynamics of monocytes and microglia in Alzheimer's disease. Alzheimers Res Ther. 2015;7(1):41.

35. Fan Z, Brooks DJ, Okello A, Edison P. An early and late peak in microglial activation in Alzheimer's disease trajectory. Brain. 2017;140(3):792–803.

36. Surmeier DJ, Obeso JA, Halliday GM. Selective neuronal vulnerability in Parkinson disease. Nat Rev Neurosci. 2017;18(2):101–13.

37. Gianaros PJ, Jennings JR, Sheu LK, Greer PJ, Kuller LH, Matthews KA. Prospective reports of chronic life stress predict decreased grey matter volume in the hippocampus. NeuroImage. 2007;35(2):795–803.

38. Di Paola M, Caltagirone C, Fadda L, Sabatini U, Serra L, Carlesimo GA. Hippocampal atrophy is the critical brain change in patients with hypoxic amnesia. Hippocampus. 2008;18(7):719–28.

39. Weng HH, Tsai YH, Chen CF, Lin YC, Yang CT, Tsai YH, Yang CY. Mapping gray matter reductions in obstructive sleep apnea: an activation likelihood estimation meta-analysis. Sleep. 2014;37(1):167–75.

40. Mosconi L, Pupi A, De Leon MJ. Brain glucose hypometabolism and oxidative stress in preclinical Alzheimer's disease. Ann N Y Acad Sci. 2008; 1147:180–95.

41. Kehagia AA, Barker RA, Robbins TW. Neuropsychological and clinical heterogeneity of cognitive impairment and dementia in patients with Parkinson's disease. Lancet Neurol. 2010;9(12):1200–13.

42. Baba M, Nakajo S, Tu PH, Tomita T, Nakaya K, Lee VM, Trojanowski JQ, Iwatsubo T. Aggregation of alpha-synuclein in Lewy bodies of sporadic Parkinson's disease and dementia with Lewy bodies. Am J Pathol. 1998; 152(4):879–84.

Preemptive intrathecal administration of endomorphins relieves inflammatory pain in male mice via inhibition of p38 MAPK signaling and regulation of inflammatory cytokines

Ting Zhang[1†], Nan Zhang[1†], Run Zhang[1], Weidong Zhao[1], Yong Chen[2], Zilong Wang[1], Biao Xu[1], Mengna Zhang[1], Xuerui Shi[1], Qinqin Zhang[1], Yuanyuan Guo[1], Jian Xiao[1], Dan Chen[1] and Quan Fang[1*]

Abstract

Background: Preemptive administration of analgesic drugs reduces perceived pain and prolongs duration of antinociceptive action. Whereas several lines of evidence suggest that endomorphins, the endogenous mu-opioid agonists, attenuate acute and chronic pain at the spinal level, their preemptive analgesic effects remain to be determined. In this study, we evaluated the anti-allodynic activities of endomorphins and explored their mechanisms of action after preemptive administration in a mouse model of inflammatory pain.

Methods: The anti-allodynic activities of preemptive intrathecal administration of endomorphin-1 and endomorphin-2 were investigated in complete Freund's adjuvant (CFA)-induced inflammatory pain model and paw incision-induced postoperative pain model. The modulating effects of endomorphins on the expression of p38 mitogen-activated protein kinase (p38 MAPK) and inflammatory mediators in dorsal root ganglion (DRG) of CFA-treated mice were assayed by real-time reverse transcription-polymerase chain reaction (RT-PCR), Western blotting, or immunofluorescence staining.

Results: Preemptive intrathecal injection of endomorphins dose-dependently attenuated CFA-induced mechanical allodynia via the mu-opioid receptor and significantly reversed paw incision-induced allodynia. In addition, CFA-caused increase of phosphorylated p38 MAPK in DRG was dramatically reduced by preemptive administration of endomorphins. Repeated intrathecal application of the specific p38 MAPK inhibitor SB203580 reduced CFA-induced mechanical allodynia as well. Further RT-PCR assay showed that endomorphins regulated the mRNA expression of inflammatory cytokines in DRGs induced by peripheral inflammation.

Conclusions: Our findings reveal a novel mechanism by which preemptive treatment of endomorphins attenuates inflammatory pain through regulating the production of inflammatory cytokines in DRG neurons via inhibition of p38 MAPK phosphorylation.

Keywords: Endomorphin, Preemptive analgesic, Inflammatory pain, p38 MAPK, Inflammatory cytokines

* Correspondence: fangq@lzu.edu.cn
†Ting Zhang and Nan Zhang contributed equally to this work.
[1]Key Laboratory of Preclinical Study for New Drugs of Gansu Province, and Institute of Physiology, School of Basic Medical Sciences, Lanzhou University, 199 Donggang West Road, Lanzhou 730000, People's Republic of China
Full list of author information is available at the end of the article

Background

Endomorphin-1 (EM-1) and endomorphin-2 (EM-2) were firstly isolated from bovine brain and exhibited high affinity and selectivity towards the mu-opioid receptor (MOR) [1]. It has been demonstrated that both EM-1 and EM-2 produced potent analgesic actions in inflammatory pain, which were reversed by the opioid receptor antagonist naloxone or β-funaltrexamine (β-FNA) [2–4]. For example, central administration of endomorphins alleviated formalin-induced nocifensive behaviors [4, 5]. Peripherally administered EM-1 significantly reduced the synovial vascular permeability in acute joint inflammation [6]. Moreover, Feehan et al. reported that the cyclized analogs of endomorphins produced potent and long-lasting analgesia in a rat model of inflammatory pain after intravenous or intrathecal administration [7]. In addition, histological studies elucidated that both EM-1 and EM-2 were expressed in macrophages and monocytes in lymph nodes during peripheral inflammation, suggesting the involvement of endomorphins in inflammatory pain [8].

Notably, compared with the opioid analgesic morphine, endomorphins induced more potent analgesia in neuropathic pain [9, 10] and had fewer side effects on reward, respiratory depression, and cardiovascular effects [11, 12]. However, central injection of endomorphins caused a short duration of antinociceptive action (less than 30 min) because of their poor enzymatic stability [13, 14]. It has been largely implicated that preemptive treatment with analgesics attenuates perceived pain for a prolonged duration, which might be explained by its ability to block the pathophysiological development of pain, including peripheral and central sensitizations. Briefly, peripheral sensitization is often accompanied by release of inflammatory mediators and decreases the threshold of terminal nerve endings, which leads to the enhancement of nociceptive pain [15]. Central sensitization results from an enhanced response which is provoked by hyperexcitability of the neurons in the dorsal horn of the spinal cord [16]. Both central and peripheral sensitizations are therefore the major causes of pain hypersensitivity. In theory, preemptive treatment with analgesics could block the noxious impulses and prevent central nervous system sensitization, contributing to more effective reduction of the nociceptive signals in a manner different to the treatment with analgesics after injury. Indeed, opioid analgesics, such as morphine and fentanyl, have well-demonstrated preemptive analgesic action in clinical and pre-clinical studies [17, 18]. To date, however, very little is known about the influence of preemptive administration of endomorphins on pain management.

Although the above evidences suggest endomorphins are potential pain therapeutics, their mechanisms await

further elucidation. Immunohistochemical analysis revealed that the mu-opioid receptor was co-expressed with substance P (SP) and calcitonin gene-related peptide (CGRP) in DRG neurons [19, 20], and EM-1 diminished the release of SP and CGRP from primary afferent terminals [21], implying endomorphins may modulate stimulation-evoked release of SP and CGRP to alleviate pain. Accumulated evidence indicates that various inflammatory mediators including pro-inflammatory cytokines and chemokines in dorsal root ganglion (DRG) and spinal cord tissues are involved in the generation and maintenance of chronic pain [22–24]. In addition, extracellular pain stimuli aggravate the activation of mitogen-activated protein kinase (MAPK) pathways and transcription factors, which plays important roles in pain sensitization through regulating inflammatory mediators [25, 26]. Effects of endomorphins on inflammatory mediators have been documented in in vitro studies. Both EM-1 and EM-2 inhibited the release of inflammatory mediators, such as interleukin-12 (IL-12) and tumor necrosis factor-α (TNF-α) from macrophage cell line THP-1 [27, 28]. Opposite effects of endomorphins on the release of interleukin-1beta (IL-1β) have been observed, with a inhibitory effect reported in cultured rat peritoneal macrophages [29], but a stimulatory effect in macrophage cells line THP-1 [27]. Moreover, previous reports found that endomorphins can inhibit the phosphorylation of p38 MAPK induced by advanced glycation end products in cultured human umbilical vein endothelial cells, and similar results were also found in LPS-stimulated murine dendritic cells [30, 31]. These in vitro studies implicate that p38 MAPK and its possible downstream targets inflammatory mediators might contribute to the pain modulation of endomorphins.

In this study, we employed a chronic inflammatory pain model-induced by complete Freund's adjuvant (CFA) to investigate the effects of preemptive intrathecal administration of EM-1 and EM-2 on the development of mechanical allodynia. We then determined the expression of the mu-opioid receptor in DRG neurons after inflammation and explored whether the MAPK signaling and inflammatory mediators in DRGs are downstream targets of preemptive analgesia of endomorphins. In addition, the preemptive analgesic effects of EM-1 and EM-2 were also evaluated at the spinal level in a postoperative pain model-induced by paw incision.

Methods

Drugs and reagents

EM-1 and EM-2 were prepared by manual solid-phase synthesis using standard N-fluorenylmethoxycarbonyl (Fmoc) chemistry as reported in our previous study [32]. Fmoc-protected amino acids (GL Biochem Ltd., China) were coupled with Rink amide 4-methybenzhydrylamine

(MBHA) resin (Tianjin Nankai Hecheng Science & Technology Co., Ltd., China). The crude peptides were purified by preparative reversed-phase HPLC (RP-HPLC) and determined by electrospray ionization mass spectrometer (ESI-Q-TOF maXis-4G, Bruker Daltonics).

Naloxone, β-FNA, nor-binaltorphimine (nor-BNI), and naltrindole (NTI) were obtained from Sigma-Aldrich. The selective p38 MAPK inhibitor SB203580 was purchased from Beyotime Institute of Biotechnology and dissolved in 1% DMSO in saline. All other drugs were dissolved in sterilized saline and stored at − 20 °C.

Experimental animals

Male Kunming mice (23 ± 2 g) were purchased from the Experimental Animal Center of Lanzhou University. Mice were housed in 12-h light-dark cycle and climate-controlled rooms at 22–24 °C with water and foods available. All behavioral tests were performed between 8:00 am and 6:00 pm, and all animals were used only once. Best efforts were made to minimize numbers of animals used and their suffering. The animal experimentation protocols were in compliance with the AR-RIVE guidelines [33] and approved by the Ethics Committee of Lanzhou University and carried out in accordance with the European Community guidelines for the use of experimental animals (2010/63/EU).

Drug administration

Intrathecal (i.t.) injection procedure was performed as previously described [34]. Briefly, a 25-μl microsyringe was inserted between L5 and L6 segment, and the flick or formation of an 'S' shape by the tail was considered as a successful injection. Drugs were injected into subarachnoid space with a total volume of 5 μl at a constant rate of 10 μl/min.

The opioid antagonists naloxone, β-FNA, nor-BNI, and NTI were injected 10 min, 4 h, 30 min, and 10 min prior to the administration of endomorphins, respectively. The doses and time of administration of these antagonists were chosen on the basis of our previous report [32].

Inflammatory pain model and behavior test

CFA inflammatory pain was conducted following previous protocol [35]. Briefly, intraplantar (i.pl.) injection of 20 μl CFA (1 mg/ml, Sigma Aldrich, USA) was performed to induce chronic inflammation. In order to evaluate the effects of preemptive administration of endomorphins, animals received an intrathecal injection of saline or endomorphins (7.5, 15, and 30 nmol) 10 min prior to CFA administration. The force (g) at which mice withdrew the hindpaw was recorded automatically using electronic von Frey apparatus (Ugo Basile, Italy), and a cutoff value of 10 g was used to prevent tissue damage. The baseline withdrawal threshold of naïve mice was measured

prior to drugs administration, and mechanical allodynia was measured at 4 h and daily for 7 days after CFA injection. To evaluate the role of p38 MAPK signal pathway in CFA-induced inflammatory pain, mice were received intrathecal injection of saline or SB203580 once a day, and mechanical allodynia was measured at 30-min and 90-min post-injection. Each time point was measured three times at 2-min intervals. The raw data from CFA-induced inflammatory pain assays were converted to area under the curve (AUC). The AUC depicting total paw withdrawal threshold versus time was computed by trapezoidal approximation. Upon termination of the experiment, all animals were subjected to euthanasia using CO_2.

Paw incision-induced post-operative pain model

We followed the procedure for the paw incision model as previously described [36–38]. Briefly, mice were anesthetized with isoflurane, and a 5-mm longitudinal incision was made though skin, fascia, and muscle on the plantar surface of the right hindpaw. The plantaris muscle was elevated and incised longitudinally. After gentle pressure for hemostasis, the skin was sutured and coated with antibiotic ointment. The effects of preemptive endomorphins were measured by von Frey test 2 h to 4 days after incision as indicated in Fig. 2.

Protein extraction and Western blot analysis

For Western blot analysis, routine procedures were followed as previously described [39]. Briefly, ipsilateral L4-L6 DRG tissues were removed from CO_2 euthanized mice, and homogenized in cell lysis buffer containing 0.1 M phenylmethylsulfonyl fluoride (PMSF). The protein concentration of each sample was estimated by BCA assay (Beijing Solarbio Science & Technology Co., Ltd., China). Equal content of proteins (80 μg) were separated by 12% SDS-polyacrylamide gelelectrophoresis and then transferred onto PVDF membrane (Bio-Rad Laboratories, China). A blocking step for 90 min at room temperature with 6% skim milk was followed by incubation with primary antibodies: rabbit anti-phosphorylated ERK1/2 antibody (P-ERK1/2) (1:1000, Cell Signaling Technology #9101, China), rabbit anti-ERK1/2 antibody (1:1000, Cell Signaling Technology #9102, China), mouse anti-p38 MAPK antibody (1:1000, Beyotime Biotechnology, AM065, China), or rabbit anti-phosphorylated p38 MAPK antibody (P-p38 MAPK) (1:1000, Cell Signaling Technology #4511, China) overnight at 4 °C. Afterwards, PVDF membranes were washed with TBST (50 mM Tris (pH 7.5), 100 mM NaCl, and 0.1% Tween 20) and incubated with secondary antibody (1:1000; HRP-labeled goat anti-mouse LgG (H + L), A0216 and HRP-labeled goat anti-rabbit LgG (H + L), A0208; Beyotime Institute of Biotechnology, China) for 2 h at room temperature. Protein signals were then visualized with enhanced chemiluminescence (Amersham Pharmacia

Biotech, UK) and quantified by Image J software. The levels of P-p38 MAPK and P-ERK1/2 were normalized against corresponding total p38 MAPK and ERK1/2 level.

Immunofluorescence staining

Immunofluorescence staining was performed following the previous report [39]. Mice were deeply anesthetized with pentobarbital sodium (100 mg/kg, intraperitoneal) and transcardially perfused with PBS followed by ice-cold 4% paraformaldehyde (PFA, Sigma-Aldrich, China). The ipsilateral L4 DRGs were dissected, post-fixed in 4% PFA, cryoprotected with 20% sucrose solutions, and then embedded in Tissue-Tek O.C.T. (Tissue-Tek, Sakura Finetek USA, CA). Immunohistochemistry staining was performed on 12-μm thickness sections. Briefly, sections were pre-incubated with 5% normal donkey serum to block the unspecific binding at room temperature for 45 min. Then, sections were incubated with the primary antibodies (Additional file 1: Table S1), including rabbit monoclonal P-p38 MAPK antibody or guinea pig monoclonal mu-opioid receptor antibody, overnight at 4 °C. This was followed by incubation with the corresponding secondary antibodies for 2 h at room temperature. For double immunofluorescence labeling, the two primary antibodies were applied simultaneously, followed by incubation with the corresponding secondary antibodies. Sections were examined using an Olympus fluorescence microscope equipped with high-resolution CCD Spot camera.

For each animal, four to six DRG sections were analyzed. Each group has at least four mice. The density threshold for the positive immunoreactivity (IR) was determined by averaging two or three cell bodies in each section that were judged to be minimally positive. All neurons for which the mean density exceeded the threshold were counted as positive, and the positive cells were expressed as a percentage of total DRG neurons.

Co-localization images were made into figures using Adobe Photoshop (Adobe Systems Incorporated, USA), and only minor adjustments to the contrast and brightness settings were applied where necessary. For evaluating co-localization of markers, six randomly selected DRG sections from each mouse were chosen for each pair of markers. Counts were made of the number of positive for each marker (P-p38 MAPK or the mu-opioid receptor), the number of the expression of both antigens and the total number of neurons. Result was presented as a percentage of total DRG neurons.

RNA extraction, reverse transcription and real-time quantitative PCR

The L4-L6 ipsilateral DRGs were quickly removed from CO_2 euthanized mice and homogenized in Trizol reagent (TaKaRa, China). Two micrograms of total RNA was reversed transcribed using a manufacturer's protocol (TaKaRa, China). Real-time quantitative PCR reactions were performed using the SYBR Premix Ex Taq™II kit (TaKaRa, China) and an Agilent MX3005P (Agilent, USA) detection system. Primer sequences used for RT-PCR (Genbank, National Center for Biotechnology Information; www.ncbi.nlm.nih.gov) were displayed in Table 1. The PCR amplifications conditions were as follows: hold: 95 °C for 60 s; cycling: 95 °C for 5 s, 60 °C for 60 s, 40 cycles; and melt from 60 to 95 °C, and the relative expressions of genes were normalized to the internal reference GAPDH and analyzed using $2^{-\Delta\Delta CT}$ method. In addition, the detection timing was chosen on the basis of the previous report [40].

Statistical analysis

All data were presented as means ± S.E.M. The effective dose 50% of maximum response (ED_{50}) values for antinociception 1 day after CFA were calculated using Graphpad Prism 5. For the time-course effects of endomorphins, data were analyzed using two-way ANOVA followed by Bonferroni post-hoc analysis, and corresponding AUC data were analyzed using one-way ANOVA followed by Dunnett or Bonferroni post-hoc test. For Western blot and immunohistochemistry assays, data were analyzed using two-tailed t test for the two groups' comparison and one-way ANOVA for multi-group comparisons. For RT-PCR, data were analyzed using Mann-Whitney test. Probabilities of less than 5% ($P < 0.05$) were considered statistically significant.

Results

Preemptive intrathecal administration of EM-1 and EM-2 robustly reduced the development of mechanical allodynia

Intraplantar injection of CFA induced a strong mechanical allodynia during the whole experimental period. As shown

Table 1 Primer sequences

Gene	Primer sequence(5'-3')	GenBank accession no.
GAPDH	GGTTGTCTCCTGCGACTTCA (forward)	NM_001115114.1
	GGGTGGTCCAGGGTTTCTTA(reverse)	
IL-1β	ACTGGTACATCAGCACCTCAC (forward)	NM_008361.4
	TAGAAACAGTCCAGCCCATAC (reverse)	
IL-10	CACTACCAAAGCCACAAG (forward)	NM_010548.2
	GGAGTCGGTTAGCAGTATG (reverse)	
TNF-α	GAGAAGTTCCCAAATGGC (forward)	NM_013693.3
	ACTTGGTGGTTTGCTACG (reverse)	
CCL2	CAGCAAGATGATCCCAATG (forward)	NM_011333.3
	TGGTTCCGATCCAGGTTT (reverse)	
CCL3	ACTGACCTGGAACTGAATG (forward)	NM_011337.2
	GAAGAGTCCCTCGATGTG (reverse)	

in Fig. 1a, c, both EM-1 and EM-2 dose-dependently attenuated mechanical sensitivity in male mice for 6 days when injected intrathecally 10 min before CFA treatment ($F_{24, 287} = 11.4$, $P < 0.001$; $F_{24, 287} = 12.0$, $P < 0.001$, respectively). The ED_{50} values for EM-1- and EM-2-induced preemptive antinociception 1 day after CFA were 10.11 (7.70–13.28) and 7.44 (0.68–81.80) nmol, respectively. Moreover, in paw incision-induced postoperative pain model, preemptive intrathecal administration of EM-1 (30 nmol) and EM-2 (30 nmol) also reversed the development of mechanical allodynia in male mice for 2 days (Fig. 2, $F_{16, 206} = 8.12$, $P < 0.001$).

Effects of intrathecal administration of opioid antagonists on preemptive anti-allodynia induced by EM-1 and EM-2

As shown in Figs. 3a and 4a, in CFA-induced inflammatory pain model, pretreatment with the nonselective opioid receptor antagonist naloxone (5 nmol, i.t.) completely reversed the anti-allodynic effects of EM-1 (30 nmol, i.t.) and EM-2 (30 nmol, i.t.) from 4 h to 4 days (Fig. 3a, $F_{24, 287} = 18.7$, $P < 0.001$; Fig. 4a, $F_{24, 287} = 18.6$, $P < 0.001$, respectively). In addition, the anti-allodynic effects of EM-1 and EM-2 from 4 h to 4 days were significantly blocked by the selective mu-opioid receptor antagonist β-FNA

(10 nmol, i.t.) (Fig. 3b, $F_{24, 269} = 15.5$, $P < 0.001$; Fig. 4b, $F_{24, 269} = 10.8$, $P < 0.001$, respectively). Interestingly, the selective delta-opioid receptor antagonist NTI (10 nmol, i.t.) only partially inhibited the preemptive antinociceptive effects of EM-1 and EM-2 during 4 h to 4 days (Fig. 3c, $F_{24, 287} = 23.3$, $P < 0.001$; Fig. 4c, $F_{24, 284} = 23.7$, $P < 0.001$, respectively). The selective kappa-opioid receptor antagonist nor-BNI (10 nmol, i.t.) significantly reduced the preemptive anti-allodynia of EM-2 from 4 h to 4 days (Fig. 4d, $F_{24, 269} = 12.8$, $P < 0.001$), but was ineffective in the response to preemptive intrathecal administration of EM-1 (Fig. 3d). As expected, at the same doses, i.t. administration of these opioid antagonists alone had no significant effects in the present pain model.

The mu-opioid receptor immunoreactivity was increased in DRG neurons after CFA treatment

In line with previous studies [41, 42], our immunostaining also showed that the mu-opioid receptor was expressed in DRG neurons (Fig. 5), which is further confirmed with a co-labeling of NeuN (a pan-neuronal marker) (Additional file 2: Figure S1A). More importantly, an increased expression of the mu-opioid receptor

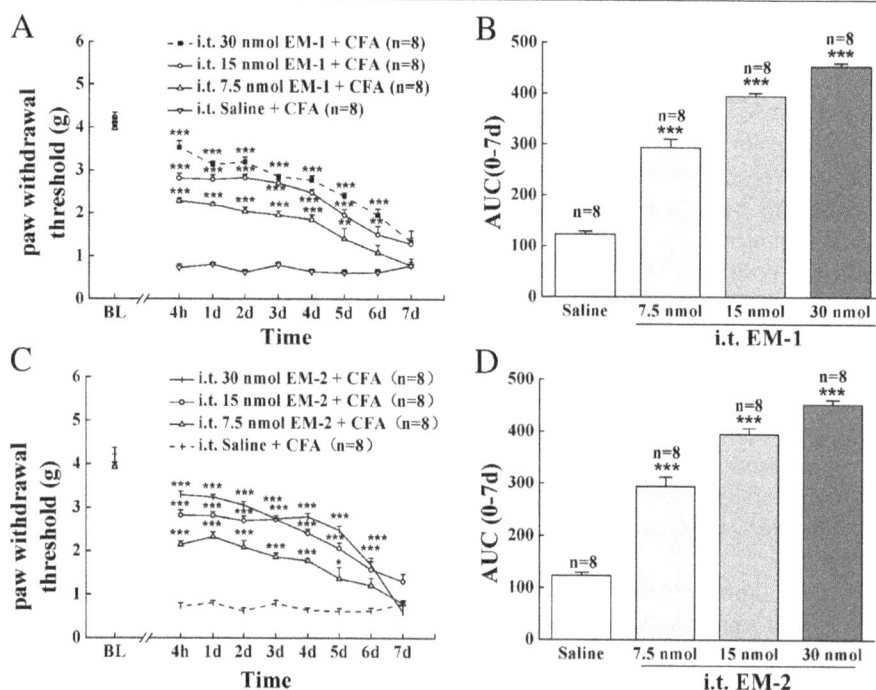

Fig. 1 Preemptive intrathecal administration of EM-1 and EM-2 attenuated CFA-induced mechanical allodynia. Preemptive intrathecal administration of EM-1 (**a**, 7.5, 15, and 30 nmol) and EM-2 (**c**, 7.5, 15, and 30 nmol) dose- and time-dependently attenuated mechanical allodynia in male mice. Each value represents mean ± S.E.M. Group size is indicated in figures. $^*P < 0.05$, $^{**}P < 0.01$, and $^{***}P < 0.001$ indicate significant differences compared with the Saline + CFA group according to two-way ANOVA followed by Bonferroni post-hoc analysis. **b**, **d** AUC was calculated during 0–7 days from dose-response curve of EM-1 or EM-2, $^*P < 0.05$, $^{**}P < 0.01$, and $^{***}P < 0.001$ indicate significant differences compared with saline according to one-way ANOVA followed by Bonferroni post-hoc analysis

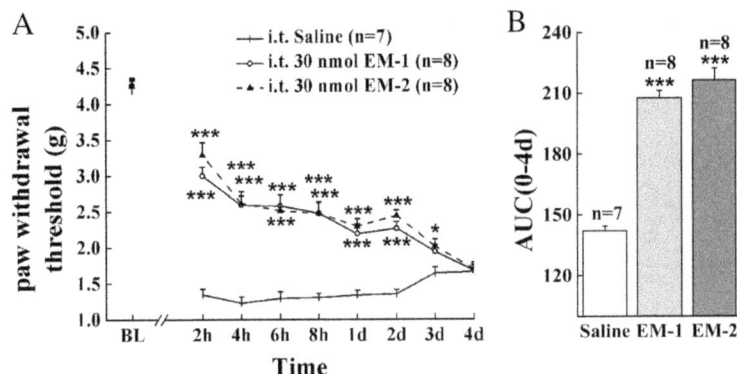

Fig. 2 Preemptive administration of EM-1 and EM-2 robustly reduced the development of paw incision-induced mechanical allodynia. **a** Preemptive intrathecal administration of EM-1 (30 nmol, i.t.) and EM-2 (30 nmol, i.t.) 10 min before paw incision time-dependently attenuated mechanical allodynia in male mice. Each value represents mean ± S.E.M. Group size is indicated in figures. *$P < 0.05$ and ***$P < 0.001$ indicate significant differences compared with the Saline group according to two-way ANOVA followed by Bonferroni post-hoc analysis. **b** AUC was calculated during 0–4 days from time-response curve of EM-1 and EM-2, and ***$P < 0.001$ indicates significant differences compared with the Saline group according to one-way ANOVA followed by Bonferroni post-hoc analysis

in DRG neurons was detected after CFA. In control mice, the percentage of the mu-opioid receptor-positive profiles among all neurons in L4 DRG was $11.76 \pm 1.73\%$ (922 positive neurons among a total of 8096 neurons derived from six sections/mouse, $n = 9$ mice). One day after CFA, a significant increase of the mu-opioid receptor-positive neurons ($28.88 \pm 3.09\%$, 2857 positive neurons among a total of 8632 neurons derived from six sections/mouse, $n = 10$ mice) was observed ($t_{17} = -4.69$, $P < 0.001$ relative to control).

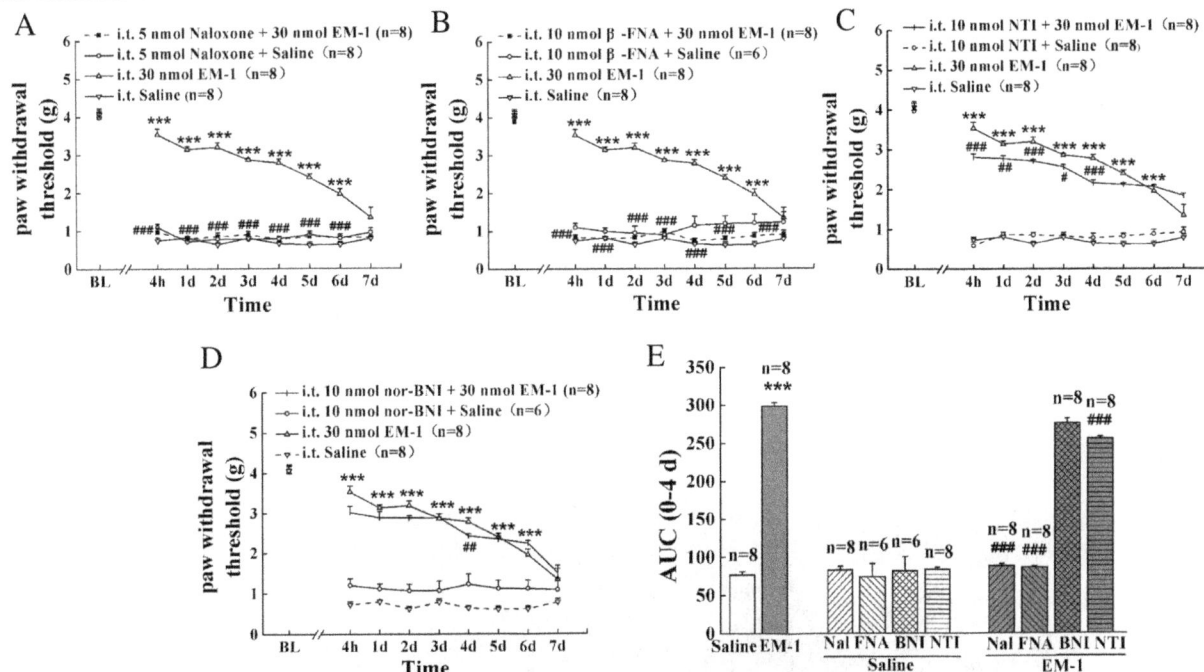

Fig. 3 Effects of the opioid antagonists on the anti-allodynic activities of preemptive administration of EM-1. The opioid antagonists naloxone (5 nmol, i.t., (**a**)), β-FNA (10 nmol, i.t., (**b**)), NTI (10 nmol, i.t., (**c**)), and nor-BNI (10 nmol, i.t., (**d**)) were administered 10 min, 4 h, 10 min, and 30 min prior to EM-1 (30 nmol, i.t.) injection, respectively. Each value represents mean ± S.E.M. Group size is indicated in figures. *$P < 0.05$, **$P < 0.01$, and ***$P < 0.001$ indicate significant differences compared with the Saline group according to two-way ANOVA followed by Bonferroni post-hoc analysis, #$P < 0.05$, ##$P < 0.01$, and ###$P < 0.001$ indicate significant differences compared with EM-1 group according to two-way ANOVA followed by Bonferroni post-hoc analysis. **e** AUC data were calculated during 0–4 days; *$P < 0.05$, **$P < 0.01$, and ***$P < 0.001$ indicate significant differences compared with the Saline group according to one-way ANOVA followed by Bonferroni post-hoc analysis. #$P < 0.05$, ##$P < 0.01$, and ###$P < 0.001$ indicate significant differences compared with EM-1 group according to one-way ANOVA followed by Bonferroni post-hoc analysis

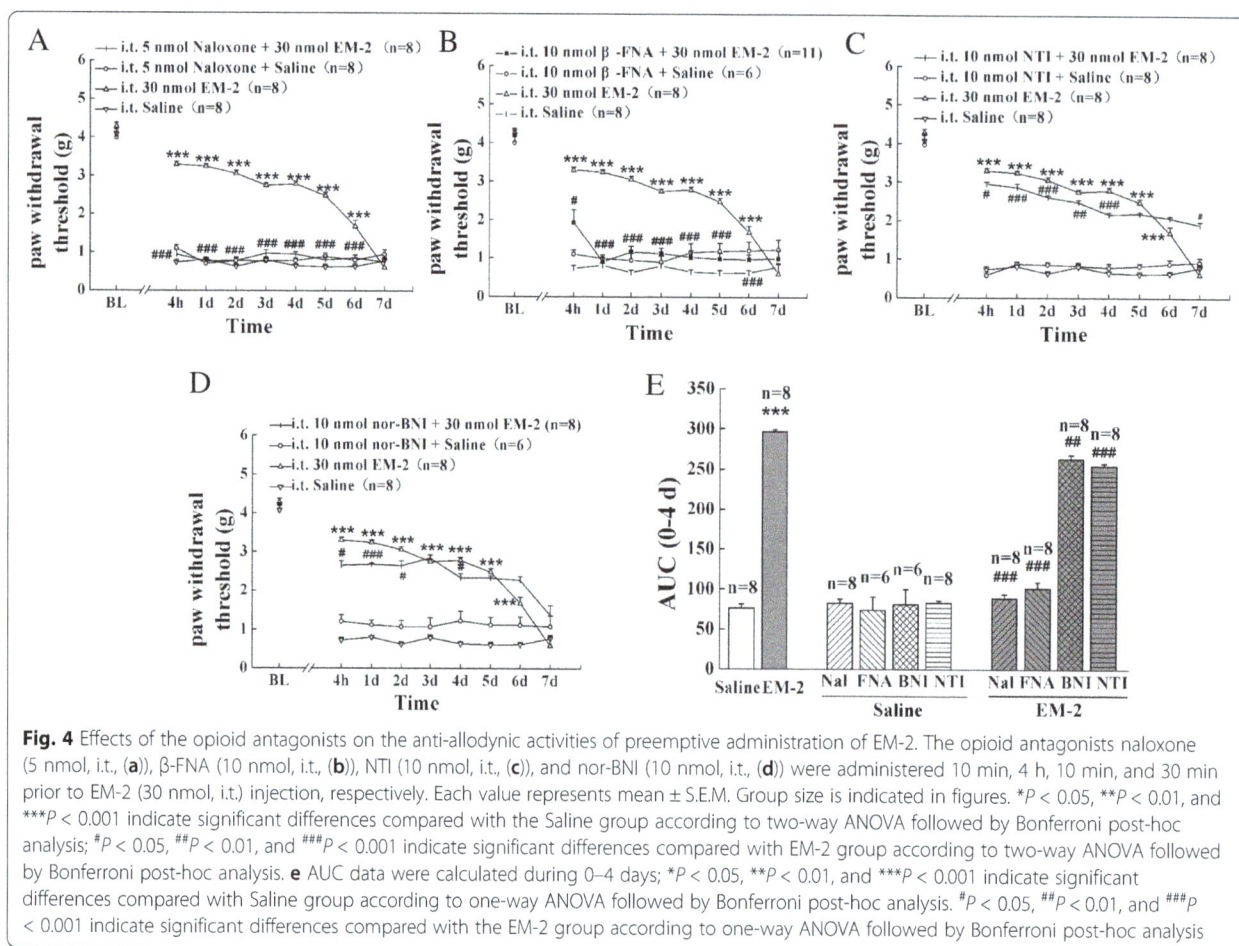

Fig. 4 Effects of the opioid antagonists on the anti-allodynic activities of preemptive administration of EM-2. The opioid antagonists naloxone (5 nmol, i.t., (**a**)), β-FNA (10 nmol, i.t., (**b**)), NTI (10 nmol, i.t., (**c**)), and nor-BNI (10 nmol, i.t., (**d**)) were administered 10 min, 4 h, 10 min, and 30 min prior to EM-2 (30 nmol, i.t.) injection, respectively. Each value represents mean ± S.E.M. Group size is indicated in figures. *$P < 0.05$, **$P < 0.01$, and ***$P < 0.001$ indicate significant differences compared with the Saline group according to two-way ANOVA followed by Bonferroni post-hoc analysis; #$P < 0.05$, ##$P < 0.01$, and ###$P < 0.001$ indicate significant differences compared with EM-2 group according to two-way ANOVA followed by Bonferroni post-hoc analysis. **e** AUC data were calculated during 0–4 days; *$P < 0.05$, **$P < 0.01$, and ***$P < 0.001$ indicate significant differences compared with Saline group according to one-way ANOVA followed by Bonferroni post-hoc analysis. #$P < 0.05$, ##$P < 0.01$, and ###$P < 0.001$ indicate significant differences compared with the EM-2 group according to one-way ANOVA followed by Bonferroni post-hoc analysis

Effects of preemptive intrathecal administration of EM-1 and EM-2 on p38 MAPK in DRG

Previous studies have shown that MAPK pathways, in particular ERK1/2 and p38 MAPK, play an important role in pain hypersensitivity [25]. Thus, to investigate whether MAPK signaling is involved in the preemptive analgesia of endomorphins in inflammatory pain model,

we further examined the effects of EM-1 and EM-2 on CFA-induced activation of p38 MAPK and ERK1/2 in DRG neurons. As shown in Fig. 6a, b, Western blot analysis revealed that the phosphorylation of ERK1/2 and p38 MAPK was dramatically increased 1 day after CFA compared with control animals ($F_{3, 19} = 2.31$, $P = 0.115$; $F_{3, 23} = 5.20$, $P = 0.008$, respectively). Notably, preemptive

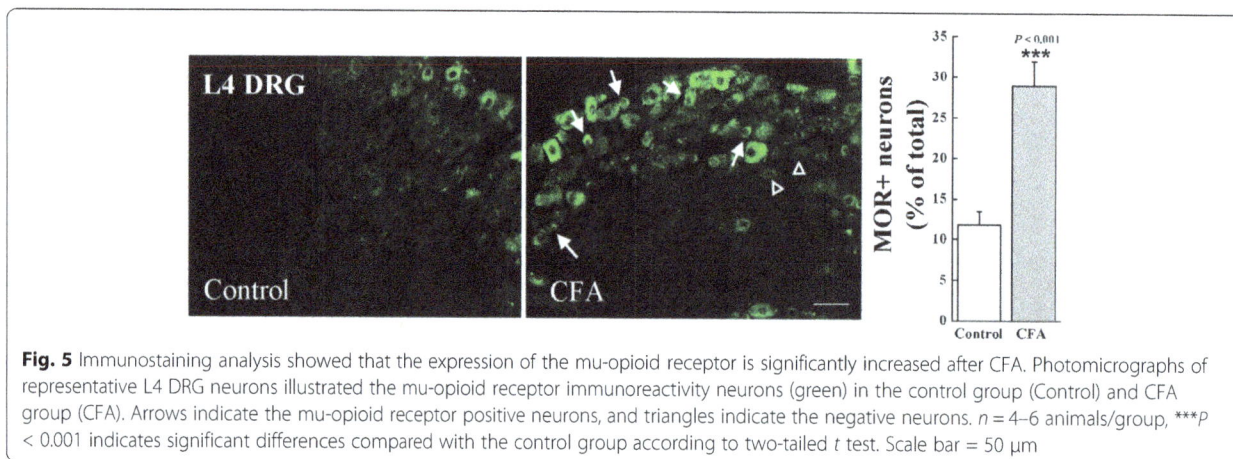

Fig. 5 Immunostaining analysis showed that the expression of the mu-opioid receptor is significantly increased after CFA. Photomicrographs of representative L4 DRG neurons illustrated the mu-opioid receptor immunoreactivity neurons (green) in the control group (Control) and CFA group (CFA). Arrows indicate the mu-opioid receptor positive neurons, and triangles indicate the negative neurons. $n = 4$–6 animals/group, ***$P < 0.001$ indicates significant differences compared with the control group according to two-tailed t test. Scale bar = 50 μm

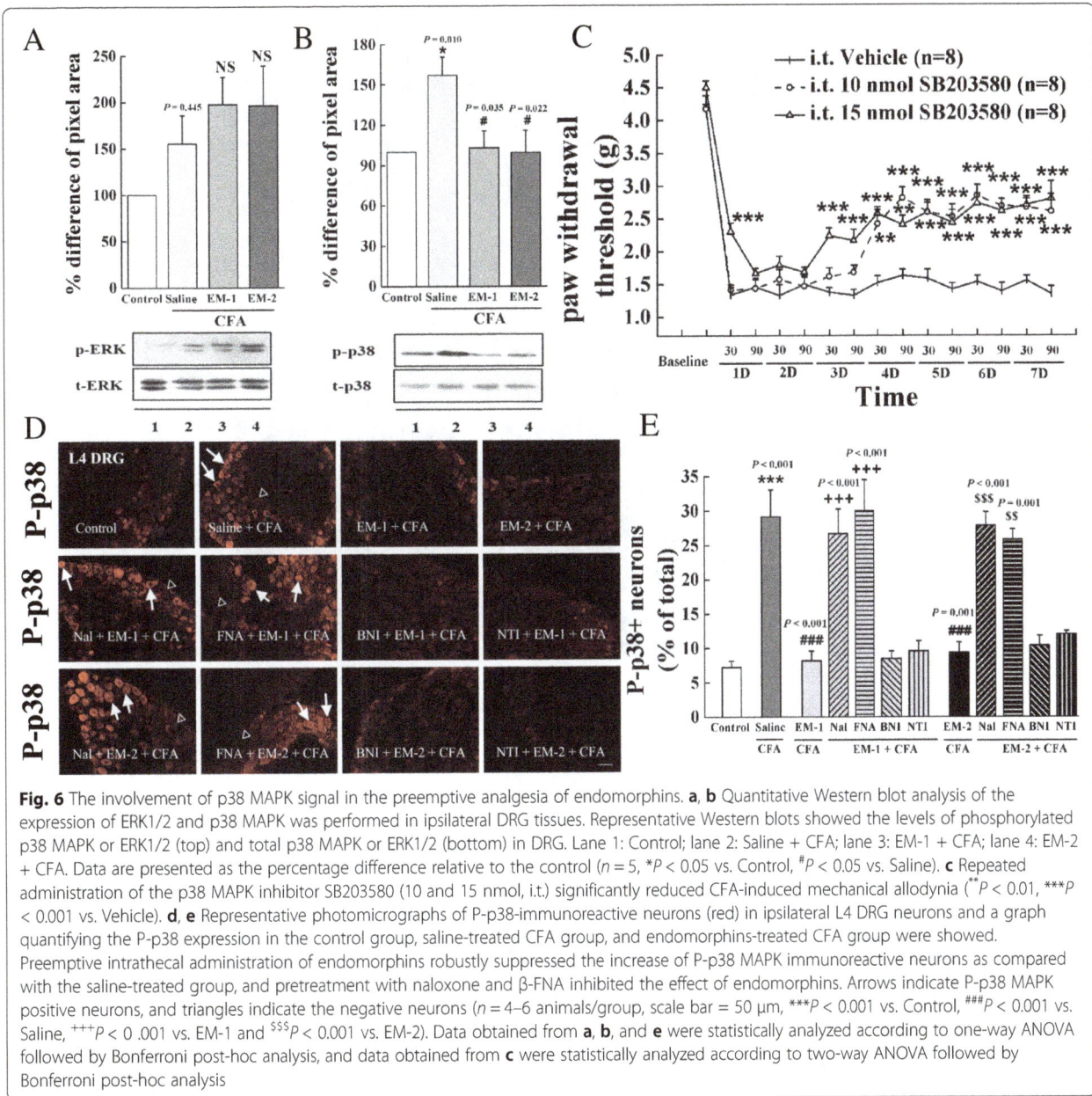

Fig. 6 The involvement of p38 MAPK signal in the preemptive analgesia of endomorphins. **a, b** Quantitative Western blot analysis of the expression of ERK1/2 and p38 MAPK was performed in ipsilateral DRG tissues. Representative Western blots showed the levels of phosphorylated p38 MAPK or ERK1/2 (top) and total p38 MAPK or ERK1/2 (bottom) in DRG. Lane 1: Control; lane 2: Saline + CFA; lane 3: EM-1 + CFA; lane 4: EM-2 + CFA. Data are presented as the percentage difference relative to the control ($n = 5$, $*P < 0.05$ vs. Control, $^{\#}P < 0.05$ vs. Saline). **c** Repeated administration of the p38 MAPK inhibitor SB203580 (10 and 15 nmol, i.t.) significantly reduced CFA-induced mechanical allodynia ($^{**}P < 0.01$, $^{***}P < 0.001$ vs. Vehicle). **d, e** Representative photomicrographs of P-p38-immunoreactive neurons (red) in ipsilateral L4 DRG neurons and a graph quantifying the P-p38 expression in the control group, saline-treated CFA group, and endomorphins-treated CFA group were showed. Preemptive intrathecal administration of endomorphins robustly suppressed the increase of P-p38 MAPK immunoreactive neurons as compared with the saline-treated group, and pretreatment with naloxone and β-FNA inhibited the effect of endomorphins. Arrows indicate P-p38 MAPK positive neurons, and triangles indicate the negative neurons ($n = 4$–6 animals/group, scale bar = 50 μm, $^{***}P < 0.001$ vs. Control, $^{\#\#\#}P < 0.001$ vs. Saline, $^{+++}P < 0.001$ vs. EM-1 and $^{\$\$\$}P < 0.001$ vs. EM-2). Data obtained from **a, b**, and **e** were statistically analyzed according to one-way ANOVA followed by Bonferroni post-hoc analysis, and data obtained from **c** were statistically analyzed according to two-way ANOVA followed by Bonferroni post-hoc analysis

intrathecal administration of EM-1 or EM-2 significantly prevented CFA-induced activation of p38 MAPK (EM-1, $P = 0.035$; EM-2, $P = 0.022$, respectively), but did not modify the upregulation of ERK1/2 phosphorylation.

Consistent with the previous study [42], the co-labeling of P-p38 MAPK and NeuN revealed P-p38 MAPK immunoreactivity in DRG neurons (Additional file 2: Figure S1B). Immunofluorescence staining data further demonstrated that a larger number of DRG neurons exhibited immunoreactivity to phosphorylated p38 MAPK 1 day after CFA (Fig. 6d, $F_{11, 47} = 17.5$, $P < 0.001$; 1205 positive neurons among a total of 4268 neurons derived from six sections/mouse, $n = 4$ mice). Preemptive intrathecal administration of EM-1 or EM-2 significantly decreased CFA-induced upregulation of phosphorylated p38 MAPK in DRG (254 positive neurons among a total of 3302 neurons derived from 4 sections/mouse, $n = 4$ mice, $P < 0.001$; 300 positive neurons among a total of 3156 neurons derived from four sections/mouse, $n = 4$ mice, $P < 0.001$, respectively). In addition, pretreatment with naloxone and β-FNA, but not nor-BNI or NTI, significantly reversed the effect of endomorphins on phosphorylated p38 MAPK signal (for EM-1, naloxone, $P < 0.001$; β-FNA, $P < 0.001$; for EM-2, naloxone, $P < 0.001$; β-FNA, $P = 0.001$).

Next, we performed co-immunolabeling of phosphorylated p38 MAPK with the mu-opioid receptor in DRG neurons from CFA-treated mice. As shown in Fig. 7 and

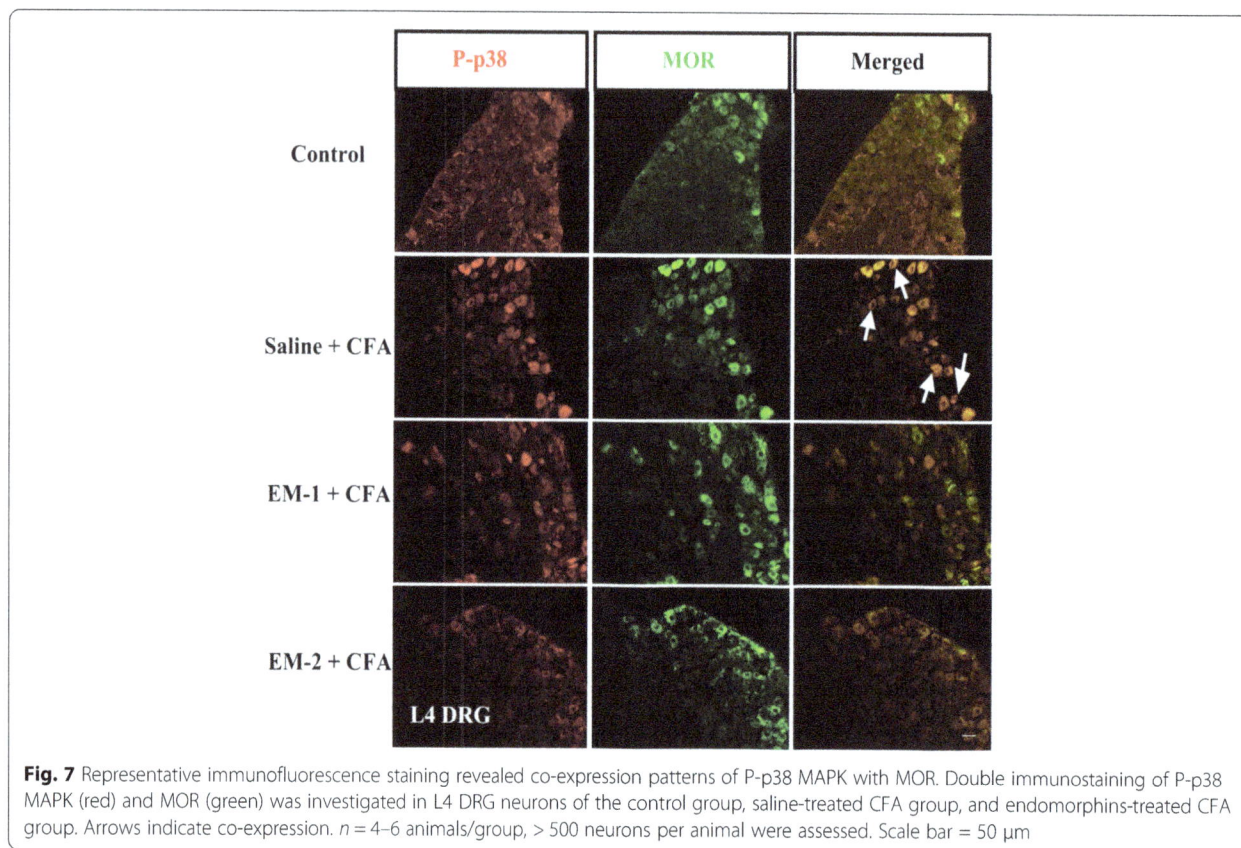

Fig. 7 Representative immunofluorescence staining revealed co-expression patterns of P-p38 MAPK with MOR. Double immunostaining of P-p38 MAPK (red) and MOR (green) was investigated in L4 DRG neurons of the control group, saline-treated CFA group, and endomorphins-treated CFA group. Arrows indicate co-expression. $n = 4$–6 animals/group, > 500 neurons per animal were assessed. Scale bar = 50 μm

Table 2, the proportion of phosphorylated p38 MAPK and the mu-opioid receptor co-localized neurons was $17.62 \pm 0.77\%$ among all DRG neurons in saline-treated CFA mice ($F_{3, 15} = 40.5$, $P < 0.001$, 469 positive neurons among a total of 3367 neurons derived from 6 sections/mouse, $n = 4$ mice), suggesting a significant increase compared with that of control mice ($2.62 \pm 0.39\%$, 64 positive neurons among a total of 3570 neurons derived from 6 sections/mouse, $n = 4$ mice). In addition, compared with saline-treated CFA group, preemptive intrathecal administration of EM-1 or EM-2 significantly reduced co-expression of phosphorylated p38 MAPK with the mu-opioid receptor (207 positive neurons among a total of 2814 neurons derived from 6 sections/mouse, n = 4 mice, $P < 0.001$; 209 positive neurons among a total of 2152 neurons derived from 6 sections/mouse, $n = 4$ mice, $P < 0.001$, respectively).

Intrathecal injection of the p38 MAPK inhibitor SB203580 attenuated CFA-induced mechanical allodynia

To evaluate the functional role of p38 MAPK signaling pathway in CFA-induced inflammatory pain, the selective p38 MAPK inhibitor SB203580 was repeatedly administered once daily for 7 days. Figure 6c showed that repetitive saline-treated mice had the intact development of mechanical allodynia after CFA treatment, while

repeated administration of SB203580 (10 and 15 nmol, i.t.) inhibited the activation of p38 MAPK and resulted in a significant anti-allodynic effect ($F_{22, 359} = 5.72$, $P < 0.001$).

Effects of preemptive intrathecal administration of EM-1 and EM-2 on CFA-induced gene expressions of inflammatory cytokines and chemokines in DRG

Pro-inflammatory cytokines and chemokines were reported to play important roles in the generation and maintenance of chronic pain. To determine the effects of preemptive intrathecal administration of endomorphins on the production of pro-inflammatory mediators, the mRNA levels of IL-1β, TNF-α, CCL2, and CCL3 in ipsilateral DRG tissues were measured by real-time PCR experiments. As shown in Fig. 8 and Table 3, CFA-induced peripheral inflammation substantially increased the expressions of pro-inflammatory mediators, including IL-1β ($P = 0.024$), TNF-α ($P = 0.024$), CCL2 ($P = 0.036$), and CCL3 ($P = 0.024$). Pretreatment with EM-1 produced a slight, but not statistically significant, decrease in CFA-induced upregulation of IL-1β ($P = 0.057$). In addition, preemptive administration of EM-2 substantially reduced the upregulation of TNF-α ($P = 0.057$) induced by CFA. However, neither EM-1 nor EM-2 had significant effects on the expressions of CCL2

Table 2 Expression or co-expression of MOR and P-p38 MAPK in DRG neurons (%: immunoreactive neurons relative to total DRG neurons)

	Control	Saline + CFA	EM-1 + CFA	EM-2 + CFA
P-p38	7.3 ± 0.9	29.2 ± 3.9 ***	8.2 ± 1.4 ###	9.4 ± 1.5 ###
MOR	11.8 ± 1.7	28.9 ± 3.1 ***	—	—
MOR + P-p38	2.6 ± 0.4	17.6 ± 0.8 ***	7.4 ± 0.9 ###	9.8 ± 0.7 ###

Quantification illustrates the expression of MOR and P-p38 MAPK and their co-expression in DRG neurons in response to CFA
***$P < 0.001$ indicates significant differences compared with Control samples according to one-way ANOVA followed by Bonferroni post-hoc analysis or two-tailed t test
###$P < 0.001$ indicates significant differences compared with Saline + CFA samples according to one-way ANOVA followed by Bonferroni post-hoc analysis

(EM-1, $P = 0.100$; EM-2, $P = 0.400$) and CCL3 (EM-1, $P = 0.100$; EM-2, $P = 1.000$) in inflammatory animals.

IL-10 is an anti-inflammatory cytokine and has a crucial role in the prevention of inflammatory diseases since it reduces the production of pro-inflammation mediators [43]. In Fig. 8b, our results indicated that the mRNA level of IL-10 in ipsilateral DRG 1 day after CFA treatment was significantly lower than that of control animals ($P = 0.036$). Moreover, pretreatment with EM-2 produced a slight, but not statistically significant, increase in CFA-induced downregulation of IL-10 expression ($P = 0.057$).

Discussion

Endomorphins were characterized as the selective mu-opioid agonists and held great promise in the design of new candidate drugs [18, 44]. Recently, several series of endomorphin analogs with potent and long-lasting antinociception provide lead compounds for the development of novel analgesics [7, 44]. Our results demonstrated that preemptive intrathecal administration of endomorphins produced potent anti-allodynic effects in CFA-induced inflammatory pain model. As a result of inflammation, mice exhibited a significant activation of p38 MAPK pathway and an increased expression of inflammatory cytokines in DRG tissues, which were partially reconciled by preemptive administration of endomorphins. In conclusion, our data implicate that preemptive intrathecal administration of endomorphins reduces inflammatory pain via inhibition of p38 MAPK phosphorylation and regulation levels of inflammatory cytokines in DRG.

Endomorphins and their analogs were reported to produce potent analgesic activities in acute and chronic pain models [2–4, 7]. However, the preemptive analgesic effects of endomorphins on chronic pain were poorly uncovered. Here, our research for the first time showed that in a mouse model of CFA inflammatory pain, endomorphins dose-dependently produced preemptive analgesic effects after i.t. administration in a manner similar

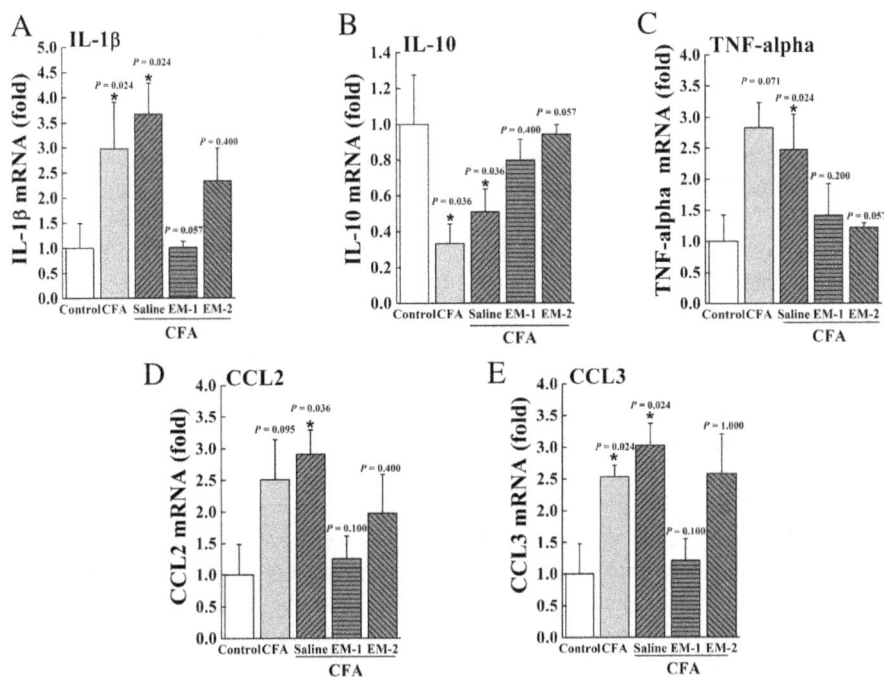

Fig. 8 Effects of preemptive intrathecal administration of endomorphins on gene expression of inflammatory cytokines and chemokines. EM-1 and EM-2 differently reversed CFA-induced regulation of mRNA expression of IL-1β (**a**), IL-10 (**b**), TNF-alpha (**c**), CCL2 (**d**), and CCL3 (**e**) in the ipsilateral DRG tissues 1 day after CFA. Results are shown as the fold expression relative to control ($n = 8$–10 animals/group). *$P < 0.05$ indicates significant differences compared with Control group according to Mann-Whitney test

Table 3 Relative mRNA levels of inflammatory mediators in DRG tissues

Gene	CFA	Saline + CFA	EM-1 + CFA	EM-2 + CFA
IL-1β	2.46 ± 0.70	3.67 ± 0.61*	1.08 ± 0.16 #	2.33 ± 0.57
IL-10	0.33 ± 0.11**	0.51 ± 0.13*	0.80 ± 0.12	0.77 ± 0.23
TNF-α	2.84 ± 0.41*	2.07 ± 0.60	1.41 ± 0.51	1.21 ± 0.08
CCL2	2.51 ± 0.63	2.91 ± 0.38*	1.25 ± 0.37	1.97 ± 0.61
CCL3	2.20 ± 0.44**	3.03 ± 0.34**	1.21 ± 0.35	2.58 ± 0.63

Inflammatory mediators mRNA levels are assessed by RT-PCR assay and normalized to GAPDH-expression
*P < 0.05 and **P < 0.01 indicates significant differences compared with Control samples according to one-way ANOVA followed by Bonferroni post-hoc analysis
#P < 0.05 indicates significant differences compared with Saline + CFA samples according to one-way ANOVA followed by Bonferroni post-hoc analysis

to the endogenous opioid ligand nociceptin/orphanin FQ (N/OFQ) [17, 45]. Of note, central administration of endomorphins produced acute antinociceptive actions which only sustained for 20–30 min [13, 14]. Mizoguchi et al. reported that i.t. administration of EM-1 and EM-2 effectively inhibited the paw-withdrawal responses within 30 min [13]. In striking contrast, we found that preemptive intrathecal administration of EM-1 and EM-2 relieved CFA-induced inflammatory pain for 6 days. Moreover, endomorphins also produced preemptive anti-allodynia for 2 days in postoperative pain model. Our findings suggest the prolonged anti-allodynic effects produced by preemptive antinociception of endomorphins might be due to their abilities of blocking the development of pain. In fact, preemptive treatment with analgesics prevents or blunts spinal facilitation evoked by nociceptive input to the spinal cord and attenuates perceived pain in a long-lasting manner [42, 45, 46]. The preemptive administration of analgesics might be an attractive strategy for the treatment of chronic pain.

Furthermore, the preemptive analgesic effects of EM-1 and EM-2 were completely blocked by the opioid receptor antagonist naloxone, suggesting the involvement of opioid system. Our present data indicated the significant antagonism with the selective mu-opioid receptor antagonist β-FNA, which further implies that both EM-1 and EM-2 produce preemptive analgesic effects via the mu-opioid receptor. These findings are consistent with the previous results that both EM-1 and EM-2 activated the mu-opioid receptor with high affinity and selectivity [1]. Previous research found that the endogenous delta-opioid ligand met-enkephalin was expressed in inflamed subcutaneous tissue [47]. Our results showed that EM-1- and EM-2-induced preemptive analgesia were partially reduced by the selective delta-opioid receptor antagonist NTI. However, i.t. administration of the selective kappa-opioid receptor antagonist nor-BNI partially attenuated the preemptive analgesic effect of EM-2, but not

that of EM-1. The different pharmacological profiles of EM-1 and EM-2 in this study are in line with the previous report that spinal antinociception of EM-1 and EM-2 is mediated by different subtypes of the mu-opioid receptor [48]. Spinal antinociception of EM-2 is mediated through activation of the mu(1)-opioid receptor which subsequently induced the release of the endogenous kappa-opioid peptide dynorphin A-(1-17) in the spinal cord [48]. Based on these results, we speculate that endomorphins-induced preemptive analgesia might be partially mediated by release of endogenous opioid peptides.

Previous studies have shown that the expression of the mu-opioid receptor mRNA is upregulated in DRG tissues by painful peripheral inflammation [49]. Here, we extended this study and found that the mu-opioid receptor at the protein level was significantly increased in ipsilateral DRG neurons 1 day after CFA injection. Considering the antinociceptive effects of endomorphins in the present study, CFA-induced activation of the mu-opioid receptor system in DRG may be associated with the suppression of nociceptive hypersensitivity in CFA-induced inflammatory pain model.

It is well known that MAPK pathways, especially ERK1/2 and p38 MAPK, modify neuronal plasticity and contribute to pain hypersensitivity [25]. A remarkable increase of phosphorylated p38 MAPK and ERK1/2 was detected in spinal cord and DRG tissues in acute and persistent inflammatory pain models [26, 50–52]. In addition, intrathecal injection of the selective inhibitors of MAPK pathways produced analgesic activities in rodent models of inflammatory, neuropathic and cancer pain [25]. The present study showed that the levels of phosphorylated ERK1/2 and p38 MAPK in DRG tissues were increased 1 day after CFA treatment, corroborating the previous findings [26, 52]. In addition, pretreatment with endomorphins selectively attenuated CFA-induced phosphorylation of p38 MAPK, which was reversed by pretreatment with the mu-opioid receptor antagonist. Furthermore, our results demonstrated that repeated i.t. injection of the p38 MAPK inhibitor SB203580 partially prevented the development of mechanical hypersensitivity induced by CFA. Taken together, our current data suggest the preemptive analgesic effects of endomorphins might be mediated by suppression of p38 MAPK pathway, but independent of ERK1/2.

To date, several studies have reported a functional interaction between the activation of the mu-opioid receptor and the phosphorylation of MAPK signaling in both in vivo and in vitro assays. For example, fentanyl selectively activated ERK1/2 signal, but not p38 MAPK signal in striatal neurons [53]. In vitro study found that EM-1 could elicit rapid activation of ERK1/2 in rat C6 glioma cells [54], and morphine induced a decrease of IL-10 and an increase of IL-12 secretion via p38 MAPK pathway in monocyte-derived human dendritic cells [55]. Furthermore, Li et al. found that endomorphins decreased the activation of p38 MAPK induced by LPS, but not that of ERK1/2 in murine dendritic cells [30]. Therefore, it is possible that the mu-opioid system might have a differential modulation on the activity of p38 MAPK or ERK1/2, depending on cell types, treatments, or in vitro or in vivo studies, etc.

Neuroinflammation is crucial pathogenesis of chronic pain [56, 57]. Numerous studies provided evidence that pro-inflammatory cytokines, such as TNF-α, IL-1β, and IL-6, were upregulated in the spinal cord after nerve injury, inflammation, and chronic opioid exposure, which contribute in inducing or facilitating inflammatory responses as well as mechanical allodynia [58]. Both TNF-α and IL-1β played essential roles in the generation of central sensitization and modulation of peripheral sensitization [59, 60]. The inhibition of IL-1β signaling was reported to block the development of inflammatory, neuropathic, and cancer pain [61]. Here, we found that intraplantar injection of CFA significantly upregulated the mRNA expressions of IL-1β and TNF-α on day 1 post-injection, which is consistent with the previous report [58]. Importantly, we found that the upregulation of IL-1β was substantially reduced by EM-1, while the activation of TNF-α was regulated by EM-2. IL-10 is an anti-inflammatory cytokine which suppresses the production of pro-inflammatory cytokines and the induction of hyperalgesia and allodynia in different pain models [43]. Although it did not achieve a significant difference, EM-2 substantially reduced the downregulation of IL-10 induced by CFA. Thus, the regulation of IL-1β, TNF-α, and IL-10 levels might be involved in EM-1- and EM-2-induced preemptive anti-allodynia, respectively. At present, there is no evidence to document the differential effects of EM-1 and EM-2 on the expressions of inflammatory cytokines. Of note, previous studies found that spinal antinociception of EM-1 and EM-2 are mediated by different mu-opioid receptor subtypes [13, 48]. Whether this could account for the differential effects of EM-1 and EM-2 on the expression of inflammatory cytokines needs further studies.

Chemokines can regulate chronic pain by modulating the signaling interactions between neurons and glial cells [62]. Previous studies have shown that nerve injury and inflammation upregulated the expressions of CCL2, CCL3, and CCL21 in DRG tissues [63, 64]. A great number of studies found that the mu-opioid receptor and chemokine receptors, such as CCR5, CCR1, CXCR4, and CX3CR1, are co-expressed on the same population of DRG neurons [65]. Moreover, chemokines also participated in the analgesic effects of opioids [65]. Our results demonstrated that CCL2 and CCL3 mRNAs were dramatically increased 1 day after CFA. Interestingly, we found that EM-1 and EM-2 had no significant effects on the gene expressions of CCL2 and CCL3 in the present study.

In addition, accumulating evidence has indicated that various inflammatory cytokines and chemokines produced by DRG satellite glial cells and released to the extracellular space contribute to the development and maintenance of chronic pain [59]. Our results showed that intrathecal pretreatment with endomorphins inhibited the activation of satellite glial cells in DRG tissues (Additional file 3: Figure S2), suggesting a possible involvement of non-neuronal mechanism in analgesia of preemptive treatment of endomorphins. Further mechanistic studies are under investigation in our lab.

Conclusions

In summary, our research provides, for the first time, preemptive analgesic effects of spinal endomorphins in CFA-induced inflammatory pain. Several lines of evidence suggest that the preemptive analgesic effects of endomorphins are associated with the regulation of inflammatory mediators via inhibiting p38 MAPK signal in DRGs. In brief, (1) peripheral inflammation increases the expression of phosphorylated p38 MAPK, which is attenuated by preemptive intrathecal administration of endomorphins, (2) pretreatment with the opioid receptor antagonists naloxone and β-FNA significantly reverses endomorphins-induced effects on phosphorylated p38 MAPK signal in DRG, (3) repeated application of the p38 MAPK inhibitor SB203580 significantly reduces CFA-induced mechanical allodynia, (4) co-localization of phosphorylated p38 MAPK with the mu-opioid receptor in DRG neurons is increased after inflammation, which is attenuated by preemptive intrathecal administration of endomorphins. These findings support the involvement of p38 MAPK signal in the preemptive analgesia of endomorphins. Moreover, preemptive intrathecal administration of endomorphins regulates the expressions of cytokines in ipsilateral DRG tissues. Therefore, our study indicates that the preemptive analgesia of endomorphins may be helpful for chronic pain treatment.

Additional files

Additional file 1: Supplemental methods. Table S1 Primary and secondary antibody information. (DOCX 25 kb)

Additional file 2: Figure S1. Phosphorylated p38 MAPK and the mu-opioid receptor were expressed in mouse ipsilateral L4 DRG neurons. (**A**) Double immunostaining of MOR (green) and NeuN (red) was investigated in L4 DRG tissues of control group and saline-treated CFA group. (**B**) Double immunostaining of P-p38 MAPK (red) and NeuN (green) was conducted in L4 DRG tissues of control group and saline-treated CFA group. Arrows indicate co-expression. n = 4 animals/group, > 500 neurons per animal were assessed. Scale bar = 50 μm. (PPTX 2054 kb)

Additional file 3: Figure S2. Preemptive administration of EM-1 and EM-2 inhibited the activation of glial cells induced by CFA. Representative photomicrographs of the immunoreactivity of GFAP (a marker of satellite glial cells) in ipsilateral L4 DRG and a graph quantifying the expression of GFAP was showed. Immunostaining analysis indicated that the expression of GFAP was significantly increased 1 day after CFA treatment. Preemptive intrathecal administration of endomorphins robustly suppressed the immunoreactivity of GFAP in ipsilateral L4 DRG tissues as compared with the saline-treated group. $n = 4$–6 animals/group, one-way ANOVA followed by Bonferroni post-hoc analysis was used. Scale bar = 50 μm. (PPTX 1192 kb)

Abbreviations
ANOVA: Analysis of variance; AUC: Area under the curve; ED_{50}: Effective dose 50% of maximum response; EM-1: Endomorphin-1; EM-2: Endomorphin-2; i.t.: Intrathecal; IL-1β: Interleukin-1beta; MOR: Mu-opioid receptor; nor-BNI: Nor-binaltorphimine; NTI: Naltrindole; S.E.M.: Standard error of the mean; TNF-α: Tumor necrosis factor-α; β-FNA: Beta-funaltrexamine

Acknowledgements
Not applicable

Funding
This study was supported by grants from the National Natural Science Foundation of China (Nos. 81673282), the Fundamental Research Funds for the Central Universities (lzujbky-2018-ot02), and the National Institute of Dental and Craniofacial Research (R01, DE027454-01A1 to YC).

Authors' contributions
ZT, ZN, ZR, ZWD, CY, WZL, XB, ZMN, SXR, ZQQ, GYY, XJ, and CD performed the research. FQ designed the research study. ZT and ZMN analyzed the data. ZT, ZN, CY, and FQ wrote the paper. All authors read and approved the final manuscript.

Competing interests
The authors declare that they have no competing interests.

Author details
[1]Key Laboratory of Preclinical Study for New Drugs of Gansu Province, and Institute of Physiology, School of Basic Medical Sciences, Lanzhou University, 199 Donggang West Road, Lanzhou 730000, People's Republic of China. [2]Department of Neurology, School of Medicine, Duke University, Durham, North Carolina 27710, USA.

References
1. Zadina JE, Hackler L, Ge LJ, Kastin AJ. A potent and selective endogenous agonist for the mu-opiate receptor. Nature. 1997;386:499–502.
2. Hao S, Wolfe D, Glorioso JC, Mata M, Fink DJ. Effects of transgene-mediated endomorphin-2 in inflammatory pain. Eur J Pain. 2009;13:380–6.
3. Xie H, Woods JH, Traynor JR, Ko MC. The spinal antinociceptive effects of endomorphins in rats: behavioral and G protein functional studies. Anesth Analg. 2008;106:1873–81.
4. Przewlocka B, Mika J, Labuz D, Toth G, Przewlocki R. Spinal analgesic action of endomorphins in acute, inflammatory and neuropathic pain in rats. Eur J Pharmacol. 1999;367:189–96.
5. Soignier RD, Vaccarino AL, Brennan AM, Kastin AJ, Zadina JE. Analgesic effects of endomorphin-1 and endomorphin-2 in the formalin test in mice. Life Sci. 2000;67:907–12.
6. McDougall JJ, Baker CL, Hermann PM. Attenuation of knee joint inflammation by peripherally administered endomorphin-1. J Mol Neurosci. 2004;22:125–37.
7. Feehan AK, Morgenweck J, Zhang X, Amgott-Kwan AT, Zadina JE. Novel endomorphin analogs are more potent and longer-lasting analgesics in neuropathic, inflammatory, postoperative, and visceral pain relative to morphine. J Pain. 2017;18:1526–41.
8. Mousa SA, Machelska H, Schafer M, Stein C. Immunohistochemical localization of endomorphin-1 and endomorphin-2 in immune cells and spinal cord in a model of inflammatory pain. J Neuroimmunol. 2002;126:5–15.
9. Obara I, Przewlocki R, Przewlocka B. Local peripheral effects of mu-opioid receptor agonists in neuropathic pain in rats. Neurosci Lett. 2004;360:85–9.
10. Przewlocki R, Labuz D, Mika J, Przewlocka B, Tomboly C, Toth G. Pain inhibition by endomorphins. Ann N Y Acad Sci. 1999;897:154–64.
11. Czapla MA, Gozal D, Alea OA, Beckerman RC, Zadina JE. Differential cardiorespiratory effects of endomorphin 1, endomorphin 2, DAMGO, and morphine. Am J Respir Crit Care Med. 2000;162:994–9.
12. Wilson AM, Soignier RD, Zadina JE, Kastin AJ, Nores WL, Olson RD, Olson GA. Dissociation of analgesic and rewarding effects of endomorphin-1 in rats. Peptides. 2000;21:1871–4.
13. Mizoguchi H, Watanabe H, Hayashi T, Sakurada W, Sawai T, Fujimura T, Sakurada T, Sakurada S. Possible involvement of dynorphin A-(1-17) release via mu1-opioid receptors in spinal antinociception by endomorphin-2. J Pharmacol Exp Ther. 2006;317:362–8.
14. Wu HE, Hung KC, Mizoguchi H, Fujimoto JM, Tseng LF. Acute antinociceptive tolerance and asymmetric cross-tolerance between endomorphin-1 and endomorphin-2 given intracerebroventricularly in the mouse. J Pharmacol Exp Ther. 2001;299:1120–5.
15. Basbaum AI, Bautista DM, Scherrer G, Julius D. Cellular and molecular mechanisms of pain. Cell. 2009;139:267–84.
16. Woolf CJ. Evidence for a central component of post-injury pain hypersensitivity. Nature. 1983;306:686–8.
17. Chen Y, Sommer C. Activation of the nociceptin opioid system in rat sensory neurons produces antinociceptive effects in inflammatory pain: involvement of inflammatory mediators. J Neurosci Res. 2007;85:1478–88.
18. Gu ZH, Wang B, Kou ZZ, Bai Y, Chen T, Dong YL, Li H, Li YQ. Endomorphins: promising endogenous opioid peptides for the development of novel analgesics. Neurosignals. 2017;25:98–116.
19. Li JL, Ding YQ, Li YQ, Li JS, Nomura S, Kaneko T, Mizuno N. Immunocytochemical localization of mu-opioid receptor in primary afferent neurons containing substance P or calcitonin gene-related peptide. A light and electron microscope study in the rat. Brain Res. 1998;794:347–52.
20. Greenwell TN, Martin-Schild S, Inglis FM, Zadina JE. Colocalization and shared distribution of endomorphins with substance P, calcitonin gene-related peptide, gamma-aminobutyric acid, and the mu opioid receptor. J Comp Neurol. 2007;503:319–33.
21. Borzsei R, Pozsgai G, Bagoly T, Elekes K, Pinter E, Szolcsanyi J, Helyes Z. Inhibitory action of endomorphin-1 on sensory neuropeptide release and neurogenic inflammation in rats and mice. Neuroscience. 2008;152:82–8.
22. Abbadie C, Bhangoo S, De Koninck Y, Malcangio M, Melik-Parsadaniantz S, White FA. Chemokines and pain mechanisms. Brain Res Rev. 2009;60:125–34.
23. DeLeo JAY, Yezierski RP. The role of neuroinflammation and neuroimmune activation in persistent pain. Pain. 2001;90:1–6.
24. Kawasaki Y, Zhang L, Cheng JK, Ji RR. Cytokine mechanisms of central sensitization: distinct and overlapping role of interleukin-1beta, interleukin-6, and tumor necrosis factor-alpha in regulating synaptic and neuronal activity in the superficial spinal cord. J Neurosci. 2008;28:5189–94.
25. Ji RR, Gereau RWT, Malcangio M, Strichartz GR. MAP kinase and pain. Brain Res Rev. 2009;60:135–48.
26. Svensson CI, Marsala M, Westerlund A, Calcutt NA, Campana WM, Freshwater JD, Catalano R, Feng Y, Protter AA, Scott B, Yaksh TL. Activation of p38 mitogen-activated protein kinase in spinal microglia is a critical link in inflammation-induced spinal pain processing. J Neurochem. 2003;86:1534–44.
27. Azuma Y, Ohura K. Endomorphin-2 modulates productions of TNF-alpha, IL-1beta, IL-10, and IL-12, and alters functions related to innate immune of macrophages. Inflammation. 2002;26:223–32.

28. Azuma Y, Ohura K. Endomorphins 1 and 2 inhibit IL-10 and IL-12 production and innate immune functions, and potentiate NF-kappa B DNA binding in THP-1 differentiated to macrophage-like cells. Scand J Immunol. 2002;56:260–9.

29. Li WY, Yang JJ, Zhu SH, Liu HJ, Xu JG. Endomorphins and ohmefentanyl in the inhibition of immunosuppressant function in rat peritoneal macrophages: an experimental in vitro study. Curr Ther Res Clin Exp. 2008;69:56–64.

30. Li ZH, Chu NS, Shan LD, Gong S, Yin QZ, Jiang XH. Inducible expression of functional mu opioid receptors in murine dendritic cells. J NeuroImmune Pharmacol. 2009;4:359–67.

31. Liu J, Yan L, Niu R, Tian L, Zhang Q, Quan J, Liu H, Wei S, Guo Q. Protection effect of endomorphins on advanced glycation end products induced injury in endothelial cells. J Diabetes Res. 2013; 2013:105780.

32. Wang ZL, Li N, Wang P, Tang HH, Han ZL, Song JJ, Li XH, Yu HP, Zhang T, Zhang R, et al. Pharmacological characterization of EN-9, a novel chimeric peptide of endomorphin-2 and neuropeptide FF that produces potent antinociceptive activity and limited tolerance. Neuropharmacology. 2016;108:364–72.

33. Kilkenny C, Browne W, Cuthill IC, Emerson M, Altman DG, Group NCRRGW. Animal research: reporting in vivo experiments: the ARRIVE guidelines. Br J Pharmacol. 2010;160:1577–9.

34. Hylden JL, Wilcox GL. Intrathecal morphine in mice: a new technique. Eur J Pharmacol. 1980;67:313–6.

35. Stein C, Millan MJ, Herz A. Unilateral inflammation of the hindpaw in rats as a model of prolonged noxious-stimulation - alterations in behavior and nociceptive thresholds. Pharmacol Biochem Behav. 1988;31:445–51.

36. Clark JD, Qiao YL, Li XQ, Shi XY, Angst MS, Yeomans DC. Blockade of the complement C5a receptor reduces incisional allodynia, edema, and cytokine expression. Anesthesiology. 2006;104:1274–82.

37. Liang DY, Li X, Shi X, Sun Y, Sahbaie P, Li WW, Clark JD. The complement component C5a receptor mediates pain and inflammation in a postsurgical pain model. Pain. 2012;153:366–72.

38. Sun Y, Li XQ, Sahbaie P, Shi XY, Li WW, Liang DY, Clark JD. miR-203 regulates nociceptive sensitization after incision by controlling phospholipase A2 activating protein expression. Anesthesiology. 2012;117:626–38.

39. Chen Y, Kanju P, Fang Q, Lee SH, Parekh PK, Lee W, Moore C, Brenner D, Gereau RWT, Wang F, Liedtke W. TRPV4 is necessary for trigeminal irritant pain and functions as a cellular formalin receptor. Pain. 2014;155:2662–72.

40. Chen JJ, Dai L, Zhao LX, Zhu X, Cao S, Gao YJ. Intrathecal curcumin attenuates pain hypersensitivity and decreases spinal neuroinflammation in rat model of monoarthritis. Sci Rep. 2015;5:10278.

41. Ji RR, Zhang Q, Law PY, Low HH, Elde R, Hokfelt T. Expression of mu-, delta-, and kappa-opioid receptor-like immunoreactivities in rat dorsal root ganglia after carrageenan-induced inflammation. J Neurosci. 1995;15:8156–66.

42. Chen Y, Geis C, Sommer C. Activation of TRPV1 contributes to morphine tolerance: involvement of the mitogen-activated protein kinase signaling pathway. J Neurosci. 2008;28:5836–45.

43. Zhang JM, An J. Cytokines, inflammation, and pain. Int Anesthesiol Clin. 2007;45:27–37.

44. Zadina JE, Nilges MR, Morgenweck J, Zhang X, Hackler L, Fasold MB. Endomorphin analog analgesics with reduced abuse liability, respiratory depression, motor impairment, tolerance, and glial activation relative to morphine. Neuropharmacology. 2016;105:215–27.

45. Yamamoto T, Ohtori S, Chiba T. Effects of pre-emptively administered nociceptin on the development of thermal hyperalgesia induced by two models of experimental mononeuropathy in the rat. Brain Res. 2000;871:192–200.

46. Woolf CJ, Chong MS. Preemptive analgesia--treating postoperative pain by preventing the establishment of central sensitization. Anesth Analg. 1993;77:362–79.

47. Przewlocki R, Hassan AH, Lason W, Epplen C, Herz A, Stein C. Gene expression and localization of opioid peptides in immune cells of inflamed tissue: functional role in antinociception. Neuroscience. 1992;48:491–500.

48. Sakurada S, Hayashi T, Yuhki M, Orito T, Zadina JE, Kastin AJ, Fujimura T, Murayama K, Sakurada C, Sakurada T, et al. Differential antinociceptive effects induced by intrathecally administered endomorphin-1 and endomorphin-2 in the mouse. Eur J Pharmacol. 2001;427:203–10.

49. Puehler W, Zollner C, Brack A, Shaqura MA, Krause H, Schafer M, Stein C. Rapid upregulation of mu opioid receptor mRNA in dorsal root ganglia in response to peripheral inflammation depends on neuronal conduction. Neuroscience. 2004;129:473–9.

50. Jin SX, Zhuang ZY, Woolf CJ, Ji RR. p38 mitogen-activated protein kinase is activated after a spinal nerve ligation in spinal cord microglia and dorsal root ganglion neurons and contributes to the generation of neuropathic pain. J Neurosci. 2003;23:4017–22.

51. Tsuda M, Mizokoshi A, Shigemoto-Mogami Y, Koizumi S, Inoue K. Activation of p38 mitogen-activated protein kinase in spinal hyperactive microglia contributes to pain hypersensitivity following peripheral nerve injury. Glia. 2004;45:89–95.

52. Zhuang ZY, Gerner P, Woolf CJ, Ji RR. ERK is sequentially activated in neurons, microglia, and astrocytes by spinal nerve ligation and contributes to mechanical allodynia in this neuropathic pain model. Pain. 2005;114:149–59.

53. Macey TA, Lowe JD, Chavkin C. Mu opioid receptor activation of ERK1/2 is GRK3 and arrestin dependent in striatal neurons. J Biol Chem. 2006;281:34515–24.

54. Belcheva MM, Haas PD, Tan Y, Heaton VM, Coscia CJ. The fibroblast growth factor receptor is at the site of convergence between mu-opioid receptor and growth factor signaling pathways in rat C6 glioma cells. J Pharmacol Exp Ther. 2002;303:909–18.

55. Messmer D, Hatsukari I, Hitosugi N, Schmidt-Wolf IGH, Singhal PC. Morphine reciprocally regulates IL-10 and IL-12 production by monocyte-derived human dendritic cells and enhances T cell activation. Mol Med. 2006;12:284–90.

56. Ji RR, Nackley A, Huh Y, Terrando N, Maixner W. Neuroinflammation and central sensitization in chronic and widespread pain. Anesthesiology. 2018;129:343–66.

57. Ji RR, Xu ZZ, Gao YJ. Emerging targets in neuroinflammation-driven chronic pain. Nat Rev Drug Discov. 2014;13:533–48.

58. DeLeo JA, Yezierski RP. The role of neuroinflammation and neuroimmune activation in persistent pain. Pain. 2001;90:1–6.

59. Hanisch UK. Microglia as a source and target of cytokines. Glia. 2002;40:140–55.

60. Xu JT, Xin WJ, Zang Y, Wu CY, Liu XG. The role of tumor necrosis factor-alpha in the neuropathic pain induced by lumbar 5 ventral root transection in rat. Pain. 2006;123:306–21.

61. Sweitzer S, Martin D, DeLeo JA. Intrathecal interleukin-1 receptor antagonist in combination with soluble tumor necrosis factor receptor exhibits an anti-allodynic action in a rat model of neuropathic pain. Neuroscience. 2001;103:529–39.

62. Ji RR, Berta T, Nedergaard M. Glia and pain: is chronic pain a gliopathy? Pain. 2013;154(Suppl 1):S10–28.

63. Kiguchi N, Maeda T, Kobayashi Y, Fukazawa Y, Kishioka S. Macrophage inflammatory protein-1alpha mediates the development of neuropathic pain following peripheral nerve injury through interleukin-1beta up-regulation. Pain. 2010;149:305–15.

64. Old EA, Nadkarni S, Grist J, Gentry C, Bevan S, Kim KW, Mogg AJ, Perretti M, Malcangio M. Monocytes expressing CX3CR1 orchestrate the development of vincristine-induced pain. J Clin Invest. 2014;124:2023–36.

65. Melik Parsadaniantz S, Rivat C, Rostene W, Reaux-Le Goazigo A. Opioid and chemokine receptor crosstalk: a promising target for pain therapy? Nat Rev Neurosci. 2015;16:69–78.

13

Innate immune activation of astrocytes impairs neurodevelopment via upregulation of follistatin-like 1 and interferon-induced transmembrane protein 3

Shinnosuke Yamada[1][†], Norimichi Itoh[1][†], Taku Nagai[1][†], Tsuyoshi Nakai[1], Daisuke Ibi[2], Akira Nakajima[3], Toshitaka Nabeshima[4] and Kiyofumi Yamada[1]*

Abstract

Background: Polyriboinosinic-polyribocytidylic acid (polyI:C) triggers a strong innate immune response that mimics immune activation by viral infections. Induction of interferon-induced transmembrane protein 3 (Ifitm3) in astrocytes has a crucial role in polyI:C-induced neurodevelopmental abnormalities. Through a quantitative proteomic screen, we previously identified candidate astroglial factors, such as matrix metalloproteinase-3 (Mmp3) and follistatin-like 1 (Fstl1), in polyI:C-induced neurodevelopmental impairment. Here, we characterized the Ifitm3-dependent inflammatory processes focusing on astrocyte-derived Fstl1 following polyI:C treatment to assess the neuropathologic role of Fstl1.

Methods: Astrocytes were treated with PBS (control) or polyI:C (10 μg/mL). The conditioned medium was collected 24 h after the polyI:C treatment and used as astrocyte condition medium (ACM). The expression of Fstl1 mRNA and extracellular Fstl1 protein levels were analyzed by quantitative PCR and western blotting, respectively. For functional studies, neurons were treated with ACM and the effects of ACM on dendritic elongation were assayed. To examine the role of Fstl1, recombinant Fstl1 protein and siRNA for Fstl1 were used. To investigate the expression of Fstl1 in vivo, neonatal mice were treated with vehicle or polyI:C on postnatal day 2 to 6.

Results: ACM prepared with polyI:C (polyI:C ACM) contained significantly higher Fstl1 protein than control ACM, but no increase in Fstl1 was observed in polyI:C ACM derived from Ifitm3-deficient astrocytes. We found that the production of Fstl1 involves the inflammatory responsive molecule Ifitm3 in astrocytes and influences neuronal differentiation. In agreement, the levels of Fstl1 increased in the hippocampus of polyI:C-treated neonatal mice. COS7 cells co-transfected with both Fstl1 and Ifitm3 had higher extracellular levels of Fstl1 than the cells transfected with Fstl1 alone. Treatment of primary cultured hippocampal neurons with recombinant Fstl1 impaired dendritic elongation, and the deleterious effect of polyI:C ACM on dendritic elongation was attenuated by knockdown of Fstl1 in astrocytes.

Conclusions: The extracellular level of Fstl1 is regulated by Ifitm3 in astrocytes, which could be involved in polyI:C-induced neurodevelopmental impairment.

Keywords: Astrocyte, Fstl1, Ifitm3, Immune response, Neuron, polyI:C, Schizophrenia, Viral infection

* Correspondence: kyamada@med.nagoya-u.ac.jp
[†]Shinnosuke Yamada, Norimichi Itoh and Taku Nagai contributed equally to this work.
[1]Department of Neuropsychopharmacology and Hospital Pharmacy, Nagoya University Graduate School of Medicine, 65 Turumai-cho, Showa-ku, Nagoya, Aichi 466-8560, Japan
Full list of author information is available at the end of the article

Background

Immune activation in the CNS is associated with the pathophysiology and/or etiology of psychiatric disorders. For example, inflammatory cytokine levels are altered in the serum of schizophrenia patients [1, 2]. Pro- and anti-inflammatory cytokines in patients with major depressive disorders are inversely correlated with severity and symptoms of major depression [3]. Epidemiological evidence also indicates that the risk of schizophrenia increases in offspring born from mothers infected during pregnancy [4–6]. Although much evidence suggests that reactive astrocytes induced by inflammatory cytokines are involved in neurodevelopmental disorders [7, 8], the underlying molecular mechanism is largely unknown.

Interferon-induced transmembrane protein 3 (Ifitm3) is induced by inflammatory cytokines such as interferon-β, interleukin (IL)-6, and tumor necrosis factor (TNF)-α. Ifitm3 acts as an antiviral factor by restricting virus entry [9–12]. Recent studies have indicated that Ifitm3 expression is increased in patients with schizophrenia [13–15]. Previously, we have reported that Ifitm3 expression in astrocytes is associated with neurodevelopmental impairment and contributes to brain dysfunction in mice that received daily polyI:C injection from postnatal day 2 to day 6 [16]. We also found that humoral factors released from polyI:C-treated astrocytes have crucial roles in Ifitm3-dependent impairment of neuronal maturation of cultured neurons [17]. For instance, matrix metalloprotease-3 (Mmp3) is released by polyI:C-treated astrocytes and impairs neuronal maturation [18]. In addition to Mmp3, we have identified several candidates of humoral factors including follistatin like-1 (Fstl1) by proteomic analysis [18].

To investigate the regulation of Fstl1 production and release, we monitored extracellular levels of Fstl1 protein in astrocyte cultures, which were stimulated with polyI:C or prepared from Ifitm3 knockout (KO) mice. We found that an immune activation induced by polyI:C upregulates Fstl1 mRNA expression in astrocytes, and that polyI:C-treated astrocytes have increased extracellular protein levels of Fstl1. Notably, in astrocytes from Ifitm3 KO mice, polyI:C treatment failed to increase the extracellular Fstl1 level. We also demonstrated that recombinant Fstl1 impaired dendritic neurite outgrowth of cultured hippocampal neurons, but knockdown of Fstl1 partially rescued polyI:C-induced impairment of neurite elongation. These results suggest that Fstl1 has an important role in Ifitm3-dependent neuronal impairment.

Methods

Animals

C57BL/6J mice were purchased from Japan SLC Inc. (Hamamatsu, Japan). Homozygous *Ifitm3*$^{-/-}$ [Ifitm3 KO] mice were generated and characterized as described previously [19]. The animals had free access to food (CE-2, Clea Japan, Tokyo, Japan) and water and were kept under controlled conditions (23 ± 1 °C) with a constant light-dark cycle (light 9:00–21:00). All animals were handled in accordance with the guidelines established by the Institutional Animal Care and Use Committee of Nagoya University, the Guiding Principles for the Care and Use of Laboratory Animals approved by the Japanese Pharmacological Society, and the National Institutes of Health Guide for the Care and Use of Laboratory Animals.

Astrocyte culture and astrocyte-conditioned medium (ACM) preparation

Secondary astrocyte cultures were prepared as described previously [18]. Briefly, cortices and hippocampi of neonatal mice at postnatal day (PD) 1–2 were mechanically dissociated and digested with 0.3% dispase (Roche Diagnostics GmbH, Mannheim, Germany) and 0.4% DNase (Roche Diagnostics GmbH). The cells were suspended in Dulbecco's modified Eagle's medium (DMEM, Sigma-Aldrich, St. Louis, MO) containing 10% fetal bovine serum (FBS, Gibco-BRL, Gaithersburg, MD) and filtered through a 40 μm nylon cell strainer (Falcon-Becton Dickinson, Le Pont de Claix, France). The cell suspension was cultured in a T150 flask at a density of six neonate brains per flask at 37 °C with 5% CO_2. Confluent primary astrocyte cultures were purified by shaking, plated onto 6-well plates, and grown to confluence in all experiments. Under these conditions, more than 95% of cells were glial fibrillary acidic protein (GFAP)-positive (a marker for astrocytes) and negative for tau/MAP2 and CD11b (neuronal and microglial markers, respectively). Culture medium was replaced with Neurobasal Medium (Invitrogen, Eugene, OR) supplemented with B-27 (Invitrogen) and 1 mM glutamine (Sigma-Aldrich) 6 days before treatment with polyI:C (Sigma-Aldrich). This medium was replaced 3 days before and 24 h before treatment with polyI:C. For western blotting, B-27 was excluded from the last medium. Astrocytes were treated with PBS (control) or polyI:C (10 μg/mL), and conditioned medium was collected 24 h after the polyI:C treatment. For the time course analysis, conditioned medium was collected 6 h and 12 h after polyI:C treatment. Conditioned media were centrifuged at 1000×g for 10 min at 4 °C, and the supernatants were used as ACM.

Microglia culture and microglia-conditioned medium (MCM) preparation

2 weeks after seeding primary astrocyte cultures, microglia were separated from the underlying astrocytic monolayer by shaking for 3 h at 150 rpm. The supernatants, including floating microglia, were centrifuged at 1000 rpm for 10 min and the pellet was resuspended in

fresh culture medium. Microglia were plated at 1×10^6 cells/well in a 6-well plate and culture medium was replaced with neurobasal medium supplemented with 1 mM glutamine 1 h after plating. The microglial cultures were > 98% pure as assessed by immunocytochemistry with an anti-Iba1 antibody (Wako, Osaka, Japan) in combination with an anti-GFAP antibody (Sigma-Aldrich) as markers for microglia and astrocytes, respectively. PBS (control) or polyI:C (10 μg/mL) were added 24 h after medium change, and conditioned media were collected 24 h after polyI:C treatment. Conditioned media were centrifuged at 1000×g for 10 min at 4 °C, and the supernatants were used as MCM.

Fstl1 and Ifitm3 transfection for COS7 cells

Myc-tagged mouse Fstl1 expression vector was purchased from OriGene Technologies (Rockville, MD), and myc-tagged mouse Ifitm3 vector was generated as described previously [17]. Control (mock) vector was generated by the removal of cDNA sequence from the cloning site of the expression vector using the appropriate restriction enzyme, then blunt-ended and ligated. The day before transfection, trypsinized COS7 cells were plated at 40×10^4 cells per well (6-well plate). Each well was transfected with 1.25 μg myc-tagged mouse Ifitm3 and Fstl1 or control vectors using Lipofectamine LTX (Invitrogen) and Opti-MEM I Reduced Serum Medium (Invitrogen). 6 h after transfection, growth medium was replaced with 2 mL of MEM without FBS and antibiotics. Conditioned medium and cell lysate samples for western blotting were prepared 30 h after transfection as described in the "Astrocyte culture and astrocyte-conditioned medium (ACM) preparation" section. Recombinant mouse Fstl1 (rmFstl1) was prepared from conditioned medium after transfection of 2.5 μg myc-tagged mouse Fstl1 expression vector. 30 h after transfection, secreted Fstl1 was purified using c-myc tagged Protein Mild Purification Kit ver.2 (MBL, Nagoya, Japan) according to the manufacturer's instructions. Protein concentration was determined using a protein assay kit (Bio-Rad Laboratories, Hercules, CA, USA).

Primary cultured neurons and ACM treatment

Primary cultured hippocampal neurons were prepared from C57BL/6J mice on gestational day 15–16 as described previously [18]. Briefly, embryo hippocampi were trypsinized (with 0.25% trypsin and 0.01% DNase) followed by trituration and seeded on coverslips precoated with 0.1 mg/mL poly-D-lysine at a low density (1.0×10^4 cells/well in a 24-well plate). Cells were cultured in Neurobasal Medium with B-27 and 1 mM glutamine. The medium was replaced with polyI:C ACM or control ACM and supplemented with 0.75 μm cytosine β-D-arabinofuranoside (Ara-C, Sigma-Aldrich) on DIV2.

For functional studies, rmFstl1 was added to control ACM or culture medium (Neurobasal Medium supplemented with B-27 and 1 mM glutamine) at the final concentrations of 10 nM, 50 nM, 100 nM, or 300 nM on DIV2. The effects of ACM on dendritic elongation were assayed on DIV7. More than 99% pure neurons, as evaluated by anti-tau or anti-MAP2 immunostaining, were obtained from this preparation.

Knockdown assay

siRNA transfection was performed 6 h before the last medium change. Astrocytes were transfected with Stealth siRNA for Fstl1 (#1 sense: GCCCAGUUGUCUGCUAUCAAGCUAA, #1 antisense: UUAGCUUGAUAGCAGACAACUGGGC; #2 sense: CCUAGACAAGUACUUUAAGAGCUUU, #2 antisense: AAAGCUCUUAAAGUACUUGUCUAGG) or Stealth RNAi siRNA negative control (control siRNA) using Lipofectamine RNAiMAX transfection reagent (all from Invitrogen).

Western blotting

ACM and MCM were concentrated using Vivaspin 2 Hydrosart 5000 MWCO (Sartorius Stedim Biotech GmbH). After removing the conditioned medium, the remaining cells were washed with ice-cold PBS and collected in lysis buffer [20 mM Tris-HCl (pH 7.4), 150 mM NaCl, 50 mM NaF, 2 mM EDTA, 1% Triton X-100, 1 mM sodium orthovanadate, 0.1% SDS, 1% sodium deoxycholate and protease inhibitor cocktail (Sigma-Aldrich)]. Protein lysates were centrifuged at 15,000×g for 20 min. ACM or cell lysates were denatured in Laemmli sample buffer containing 20% β-mercaptoethanol at 95 °C for 5 min. An equal amount of protein for each sample was separated by 10% SDS-PAGE and transferred to a polyvinylidene fluoride (PVDF) membrane (Millipore). The membrane was blocked with detector block solution (KPL, Gaithersburg, MD). The membrane was incubated with goat anti-Fstl1 antibody (R&D Systems, Minneapolis, MN) or goat anti-actin antibody (Santa Cruz Biotechnology, Santa Cruz, CA) at 4 °C overnight. After incubation with horseradish peroxidase-conjugated secondary anti-goat antibody (R&D Systems) for 2 h, the membrane was incubated with ECL prime western blotting detection reagents (GE Healthcare) and protein bands were detected using a luminescent image analyzer (Atto, Tokyo, Japan).

Total RNA isolation and real-time RT-PCR

After removing the conditioned medium, total RNA of astrocytes and microglia were prepared using RNeasy Mini Kit (Qiagen, Hilden, Germany) and converted into complementary DNA (cDNA) using the SuperScript III First-Strand Synthesis Kit (Invitrogen). Quantitative real-time PCR was performed on a 7300 Real-Time PCR

System (Applied Biosystems, Foster City, CA) using Power SYBR Green Master Mix (Applied Biosystems) according to the manufacturer's protocol. The primers used were as follows: forward, GCCTATGCCTACTCCGTGAAGT and reverse, GCCTGGGCTCCAGTCACAT for Ifitm3; forward, CACCAGGGCACAGCAGAAA and reverse, GTGCTCTGTGCCTCTTCTTAGATCT for Fstl1; and forward, CGATGCCCTGAGGCTCTTT and reverse, TGGATGCCACAGGATTCCA for β-actin used as an internal control. Real-time PCR reactions were conducted as follows: initial 2 min incubation at 50 °C and 10 min incubation at 95 °C, followed by 40 reaction cycles of 95 °C for 15 s and 60 °C for 1 min. Fluorescent signals were monitored at the extension step of 60 °C in each cycle. For each sample test, each PCR reaction had two replicates and the relative gene expression differences were quantified using the comparative Ct method ($^{\Delta\Delta}$Ct).

Immunocytochemistry

Cells were fixed in 4% paraformaldehyde in 0.1 M phosphate buffer (pH 7.4) for 20 min and then permeabilized with 0.1% Triton X-100 for 10 min. After incubation in blocking solution (1% goat and 1% donkey serum in PBS) for 30 min, mouse anti-tau (1:500, Santa Cruz Biotechnology) and rabbit anti-MAP2 (1:1000, Millipore) antibodies diluted in blocking solution were added to the cells. After overnight incubation with primary antibodies at 4 °C, the cells were treated with goat anti-mouse Alexa Fluor (AF) 488 and anti-rabbit AF568 antibodies (1:1,000, Invitrogen) for 2 h at room temperature. The cells were mounted in fluorescence mounting medium (Dako, Glostrup, Denmark) and photographed under a fluorescence microscope (Zeiss, Jena, Germany) using AxioCam MRc5 (Zeiss).

Dendritic elongation assay

Dendritic elongation of cultured hippocampal neurons was analyzed in accordance with a previous study [18]. Axons were identified by double immunostaining in terms of tau-positive (axonal marker) and MAP2-negative (dendritic marker), and only MAP2-positive neurites were defined as dendrites. Neurons that clearly had tau- or MAP2-positive neurites were selected randomly by an expert researcher who was blinded to the experimental groups. Dendrites were traced automatically with the same configuration using Neurolucida software (MicroBrightField, Williston, VT) and total dendritic length in a single neuron was calculated using Neuroexplorer (MicroBrightField). This assay was performed for three independent experiments.

Immunohistochemistry (IHC) for polyI:C-treated neonatal mice

All litters from C57BL/6J mice were randomly divided into two groups: vehicle- and polyI:C-treated. Neonatal C57BL/6J mice were administered with a daily subcutaneous injection of saline (control) or polyI:C (5 mg/kg, Sigma-Aldrich) between PD2 and PD6. Immunohistochemistry was conducted as described previously [17]. Neonatal mice were deeply anesthetized with diethyl ether 24 h after the final polyI:C treatment and perfused transcardially with saline, followed by 4% paraformaldehyde in phosphate-buffered saline (PBS, pH 7.4). The brains were removed and cryoprotected. 20-μm-thick coronal brain sections were cut on a cryostat and mounted on slides. The sections were denatured in a microwave oven in 0.01 M citrate buffer (pH 6.0). After blocking with 5% donkey and 5% goat serum/PBS, mouse anti-glial fibrillary acidic protein (GFAP, a marker for astrocytes, 1:1,000, Sigma-Aldrich) and rat anti-Fstl1 (1:100, R&D systems) were added to the sections. After washing in PBS, goat anti-mouse Alexa Fluor (AF) 568 and anti-rat AF488 antibodies (1:1,000, Invitrogen) were added to the sections. The samples were observed using a confocal-laser scanning microscope (LSM 700 Axio Imager; Zeiss).

Statistical analysis

Data are shown as the mean ± SE. Differences between two groups were analyzed by two-tailed Student's t test and the data distribution was tested for normality with Shapiro-Wilk test. One-way and two-way analyses of variance (ANOVA) followed by Bonferroni post hoc test was applied for differences in three or more groups.

Results

We previously reported that Fstl1 was a candidate molecule responsible for polyI:C-induced neurodevelopmental impairment, and that depletion of Ifitm3 in astrocytes attenuated polyI:C ACM-induced neurodevelopmental impairment [17, 18]. We compared changes in Fstl1 protein levels between WT and Ifitm3 KO astrocytes after polyI:C treatment (Fig. 1a). Two-way ANOVA revealed significant main effects of polyI:C treatment on Fstl1 protein levels in both cell lysates (polyI:C treatment: $F(1,8) = 28.80$, $p < 0.01$; genotype: $F(1,8) = 0.22$, $p = 0.65$; interaction of polyI:C treatment and genotype: $F(1,8) = 0.01$, $p = 0.94$, Fig. 1b) and ACM (polyI:C treatment: $F(1,8) = 66.09$, $p < 0.01$; genotype: $F(1,8) = 37.21$, $p < 0.01$); with an interaction of polyI:C treatment and genotype: ($F(1,8) = 23.77$, $p < 0.01$, Fig. 1c). PolyI:C treatment significantly increased Fstl1 protein levels in the cell lysates of both WT and Ifitm3 KO astrocytes ($p < 0.05$) (Fig. 1b). Notably, polyI:C treatment significantly increased Fstl1 levels in ACM from WT astrocytes but had no effect on extracellular Fstl1 levels in ACM from Ifitm3 KO astrocytes (Fig. 1c). To examine the influence of Ifitm3 expression on extracellular Fstl1 levels, COS7 cells were co-transfected with Fstl1 and Ifitm3. Fstl1 in COS7 cell lysates was not affected by

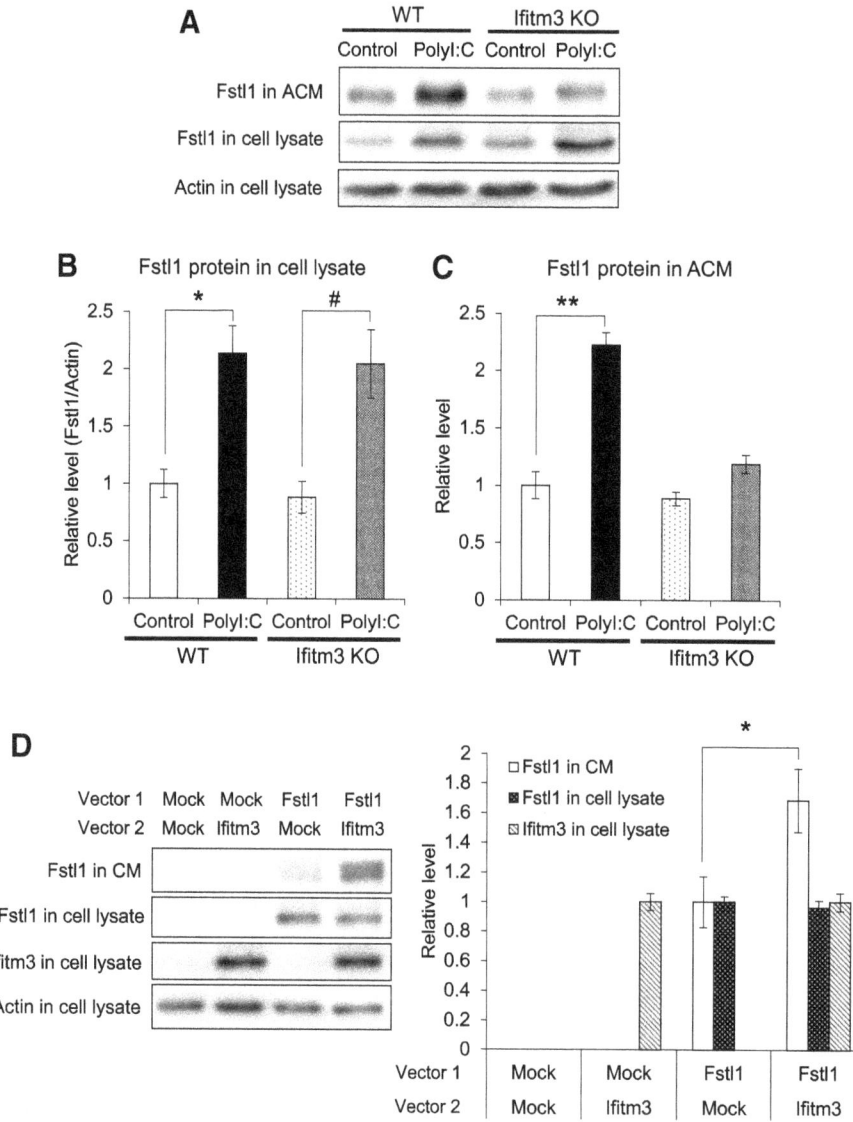

Fig. 1 Ifitm3 regulates the extracellular level of Fstl1. **a** Representative western blot images of Fstl1 protein expression in cell lysates and ACM derived from WT and Ifitm3 KO astrocytes 24 h after polyI:C treatment. **b, c** Fstl1 protein levels in cell lysates (**b**) and ACM (**c**) derived from WT and Ifitm3 KO astrocytes after polyI:C treatment. Values indicate the means ± SE ($n = 3$). *$p < 0.05$, #$p < 0.05$, and **$p < 0.01$ versus the respective control treatment. **d** The extracellular level of Fstl1 in conditioned medium after Fstl1 and Ifitm3 overexpression. COS7 cells were co-transfected with Fstl1, Ifitm3, and control vectors (mock) as indicated respectively. Overexpression of Ifitm3 increased Fstl1 protein in CM without affecting Fstl1 expression in COS7 cell lysates. Data show the mean ± SE ($n = 6$). *$p < 0.05$ versus Fstl1/mock. CM, conditioned medium

overexpression of Ifitm3. On the other hand, Fstl1 levels in conditioned medium (CM) from COS7 cells co-transfected with Fstl1 and Ifitm3 were markedly higher than the levels from Fstl1 alone transfection ($p < 0.05$, Fig. 1d). These results suggest that the Fstl1 release is regulated by Ifitm3.

Because microglia are immunocompetent cells in the CNS, it is possible that microglia also play a similar role in the polyI:C-triggered glial inflammatory response. Accordingly, we examined the mRNA expression of Fstl1 and Ifitm3 in astrocytes and microglia. A two-way ANOVA revealed significant effects of polyI:C treatment on Ifitm3 mRNA levels in astrocyte and microglia cell lysates

(polyI:C treatment: $F(1,12) = 188.0$, $p < 0.01$; cell type: $F(1,12) = 19.91$, $p < 0.01$; interaction of polyI:C treatment and cell type: $F(1,12) = 0.36$, $p = 0.56$, Fig. 2a). In contrast, there were significant interactions between cell type and polyI:C treatment on Fstl1 mRNA levels (polyI:C treatment: $F(1,12) = 25.84$, $p < 0.01$; cell type: $F(1,12) = 127.8$, $p < 0.01$; interaction of polyI:C treatment and cell type: $F(1,12) = 28.04$, $p < 0.01$, Fig. 2b). A multiple-comparison test with Bonferroni post hoc tests indicated that polyI:C treatment induced the expression of Fstl1 mRNA in astrocytes, but not in microglia ($p < 0.01$, Fig. 2b). Furthermore, Fstl1 protein was not detected in MCM with or without

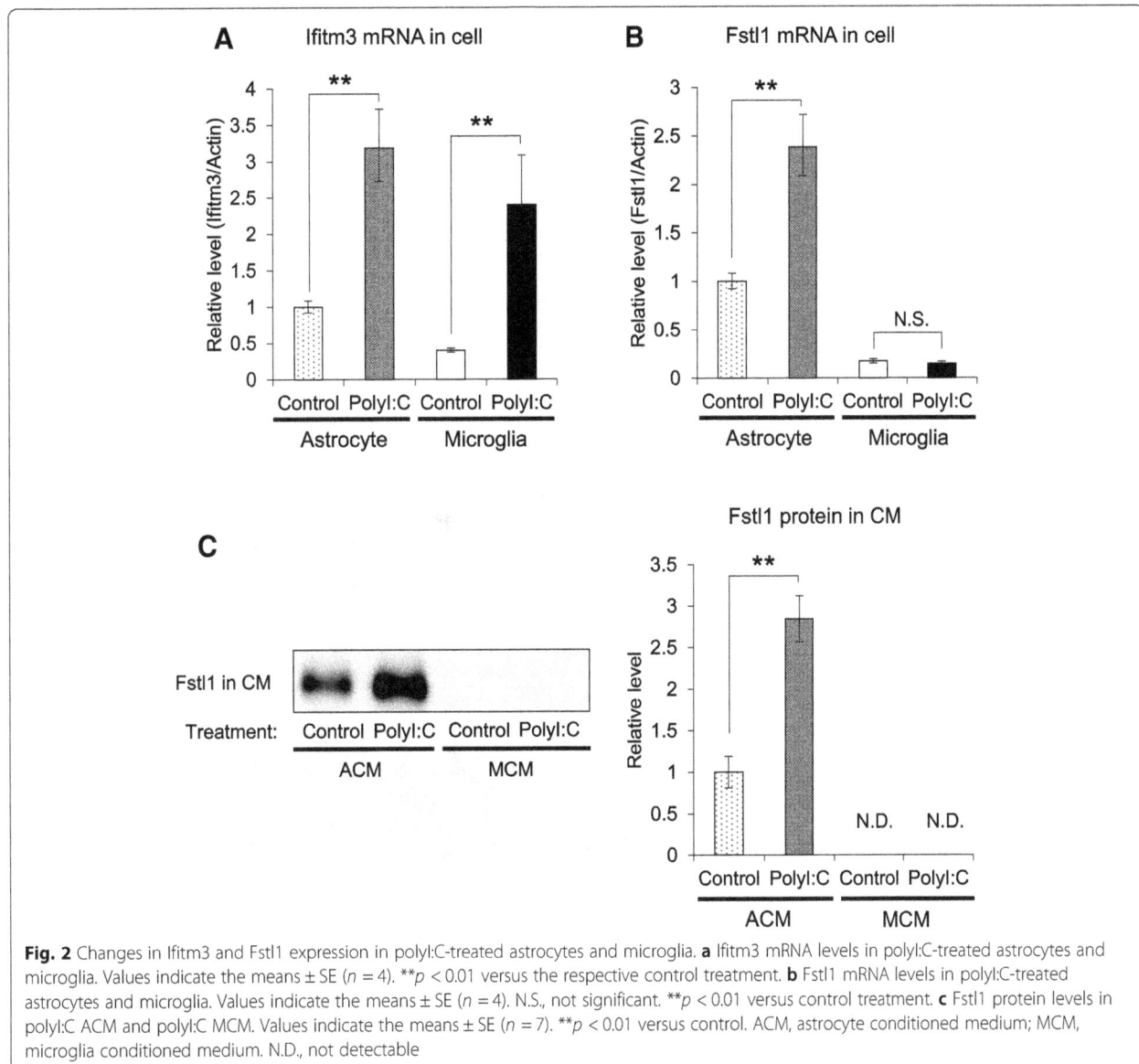

Fig. 2 Changes in Ifitm3 and Fstl1 expression in polyI:C-treated astrocytes and microglia. **a** Ifitm3 mRNA levels in polyI:C-treated astrocytes and microglia. Values indicate the means ± SE ($n = 4$). **$p < 0.01$ versus the respective control treatment. **b** Fstl1 mRNA levels in polyI:C-treated astrocytes and microglia. Values indicate the means ± SE ($n = 4$). N.S., not significant. **$p < 0.01$ versus control treatment. **c** Fstl1 protein levels in polyI:C ACM and polyI:C MCM. Values indicate the means ± SE ($n = 7$). **$p < 0.01$ versus control. ACM, astrocyte conditioned medium; MCM, microglia conditioned medium. N.D., not detectable

polyI:C treatment, while Fstl1 protein levels were significantly increased in polyI:C ACM compared to that of the control ($p < 0.01$, Fig. 2c). These results suggest that Fstl1 is induced by polyI:C treatment in astrocytes but not in microglia, and thereby microglia may not play a role in the regulation of extracellular Fstl1 level.

We previously found that polyI:C-treated ACM impairs dendritic elongation of cultured hippocampal neurons [17]. Therefore, the role of Fstl1 in dendritic elongation was assessed using an RNA interference method. The effect of siRNA was confirmed by western blotting. When primary cultured astrocytes were transfected with control, Fstl1 #1 or #2 siRNA, the expression levels of Fstl1 in #1 or #2 siRNA were significantly decreased to 34% and 22% of control siRNA transfected cell (Additional file 1: Figure S1). Under this condition,

Fstl1 protein levels in ACM were significantly increased by polyI:C treatment ($F(3,12) = 14.09$, $p < 0.01$, Fig. 3a). When astrocytes were transfected with either Fstl1 siRNA #1 or #2 to down-regulate Fstl1 expression, polyI:C failed to increase extracellular Fstl1 protein levels in ACM, and the levels were similar to those in control ACM ($F(3,12) = 14.09$, $p < 0.01$, Fig. 3a). To assess whether Fstl1 plays a negative role in neurite elongation, we measured dendrite length of primary cultured hippocampal neurons which were cultured with the ACM derived from either control or siRNA-treated astrocytes. PolyI:C-treated ACM impaired the dendritic elongation of cultured hippocampal neurons in control siRNA-transfected groups. This impairment was partially attenuated when astrocytes were transfected with either Fstl1 siRNA #1 or #2 ($F(3,174) = 92.53$, $p < 0.01$, Fig. 3b).

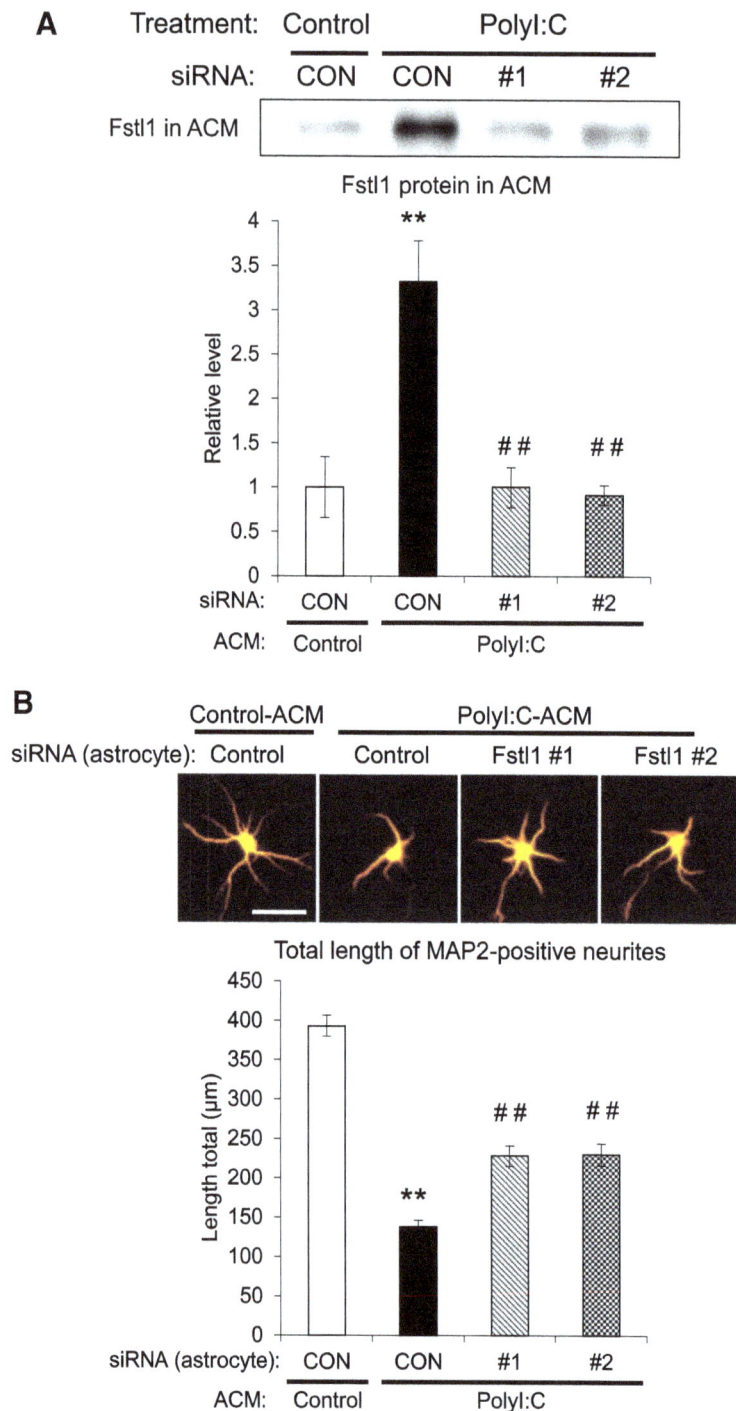

Fig. 3 Effect of Fstl1 knockdown in astrocytes on polyI:C ACM-induced impairment of neuronal development. Astrocytes were transfected with control siRNA (CON), Fstl1 siRNA #1 (#1), or Fstl1 siRNA #2 (#2) before polyI:C or vehicle treatment, and then ACM and cell lysate samples were prepared 24 h after polyI:C treatment. **a** Representative western blot images of Fstl1 protein levels in ACM derived from siRNA-treated astrocytes. Values indicate the means ± SE ($n = 4$). **$p < 0.01$ versus control ACM, ##$p < 0.01$ versus control siRNA-treated polyI:C ACM. **b** Effect of polyI:C ACM derived from Fstl1 knockdown astrocytes on MAP2-positive dendrite length of primary cultured neurons (DIV7). Neurons were cultured for 5 days (DIV2-7) with control ACM or polyI:C ACM derived from astrocytes transfected with control siRNA (CON) or Fstl1 siRNA (#1 or #2). Values indicate the means ± SE of more than three independent experiments ($n = 28$–59 neurons). **$p < 0.01$ versus control ACM, ##$p < 0.01$ versus control siRNA-treated polyI:C ACM. Scale bar, 50 µm

We further examined whether Fstl1 protein could mimic the above deleterious effect of polyI:C ACM. Addition of recombinant mouse Fstl1 protein to control ACM on DIV2 resulted in a concentration-dependent decrease in dendrite length of primary cultured neurons assayed on DIV7 ($F(3,203) = 22.08$, $p < 0.01$, Fig. 4a). The decrease in dendrite length induced by rmFstl1 treatment was 12% (50 nM), 32% (100 nM), and 35% (300 nM) compared to that treated with control ACM alone, and a significant decrease of dendritic length was observed at more than 100 nM rmFstl1 ($p < 0.01$, Fig. 4a). Of note, the addition of 300 nM rmFstl1 to normal culture medium on DIV2 had no effect on dendritic elongation of primary cultured hippocampal neurons assayed on DIV7 (Fig. 4b). rmFstl1 treatment had no effect on branched number of neurites and viability of neurons (Additional files 2 and 3: Figures S2 and S3). These results suggest that Fstl1 itself may not directly inhibit the dendritic elongation of neurons but interrupt neurite elongation by cooperating with some factors in ACM.

Finally, the in vivo expression of Fstl1 in the hippocampus 24 h after neonatal polyI:C treatment was analyzed by IHC. The expression of Fstl1 was hardly detected in vehicle-treated control mice under the same experimental conditions (Fig. 5a). Fstl1 immunofluorescence was clearly observed in the hippocampus of polyI:C-treated mice, and the signal coincided with GFAP, a marker for astrocytes (Fig. 5a). Approximately, 60% of astrocytes were positive for Fstl1 in the hippocampus of polyI:C-treated mice (Fig. 5b). The co-expression of Fstl1 with Iftim3 in astrocyte was observed in the hippocampus of polyI:C-treated neonatal mice (Additional file 4: Figure S4). The expression level of Fstl1 in polyI:C-treated Ifitm3 KO mice was comparable to the level in polyI:C-treated WT mice (Additional file 5: Figure S5).

Discussion

We have previously demonstrated that mice received neonatal polyI:C treatment exhibit some characteristics of neurodevelopmental disorders including cognitive and emotional impairments in adulthood, which is accompanied by the decrease in spine density and dendrite complexity of pyramidal neurons in the frontal cortex [16, 17, 20]. PolyI:C treatment induces expression of several inflammation-related genes, and induction of these molecules plays a pivotal role in polyI:C-induced neuronal impairment. We have already demonstrated that Ifitm3 expression is increased by polyI:C treatment in astrocytes. Ifitm3 protein localizes to the early endosomes and reduces the endocytic activity of astrocytes, which may change the composition of the extracellular humoral factors. Ifitm3-mediated accumulation of humoral factors released from astrocytes is a determinant in polyI:C-induced neurodevelopmental impairment [17]. Mmp-3 is one of such humoral factors that contribute to the polyI:C-induced neuronal impairment [18].

In the present study, we demonstrated that extracellular Fstl1 level was also dramatically increased in

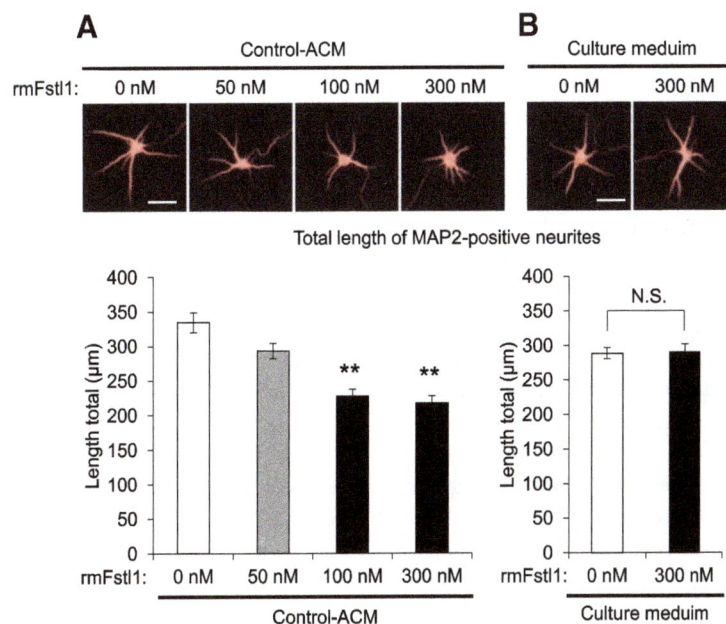

Fig. 4 Effect of Fstl1 on dendritic elongation of primary cultured neurons. Neurons were cultured for 5 days (DIV2–7) with control ACM or culture medium supplemented with the indicated concentration of rmFstl1 or vehicle. **a**, **b** MAP2-positive dendrite length of neurons cultured with control ACM (**a**) and culture medium (**b**) supplemented with the indicated doses of rmFstl1 or vehicle (DIV7). Values indicate the means ± SE of three independent experiments ($n = 49$–55 for control ACM and $n = 52$ for culture medium). **$p < 0.01$ versus vehicle-treated control ACM. Scale bar, 50 μm

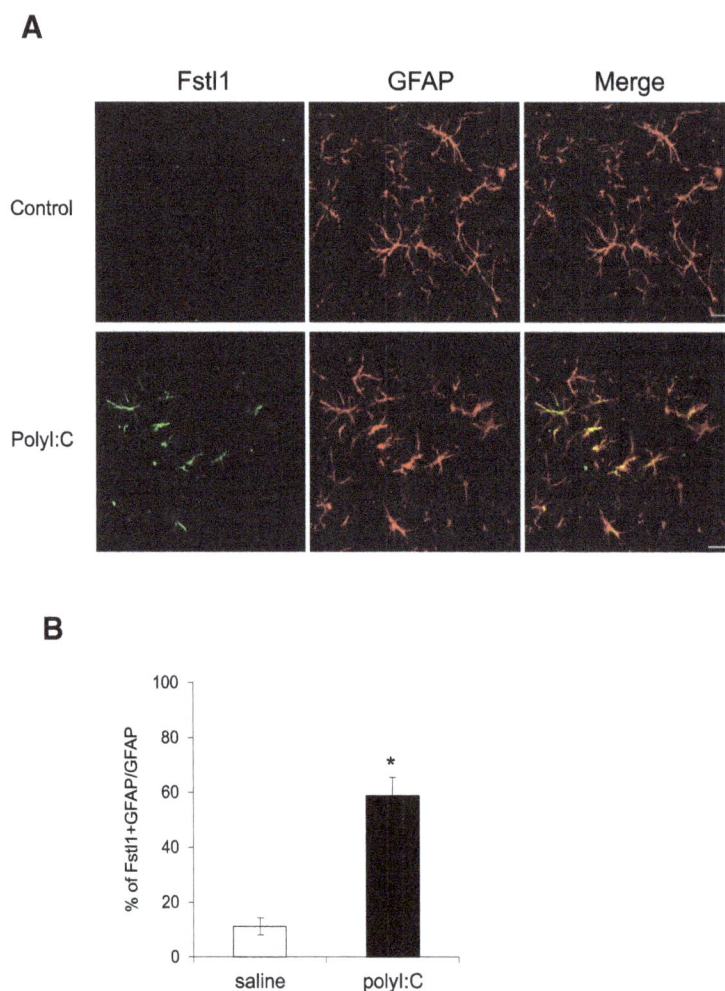

Fig. 5 In vivo expression of Fstl1 protein in PD7 neonates. Neonatal C57BL/6J mice were administered with a daily subcutaneous injection of saline (control) or polyl:C (5 mg/kg) between PD2 and PD6. **a** Hippocampal sections were isolated 24 h after the final drug treatment and Fstl1 (green) and GFAP (red, a marker for astrocytes) protein expressions were assessed by IHC. Scale bar, 10 μm. **b** Ratio of Fstl1- and GFAP-double positive cells versus GFAP positive cells was quantified. Values indicate the means ± SE of three independent experiments. *$p < 0.05$ versus control

polyI:C-treated astrocytes. We confirmed that Fstl1 is upregulated in polyI:C-treated astrocytes and acts as a humoral factor to impair neurite elongation of cultured neurons. PolyI:C stimulates toll-like receptor 3 (TLR3) signaling, which leads to production of inflammatory cytokines [17, 21], while the expression level of Fstl1 mRNA increases in response to inflammatory cytokines such as IL-1, IL-6, and TNF-α [22, 23]. Therefore, polyI:C may upregulate Fstl1 mRNA levels through the production of inflammatory cytokines.

Fstl1 is a glycoprotein that is secreted in response to inflammatory signals. Lipopolysaccharide (LPS) increases Fstl1 expression [24, 25]. In the present study, we demonstrated that the extracellular level of Fstl1 in cultured astrocytes was increased by polyI:C treatment, but such increase was attenuated in Ifitm3 KO astrocytes. Moreover, co-expression of Fstl1 and Ifitm3 in COS7 cells significantly increased the extracellular level of Fstl1 compared to the level in COS7 cells only expressing Fstl1 but not Ifitm3. We speculate that polyI:C treatment may increase the extracellular level of Fstl1 through the inhibitory effect of Ifitm3 of endocytic activity [17]. An alternative explanation is that Ifitm3 may affect membrane vesicle trafficking and secretion in astrocytes. Because neither the mRNA expression level nor were the intracellular protein level of Fstl1 affected by Ifitm3 expression, regulation of Fstl1 expression may be independent on Ifitm3 expression. Ifitm3-independent expression of Fstl1 was also demonstrated in vivo. Although we attempted to measure extracellular Fstl1 in mice, it has not been detected yet because of analytical limitation. Further study is needed to directly show that the increased extracellular Fstl1 is responsible for the polyI:C-induced neuronal impairment.

In addition to astrocytes, microglia are involved in the inflammation-related neuronal impairment [26, 27]. PolyI:C activates both astrocytes and microglia through activation of TLR3 [28, 29], which led us to hypothesize that Fstl1 expression would be increased not only in astrocytes but also in microglia, in response to polyI:C stimulation. The expression level of Ifitm3 mRNA was significantly increased by treatment with polyI:C both in cultured astrocytes and in cultured microglia. On the other hand, the expression level of Fstl1 mRNA was very limited in microglia compared to astrocytes, and not increased by polyI:C treatment in microglia. Furthermore, the extracellular Fstl1 protein of cultured microglia could not be detected either in the presence or absence of polyI:C treatment. These results suggest that the induction of Fstl1 in response to TLR3 activation by polyI:C may be a specific event in astrocytes, but not occur in microglia.

How does Fstl1 impair morphologic neuronal development? The role of Fstl1 is controversial because some findings suggest that Fstl1 functions as a pro-inflammation cytokine [24, 30–32], but others suggest a role as an anti-inflammatory cytokines [25, 33, 34]. Fstl1 protects cells from apoptosis in heat failure through Fstl1 receptor disco-interacting protein 2 (DIP2), which activates the Akt signaling pathway [35, 36]. Some reports suggest that Fstl1 works as a scavenger by sequestering bone morphogenetic protein (Bmp)-4, which results in blockage of BMP signaling during development [37–39]. The addition of both Fstl1 and ACM suppressed neurite outgrowth, but addition of Fstl1 alone did not. Co-treatment of Fstl1 with Bmp-4 unaffected to neurites elongation (Additional file 6: Figure S6). A possible explanation is that secreted Fstl1 from astrocytes may inhibit signals promoting neurite outgrowth BMP-independent manner. In DRG neurons, Fstl1 impairs neurite elongation through activation of Na/K-ATPase [40]. The similar mechanism might operate in the hippocampal neurons. In this study, we could not address the role of Fstl1 in vivo because of technical limitation; it is hard to manipulate gene expression specifically in astrocytes of neonatal mice. Thus, further studies are needed to disclose the role of Fstl1 in polyI:C-induced neuronal impairment.

The association of Fstl1 with neuropsychiatric disorders is unclear. Recently, a SNP in miR-198, whose expression is mutually exclusive to Fstl1, was found to be associated with schizophrenia [41–43]. We found that the expression of Ifitm3 increased the extracellular level of Fstl1, while other studies reported the increased expression of Ifitm3 in the brains of schizophrenia patients [13–15]. Taken together with our present findings, it is possible that Fstl1 may play a role in the pathophysiology of psychiatric disorders on downstream of Ifitm3.

Conclusions

From our findings, we conclude that the extracellular level of Fstl1 is regulated by Ifitm3 in astrocytes. However, Fstl1 itself may not directly inhibit the dendritic elongation of neurons but interrupt neurite elongation by cooperating with some factors in ACM.

Additional files

Additional file 1: Figure S1. Validation of Fslt1 knockdown, related to Fig. 3. Culture astrocytes were transfected with siRNA targeting for Fstl1 or control siRNA. Western blotting was performed with indicated antibodies. (PPTX 66 kb)

Additional file 2: Figure S2. Effect of rFstl1 treatment on neurite branch, related to Fig. 4. Neurons were treated with indicated concentration of rmFstl1 or vehicle. Branched number of neurites was counted. Values indicate the means ± SE (n = 26–36). (PPTX 46 kb)

Additional file 3: Figure S3. Effect of rFstl1 treatment on cell viability, related to Fig. 4. Neurons were treated with indicated concentration of rmFstl1 or vehicle. The cell viability of neurons was measured. Values indicate the means ± SE (n = 3). (PPTX 43 kb)

Additional file 4: Figure S4. Co-expression of Fstl1 with Ifitm3 in the hippocampus of polyI:C-treated neonatal mice, related to Fig. 5. Hippocampal sections prepared from mice treated with vehicle or polyI:C were immunostained with indicated antibodies. Scale bar, 20 μm. (PPTX 470 kb)

Additional file 5: Figure S5. Expression of Fstl1 in polyI:C-treated Ifitm3 KO mice, related to Fig. 5. Hippocampal brain slices prepared from vehicle- or polyI:C-treated Ifitm3 KO mice were immunostained with indicated antibodies. Scale bar, 20 μm. (PPTX 23832 kb)

Additional file 6: Figure S6. Combinatory treatment of rBmp4 with rFstl1, related to Fig. 4. Neurons were cultured for 5 days (DIV2-7) with culture medium supplemented with the indicated concentration of rmFstl1 and/or rBmp-4. MAP2-positive dendrite length of neurons was measured. Values indicate the means ± SE of three independent experiments. Scale bar, 50 μm. (PPTX 120 kb)

Abbreviations
ACM: Astrocyte conditioned medium; Bmp-4: Bone morphogenetic protein-4; CNS: Central nervous system; DIP2: Disco-interacting protein 2; Fstl1: Follistatin-like 1; GFAP: Glial fibrillary acidic protein; Ifitm3: Interferon-induced transmembrane protein 3; IHC: Immunohistochemistry; IL-6: Interleukin-6; LPS: Lipopolysaccharide; MCM: Microglia-conditioned medium; Mmp3: Matrix metalloproteinase 3; PolyI:C: Polyriboinosinic-polyribocytidylic acid; TLR3: Toll-like receptor 3; TNF-α: Tumor necrosis factor-α

Acknowledgements
We thank Dr. Ulrike C. Lange, David J. Adams, and Azim Surani for providing the Ifitm3 KO mouse. We also thank all members of Yamada Lab for their helpful discussions and support of this work.

Funding
This work was supported by the Japan Society for the Promotion of Science (JSPS) KAKENHI (Grant-in Aid for Scientific Research (B) 17H04031 to K.Y., 17H04252 to T. Nabeshima, 17H02220 to T. Nagai, Grant-in Aid for Challenging Exploratory Research 16K15201 to K.Y., 17K19483 to T. Nagai, Grant-in Aid for Scientific Research on Innovative Areas 24111518 to K.Y., Grant-in Aid for Young Scientists (B) 16K21080 to N.I.) and the Private University Research Branding Project from the Ministry of Education, Culture, Sports, Science, and Technology (MEXT), the Astellas Foundation for Research on Metabolic Disorders, The Hori Science and Arts Foundation, Grant for Biomedical Research from Smoking Research Foundation (SRF), the Uehara Memorial Foundation and partially supported by the Strategic Research Program for Brain Sciences, and Research on Regulatory Science of Pharmaceuticals and Medical Devices from Japan Agency for Medical Research and Development, AMED. The Pharmacological Research Foundation, Tokyo.

Authors' contributions

SY, TNagai, NI, and KY designed the study. SY, TNagai, and NI performed experiments and analyzed the data. SY, TNagai, NI, TNakai, DI, AN, TNabeshima, and KY analyzed and interpreted the data. SY, NI, TNagai, TNabeshima, and KY wrote the manuscript. All of the authors discussed the results and agreed on the content of the manuscript.

Competing interests

The authors declare that they have no competing interests.

Author details

[1]Department of Neuropsychopharmacology and Hospital Pharmacy, Nagoya University Graduate School of Medicine, 65 Turumai-cho, Showa-ku, Nagoya, Aichi 466-8560, Japan. [2]Department of Chemical Pharmacology, Faculty of Pharmaceutical Science, Meijo University, 150 Yagotoyama, Tenpaku-ku, Nagoya, Japan. [3]Faculty of Agriculture and Life Science, Hirosaki University, 3 Bunkyo-cho, Hirosaki, Aomori 036-8561, Japan. [4]Advanced Diagnostic System Research Laboratory, Fujita Health University, Graduate School of Health Science and Aino University, 1-98 Dengakugakubo, Kutsukake-cho, Toyoake, Aichi 470-1192, Japan.

References

1. Luo Y, He H, Zhang M, Huang X, Zhang J, Zhou Y, Liu X, Fan N. Elevated serum levels of TNF-alpha, IL-6 and IL-18 in chronic schizophrenic patients. Schizophr Res. 2014;159:556–7.
2. Stojanovic A, Martorell L, Montalvo I, Ortega L, Monseny R, Vilella E, Labad J. Increased serum interleukin-6 levels in early stages of psychosis: associations with at-risk mental states and the severity of psychotic symptoms. Psychoneuroendocrinology. 2014;41:23–32.
3. Schmidt FM, Schroder T, Kirkby KC, Sander C, Suslow T, Holdt LM, Teupser D, Hegerl U, Himmerich H. Pro- and anti-inflammatory cytokines, but not CRP, are inversely correlated with severity and symptoms of major depression. Psychiatry Res. 2016;239:85–91.
4. Brown AS, Begg MD, Gravenstein S, Schaefer CA, Wyatt RJ, Bresnahan M, Babulas VP, Susser ES. Serologic evidence of prenatal influenza in the etiology of schizophrenia. Arch Gen Psychiatry. 2004;61:774–80.
5. Khandaker GM, Zimbron J, Dalman C, Lewis G, Jones PB. Childhood infection and adult schizophrenia: a meta-analysis of population-based studies. Schizophr Res. 2012;139:161–8.
6. Khandaker GM, Zimbron J, Lewis G, Jones PB. Prenatal maternal infection, neurodevelopment and adult schizophrenia: a systematic review of population-based studies. Psychol Med. 2013;43:239–57.
7. Ibi D, Yamada K. Therapeutic targets for neurodevelopmental disorders emerging from animal models with perinatal immune activation. Int J Mol Sci. 2015;16:28218–29.
8. Koyama Y. Functional alterations of astrocytes in mental disorders: pharmacological significance as a drug target. Front Cell Neurosci. 2015;9:261.
9. Bailey CC, Zhong G, Huang IC, Farzan M. IFITM-family proteins: the cell's first line of antiviral defense. Annu Rev Virol. 2014;1:261–83.
10. Chesarino NM, McMichael TM, Yount JS. Regulation of the trafficking and antiviral activity of IFITM3 by post-translational modifications. Future Microbiol. 2014;9:1151–63.
11. Everitt AR, Clare S, Pertel T, John SP, Wash RS, Smith SE, Chin CR, Feeley EM, Sims JS, Adams DJ, Wise HM, Kane L, Goulding D, Digard P, Anttila V, Baillie JK, Walsh TS, Hume DA, Palotie A, Xue Y, Colonna V, Tyler-Smith C, Dunning J, Gordon SB, Gen II, Investigators M, Smyth RL, Openshaw PJ, Dougan G, Brass AL, Kellam P. IFITM3 restricts the morbidity and mortality associated with influenza. Nature. 2012;484:519–23.
12. Brass AL, Huang IC, Benita Y, John SP, Krishnan MN, Feeley EM, Ryan BJ, Weyer JL, van der Weyden L, Fikrig E, Adams DJ, Xavier RJ, Farzan M, Elledge SJ. The IFITM proteins mediate cellular resistance to influenza A H1N1 virus, West Nile virus, and dengue virus. Cell. 2009;139:1243–54.
13. Hwang Y, Kim J, Shin JY, Kim JI, Seo JS, Webster MJ, Lee D, Kim S. Gene expression profiling by mRNA sequencing reveals increased expression of immune/inflammation-related genes in the hippocampus of individuals with schizophrenia. Transl Psychiatry. 2013;3:e321.
14. Horvath S, Mirnics K. Immune system disturbances in schizophrenia. Biol Psychiatry. 2014;75:316–23.
15. Saetre P, Emilsson L, Axelsson E, Kreuger J, Lindholm E, Jazin E. Inflammation-related genes up-regulated in schizophrenia brains. BMC Psychiatry. 2007;7:46.
16. Ibi D, Nagai T, Kitahara Y, Mizoguchi H, Koike H, Shiraki A, Takuma K, Kamei H, Noda Y, Nitta A, Nabeshima T, Yoneda Y, Yamada K. Neonatal polyI:C treatment in mice results in schizophrenia-like behavioral and neurochemical abnormalities in adulthood. Neurosci Res. 2009;64:297–305.
17. Ibi D, Nagai T, Nakajima A, Mizoguchi H, Kawase T, Tsuboi D, Kano S, Sato Y, Hayakawa M, Lange UC, Adams DJ, Surani MA, Satoh T, Sawa A, Kaibuchi K, Nabeshima T, Yamada K. Astroglial IFITM3 mediates neuronal impairments following neonatal immune challenge in mice. Glia. 2013;61:679–93.
18. Yamada S, Nagai T, Nakai T, Ibi D, Nakajima A, Yamada K. Matrix metalloproteinase-3 is a possible mediator of neurodevelopmental impairment due to polyI:C-induced innate immune activation of astrocytes. Brain Behav Immun. 2014;38:272–82.
19. Lange UC, Adams DJ, Lee C, Barton S, Schneider R, Bradley A, Surani MA. Normal germ line establishment in mice carrying a deletion of the Ifitm/ Fragilis gene family cluster. Mol Cell Biol. 2008;28:4688–96.
20. Ibi D, Nagai T, Koike H, Kitahara Y, Mizoguchi H, Niwa M, Jaaro-Peled H, Nitta A, Yoneda Y, Nabeshima T, Sawa A, Yamada K. Combined effect of neonatal immune activation and mutant DISC1 on phenotypic changes in adulthood. Behav Brain Res. 2010;206:32–7.
21. Sobue A, Ito N, Nagai T, Shan W, Hada K, Nakajima A, Murakami Y, Mouri A, Yamamoto Y, Nabeshima T, Saito K, Yamada K. Astroglial major histocompatibility complex class I following immune activation leads to behavioral and neuropathological changes. Glia. 2018;66:1034–52.
22. Clutter SD, Wilson DC, Marinov AD, Hirsch R. Follistatin-like protein 1 promotes arthritis by up-regulating IFN-gamma. J Immunol. 2009;182:234–9.
23. Wilson DC, Marinov AD, Blair HC, Bushnell DS, Thompson SD, Chaly Y, Hirsch R. Follistatin-like protein 1 is a mesenchyme-derived inflammatory protein and may represent a biomarker for systemic-onset juvenile rheumatoid arthritis. Arthritis Rheum. 2010;62:2510–6.
24. Murakami K, Tanaka M, Usui T, Kawabata D, Shiomi A, Iguchi-Hashimoto M, Shimizu M, Yukawa N, Yoshifuji H, Nojima T, Ohmura K, Fujii T, Umehara H, Mimori T. Follistatin-related protein/follistatin-like 1 evokes an innate immune response via CD14 and toll-like receptor 4. FEBS Lett. 2012;586:319–24.
25. Cheng KY, Liu Y, Han YG, Li JK, Jia JL, Chen B, Yao ZX, Nie L, Cheng L. Follistatin-like protein 1 suppressed pro-inflammatory cytokines expression during neuroinflammation induced by lipopolysaccharide. J Mol Histol. 2017;48:63–72.
26. Jha MK, Lee WH, Suk K. Functional polarization of neuroglia: implications in neuroinflammation and neurological disorders. Biochem Pharmacol. 2016;103:1–16.
27. Mondelli V, Vernon AC, Turkheimer F, Dazzan P, Pariante CM. Brain microglia in psychiatric disorders. Lancet Psychiatry. 2017;4:563.
28. van Noort JM, Bsibsi M. Toll-like receptors in the CNS: implications for neurodegeneration and repair. Prog Brain Res. 2009;175:139–48.
29. Ribeiro BM, do Carmo MR, Freire RS, Rocha NF, Borella VC, de Menezes AT, Monte AS, Gomes PX, de Sousa FC, Vale ML, de Lucena DF, Gama CS, Macedo D. Evidences for a progressive microglial activation and increase in iNOS expression in rats submitted to a neurodevelopmental model of schizophrenia: reversal by clozapine. Schizophr Res. 2013;151:12–9.
30. Miyamae T, Marinov AD, Sowders D, Wilson DC, Devlin J, Boudreau R, Robbins P, Hirsch R. Follistatin-like protein-1 is a novel proinflammatory molecule. J Immunol. 2006;177:4758–62.
31. Ni S, Miao K, Zhou X, Xu N, Li C, Zhu R, Sun R, Wang Y. The involvement of follistatin-like protein 1 in osteoarthritis by elevating NF-kappaB-mediated inflammatory cytokines and enhancing fibroblast like synoviocyte proliferation. Arthritis Res Ther. 2015;17:91.
32. Zhang ZM, Zhang AR, Xu M, Lou J, Qiu WQ. TLR-4/miRNA-32-5p/FSTL1 signaling regulates mycobacterial survival and inflammatory responses in mycobacterium tuberculosis-infected macrophages. Exp Cell Res. 2017;352:313–21.
33. Li D, Wang Y, Xu N, Wei Q, Wu M, Li X, Zheng P, Sun S, Jin Y, Zhang G, Liao R, Zhang P. Follistatin-like protein 1 is elevated in systemic autoimmune diseases and correlated with disease activity in patients with rheumatoid arthritis. Arthritis Res Ther. 2011;13:R17.
34. Hayakawa S, Ohashi K, Shibata R, Kataoka Y, Miyabe M, Enomoto T, Joki Y, Shimizu Y, Kambara T, Uemura Y, Yuasa D, Ogawa H, Matsuo K, Hiramatsu-Ito M, van den Hoff MJ, Walsh K, Murohara T, Ouchi N. Cardiac myocyte-

derived follistatin-like 1 prevents renal injury in a subtotal nephrectomy model. J Am Soc Nephrol. 2015;26:636–46.

35. Ouchi N, Asaumi Y, Ohashi K, Higuchi A, Sono-Romanelli S, Oshima Y, Walsh K. DIP2A functions as a FSTL1 receptor. J Biol Chem. 2010;285:7127–34.

36. Tanaka M, Murakami K, Ozaki S, Imura Y, Tong XP, Watanabe T, Sawaki T, Kawanami T, Kawabata D, Fujii T, Usui T, Masaki Y, Fukushima T, Jin ZX, Umehara H, Mimori T. DIP2 disco-interacting protein 2 homolog A (Drosophila) is a candidate receptor for follistatin-related protein/follistatin-like 1–analysis of their binding with TGF-beta superfamily proteins. FEBS J. 2010;277:4278–89.

37. Geng Y, Dong Y, Yu M, Zhang L, Yan X, Sun J, Qiao L, Geng H, Nakajima M, Furuichi T, Ikegawa S, Gao X, Chen YG, Jiang D, Ning W. Follistatin-like 1 (Fstl1) is a bone morphogenetic protein (BMP) 4 signaling antagonist in controlling mouse lung development. Proc Natl Acad Sci U S A. 2011;108:7058–63.

38. Sylva M, Li VS, Buffing AA, van Es JH, van den Born M, van der Velden S, Gunst Q, Koolstra JH, Moorman AF, Clevers H, van den Hoff MJ. The BMP antagonist follistatin-like 1 is required for skeletal and lung organogenesis. PLoS One. 2011;6:e22616.

39. Xu J, Qi X, Gong J, Yu M, Zhang F, Sha H, Gao X. Fstl1 antagonizes BMP signaling and regulates ureter development. PLoS One. 2012;7:e32554.

40. Li KC, Zhang FX, Li CL, Wang F, Yu MY, Zhong YQ, Zhang KH, Lu YJ, Wang Q, Ma XL, Yao JR, Wang JY, Lin LB, Han M, Zhang YQ, Kuner R, Xiao HS, Bao L, Gao X, Zhang X. Follistatin-like 1 suppresses sensory afferent transmission by activating Na+, K+-ATPase. Neuron. 2011;69:974–87.

41. Sundaram GM, Common JE, Gopal FE, Srikanta S, Lakshman K, Lunny DP, Lim TC, Tanavde V, Lane EB, Sampath P. 'See-saw' expression of microRNA-198 and FSTL1 from a single transcript in wound healing. Nature. 2013;495:103–6.

42. Hansen T, Olsen L, Lindow M, Jakobsen KD, Ullum H, Jonsson E, Andreassen OA, Djurovic S, Melle I, Agartz I, Hall H, Timm S, Wang AG, Werge T. Brain expressed microRNAs implicated in schizophrenia etiology. PLoS One. 2007;2:e873.

43. Beveridge NJ, Cairns MJ. MicroRNA dysregulation in schizophrenia. Neurobiol Dis. 2012;46:263–71.

14

Sphingosine 1-phosphate receptor subtype 3 (S1P₃) contributes to brain injury after transient focal cerebral ischemia via modulating microglial activation and their M1 polarization

Bhakta Prasad Gaire[1], Mi-Ryoung Song[2*] and Ji Woong Choi[1*]

Abstract

Background: The pathogenic roles of receptor-mediated sphingosine 1-phosphate (S1P) signaling in cerebral ischemia have been evidenced mainly through the efficacy of FTY720 that binds non-selectively to four of the five S1P receptors ($S1P_{1,3,4,5}$). Recently, $S1P_1$ and $S1P_2$ were identified as specific receptor subtypes that contribute to brain injury in cerebral ischemia; however, the possible involvement of other S1P receptors remains unknown. $S1P_3$ can be the candidate because of its upregulation in the ischemic brain, which was addressed in this study, along with underlying pathogenic mechanisms.

Methods: We used transient middle cerebral artery occlusion/reperfusion (tMCAO), a mouse model of transient focal cerebral ischemia. To identify $S1P_3$ as a pathogenic factor in cerebral ischemia, we employed a specific $S1P_3$ antagonist, CAY10444. Brain damages were assessed by brain infarction, neurological score, and neurodegeneration. Histological assessment was carried out to determine microglial activation, morphological transformation, and proliferation. M1/M2 polarization and relevant signaling pathways were determined by biochemical and immunohistochemical analysis.

Results: Inhibiting $S1P_3$ immediately after reperfusion with CAY10444 significantly reduced tMCAO-induced brain infarction, neurological deficit, and neurodegeneration. When $S1P_3$ activity was inhibited, the number of activated microglia was markedly decreased in both the periischemic and ischemic core regions in the ischemic brain 1 and 3 days following tMCAO. Moreover, inhibiting $S1P_3$ significantly restored the microglial shape from amoeboid to ramified microglia in the ischemic core region 3 days after tMCAO, and it attenuated microglial proliferation in the ischemic brain. In addition to these changes, $S1P_3$ signaling influenced the proinflammatory M1 polarization, but not M2. The $S1P_3$-dependent regulation of M1 polarization was clearly shown in activated microglia, which was affirmed by determining the in vivo activation of microglial NF-κB signaling that is responsible for M1 and in vitro expression levels of proinflammatory cytokines in activated microglia. As downstream effector pathways in an ischemic brain, $S1P_3$ influenced phosphorylation of ERK1/2, p38 MAPK, and Akt.

(Continued on next page)

* Correspondence: msong@gist.ac.kr; pharmchoi@gachon.ac.kr
[2]School of Life Sciences, Gwangju Institute of Science and Technology, Buk-gu, Gwangju 500-712, Republic of Korea
[1]College of Pharmacy and Gachon Institute of Pharmaceutical Sciences, Gachon University, Incheon 406-799, Republic of Korea

(Continued from previous page)

Conclusions: This study identified S1P$_3$ as a pathogenic mediator in an ischemic brain along with underlying mechanisms, involving its modulation of microglial activation and M1 polarization, further suggesting that S1P$_3$ can be a therapeutic target for cerebral ischemia.

Keywords: Transient focal cerebral ischemia, S1P$_3$, CAY10444, Microglial activation, M1 polarization, ERK1/2, p38 MAPK

Background

Sphingosine 1 phosphate (S1P), which is a bioactive sphingolipid, has been known to influence a variety of biological actions throughout the body [1]. These actions of S1P in various organs are mostly mediated by its five specific G-protein coupled receptors (S1P$_{1-5}$) [1]. Based on the identified biological actions of S1P, a considerable effort has been made to develop a drug that targets S1P receptors, leading to the first successful output, FTY720 (fingolimod, Gilenya, Novartis), that binds non-selectively to 4 of the 5 S1P receptors after being phosphorylated [1] and is currently used for treatment of multiple sclerosis [2]. In addition to this success, FTY720 is now under clinical trials for the treatment of several disease types, including acute stroke, amyotrophic lateral sclerosis, schizophrenia, Rett syndrome, and glioblastoma [2], strongly suggesting that receptor-mediated S1P signaling can be a considerable drug target in different diseases. However, the S1P receptor subtypes involved in each disease type is still unclear. Even the efficacy of FTY720 has been assumed to be primarily mediated by S1P$_1$, and no other subtypes targeted by FTY720 have been identified that mediate its efficacy.

Cerebral ischemia, which is caused by a sudden interruption of blood flow to the brain, is a disease type where S1P receptors become validated drug targets mainly due to the efficacy of FTY720. Numerous in vivo studies have been conducted to prove the neuroprotective effects of FTY720 in the brain against ischemic challenge [3–9]. FTY720 itself [10, 11] or combined with a thrombolytic agent [12] is under clinical trials for the treatment in acute stroke. Despite this validated efficacy, among the four S1P receptor subtypes targeted by FTY720, S1P$_1$ is the only identified receptor subtype to be associated with cerebral ischemia [13], indicating the possible involvement of other subtypes of FTY720-relevant S1P receptors. Besides S1P$_1$, S1P$_2$ (which is not a target for FTY720) was also revealed to influence brain injury after ischemic challenge [14]. These two independent studies identified the importance of receptor-mediated S1P signaling in cerebral ischemia and further demonstrated the pathogenic roles of both receptor subtypes in this disease. Interestingly, the pathogenic roles of S1P$_1$ in cerebral ischemia [13] demonstrated that FTY720's efficacy in this disease is via its unique action as a functional antagonist for S1P$_1$ [15, 16]. In addition to S1P$_1$, FTY720-phosphate may also antagonize S1P$_3$ because it reduced cellular responses through

S1P-S1P$_3$ signaling axis [17]. Furthermore, S1P$_3$ was reported to be upregulated at mRNA levels in the brain after ischemic challenge [6]. This notion raised the possibility that S1P$_3$ could be an additional pathogenic factor for cerebral ischemia, and FTY720's efficacy in cerebral ischemia can also be mediated via suppressing S1P$_3$. However, whether S1P$_3$ influences brain injury in focal cerebral ischemia and the role of S1P$_3$, pathogenic or neuroprotective, has not been identified.

In this study, we aimed to address the pathogenic role of S1P$_3$ in transient focal cerebral ischemia with a mouse model of transient middle cerebral artery occlusion and reperfusion (tMCAO). To identify the role, we used a selective S1P$_3$ antagonist, CAY10444, that was given to mice immediately after reperfusion. We then assessed brain damage such as brain infarction, neurological functional deficit, and neural cell death. We further assessed whether S1P$_3$ influenced microglial activation and polarization, a core pathogenic event in cerebral ischemia, along with a clarification of S1P$_3$-dependent effector pathways in the brain after tMCAO challenge.

Methods

Animals and surgical procedures

Male ICR mice (32 ± 2 g; 6 weeks old) were bought from the Orient Bio company (Korea) and housed under controlled environmental conditions of diurnal lighting (light on 07:00–19:00), temperature (22 ± 2 °C), and relative humidity ($60 \pm 10\%$). All animal handling and surgical procedures were carried out in accordance with the approved animal protocols specified by the Institutional Animal Care and Use Committee at Gachon University (Incheon, Republic of Korea) (no. of approved animal protocols: LCDI-2015–0048; LCDI-2014–0079). Following 1 week of laboratory acclimatization, the mice were challenged with tMCAO as described previously [18]. In brief, the mice were anesthetized with isoflurane (3% for induction and 1.5% for maintenance of anesthesia) in a $N_2O : O_2$ (3 : 1) mixture, and the right common carotid artery was isolated through a ventral neck incision. A silicone-coated 5–0 monofilament was introduced to the internal carotid artery from carotid bifurcation and advanced to occlude the middle cerebral artery (MCA). After 90 min of MCAO, the filament was withdrawn to allow complete reperfusion of the cerebral area. During surgery, rectal temperature was maintained at 37.0 ±

0.5 °C with a homoeothermic blanket. Sham-operated mice received similar surgical procedure except for the occlusion of MCA. After surgery, three mice were kept in a single cage; wet food and soft bedding were provided to minimize the suffering from the operation until they were sacrificed for brain sampling.

CAY10444 administration

CAY10444 (Cayman chemical, MI, USA) was dissolved in 1:1 mixture of chremophore EL and 100% ethanol, diluted in water, and injected intraperitoneally to mice at 0.1, 0.2, and 0.5 mg/kg at the time of reperfusion. For the tMCAO group, equal volumes of the vehicle were injected.

Neurological function assessment and brain infarction determination

Functional neurological deficit was assessed using modified neurological severity score (mNSS) scale to determine the motor, sensory, balance, and reflex disorder 24 h following MCAO, as described previously [18–20]. Following the neurological score assessment, the mice were sacrificed with CO_2 exposure; their brains were quickly removed and sliced in the mice brain matrix at 2 mm thickness. The obtained brain slices were incubated with 2% 2,3,5-triphenyltetrazolium chloride (TTC) in physiological saline for 20 min at 37 °C. The TTC-stained brain slices were photographed, and the infarct area was calculated using ImageJ software (National Institute of Mental Health, Bethesda, MD).

Histological analysis
Tissue preparation

Brain tissue samples for histological analysis were obtained 1 or 3 days after tMCAO. Mice were anesthetized with a mixture of Zoletil 50® (10 mg/kg, i.m.) and Rompun® (3 mg/kg, i.m.), and their brains were perfused with ice-cold phosphate-buffered saline (PBS; pH 7.4) followed by 4% paraformaldehyde. The brains were incubated in the same fixative solution overnight, cryoprotected with 30% sucrose, and cut into 20-μm sections using a microtome cryostat. To ensure anatomical similarity of brain regions, two coronal brain sections obtained from the rostral to middle portion of the striatum and the cortex of each mouse brain were used for histological evaluation. In a different set of experiments, the mice brains were transcardially washed with ice-cold PBS and the ipsilateral brain hemisphere was used for RNA and protein extraction.

Fluoro Jade B staining

In order to identify any degenerating neurons following the tMCAO challenge, Fluoro Jade B (FJB) histochemical staining was performed 1 day after tMCAO induction.

Brain sections were sequentially immersed in ethanol series (100% for 3 min, and 70% and 30% for 1 min each), rinsed in deionized water, and oxidized in 0.06% w/v $KMnO_4$. Then, sections were stained with 0.001% (w/v) FJB in 0.1% (v/v) acetic acid solution for 30 min, rinsed in deionized water, dried in a slide warmer, cleared in xylene, and then cover-slipped.

Iba1 or glial fibrillary acidic protein (GFAP) immunohistochemistry

To evaluate the effect of $S1P_3$ activity on microglia or astrocyte activation, Iba1 or GFAP immunohistochemistry was performed 1 or 3 days after tMCAO. Brain sections were oxidized with 1% H_2O_2 in PBS for 15 min and blocked with 1% fetal bovine serum (FBS) in 0.3% Triton-X100 in PBS for 1 h to block non-specific protein binding. Then, the brain sections were incubated with primary antibody against Iba1 (1:500, Wako) or GFAP (1: 500, Invitrogen) overnight at 4 °C followed by anti-rabbit secondary antibody (1:200). Sections were exposed to avidin and biotinylated horse-radish peroxidase macromolecular complex (ABC) kit (1:100, Vector Labs) and visualized with 3, 3′-diaminobenzidine tetrahydrochloride (DAB) exposure (0.02% DAB and 0.01% H_2O_2 in 0.05 M TRIS solution), dehydrated with ethanol, cleared in xylene, and mounted using mounting media.

Iba1/NF-κB double-immunohistochemistry

In order to determine whether the NF-κB pathway is triggered in activated microglia after the tMCAO challenge, cryostat brain sections were processed for double immunolabeling using antibodies against NF-κB (p65) and Iba1. The sections were incubated with TRIS-EDTA solution at 100 °C for 30 min for antigen retrieval, blocked with 1% FBS in 0.3% Triton X-100, and labeled with rabbit NF-κB (p65) (1:100) antibody overnight at 4 °C. The sections were labeled with a biotinylated secondary antibody (1:200) followed by incubation with an ABC kit. The signals were visualized with DAB staining (0.02% DAB and 0.01% H_2O_2 for 2 min). The stained sections were then washed with PBS (3 × 5 min), blocked, and incubated with primary antibodies against Iba1 (1:500) overnight at 4 °C. Sections were then labeled with appropriate secondary antibodies conjugated with Cy3 (1:1000) and mounted with VECTA SHIELD mounting medium.

Bromodeoxyuridine (BrdU)/Iba1 immunofluorescence

The role of $S1P_3$ activity on tMCAO-induced microglia proliferation was determined using Iba1/BrdU double immunofluorescence. BrdU (50 mg/kg in PBS, i.p.) was administered twice a day at 12-h intervals on the second and third day after tMCAO challenge. Brain sections were prepared for Iba1/BrdU immunofluorescence as described previously [18, 21].

Image preparation and quantification

The brain sections after staining or immunolabeling were photographed using bright-field and fluorescence microscopy (BX53T, Olympus, Japan) equipped with a DP72 camera. Representative images were prepared using Adobe Photoshop CS3. For quantification, three photographs were taken from different area of each region and the number of immunopositive cells was counted. Then, the average number of immunopositive cells from each region was expressed in per unit area (mm^2).

Western blot analysis

Ipsilateral brain hemispheres were obtained 24 h following tMCAO induction and triturated with neuronal protein extraction reagent (NPER); the obtained proteins was thus separated in a 10% SDS-PAGE system and transferred to the polyvinylidene difluoride membrane. The membrane was blocked with 5% skim milk to avoid non-specific protein bindings and incubated with primary antibodies against rabbit pAkt, Akt, pERK1/2, ERK1/2, pp38, p38 (Cell signaling, all at 1:1000 dilution), and mouse β-actin (Sigma Aldrich, 1:5000) overnight at 4 °C followed by incubation with respective secondary antibodies (Jackson ImmunoResearch, 1:10000) for 2 h at room temperature and visualized with enhanced chemiluminescence (ECL) solution. The band intensity of each protein was analyzed using ImageQuant (TM) TL software, normalized with β-actin, and then expressed as fold changes of the sham-operated group.

Mouse primary microglia culture, CAY10444 treatment, and transfection with S1P3 shRNA

Primary microglial cells were obtained from the brain cortices of 1–2-day-old mouse pups as described previously [13]. The microglial cells were seeded on 6-well plates at a density of 1×10^5 cells/well. Microglial cells were starved overnight and treated with CAY10444 (1 μM) or vehicle (0.1% DMSO in DMEM). Thirty minutes later, microglia were stimulated with lipopolysaccharides (LPS) (100 ng/ml) for additional 24 h. Alternatively, the shRNA targeted with $S1P_3$ (sh$S1P_3$) receptor or non-targeted control shRNA was transfected into the cells in serum and antibiotic-free medium. After 6 h of incubation, the media were replaced with serum and antibiotic containing media for an additional 42 h. $S1P_3$-infected microglial cells were then challenged with serum starvation for 12 h and stimulated with LPS, and then harvested for qRT-PCR analysis.

Quantitative real-time polymerase chain reaction (qRT-PCR)

Total RNA was extracted from the ipsilateral hemisphere of mice brain and cultured microglia cells using TRIzol Reagent (Invitrogen). One microgram of total RNA was reverse transcribed (RT) to synthesize cDNA. The gene expression levels of the different markers of M1- and M2-polarized microglia were determined using the StepOnePlus™ qRT-PCR system (Applied Biosystems) with the FG Power SYBR Green PCR master mix (Life Technologies) and primer sets (Additional file 1: Table S1). β-actin was used as the housekeeping gene.

Statistical analysis

All statistical tests were performed using Graph Pad Prism 5 (Graph Pad Software Inc., La Jolla, CA, USA), and the data are presented as mean ± S.E.M. One-way ANOVA followed by the Newman-Keuls post hoc test was used to compare the data among the multiple experimental groups, while comparisons between the two groups were performed using the Student's t test. $p < 0.05$ was set as statistically significant.

Results

Suppression of S1P$_3$ activity attenuates brain infarction and neurological deficit in tMCAO-challenged mice

The vehicle-administered mice developed severe brain infarction in both the ischemic cortex and striatum 24 h after the tMCAO challenge (Fig. 1a, b). However, the mice administered with $S1P_3$ antagonist (CAY10444) showed significantly decreased brain infarction in a dose-dependent manner (Fig. 1a, b). The brain infarction volume of the vehicle-administered tMCAO group was $31.20 \pm 1.65\%$, whereas that in the different dosages of CAY10444-administered mice were $28.63 \pm 0.97\%$, $25.20 \pm 1.15\%$, and $21.96 \pm 1.68\%$ at 0.1, 0.2, and 0.5 mg/kg, respectively (Fig. 1a, b). The lowest dose of CAY10444 (0.1 mg/kg) was not effective, but 0.2 and 0.5 mg/kg were effective to attenuate the brain infarction. Similarly, the neurological deficit parameters reflecting motor, sensory, reflex, and balance disorders, as evidenced by mNSS analysis, were significantly improved in the CAY10444-administered mice compared to the vehicle-administered group (Fig. 1c). Among the tested doses, 0.5 mg/kg was found to be the most effective to attenuate brain infarction and neurological deficit; this dose was therefore chosen for the remaining experiments. The neuroprotective potential of CAY10444 in tMCAO-induced brain damage was further affirmed by analyzing the extent of neurodegeneration 24 h following ischemic challenge using FJB staining. CAY10444 reduced the extent of neuronal damage compared with vehicle exposure (Additional file 1: Figure S1). These results clearly demonstrated that the suppression of S1P$_3$ activity attenuated

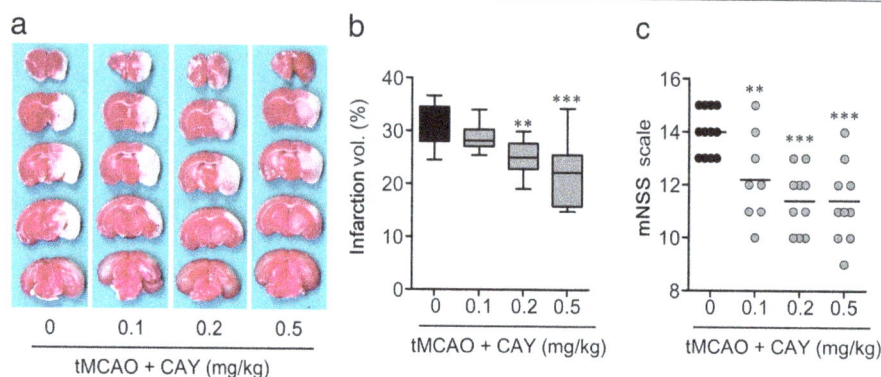

Fig. 1 CAY10444 (CAY) administration attenuates tMCAO-induced brain infarction and neurological deficit. Mice were challenged with tMCAO, and CAY (0.1. 0.2, and 0.5 mg/kg) was administered intraperitoneally immediately after reperfusion. Brain damage was ascertained 24 h after tMCAO challenge (**a–c**). Effects of different dosage of CAY on infarct volume (**a, b**) and neurological function (**c**) were determined. Representative images of TTC-stained brain tissue (**a**), quantification of brain infarction (**b**), and neurological deficit (**c**) are shown. $n = 10 \sim 12$ mice per group. $^{**}p < 0.01$ and $^{***}p < 0.001$ versus vehicle-administered tMCAO group

tMCAO-induced brain damage, indicating the pathogenic role of S1P$_3$ in cerebral ischemia.

Suppression of S1P$_3$ activity attenuates microglial activation and proliferation in the brain of tMCAO-challenged mouse

Focal cerebral ischemia-induced microglial activation was analyzed in the brain through Iba1 immunohistochemistry 1 and 3 days following tMCAO challenge. The vehicle-administered tMCAO group showed the robust activation of microglia, as demonstrated by an increased number of Iba1-immunopositive cells in the ischemic hemisphere at both time points. CAY10444 administration significantly reduced the number of Iba1-immunopositive cells in a time- and region-dependent manner compared with the vehicle administration (Figs. 2 and 3). The number of activated microglia was significantly reduced in both the periischemic and ischemic core regions of the

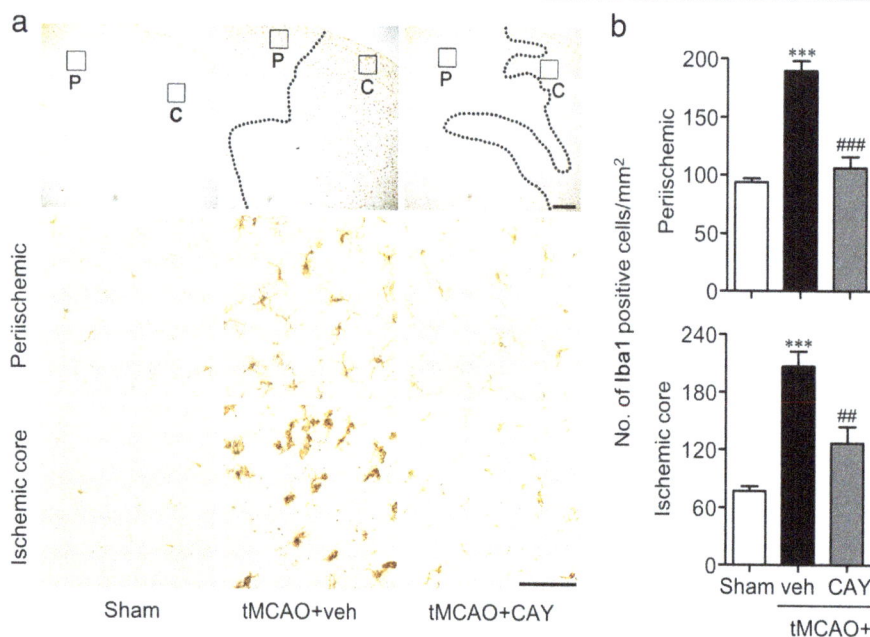

Fig. 2 CAY10444 (CAY) administration attenuates tMCAO-induced microglia activation in 1 day post-ischemic brain. Mice were challenged with tMCAO, and CAY (0.5 mg/kg) was administered intraperitoneally immediately after reperfusion. The effect of CAY on microglial activation was determined by Iba1 immunohistochemistry in 1 day post-ischemic brain. **a** Representative images of Iba1-immunopositive cells in periischemic (P) and ischemic core (C) regions. Scale bars, 200 μm (top panels) and 50 μm (middle and bottom panels). **b** Quantification of the number of Iba1-immunopositive cells in both regions. $n = 4 \sim 5$ mice per group. $^{***}p < 0.001$ versus sham. $^{##}p < 0.01$ and $^{###}p < 0.001$ versus vehicle-administered tMCAO group (tMCAO+veh)

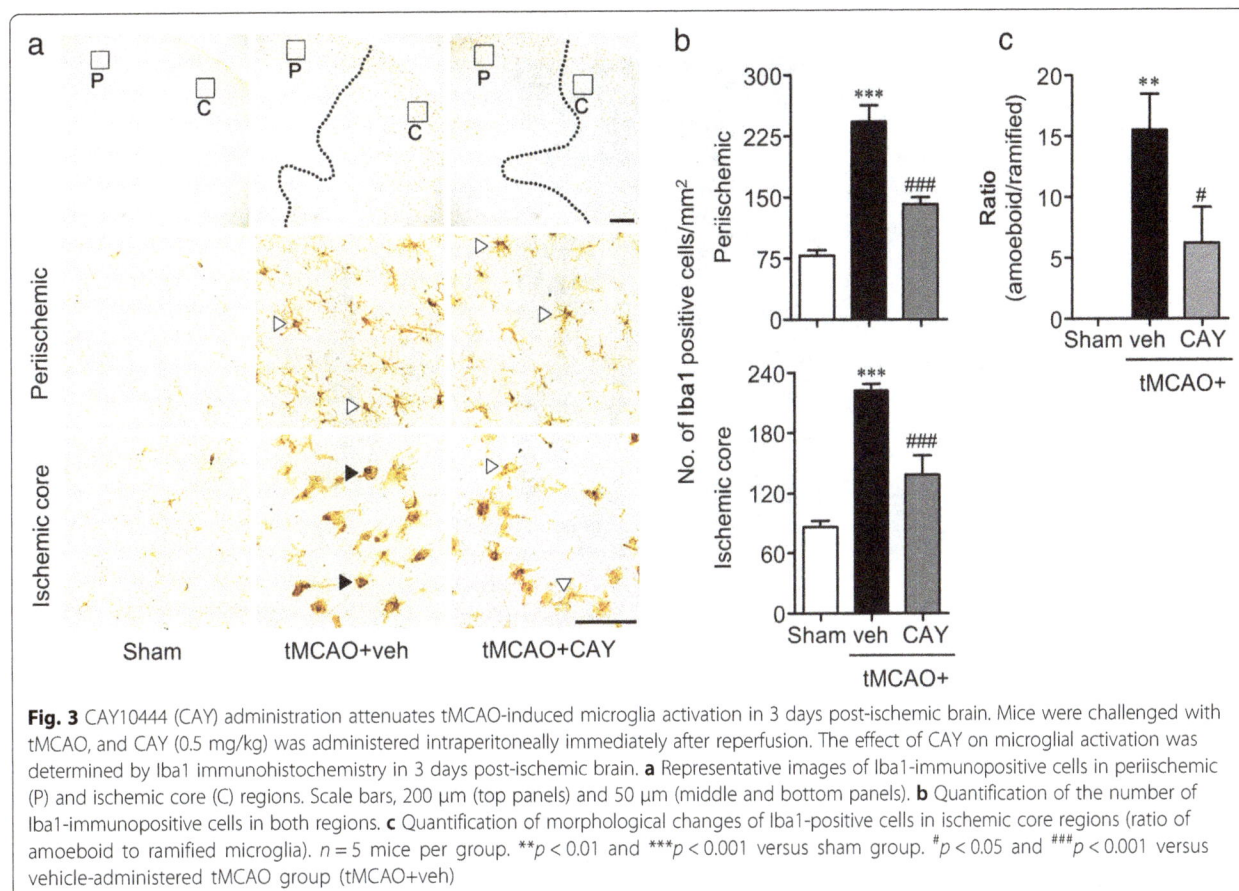

Fig. 3 CAY10444 (CAY) administration attenuates tMCAO-induced microglia activation in 3 days post-ischemic brain. Mice were challenged with tMCAO, and CAY (0.5 mg/kg) was administered intraperitoneally immediately after reperfusion. The effect of CAY on microglial activation was determined by Iba1 immunohistochemistry in 3 days post-ischemic brain. **a** Representative images of Iba1-immunopositive cells in periischemic (P) and ischemic core (C) regions. Scale bars, 200 μm (top panels) and 50 μm (middle and bottom panels). **b** Quantification of the number of Iba1-immunopositive cells in both regions. **c** Quantification of morphological changes of Iba1-positive cells in ischemic core regions (ratio of amoeboid to ramified microglia). $n = 5$ mice per group. $**p < 0.01$ and $***p < 0.001$ versus sham group. $^{#}p < 0.05$ and $^{###}p < 0.001$ versus vehicle-administered tMCAO group (tMCAO+veh)

CAY10444-administered mice compared with the vehicle-administered mice at both time points (Figs. 2 and 3). Moreover, the number of amoeboid microglia in the ischemic core region was significantly reduced in the CAY10444-administered mice, as depicted by the reduced ratio of amoeboid/ramified microglia (Fig. 3c). These data demonstrated that suppressing S1P$_3$ activity in an ischemic brain not only attenuated the activation of microglia, but also reduced the morphological transformation of ramified microglia to amoeboid microglia.

The brain resident microglia proliferated during the first week following the ischemic challenge, and these newly born microglia may participate in inflammatory responses [22]. To analyze the regulatory roles of S1P$_3$ on microglial proliferation in the ischemic brain, we performed double immunofluorescence for BrdU and Iba1 in the brain 3 days after the tMCAO challenge. Microglial proliferation was obviously observed in the ischemic penumbra region of the vehicle-administered tMCAO group as evidenced by the increased number of BrdU/Iba1 double-immunopositive cells. The administration of CAY10444 significantly decreased the number of BrdU/Iba1 double-immunopositive cells compared with the vehicle administration (Fig. 4a, b), demonstrating that S1P$_3$ is involved in microglial proliferation following ischemic challenge.

Besides microglial activation, astrogliosis is another core pathogenesis in cerebral ischemia [23], and S1P$_3$ regulates inflammatory responses in activated astrocytes [24]. In this study, we also determined whether suppressing S1P$_3$ activity reduced astrogliosis following ischemic challenge through GFAP immunohistochemistry. The vehicle-administered mice developed a significant astrogliosis in the corpus callosum as evidenced by the increased number of GFAP-immunopositive cells 1 and 3 days after the tMCAO challenge. CAY10444 administration significantly reduced the number of GFAP-immunopositive cells at both time points. In addition, the morphology of astrocytes was transformed towards reactive phenotype, particularly, 3 days after the tMCAO challenge, which was markedly attenuated by CAY10444 administration (Additional file 1: Figure S3). These results demonstrated that S1P$_3$ signaling also regulated astrogliosis in the ischemic brain.

S1P$_3$ regulates microglial M1 polarization in the brain of tMCAO-challenged mouse

Following ischemic injury, activated microglia become polarized into two distinct phenotypes, broadly known as proinflammatory M1 and anti-inflammatory M2 phenotypes [25]. In order to identify the association between

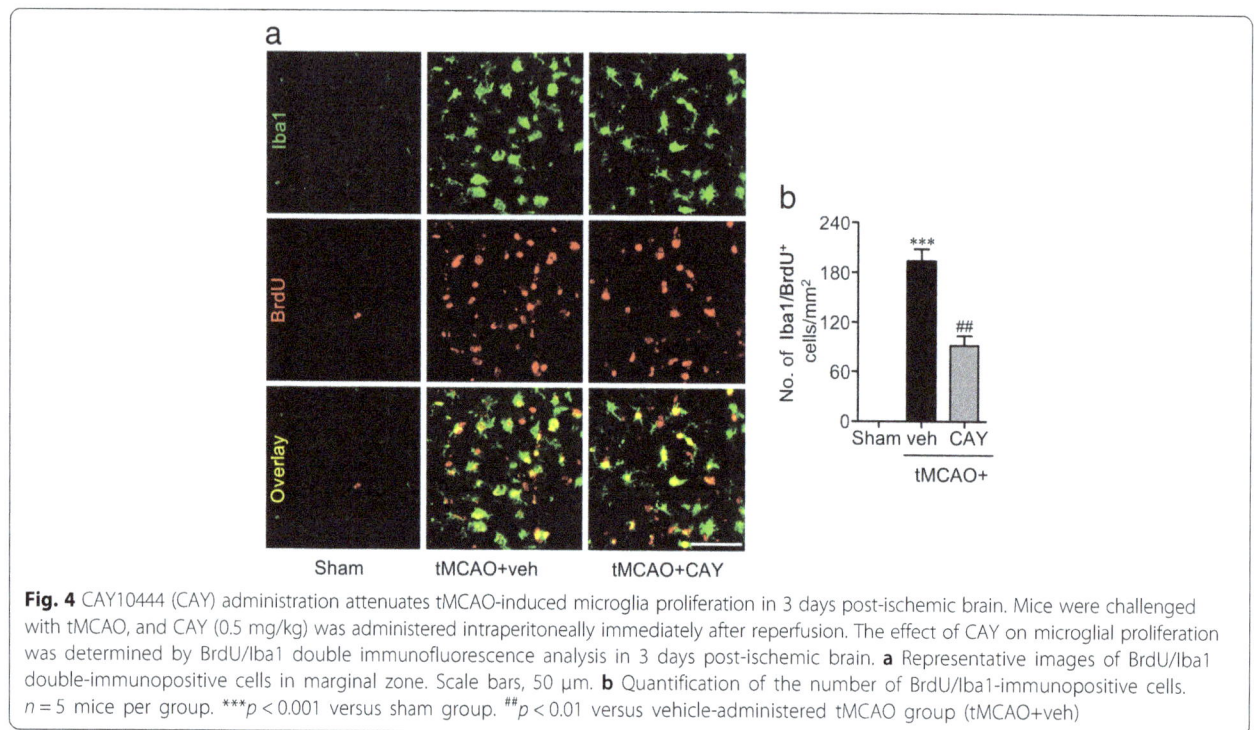

Fig. 4 CAY10444 (CAY) administration attenuates tMCAO-induced microglia proliferation in 3 days post-ischemic brain. Mice were challenged with tMCAO, and CAY (0.5 mg/kg) was administered intraperitoneally immediately after reperfusion. The effect of CAY on microglial proliferation was determined by BrdU/Iba1 double immunofluorescence analysis in 3 days post-ischemic brain. **a** Representative images of BrdU/Iba1 double-immunopositive cells in marginal zone. Scale bars, 50 μm. **b** Quantification of the number of BrdU/Iba1-immunopositive cells. $n = 5$ mice per group. ***$p < 0.001$ versus sham group. ##$p < 0.01$ versus vehicle-administered tMCAO group (tMCAO+veh)

$S1P_3$ activity and M1/M2 polarization in the ischemic brain, the mRNA expression levels of different markers, both surface and soluble, of M1 and M2 polarization were determined. The mRNA expression levels of M1 surface markers (CD11b, CD16, CD32, and CD86) were significantly upregulated 1 and 3 days following the tMCAO challenge (Fig. 5). The upregulated surface markers of M1 polarization in the ischemic brain, such as CD16 and CD32, were significantly downregulated in the CAY10444-administered mice 1 day after the ischemic challenge (Fig. 5a–d). Similarly, CAY10444 administration significantly downregulated the mRNA expression levels of M1 surface markers (CD11b, CD16, and CD32) 3 days after the tMCAO challenge (Fig. 5e–h). We then determined whether $S1P_3$ also regulated the expression of soluble markers that are functionally more important M1 markers. The administration of CAY10444 significantly reduced the mRNA expression levels of the proinflammatory cytokines, such as TNF-α and IL-1β, but not IL-6 (Fig. 6a–c) in the 1-day post-ischemic brain, which were reproduced in the 3-day post-ischemic brain (Fig. 6d–f). These data demonstrated that $S1P_3$ triggered the proinflammatory responses of M1-polarized cells in the ischemic brain. We further determined whether $S1P_3$, in the ischemic brain, had a role in the anti-inflammatory M2 polarization. However, the administration of CAY10444 did not alter the gene expression levels of the M2 markers (Arg1, CCL-22, CD206, TGF-β, and Ym-1) at both day 1 (Additional file 1: Figure S2a–e) and day 3 (Additional file 1: Figure S2f–j) following the ischemic

challenge, suggesting that $S1P_3$ in an ischemic brain is mainly associated with M1 polarization rather than M2 polarization.

The M1 polarization is closely related to NF-κB signaling as the expression of most of the soluble M1 markers are dependent on a transcriptional activation of NF-κB. $S1P_3$ was also found to regulate microglial activation and M1 polarization following ischemic injury in this study. Therefore, we tried to correlate the roles of $S1P_3$ with NF-κB activation, especially in activated microglia, which was addressed by double immunolabeling for NF-κB(p65) and Iba1 1 day after the ischemic challenge. The vehicle-administered tMCAO group showed an enhanced expression of NF-κB(p65) which are easily identified in Iba1-immunopositive cells in the ischemic core region (Fig. 7a, b). CAY10444 administration significantly decreased the number of NF-κB(p65)-immunopositive cells or NF-κB(p65)/Iba1 double-immunopositive cells (Fig. 7a, b). These data further demonstrated that $S1P_3$ in the ischemic brain mediated the M1 polarization through the activation of NF-κB signaling, in particular, in activated microglia. The regulatory role of $S1P_3$ on M1 microglial polarization was reaffirmed using LPS-stimulated mouse primary microglia. For this purpose, we used LPS because LPS is a well-known stimulus to induce M1 polarization of microglia [26, 27]. The mRNA expression levels of M1-soluble markers (TNF-α, IL-6, and IL-1β) were significantly upregulated in LPS-treated cells. Suppressing $S1P_3$ activity either pharmacologically, using CAY10444 (Fig. 8a–c), or genetically, using $S1P_3$-specific shRNA

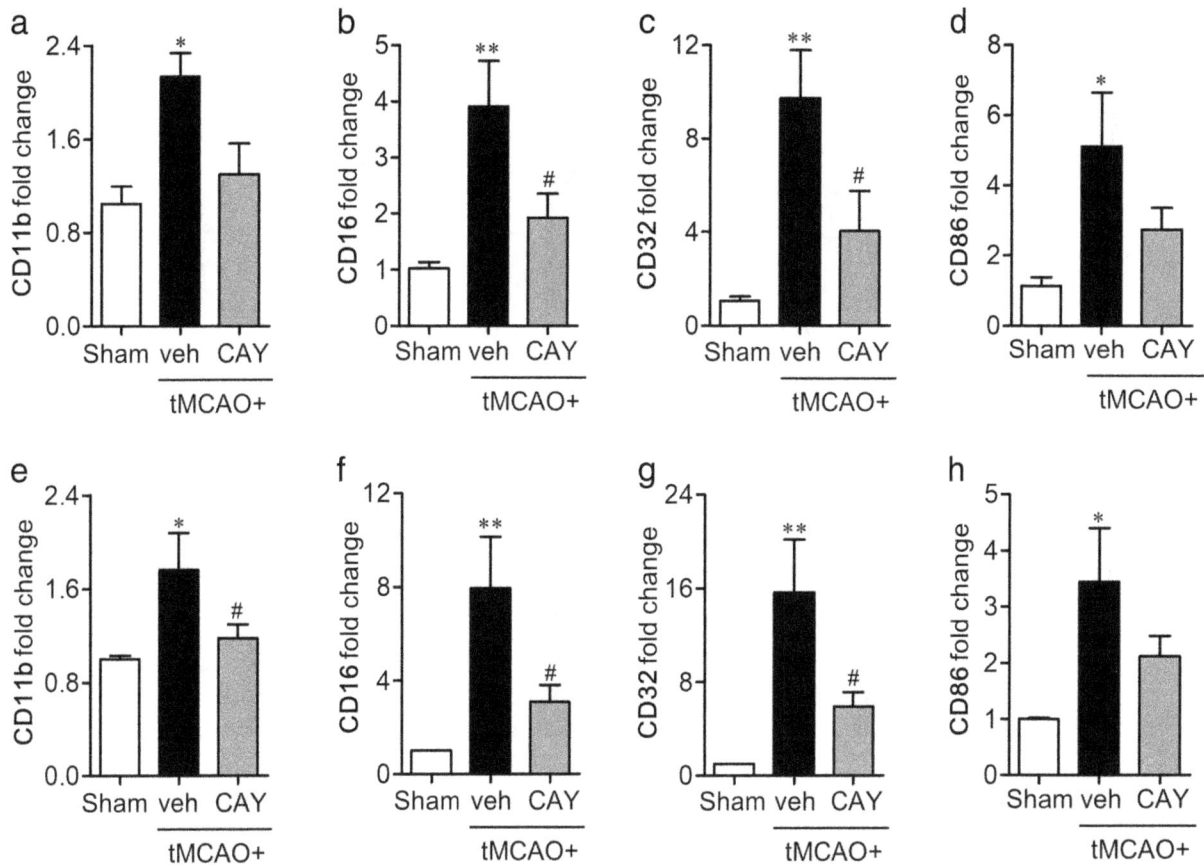

Fig. 5 CAY10444 (CAY) administration attenuates expression level of surface markers of M1 polarization in post-ischemic brain. Mice were challenged with tMCAO, and CAY (0.5 mg/kg) was administered intraperitoneally immediately after reperfusion. The effect of CAY on mRNA expression of M1 surface markers in 1 day (**a–d**) and 3 days (**e–h**) post-ischemic brain was determined by qRT-PCR analysis. $n = 5$ mice per group. *$p < 0.05$ and **$p < 0.01$ versus sham group. #$p < 0.05$ versus vehicle-administered tMCAO group (tMCAO+veh)

lentivirus (Fig. 8d–g), attenuated the expression of these M1 markers. These data ensured that S1P$_3$ in the ischemic brain might be associated with the inflammatory M1 polarization of activated microglia.

S1P$_3$ activity in ischemic brain was linked with activation of ERK1/2, p38 MAPK, and Akt effector pathways

Microglial activation and their phenotype shift towards M1 polarization are linked to several signaling molecules, including ERK1/2, p38 MAPK, and PI3K/Akt [28–31]. Additionally, these signaling pathways function as G$_i$ protein-associated effector systems under S1P$_3$ activation [1]. Therefore, we determined whether S1P$_3$ influenced the activation of these signaling components in an ischemic brain 24 h after tMCAO. In the ischemic brain, ERK1/2 and p38 MAPKs were significantly activated, as assessed by Western blotting for their phosphorylated forms (Fig. 9a, b). When S1P$_3$ activity was blocked by CAY10444 administration, the increased phosphorylation of ERK1/2 and p38 MAPKs was significantly attenuated (Fig. 9a, b). Akt phosphorylation was reduced in

the ischemic brain, and this reduction was significantly reversed by S1P$_3$ antagonism (Fig. 9a, b), further implying the neurotoxic roles of S1P$_3$ following the ischemic challenge because Akt phosphorylation is a well-known survival factor [32]. These data demonstrated that S1P$_3$ influenced the activation of ERK1/2 and p38 MAPKs as well as the inactivation of Akt as downstream signaling cascades in cerebral ischemia.

Discussion

In the current study, we identified S1P$_3$ as another S1P receptor subtype that triggers pathogenesis in transient focal cerebral ischemia along with mechanistic features, particularly in terms of microglial biology, and the effector signaling pathways after S1P$_3$ activation. Suppression of S1P$_3$ activity after tMCAO by its specific antagonist results in attenuation of brain damages. The pathogenic roles of S1P$_3$ in the ischemic brain are closely associated with microglial activation, involving an increased number of activated microglia, morphological transformation into amoeboid shape, and microglial

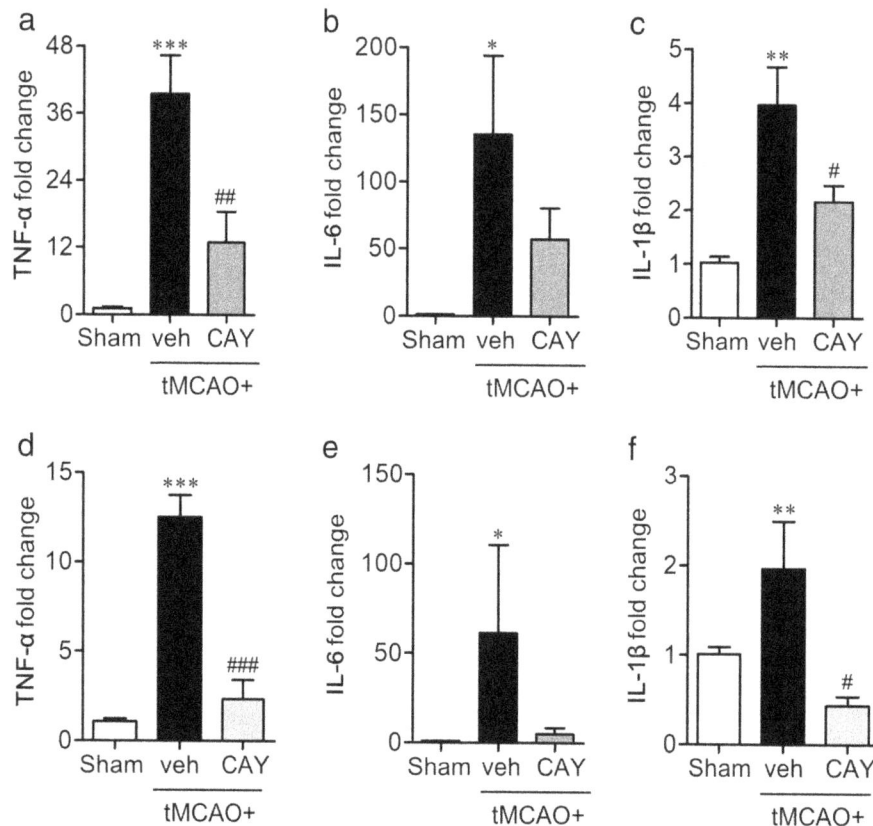

Fig. 6 CAY10444 (CAY) administration attenuates expression level of soluble markers of M1 polarization in post-ischemic brain. Mice were challenged with tMCAO, and CAY (0.5 mg/kg) was administered intraperitoneally immediately after reperfusion. The effect of CAY on mRNA expression of M1 soluble markers in 1 day (**a–d**) and 3 days (**e–h**) post-ischemic brain was determined by qRT-PCR analysis. $n = 5$ mice per group. $*p < 0.05$, $**p < 0.01$, and $***p < 0.001$ versus sham group. $\#p < 0.05$, $\#\#p < 0.01$, and $\#\#\#p < 0.001$ versus vehicle-administered tMCAO group (tMCAO+veh)

proliferation. In addition, $S1P_3$ regulates M1 microglial polarization, but not M2 polarization, in the ischemic brain because inhibiting $S1P_3$ after tMCAO weakened the characteristics of M1 polarization without any influence on the M2 markers. These biological roles were further supported in vitro using LPS-stimulated primary microglia. Finally, PI3K/Akt, ERK1/2 MAPK, and p38 MAPK pathways were identified as effector pathways after $S1P_3$ activation in the ischemic brain.

The use of receptor-mediated S1P signaling has been assumed as a possible therapeutic strategy to overcome cerebral ischemia because FTY720, which is a non-selective modulator of 4 of 5 S1P receptors after being phosphorylated, exerts neuroprotective effects in rodent models [3–8]. Currently, FTY720 is under clinical trial for the treatment of acute stroke [10, 11], and another trial for acute ischemic stroke is underway to determine its clinical efficacy in combination with a thrombolytic therapy, alteplase [12]. Despite these successful efforts, until recently, which S1P receptor subtypes are actual mediators for FTY720's efficacy has remained uncertain. Our previous report proposed the first possibility for this, demonstrating $S1P_1$ as a pathogenic factor in focal cerebral

ischemia using a mouse model for transient focal cerebral ischemia [13]. The current study identified $S1P_3$ as an additional S1P receptor subtype to mediate brain injury in cerebral ischemia. Notably, it has been discovered that FTY720-phosphate acts as a functional antagonist for $S1P_1$ [15, 16] and possibly for $S1P_3$. Even with no direct evidence for the latter, a few findings indicate that FTY720-phosphate antagonizes $S1P_3$ signaling. Either FTY720-phosphate or TY-52156 (a selective $S1P_3$ antagonist) reduced p-selectin production and leucocyte rolling via S1P-$S1P_3$ signaling axis, which was reaffirmed in $S1P_3$ knockouts [17]. FTY720-phosphate was also reported to antagonize G_q-mediated signaling pathway under $S1P_3$ activation [33]. Considering the inhibitory roles of FTY720-phosphate for $S1P_1$ and $S1P_3$, our previous and current in vivo findings strongly indicate that the reported FTY720's efficacy in cerebral ischemia may be through suppressing at least the $S1P_1$ and $S1P_3$ activities. Besides FTY720-relevant target receptors, $S1P_2$ was also identified to mediate brain injury in cerebral ischemia through the disruption of vascular integrity in the ischemic brain [14], even though it is not a target for FTY720-phosphate. Therefore, three subtypes of S1P receptors have been

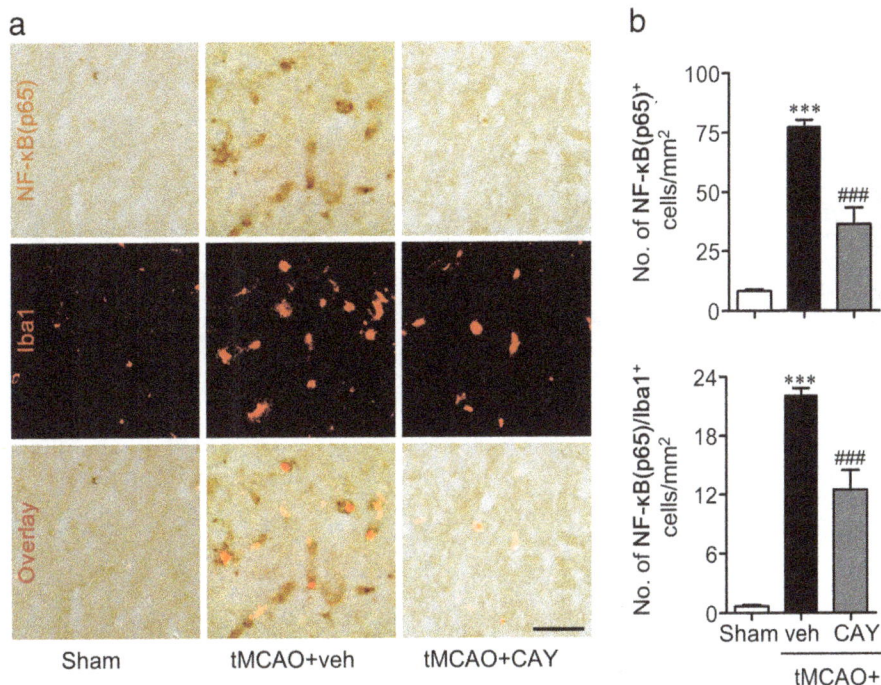

Fig. 7 CAY10444 (CAY) administration attenuates tMCAO-induced microglial NF-κB expression in post-ischemic brain. Mice were challenged with tMCAO, and CAY (0.5 mg/kg) was administered intraperitoneally immediately after reperfusion. The effect of CAY on NF-κB expression in activated microglia was determined by NF-κB(p65)/Iba1 double immunohistochemical analysis in 1 day post-ischemic brain. **a** Representative images of NF-κB(p65)/Iba1-immunopositive cells in ischemic core regions. Scale bars, 50 μm. **b** Quantification of the number of NF-κB(p65)- and NF-κB(p65)/Iba1-immunopositive cells. $n = 4 \sim 5$ mice per group. ***$p < 0.001$ versus sham group and ###$p < 0.001$ versus vehicle-administered tMCAO group (tMCAO+veh)

identified as pathogenic factors for cerebral ischemia. However, it is still unclear whether the mediation of the brain injury in the cerebral ischemia differs among the receptor subtypes and whether additional S1P receptor subtypes participate, such as $S1P_4$ or $S1P_5$.

Despite the clear pathogenic role of $S1P_3$ in the brain, its roles in ischemic conditions seem to be tissue-specific. In fact, earlier studies reported controversial roles of $S1P_3$ in non-neural ischemic models: protective or harmful. In the heart, the deletion of both $S1P_2$ and $S1P_3$ was shown to aggravate myocardial infarction in mice, which supported the cardioprotective role of $S1P_3$ [34]. In the kidneys, however, $S1P_3$ was shown to be associated with tissue injury after ischemic challenge. Deletion of bone marrow $S1P_3$ attenuated tissue damage following renal ischemia/reperfusion, in which its deletion reduced the expression levels of proinflammatory cytokines and increased the expression levels of anti-inflammatory cytokines [35, 36]. These disparate roles for S1P receptors were similarly observed in the case of $S1P_1$. Renal injury after ischemic challenge was reduced or exacerbated by exposure to an $S1P_1$ agonist [37] or endothelial $S1P_1$ deletion [38]. However, in the brain, $S1P_1$ knockdown reduced brain injury after ischemic challenge [13]. Regardless of the different roles of receptor-mediated S1P signaling in

non-neural tissues, it should be noted that all three identified S1P receptors ($S1P_1$, $S1P_2$, and $S1P_3$) mediate pathogenesis in ischemic brain.

In this study, we have used CAY10444 to address the role of $S1P_3$ in cerebral ischemia because CAY10444 has been widely used as a specific antagonist for $S1P_3$ [39–41]. But, additional possible modes of actions of CAY10444 were suggested, which included $S1P_2$, P2 receptor, or α_{1A}-adrenoceptor [42]. CAY10444 at 10 μM blocked the $S1P_2$- and $S1P_3$-mediated increase in the intracellular calcium levels in Chinese hamster ovary cells. This inhibitory effect of CAY10444 was also mediated through the stimulation of P2 receptor or α_{1A}-adrenoceptor [42]. These findings indicate that CAY10444 could also act as an antagonist for $S1P_2$ and an agonist for P2 receptor or α_{1A}-adrenoceptor. The latter agonistic property could be excluded in the protective effects of CAY10444 against cerebral ischemia: the association of α_{1A}-adrenoceptor with cerebral ischemia is unclear and suppressing P2 receptor is neuroprotective in this disease [43, 44]. Unlikely, $S1P_2$ could mediate the neuroprotective effects of CAY10444 in cerebral ischemia because $S1P_2$ was reported as a pathogenic factor in this disease [14]. However, it is also possible that CAY10444's efficacy is solely mediated through $S1P_3$ in cerebral ischemia. In renal

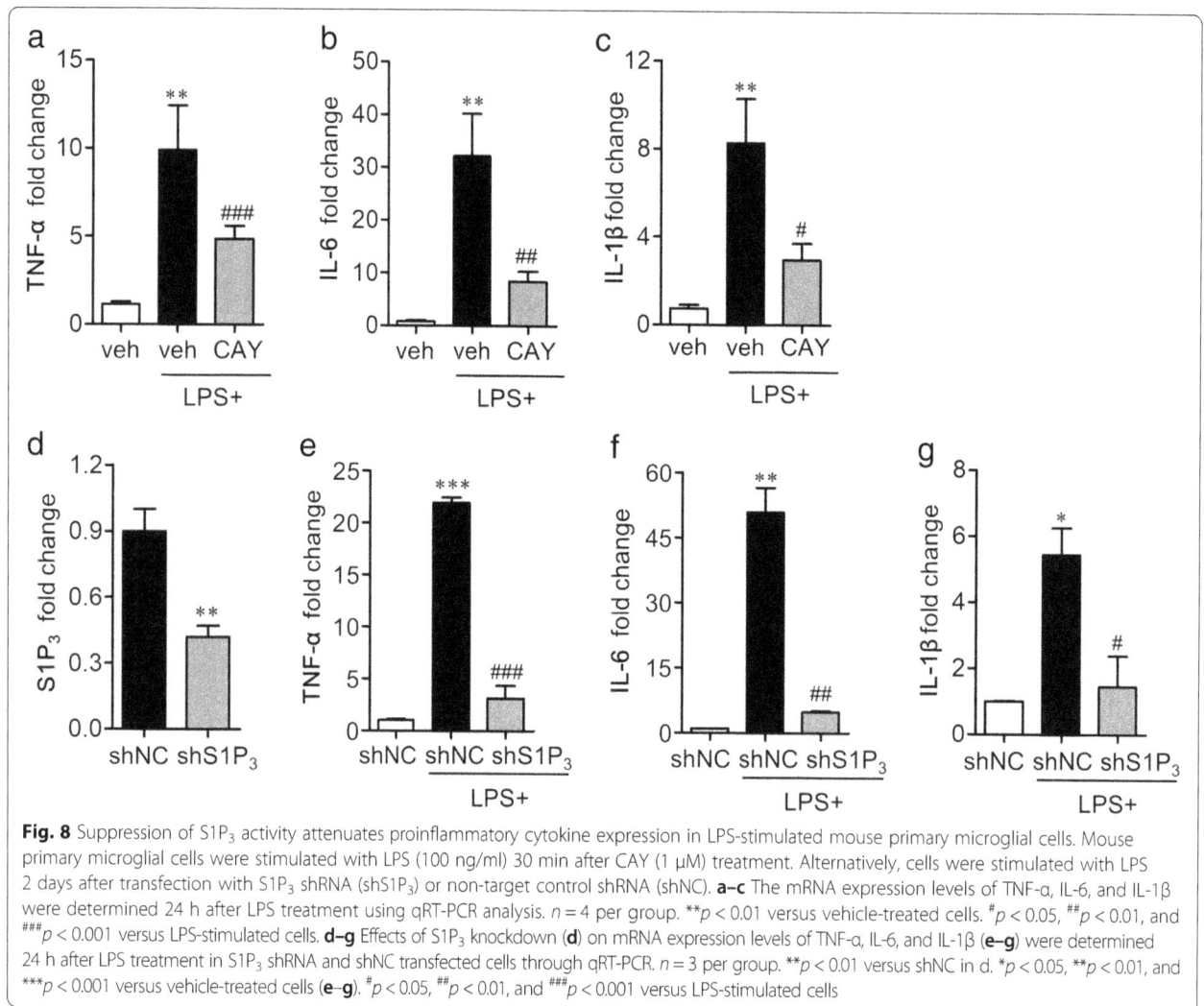

Fig. 8 Suppression of S1P$_3$ activity attenuates proinflammatory cytokine expression in LPS-stimulated mouse primary microglial cells. Mouse primary microglial cells were stimulated with LPS (100 ng/ml) 30 min after CAY (1 μM) treatment. Alternatively, cells were stimulated with LPS 2 days after transfection with S1P$_3$ shRNA (shS1P$_3$) or non-target control shRNA (shNC). **a–c** The mRNA expression levels of TNF-α, IL-6, and IL-1β were determined 24 h after LPS treatment using qRT-PCR analysis. $n = 4$ per group. **$p < 0.01$ versus vehicle-treated cells. #$p < 0.05$, ##$p < 0.01$, and ###$p < 0.001$ versus LPS-stimulated cells. **d–g** Effects of S1P$_3$ knockdown (**d**) on mRNA expression levels of TNF-α, IL-6, and IL-1β (**e–g**) were determined 24 h after LPS treatment in S1P$_3$ shRNA and shNC transfected cells through qRT-PCR. $n = 3$ per group. **$p < 0.01$ versus shNC in d. *$p < 0.05$, **$p < 0.01$, and ***$p < 0.001$ versus vehicle-treated cells (**e–g**). #$p < 0.05$, ##$p < 0.01$, and ###$p < 0.001$ versus LPS-stimulated cells

ischemic injury, blocking S1P$_2$ activity by JTE013 resulted in renoprotection, whereas CAY10444 did not [45]. The latter indicates that CAY10444 does not act as S1P$_2$ antagonist. It would be tempting to address these opposite notions using genetic tools such as knockout mice for S1P$_3$ in future studies.

The neuroharmful role of S1P$_3$ in the ischemic brain appears to be associated with the activation of brain residence microglia, which is a common pathogenic event in several central nervous system (CNS) disorders, including stroke [46, 47]. Previously, receptor-mediated S1P signaling was reported to be involved in microglial activation through both in vitro and in vivo studies [6, 48]. Recently, we identified that S1P$_1$-mediated brain damage after focal cerebral ischemia was mainly mediated through microglial activation [13]. In this study, we identified that S1P$_3$ was also associated with microglial activation: inhibiting S1P$_3$ using its specific antagonist reduced the number of activated microglia in the ischemic brain, in both a time- and region-dependent manner. Furthermore, the suppression

of S1P$_3$ activity in the ischemic brain attenuated microglial proliferation. In addition to the increase in the population, S1P$_3$ in the ischemic brain was closely associated with the morphological transformation of activated microglia. In the ischemic core regions 3 days or more after ischemic challenge, most of the activated microglia were amoeboid shaped and were mainly responsible for neuronal damage in ischemic brain by releasing several proinflammatory mediators [49, 50]. We demonstrated that inhibiting S1P$_3$ resulted in a significant attenuation of the transformation of activated microglia into an amoeboid shape.

S1P$_3$ in the ischemic brain may also link into astrogliosis, a core pathogenesis associated with inflammatory responses in cerebral ischemia [23]. In fact, S1P microinjection into the brain has been reported to cause astrogliosis [6, 51]. Recently, S1P$_3$ was identified as the receptor subtype to regulate astrogliosis, in which a pharmacological antagonism or genetic deletion of S1P$_3$ reduced S1P-triggered inflammatory responses in astrocytes [24]. These previous findings indicate that S1P$_3$-triggered

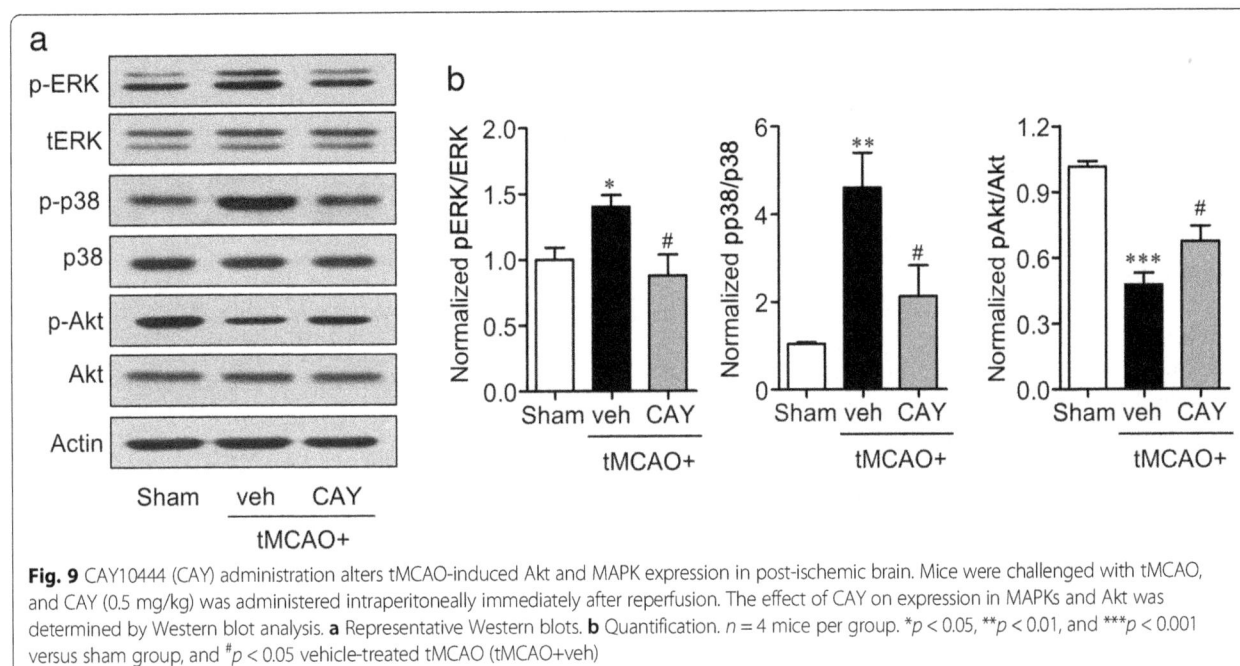

Fig. 9 CAY10444 (CAY) administration alters tMCAO-induced Akt and MAPK expression in post-ischemic brain. Mice were challenged with tMCAO, and CAY (0.5 mg/kg) was administered intraperitoneally immediately after reperfusion. The effect of CAY on expression in MAPKs and Akt was determined by Western blot analysis. **a** Representative Western blots. **b** Quantification. $n = 4$ mice per group. $*p < 0.05$, $**p < 0.01$, and $***p < 0.001$ versus sham group, and $\#p < 0.05$ vehicle-treated tMCAO (tMCAO+veh)

astrogliosis may occur in an ischemic brain. Indeed, we demonstrated that inhibiting S1P$_3$ after tMCAO challenge resulted in a significant attenuation of astrogliosis.

The phenotypical shift of activated microglia has also been extensively considered to understand the pathogenesis of cerebral ischemia [25]. Activated microglia in the ischemic brain become polarized to different phenotypes: classically activated M1- or alternatively activated M2-polarized microglia [25]. M1 microglia are considered as toxic and proinflammatory cells in diverse CNS disorders including cerebral ischemia [52], and the prevention of toxic transformation towards M1 phenotypes has been considered as a possible therapeutic strategy for cerebral ischemia [53, 54]. In contrast, M2-polarized microglia are involved in the repair and resolution phase of ischemic recovery, leading to the neuroprotection [53]. In this study, the suppression of S1P$_3$ activity in the ischemic brain attenuated M1 polarization, as evidenced by the attenuated gene expression of relative markers following tMCAO. However, S1P$_3$ suppression did not alter the expression levels of M2 polarization-relevant markers following tMCAO. These data demonstrate that S1P$_3$ in the ischemic brain is selectively associated with the M1 polarization. This unique role of S1P$_3$ in M1 polarization was obvious in activated microglia, which was confirmed by determining the expression levels of microglial NF-κB, a characteristic marker for M1 polarization [54]. Inhibiting S1P$_3$ significantly reduced the number of Iba1/p65 NF-κB double-immunopositive cells. These in vivo findings of the link between S1P$_3$ and M1 microglial polarization were further affirmed in LPS-stimulated mouse primary microglia, in which

inhibiting S1P$_3$ by both genetic and pharmacological tools ensured the attenuation of proinflammatory cytokines. Therefore, S1P$_3$ may mediate brain injury following tMCAO by altering the microglial polarization states to M1, further suggesting that S1P$_3$ is a novel and selective player in regulating M1 microglial polarization.

The underlying signaling mechanisms for the pathogenic roles of S1P$_3$ in cerebral ischemia were linked to PI3K/Akt and MAPK pathways, including ERK1/2 and p38 MAPK. Inhibiting S1P$_3$ following tMCAO increased the Akt phosphorylation in the ischemic brain, whereas it attenuated the phosphorylation of ERK1/2 and p38 MAPK. These signaling molecules are, in particular, considered to regulate the phenotype shift between M1 and M2 polarization. Akt activation in microglia is a signaling molecule that drives activated microglia towards M2 polarization. Additionally, the activation of PI3K/Akt signaling is critical for restricting inflammatory activation of microglia/macrophages and negatively regulates NF-κB signaling, whereas its inhibition drives activated microglia/macrophages towards their M1 polarization [31, 55]. In this context, Akt activation is crucial for cell phenotype shift by inhibiting M1 and activating M2 polarization. In this study, the suppression of S1P$_3$ activity in ischemic brain increased Akt phosphorylation without altering the expression markers of M2 polarization, indicating that the increased Akt phosphorylation by S1P$_3$ inhibition may be linked to the restriction of M1 polarization rather than to the enhancing of M2 polarization. Persistent activation of ERK1/2 signaling has been reported to trigger NF-κB transcriptional activity [28, 29] similar to the activation of p38 [30], both of which eventually lead to the secretion of proinflammatory mediators that are associated with the M1 polarization of activated microglia [56–58]. This further ensured that $S1P_3$ activation is closely associated with the M1 polarization of activated microglia in the ischemic brain because the suppression of $S1P_3$ activity attenuated ERK1/2 and p38 MAPK phosphorylation in the ischemic brain.

Conclusions

This study identified $S1P_3$ as a novel pathogenic factor in cerebral ischemia and provided underlying mechanisms, particularly in view of microglial activation. The medically relevant roles of the S1P receptor subtypes in cerebral ischemia have emerged through translational studies. Now, at least three subtypes have been identified to mediate brain injury in cerebral ischemia, including $S1P_1$ [13], $S1P_2$ [14], and $S1P_3$ (the current study). Even though $S1P_3$ may be limited as a therapeutic target because of its negative effects on the heart, it would be a good therapeutic strategy for cerebral ischemia if $S1P_3$-specific antagonist can act inside the CNS. In addition to the identification of novel roles of $S1P_3$, our findings also implicate that the neuroprotective effects exerted by FTY720 in cerebral ischemia in previous studies occur additionally via suppressing $S1P_3$ activity [17], similar to the case of $S1P_1$ [13, 59, 60].

Abbreviations

ABC: Avidin and biotinylated horse-radish peroxidase macromolecular complex; BrdU: Bromodeoxyuridine; CNS: Central nervous system; DAB: 3, 3′-diaminobenzidine tetrahydrochloride; ECL: Enhanced chemiluminescence; FBS: Fetal bovine serum; FJB: Fluoro Jade B; GFAP: Glial fibrillary acidic protein; LPS: Lipopolysaccharides; mNSS: Modified neurological severity score; NPER: Neuronal protein extraction reagent; PBS: Phosphate-buffered saline; S1P: Sphingosine 1-phosphate; tMCAO: Transient middle cerebral artery occlusion; TTC: 2,3,5-Triphenyltetrazolium chloride

Acknowledgements

We thank YJ Bae for the assistance with primary microglia culture and Western blot analysis.

Funding

This work was supported by grants from the National Research Foundation (NRF) to JWC (NRF-2014M3A9B6069339 and NRF-2017R1A2B4002818).

Authors' contributions

BPG, MRS, and JWC designed the research. BPG carried out the in vivo and in vitro experiments. BPG, MRS, and JWC analyzed the data and wrote the manuscript. All authors read and approved the final manuscript.

Competing interests

The authors declare that they have no competing interests.

References

1. Choi JW, Chun J. Lysophospholipids and their receptors in the central nervous system. Biochim Biophys Acta. 1831;2013:20–32.
2. O'Sullivan S, Dev KK. Sphingosine-1-phosphate receptor therapies: advances in clinical trials for CNS-related diseases. Neuropharmacology. 2017;113:597–607.
3. Czech B, Pfeilschifter W, Mazaheri-Omrani N, Strobel MA, Kahles T, Neumann-Haefelin T, Rami A, Huwiler A, Pfeilschifter J. The immunomodulatory sphingosine 1-phosphate analog FTY720 reduces lesion size and improves neurological outcome in a mouse model of cerebral ischemia. Biochem Biophys Res Commun. 2009;389:251–6.
4. Hasegawa Y, Suzuki H, Sozen T, Rolland W, Zhang JH. Activation of sphingosine 1-phosphate receptor-1 by FTY720 is neuroprotective after ischemic stroke in rats. Stroke. 2010;41:368–74.
5. Kraft P, Gob E, Schuhmann MK, Gobel K, Deppermann C, Thielmann I, Herrmann AM, Lorenz K, Brede M, Stoll G, et al. FTY720 ameliorates acute ischemic stroke in mice by reducing thrombo-inflammation but not by direct neuroprotection. Stroke. 2013;44:3202–10.
6. Moon E, Han JE, Jeon S, Ryu JH, Choi JW, Chun J. Exogenous S1P exposure potentiates ischemic stroke damage that is reduced possibly by inhibiting S1P receptor signaling. Mediat Inflamm. 2015;2015:492659.
7. Nazari M, Keshavarz S, Rafati A, Namavar MR, Haghani M. Fingolimod (FTY720) improves hippocampal synaptic plasticity and memory deficit in rats following focal cerebral ischemia. Brain Res Bull. 2016;124:95–102.
8. Shichita T, Sugiyama Y, Ooboshi H, Sugimori H, Nakagawa R, Takada I, Iwaki T, Okada Y, Iida M, Cua DJ, et al. Pivotal role of cerebral interleukin-17-producing gammadeltaT cells in the delayed phase of ischemic brain injury. Nat Med. 2009;15:946–50.
9. Wei Y, Yemisci M, Kim HH, Yung LM, Shin HK, Hwang SK, Guo S, Qin T, Alsharif N, Brinkmann V, et al. Fingolimod provides long-term protection in rodent models of cerebral ischemia. Ann Neurol. 2011;69:119–29.
10. Fu Y, Hao J, Zhang N, Ren L, Sun N, Li YJ, Yan Y, Huang D, Yu C, Shi FD. Fingolimod for the treatment of intracerebral hemorrhage: a 2-arm proof-of-concept study. JAMA Neurol. 2014;71:1092–101.
11. Fu Y, Zhang N, Ren L, Yan Y, Sun N, Li YJ, Han W, Xue R, Liu Q, Hao J, et al. Impact of an immune modulator fingolimod on acute ischemic stroke. Proc Natl Acad Sci U S A. 2014;111:18315–20.
12. Zhu Z, Fu Y, Tian D, Sun N, Han W, Chang G, Dong Y, Xu X, Liu Q, Huang D, Shi FD. Combination of the immune modulator fingolimod with alteplase in acute ischemic stroke: a pilot trial. Circulation. 2015;132:1104–12.
13. Gaire BP, Lee CH, Sapkota A, Lee SY, Chun J, Cho HJ, Nam TG, Choi JW. Identification of sphingosine 1-phosphate receptor subtype 1 (S1P1) as a pathogenic factor in transient focal cerebral ischemia. Mol Neurobiol. 2018; 55:2320–32.
14. Kim GS, Yang L, Zhang G, Zhao H, Selim M, McCullough LD, Kluk MJ, Sanchez T. Critical role of sphingosine-1-phosphate receptor-2 in the disruption of cerebrovascular integrity in experimental stroke. Nat Commun. 2015;6:7893.
15. LaMontagne K, Littlewood-Evans A, Schnell C, O'Reilly T, Wyder L, Sanchez T, Probst B, Butler J, Wood A, Liau G, et al. Antagonism of sphingosine-1-phosphate receptors by FTY720 inhibits angiogenesis and tumor vascularization. Cancer Res. 2006;66:221–31.
16. Quancard J, Bollbuck B, Janser P, Angst D, Berst F, Buehlmayer P, Streiff M, Beerli C, Brinkmann V, Guerini D, et al. A potent and selective S1P(1) antagonist with efficacy in experimental autoimmune encephalomyelitis. Chem Biol. 2012;19:1142–51.
17. Nussbaum C, Bannenberg S, Keul P, Graler MH, Goncalves-de-Albuquerque CF, Korhonen H, von Wnuck Lipinski K, Heusch G, de Castro Faria Neto HC, Rohwedder I, et al. Sphingosine-1-phosphate receptor 3 promotes leukocyte rolling by mobilizing endothelial P-selectin. Nat Commun. 2015;6:6416.
18. Gaire BP, Kwon OW, Park SH, Chun KH, Kim SY, Shin DY, Choi JW. Neuroprotective effect of 6-paradol in focal cerebral ischemia involves the attenuation of neuroinflammatory responses in activated microglia. PLoS One. 2015;10:e0120203.
19. Chen J, Sanberg PR, Li Y, Wang L, Lu M, Willing AE, Sanchez-Ramos J, Chopp M. Intravenous administration of human umbilical cord blood reduces behavioral deficits after stroke in rats. Stroke. 2001;32:2682–8.

20. Han JE, Lee EJ, Moon E, Ryu JH, Choi JW, Kim HS. Matrix metalloproteinase-8 is a novel pathogenetic factor in focal cerebral ischemia. Mol Neurobiol. 2016;53:231–9.

21. Sapkota A, Gaire BP, Cho KS, Jeon SJ, Kwon OW, Jang DS, Kim SY, Ryu JH, Choi JW. Eupatilin exerts neuroprotective effects in mice with transient focal cerebral ischemia by reducing microglial activation. PLoS One. 2017;12: e0171479.

22. Li T, Pang S, Yu Y, Wu X, Guo J, Zhang S. Proliferation of parenchymal microglia is the main source of microgliosis after ischaemic stroke. Brain. 2013;136:3578–88.

23. Takano T, Oberheim N, Cotrina ML, Nedergaard M. Astrocytes and ischemic injury. Stroke. 2009;40:S8–12.

24. Dusaban SS, Chun J, Rosen H, Purcell NH, Brown JH. Sphingosine 1-phosphate receptor 3 and RhoA signaling mediate inflammatory gene expression in astrocytes. J Neuroinflammation. 2017;14:111.

25. Hu X, Li P, Guo Y, Wang H, Leak RK, Chen S, Gao Y, Chen J. Microglia/macrophage polarization dynamics reveal novel mechanism of injury expansion after focal cerebral ischemia. Stroke. 2012;43:3063–70.

26. Chhor V, Le Charpentier T, Lebon S, Ore MV, Celador IL, Josserand J, Degos V, Jacotot E, Hagberg H, Savman K, et al. Characterization of phenotype markers and neuronotoxic potential of polarised primary microglia in vitro. Brain Behav Immun. 2013;32:70–85.

27. Orihuela R, McPherson CA, Harry GJ. Microglial M1/M2 polarization and metabolic states. Br J Pharmacol. 2016;173:649–65.

28. Jiang B, Brecher P, Cohen RA. Persistent activation of nuclear factor-kappaB by interleukin-1beta and subsequent inducible NO synthase expression requires extracellular signal-regulated kinase. Arterioscler Thromb Vasc Biol. 2001;21:1915–20.

29. Jiang B, Xu S, Hou X, Pimentel DR, Brecher P, Cohen RA. Temporal control of NF-kappaB activation by ERK differentially regulates interleukin-1beta-induced gene expression. J Biol Chem. 2004;279:1323–9.

30. Olson CM, Hedrick MN, Izadi H, Bates TC, Olivera ER, Anguita J. p38 mitogen-activated protein kinase controls NF-kappaB transcriptional activation and tumor necrosis factor alpha production through RelA phosphorylation mediated by mitogen- and stress-activated protein kinase 1 in response to Borrelia burgdorferi antigens. Infect Immun. 2007;75:270–7.

31. Vergadi E, Ieronymaki E, Lyroni K, Vaporidi K, Tsatsanis C. Akt signaling pathway in macrophage activation and M1/M2 polarization. J Immunol. 2017;198:1006–14.

32. Zhao H, Sapolsky RM, Steinberg GK. Phosphoinositide-3-kinase/akt survival signal pathways are implicated in neuronal survival after stroke. Mol Neurobiol. 2006;34:249–70.

33. Sensken SC, Staubert C, Keul P, Levkau B, Schoneberg T, Graler MH. Selective activation of G alpha i mediated signalling of S1P3 by FTY720-phosphate. Cell Signal. 2008;20:1125–33.

34. Means CK, Xiao CY, Li Z, Zhang T, Omens JH, Ishii I, Chun J, Brown JH. Sphingosine 1-phosphate S1P2 and S1P3 receptor-mediated Akt activation protects against in vivo myocardial ischemia-reperfusion injury. Am J Physiol Heart Circ Physiol. 2007;292:H2944–51.

35. Bajwa A, Huang L, Ye H, Dondeti K, Song S, Rosin DL, Lynch KR, Lobo PI, Li L, Okusa MD. Dendritic cell sphingosine 1-phosphate receptor-3 regulates Th1-Th2 polarity in kidney ischemia-reperfusion injury. J Immunol. 2012;189:2584–96.

36. Bajwa A, Huang L, Kurmaeva E, Gigliotti JC, Ye H, Miller J, Rosin DL, Lobo PI, Okusa MD. Sphingosine 1-phosphate receptor 3-deficient dendritic cells modulate splenic responses to ischemia-reperfusion injury. J Am Soc Nephrol. 2016;27:1076–90.

37. Awad AS. Selective sphingosine 1-phosphate 1 receptor activation reduces ischemia-reperfusion injury in mouse kidney. AJP: Renal Physiol. 2006;290: F1516–F24.

38. Ham A, Kim M, Kim JY, Brown KM, Fruttiger M, D'Agati VD, Thomas LH. Selective deletion of the endothelial sphingosine-1-phosphate 1 receptor exacerbates kidney ischemia–reperfusion injury. Kidney Int. 2013;85:807–23.

39. Shirakawa H, Katsumoto R, Iida S, Miyake T, Higuchi T, Nagashima T, Nagayasu K, Nakagawa T, Kaneko S. Sphingosine-1-phosphate induces Ca(2+) signaling and CXCL1 release via TRPC6 channel in astrocytes. Glia. 2017;65:1005–16.

40. Li C, Li JN, Kays J, Guerrero M, Nicol GD. Sphingosine 1-phosphate enhances the excitability of rat sensory neurons through activation of sphingosine 1-phosphate receptors 1 and/or 3. J Neuroinflammation. 2015;12:70.

41. Tang HB, Jiang XJ, Wang C, Liu SC. S1P/S1PR3 signaling mediated proliferation of pericytes via Ras/pERK pathway and CAY10444 had beneficial effects on spinal cord injury. Biochem Biophys Res Commun. 2018;498:830–6.

42. Jongsma M, Hendriks-Balk MC, Michel MC, Peters SL, Alewijnse AE. BML-241 fails to display selective antagonism at the sphingosine-1-phosphate receptor, S1P(3). Br J Pharmacol. 2006;149:277–82.

43. Pedata F, Dettori I, Coppi E, Melani A, Fusco I, Corradetti R, Pugliese AM. Purinergic signalling in brain ischemia. Neuropharmacology. 2016;104:105–30.

44. Webster CM, Hokari M, McManus A, Tang XN, Ma H, Kacimi R, Yenari MA. Microglial P2Y12 deficiency/inhibition protects against brain ischemia. PLoS One. 2013;8:e70927.

45. Park SW, Kim M, Brown KM, D'Agati VD, Lee HT. Inhibition of sphingosine 1-phosphate receptor 2 protects against renal ischemia-reperfusion injury. J Am Soc Nephrol. 2012;23:266–80.

46. Block ML, Zecca L, Hong JS. Microglia-mediated neurotoxicity: uncovering the molecular mechanisms. Nat Rev Neurosci. 2007;8:57–69.

47. Gerhard A, Schwarz J, Myers R, Wise R, Banati RB. Evolution of microglial activation in patients after ischemic stroke: a [11C](R)-PK11195 PET study. NeuroImage. 2005;24:591–5.

48. Nayak D, Huo Y, Kwang WX, Pushparaj PN, Kumar SD, Ling EA, Dheen ST. Sphingosine kinase 1 regulates the expression of proinflammatory cytokines and nitric oxide in activated microglia. Neuroscience. 2010;166:132–44.

49. Taylor RA, Sansing LH. Microglial responses after ischemic stroke and intracerebral hemorrhage. Clin Dev Immunol. 2013;2013:746068.

50. Sawano T, Watanabe F, Ishiguchi M, Doe N, Furuyama T, Inagaki S. Effect of Sema4D on microglial function in middle cerebral artery occlusion mice. Glia. 2015;63:2249–59.

51. Sorensen SD, Nicole O, Peavy RD, Montoya LM, Lee CJ, Murphy TJ, Traynelis SF, Hepler JR. Common signaling pathways link activation of murine PAR-1, LPA, and S1P receptors to proliferation of astrocytes. Mol Pharmacol. 2003; 64:1199–209.

52. London A, Cohen M, Schwartz M. Microglia and monocyte-derived macrophages: functionally distinct populations that act in concert in CNS plasticity and repair. Front Cell Neurosci. 2013;7:34.

53. Hu X, Leak RK, Shi Y, Suenaga J, Gao Y, Zheng P, Chen J. Microglial and macrophage polarization-new prospects for brain repair. Nat Rev Neurol. 2015;11:56–64.

54. Xia CY, Zhang S, Gao Y, Wang ZZ, Chen NH. Selective modulation of microglia polarization to M2 phenotype for stroke treatment. Int Immunopharmacol. 2015;25:377–82.

55. Byles V, Covarrubias AJ, Ben-Sahra I, Lamming DW, Sabatini DM, Manning BD, Horng T. The TSC-mTOR pathway regulates macrophage polarization. Nat Commun. 2013;4:2834.

56. Harari OA, Liao JK. NF-kappaB and innate immunity in ischemic stroke. Ann N Y Acad Sci. 2010;1207:32–40.

57. Gabriel C, Justicia C, Camins A, Planas AM. Activation of nuclear factor-kappaB in the rat brain after transient focal ischemia. Brain Res Mol Brain Res. 1999;65:61–9.

58. Mattson MP, Camandola S. NF-kappaB in neuronal plasticity and neurodegenerative disorders. J Clin Invest. 2001;107:247–54.

59. Choi JW, Gardell SE, Herr DR, Rivera R, Lee CW, Noguchi K, Teo ST, Yung YC, Lu M, Kennedy G, Chun J. FTY720 (fingolimod) efficacy in an animal model of multiple sclerosis requires astrocyte sphingosine 1-phosphate receptor 1 (S1P1) modulation. Proc Natl Acad Sci U S A. 2011;108:751–6.

60. Graler MH, Goetzl EJ. The immunosuppressant FTY720 down-regulates sphingosine 1-phosphate G-protein-coupled receptors. FASEB J. 2004;18:551–3.

15

Reduced AMPK activation and increased HCAR activation drive anti-inflammatory response and neuroprotection in glaucoma

Mohammad Harun-Or-Rashid and Denise M. Inman*[iD]

Abstract

Background: Glaucoma is a chronic degenerative disease for which inflammation is considered to play a pivotal role in the pathogenesis and progression. In this study, we examined the impact of a ketogenic diet on the inflammation evident in glaucoma as a follow-up to a recent set of experiments in which we determined that a ketogenic diet protected retinal ganglion cell structure and function.

Methods: Both sexes of DBA/2J (D2) mice were placed on a ketogenic diet (keto) or standard rodent chow (untreated) for 8 weeks beginning at 9 months of age. DBA/2J-$Gpnmb^+$ (D2G) mice were also used as a non-pathological genetic control for the D2 mice. Retina and optic nerve (ON) tissues were micro-dissected and used for the analysis of microglia activation, expression of pro- and anti-inflammatory molecules, and lactate- or ketone-mediated anti-inflammatory signaling. Data were analyzed by immunohistochemistry, quantitative RT-PCR, ELISA, western blot, and capillary tube-based electrophoresis techniques.

Results: Microglia activation was observed in D2 retina and ON as documented by intense microglial-specific Iba1 immunolabeling of rounded-up and enlarged microglia. Ketogenic diet treatment reduced Iba1 expression and the activated microglial phenotype. We detected low energy-induced AMP-activated protein kinase (AMPK) phosphorylation in D2 retina and ON that triggered NF-κB p65 signaling through its nuclear translocation. NF-κB induced pro-inflammatory TNF-α, IL-6, and NOS2 expression in D2 retina and ON. However, treatment with the ketogenic diet reduced AMPK phosphorylation, NF-κB p65 nuclear translocation, and expression of pro-inflammatory molecules. The ketogenic diet also induced expression of anti-inflammatory agents Il-4 and Arginase-1 in D2 retina and ON. Increased expression of hydroxycarboxylic acid receptor 1 (HCAR1) after ketogenic diet treatment was observed. HCAR1 stimulation by lactate or ketones from the ketogenic diet reduced inflammasome formation, as shown by reduced mRNA and protein expression of NLRP3 and IL-1β. We also detected increased levels of Arrestin β-2 protein, an adapter protein required for HCAR1 signaling.

Conclusion: Our data demonstrate that the AMPK activation apparent in the glaucomatous retina and ON triggers NF-κB signaling and consequently induces a pro-inflammatory response. The ketogenic diet resolves energy demand and ameliorates the inflammation by inhibition of AMPK activation and stimulation of HCAR1-ARRB2 signaling that inhibits NLRP3 inflammasome-mediated inflammation. Thus, these findings depict a neuroprotective mechanism of the ketogenic diet in controlling inflammation and suggest potential therapeutic targets for inflammatory neurodegenerative diseases, including glaucoma.

Keywords: Glaucoma, AMP-activated protein kinase, Ketogenic diet, Inflammation hydroxycarboxylic acid receptor

* Correspondence: dinman@neomed.edu
Department of Pharmaceutical Sciences, Northeast Ohio Medical University,
4209 State Route 44, Rootstown, OH 44272, USA

Background

Glaucoma is a chronic optic neuropathy that progressively damages the optic nerve (ON) and leads to retinal ganglion cell (RGC) loss [1, 2]. It is one of the leading causes of irreversible vision loss worldwide [3]. A critical risk factor for ON damage is elevated intraocular pressure (IOP), but how RGC dysfunction and degeneration occurs is not fully understood [4, 5].

Energy compromise can contribute to axon loss through axon degeneration initiated by nicotinamide mononucleotide adenylyltransferase-2 (NMNAT2) depletion [6] exacerbated by loss of membrane potential that initiates Ca^{++} dysregulation and cytoskeletal breakdown [7]. NMNAT2 loss could critically tie axon maintenance and metabolism with the optic neuropathy of glaucoma. Our recent studies in the DBA/2J (D2) model of glaucoma revealed that ONs of D2 mice are metabolically vulnerable and exhibit chronic metabolic stress [8]. The D2 ON exhibited lower ATP levels, low substrate availability, transporter downregulation, and mitochondrial defects [8–10]. Axonal metabolic decline can be reversed through increased substrate availability and upregulation of monocarboxylic transporters as a result of placing mice on a ketogenic diet [8]. A ketogenic diet is primarily composed of fat with a moderate level of protein and little to no carbohydrate. Ketogenic diet induces hepatic ketogenic metabolism and produces ketone bodies, primarily β-hydroxybutyrate (βHB) [11]. Ketogenic diet has been used as a therapy for neurological disorders, including in patients with Alzheimer's disease, and in animal models of multiple sclerosis, Parkinson's disease, and amyotrophic lateral sclerosis [12–16]. An ongoing clinical trial has used ketogenic diet to treat Alzheimer's disease (study ID: NCT02912936), leading to reduction of short-term memory loss [17]. The exact mechanism of action of ketogenic diet in neuroprotection is not entirely known. Recent studies suggested ketogenic diet attenuates oxidative stress, inhibits class I histone deacetylases, promotes Nrf2 activation to upregulate antioxidants, and inhibits NF-κB to limit inflammation [18, 19]. In the treatment of epilepsy, the ketogenic diet inhibits neuronal activation through, among other changes, increased GABAergic output and lowered presynaptic excitatory neurotransmitter release [20].

AMP-activated protein kinase (AMPK) is a ubiquitously expressed Ser/Thr kinase that acts as an energy sensor by monitoring the AMP/ATP level and regulates cellular metabolism through ATP restoration [21]. In addition to acting as a key regulator of cellular energy dynamics, AMPK signaling is involved in regulating inflammation. Studies suggest AMPK signaling regulates NF-κB activation, enabling release of pro-inflammatory cytokines [22, 23]. NF-κB is a critical regulator of inflammatory response and immunity. There are five

family members of NF-κB, including NF-κB p50, NF-κB p52, NF-κB p65, RELB, and c-REL that can form homo- and hetero-dimers [24]. The most conventional dimer form is the NF-κB p65-p50 heterodimer that remains bound to the IκB family of inhibitory proteins in the cytoplasm [25]. Phosphorylation of the NF-κB/IκB complex on IκB serine residues results in dissociation of IκB from NF-κB, leading to NF-κB p65 translocation to the nucleus. The translocated NF-κB p65 binds to DNA sequences in the promoter regions of specific genes such as tumor necrosis factor alpha (TNF-α), interleukin 1 beta (IL-1β), and interleukin 6 (IL-6), inducing their transcription [26].

Lactate or ketone bodies produced from the ketogenic diet can bind and activate hydroxycarboxylic acid receptors (HCARs). Three receptor subtypes have been identified: HCAR1 (also known as GPR81), HCAR2 (GPR109A), and HCAR3 (GPR109B). The HCAR3 subtype is evolutionary lost in rodents [27]. The HCARs are G-protein-coupled receptors (GPCRs) associated with downregulation of cyclic adenosine monophosphate (cAMP) through G_i signaling that inhibits lipolysis in adipocytes [28]. HCAR expression is not confined to adipocytes but is also present on neutrophils, on tissue macrophages, in the brain on neurons and astrocytes of the hippocampus and the cerebellum, and in the retina, including on Müller glia [27, 29, 30]. HCAR activation by lactate or ketone bodies has a direct anti-inflammatory effect. Lactate activation of HCAR1 reduces liver and pancreatic injuries via inhibition of inflammasome-mediated inflammation [31]. Stimulation of HCAR2 by βHB in a mouse model of stroke induces neuroprotection via the activity of bone marrow-derived macrophages that infiltrate the brain [32]. Studies suggested the anti-inflammatory effect of lactate is solely dependent on HCAR1 and its adapter protein Arrestin β-2 (ARRB2), which ultimately reduces the activation of the NLRP3 inflammasome [32]. Inhibition of NLRP3 inflammasome activation prevents proteolytic cleavage and activation of the pro-inflammatory cytokine IL-1β, the gatekeeper cytokine that regulates most of the inflammatory response [33].

Low energy can drive inflammation [22]. Compromised energy has been observed in glaucoma [8]; additionally, inflammation has been implicated in the mechanism of glaucomatous cell dysfunction and death [34]. In this study, we investigated whether the metabolic vulnerability observed in glaucoma contributes to an extended inflammatory response, then tested the hypothesis that the ketogenic diet resolves the inflammatory response in glaucoma. Our data indicate that low energy drives inflammation in D2 chronic glaucoma mice as shown by phosphorylation of AMPK that leads to activation of NF-κB and cytokine production and release. Treatment with the ketogenic diet ameliorates inflammation through inhibition of AMPK activation and HCAR1-mediated inhibition of the NLRP3 inflammasome.

Methods

Animals

Both sexes of DBA/2J (D2) and DBA/2J-*Gpnmb* + (D2G) mice were purchased from The Jackson Laboratory (Bar Harbor, ME, USA) and housed at Northeast Ohio Medical University. The D2 mouse has mutations in the *Tyrp1* and *Gpnmb* genes that cause iris stromal atrophy and iris pigment dispersion disease, leading to age-related elevation of intraocular pressure and ocular hypertension-related retinal ganglion cell death [35]. The D2G mouse shares the D2 genetic background but carries a wildtype allele of the *Gpnmb* gene and does not develop pigmentary glaucoma. These experiments used 34 D2 mice split across two treatment groups and 6 D2G mice (Table 1). All animal procedures were approved by the Institutional Animal Care and Use Committee and performed in accordance with the ARVO Statement for the Use of Animals in Ophthalmic and Vision Research.

Intraocular pressure measurement

The Tono-Lab rebound tonometer (Tiolat-Oy, Finland) calibrated for mice was used to measure intraocular pressure (IOP). Mice were anesthetized (2.5% isoflurane delivered by vaporizer with oxygen) prior to IOP measurement and 10–15 measures were taken, and values were averaged. Both baseline and terminal IOP were measured for untreated and keto D2 and D2G mice (Table 1). All IOP measurements were carried out within 3 min of anesthetization in order to avoid any anesthetic-induced reduction of IOP [36].

Diets

Both D2 and D2G mice were fed by standard lab chow (Formulab Diet 5008; 26.8% protein, 56.4% carbohydrate, 16.7% fat) ad libitum. At 9 months of age, D2 mice were switched from standard lab chow to a very low carbohydrate, ketogenic diet (D12369B, Research Diets) for 8 weeks. The composition of the ketogenic diet was 10.4% protein, 0.1% carbohydrate, and 89.5% fat. The ketogenic diet was a soft dough, given to the mice in small stainless-steel bowl. A nylon chew bar (I-Chews from Animal Specialties & Provisions) was placed in the cage in order to provide a non-nutritive chewing surface to compensate for potential tooth overgrowth anticipated in mice provided the ketogenic diet. All mice and their food intake were weighed once weekly over 8 weeks (Table 1). Ketone levels were measured from tail vein blood using a Nova Max Plus hand-held ketone testing device once weekly from a random sample of untreated and ketogenic diet (keto) D2 mice. Final measurements of serum βHB levels were measured using a βHB assay kit (700190, Cayman Chemical, Ann Arbor, MI, USA) from blood collected at euthanasia (Table 1).

Immunohistochemistry

Freshly enucleated eyes were immersion fixed in 4% paraformaldehyde for 1 h then cryoprotected in 30% sucrose with 0.02% sodium azide. Lenses were removed from the globes that were then embedded in OCT (Sakura Finetek, Torrance, CA, USA) and frozen on dry ice. Optic nerves were fine-dissected from the brain and similarly cryoprotected and embedded in OCT. Both eyes and optic nerves were sectioned at 10 μm on a cryostat. For immunohistochemistry, all tissues were washed in 0.1 M PBS, then incubated in blocking solution (5% donkey serum, 0.5% Triton X-100 in 0.1 M PBS) for 1 h, incubated with primary antibody (diluted in 0.5% BSA, 0.9% NaCl, 0.5% Triton X-100 in 0.1 M PBS) for 24 h at 4 °C, then washed and incubated with secondary antibody for 2 h at room temperature, washed, then cover slipped with DAPI Fluoromount-G (Southern Biotech). Primary antibodies were rabbit anti-Iba1 (1:300, 019-19741, WAKO, Richmond, VA, USA), mouse anti-TNF-α (1:50, ab1793, Abcam, Cambridge, MA, USA), rabbit anti-NF-κB p65 (1:100, SAB4502610, Sigma-Aldrich, St. Louis, MO, USA), mouse anti-NOS2 (1:50, sc-7271, Santa Cruz Biotechnology, Dallas, TX, USA), mouse anti-Arginase 1 (1:50, sc-271430, Santa Cruz), mouse anti-HCAR1 (1:200, SAB1300090, Sigma-Aldrich), and goat anti-GFAP (1:250, ab53554, Abcam). Secondary antibodies were obtained from Jackson ImmunoResearch, used at 1:250 dilution, and raised in donkey against the species appropriate to the primary antibody: anti-mouse Alexa Fluor 488 (715-545-150), anti-mouse Alexa Fluor 594 (711-585-150), anti-goat Alexa Fluor 488 (705545-147), anti-rabbit Alexa Fluor 647 (711-605-152), and anti-rabbit Alexa Fluor 594 (711-545-152).

Microscopy

A Leica DMi8 confocal microscope integrated with Leica application Suite X 3.1.1.15751 (Leica Microsystems, Buffalo Grove, IL, USA) was used for microscopy. The same exposure time settings were used for capturing all the photomicrographs among all groups. Photomicrographs were obtained from the central part of retina and from proximal region of optic nerves. Immunoreactivity was quantified by using an optical density measurement within regions of interest (ROIs) using Fiji-ImageJ [37]. Minimum eight ROIs were used per antigen for quantification. For microglial quantification, five sections per retina and ON and five retinas and ONs for each group (a total of 25 sections per tissue) were used. Microglia were only counted if the DAPI-stained nucleus could be identified.

RNA analysis

Retina was dissected from freshly enucleated eyes, and total RNA was isolated using the Trizol extraction kit

Table 1 Ketogenic and control mouse indices

Mice		Baseline IOP (mmHg)	Terminal IOP (mmHg)	Baseline weight (g)	Terminal weight (g)	Food intake by week (g)	kCal by week	Plasma βHB levels (mM)
Keto D2	Male (n = 10)	17.2 ± 1.3	18.5 ± 1.3	33.2 ± 1.7	40.2 ± 2.1	18.5 ± 0.7	116.5 ± 0.8	0.53 ± 0.042
	Female (n = 8)	16.5 ± 0.8	17.4 ± 1.2	26.6 ± 0.8	29.5 ± 1.5	12.5 ± 0.4	78.7 ± 1.5	0.40 ± 0.03
Control D2	Male (n = 10)	17.5 ± 0.2	18.1 ± 0.8	32.2 ± 1.4	32.0 ± 1.2	30.5 ± 1.2	119.8 ± 1.1	0.102 ± 0.01
	Female (n = 6)	16.4 ± 1.0	17.5 ± 1.0	26.5 ± 0.9	26.1 ± 1.2	24.5 ± 1.6	95.5 ± 1.2	0.090 ± 0.04
D2G	Male (n = 3)	12.5 ± 0.1	12.2 ± 0.1	30.5 ± 1.5	31.0 ± 1.5	29.5 ± 1.5	115.5 ± 1.4	0.07 ± 0.01
	Female (n = 3)	12.1 ± 0.2	11.8 ± 0.2	25.5 ± 1.0	26.2 ± 1.1	22.1 ± 1.2	86.2 ± 1.3	0.06 ± 0.02

All values ± SEM

n number of mice

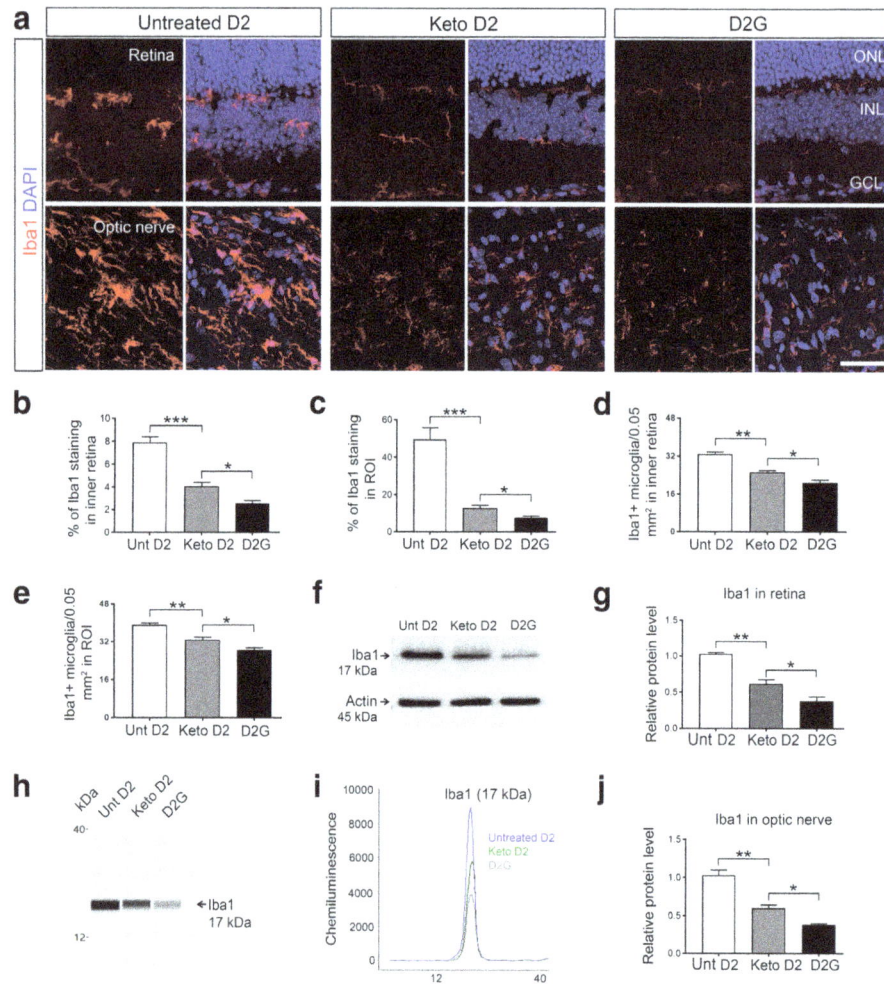

Fig. 1 Iba1 expression in the retina and ON of D2 and D2G mice. **a** Immunohistochemical analysis of Iba1 (red) expression in untreated (Unt) and keto D2 and D2G retinas and ONs. DAPI (blue) stains nuclei. **b**, **c** Percentage of mean fluorescence of Iba1 in the inner retina (**b**), *p = 0.0369, ***p = 0.0001, and in the region of interest (ROI) of the proximal ON (**c**), *p = 0.0415, ***p = 0.0001. **d**, **e** Quantification of Iba1+ microglia in the inner retina (**d**), *p = 0.0341, ***p = 0.0001, and in the ROI of the proximal ON (**e**), *p = 0.0245, ***p = 0.0001. For **b**–**e**, five retinas and ON from each group were analyzed, with five sections from each individual retina or ON. **f** Western blot analysis of Iba1 protein expression in retinas. **g** Bar graph with densitometry of Iba1 levels normalized to actin (β isoform) levels, *p = 0.0293, **p = 0.0022; n = 3 blots per group, each with independent samples. **h**–**j** Capillary tube electrophoresis of Iba1 protein in ON, normalized to actin levels. Typical capillary electrophoresis output, showing digital view of bands within capillary tube (**h**), digital graphical plot of HRP signal produced by HRP-conjugated secondary antibody that is bound to the antigen of interest (**i**); bar graph represents the areas of HRP signal normalized to areas of actin HRP signal (**j**), *p = 0.0310, ***p = 0.0013; n = 3 biological replicates per group. All bar graphs are the mean ± SEM, n = 5, analyzed by two-way, unpaired t test. Scale bar, 20 μm

(Thermo-Fisher Scientific, Waltham, MA, USA). cDNA was synthesized from 1 μg DNase-treated RNA by using cDNA synthesis kit (Verso cDNA Synthesis Kit, Thermo-Fisher Scientific) then analyzed using real-time quantitative PCR with a QuantStudio™ 6 Flex Real-Time PCR System instrument (Applied Biosystems). Both Taq-Man and SYBR Green assays were used for mRNA analysis. TaqMan Gene Expression Assays from Thermo-Fisher Scientific with a FAM reporter dye at the 5′ end of the TaqMan MGB probe were used; TaqMan assay probes were *Hcar1* (Mm00558586_s1), *Hcar2* (Mm01199527_s1), and *Hprt* (Mm00446968_m1). SYBR Green assays were performed using previously published primers [38] including *Il-6* For-TCCATCCAGTTGCCT TCTT G and Rev-ATTGCCATTGCACAACTCTTTT, *Nos2* For-TCACGCTTGGGTCTTGTT and Rev-CAGG TCACTTTGGTAGGATTT, *Il-4* For ACCACAGAGA GTGAGCTCGT and Rev-AGGCATCGAAAAGCCCG AAA, *Arg1* For-GGACCTGGCCTTTGTTGATG and Rev-AGACCGTGGGTTCTTCACAATT, *Nlrp3* For-TGCTCTTCACTGCTATCAAGCCCT and Rev-ACAA GCCTTTGCTCCAGACCCTAT, *Il-1β* For-TGGACCT

TCCAGGATGAGGACA and Rev-GTTCATCTCGGAGC CTGTAGTG, and *Hprt* For-CAGTCAACGGGGGA CATAAA and Rev-AGAGGTCCTTTTCACCAGCAA. All primers were obtained from Thermo-Fisher Scientific. *Hprt* was used as the housekeeping gene, chosen after a comparison of *Actb*, *Rpl*, *Hprt*, and *GlucB*, which showed *Hprt* had the most stable gene expression across age and strain using retina and optic nerve mRNA.

Protein analysis

Fresh retina and optic nerve tissues from D2 and D2G retina and ON were isolated and flash frozen in liquid nitrogen until homogenization in T-PER buffer (Thermo-Fisher Scientific) with HALT protease and phosphatase inhibitors (78442, Thermo-Fisher Scientific) to prevent enzymatic degradation of protein. A Branson Sonicator using three 3-s pulses at 10% amplitude was used for sonicating tissues. All protein samples were spun down at 10,000g for 10 min; supernatants were collected, and the nuclear protein fraction was extracted using the EpiQuik total histone extraction kit (# OP-0006, EpiGentek, Farmingdale, NY, USA). Both cell lysate and nuclear protein fractions were analyzed by western blot (WB) and capillary tube-based electrophoresis immunoassay using the Wes, a ProteinSimple instrument (San Jose, CA, USA) that separates proteins by electrical charge in capillary tubes and allows binding of antibodies and detection within the capillary. The Wes is suitable for analysis of very small amounts of protein, allowing us to assay individual optic nerve and quantify specific proteins within a lysate. All the Wes results (see Fig. 1f–h) were normalized to β-actin protein level. Primary antibodies used were rabbit anti-Iba1 (1:1000 for WB, 1:50 for Wes; 019-19741, WAKO), mouse anti-AMPK α1 2B7 (1:200 for Wes, NBP2-2217, Novus Biological, Littleton, CO, USA), anti-mouse AMPK α1$_{Thr172}$ (1:50 for Wes, NBP1-74502, Novus Biological), mouse anti-TNF-α (1:1000 for WB, 1:50 for Wes; ab1793, Abcam), mouse anti-NF-κB p65 (1:1000 for WB, 1:25 for Wes; 6956, Cell signaling, Danvers, MA, USA), mouse anti-Histone H3 (1:1000 for WB, 1:25 for Wes; 61473, Active Motif Carlsbad, CA, USA), mouse anti-Actin (β isoform) (1:1000 for WB, 1:25 for Wes; NB600-501, Novus Biological), mouse anti-Arginase 1 (1:100 for WB, 1:25 for Wes; sc-271430, Santa Cruz), mouse anti-HCAR1 (1:1000 for WB, 1:25 for Wes; SAB1300090, Sigma-Aldrich), mouse anti-NLRP3 (1:1000 for WB, AG-20B-0014-C100, AdipoGen, San Diego, CA, USA), rabbit anti-IL-1β (1:1000, AB1413-I, Millipore Sigma, Burlington, MA, USA), and mouse anti-ARRB2 (1:100 for WB, 1:25 for Wes; sc-365445, Santa Cruz). Secondary antibodies used were donkey anti-rabbit IgG, HRP conjugated (1:5000, 711-035-152, Jackson ImmunoResearch), and goat anti-mouse IgG, HRP conjugated (1:5000, sc-2031, Santa Cruz Biotechnology).

Enzyme-linked immunosorbent assay (ELISA)

Optic nerve protein samples were extracted as described above, and ELISA was performed using the mouse cytokine ELISA plate array I (EA-4005, Signosis, Santa Clara, CA, USA). ON protein lysate (100 μL per well) was added to the plate and incubated 24 h at 4 °C with gentle shaking. Two wells were designated blanks by adding diluent buffer instead of protein sample. After incubation, each well was aspirated and washed with washing buffer and then incubated with 100 μl biotin-labeled antibody mixture for 2 h at room temperature, then aspirated, washed, and incubated with 100 μl streptavidin-HRP conjugate for 1 h at room temperature with gentle shaking. After aspiration and wash, the plate was incubated with 100 μl substrate for 45 min at room temperature. The substrate reaction was stopped by adding 50 μl stop solution that changed color from blue to yellow, and then optical density was determined with a microtiter plate reader at 450 nm. Output of ELISA was normalized by total protein level as quantified by the Pierce™ BCA Protein Assay Kit (23225, Thermo-Fisher Scientific).

Statistical analysis

All statistical analyses were performed by GraphPad Prism Version 7.02 (GraphPad software, Inc., La Jolla, CA, 92037 USA). Data were analyzed by unpaired, two-tailed t test when comparing two groups. One-way ANOVA and Tukey's multiple comparison post hoc test was used when comparing across multiple groups. All data were presented as the mean ± SEM, and $p < 0.05$ was considered significant difference. In the text and figure legends, "n" represents number of samples, either retina or ON.

Results

At 9 months of age, D2 mice have significant IOP elevation (D2 average IOP 18.1 ± 1.3 mmHg versus D2G average IOP 11.9 ± 0.2 mmHg, as shown in Table 1), but have not yet undergone significant optic nerve degeneration and retinal ganglion cell loss [1, 8]. The D2 mice were placed on the ketogenic diet at 9 months of age to probe the role of inflammation in the neuroprotection observed with ketogenic diet treatment [8].

Ketogenic diet reduces microglia number

Microglia monitor the microenvironment in the central nervous system (CNS) and display small somata and ramified morphology with many complex processes in their resting stage. During injury or any kind of CNS pathology, microglia become activated and change their morphology [39]. We used the microglia-specific marker Iba1 [40] to monitor the activation of microglia in the retina and optic nerve (ON) of D2 glaucoma mice and investigated whether feeding D2 glaucoma mice a ketogenic diet affected microglia activation or number. Using immunohistochemistry, we detected Iba1-positive (+) microglia in the retina and ON tissues. We observed highly intense Iba1+ microglia in untreated D2 retina and ONs, whereas in the ketogenic diet-fed D2 retina and ON, Iba1 staining intensity was reduced (Fig. 1a–c). Quantification of Iba1+ microglia showed significantly increased numbers of Iba1+ microglia in untreated D2 retina and ON compared to keto D2 retina and ON (Fig. 1d, e), though microglial numbers in keto D2 retina and ON were also significantly higher than age-matched D2G tissue. We quantified Iba1 protein level in the retina and ON by western blot analysis and capillary tube electrophoresis respectively, detecting significantly decreased Iba1 protein in keto D2 retina and ON compared to untreated D2 retina (Fig. 1f, g) and ON (Fig. 1h–j). Thus, these results indicate that the ketogenic diet limits microglia activation in D2 retina and ON.

Ketogenic diet regulates AMPK activation, TNF-α release, and nuclear translocation of NF-κB p65

AMPK is a major energy sensor and regulator that promotes ATP production and inhibits ATP consumption during energy shortage [41]. In addition to its key role in energy balance, it can stimulate a variety of transcription factors and signal transduction molecules, including inflammatory cytokine release and activation of NF-κB signaling [22, 23]. We examined whether the ketogenic diet impacted AMPK signaling, cytokine release, and NF-κB activation in D2 mice. We detected significantly lower protein levels of pAMPK from the retina (Fig. 2a) and ON (Fig. 2b) from D2 mice on the ketogenic diet as compared to D2 mice on the control diet. We measured expression of the cytokine TNF-α in the retina and ON of D2 mice, revealing increased levels of TNF-α staining in D2 control diet retina (Fig. 2c, d) and ON (Fig. 2c, e) that were significantly reduced by the ketogenic diet (Fig. 2c–e). TNF-α levels in D2 retina quantified by western blot and in the ON by enzyme-linked immunosorbent assay (ELISA) showed increased levels of TNF-α in both D2 control diet retina (Fig. 2f, g) and ON (Fig. 2h) that were significantly reduced in D2 mice on the ketogenic diet (Fig. 2f–h).

TNF-α and interleukin 1-beta (IL-1β) can induce NF-κB p65, leading to its nuclear translocation and promotion of many inflammatory genes [42]. We extracted nuclear protein fractions from the retina and ON then measured NF-κB p65 levels, detecting elevated levels of nuclear NF-κB p65 in control diet D2 retina and ON that were significantly decreased in keto D2 retina (Fig. 2i, j) and ON (Fig. 2k), but still significantly higher than levels observed in the D2G retina and ON (Fig. 2j, k). Immunohistochemistry analysis of ON sections showed increased NF-κB

p65 immunostaining and nuclear translocation in untreated D2 ON compared to keto D2 ON (Fig. 2l). Collectively, these results suggest that the ketogenic diet satisfies energy demand, thereby inhibiting AMPK activation and preventing AMPK-induced TNF-α release and subsequent NF-κB p65 transcriptional activity.

Ketogenic diet reduces pro-inflammatory response and enhances anti-inflammatory signals

To further understand the consequences of the ketogenic diet on inflammation, we examined the expression of pro-inflammatory cytokine IL-6 and NOS2 in D2 glaucoma mice with or without the ketogenic diet. Quantitative RT-PCR analysis showed increased Il-6 and Nos2 mRNA expression in D2 retina, both of which are reduced after ketogenic diet treatment (Fig. 3a, d). Elevated IL-6 protein levels were detected in untreated D2 mice compared to the keto D2, in both the retina (Fig. 3b) and ON (Fig. 3c) by ELISA. Immunohistochemistry analysis of NOS2 showed intense immunolabeling in untreated D2 retina (Fig. 3e, f) and ON (Fig. 3e, g), whereas NOS2 labeling was very low in keto D2 retina and ON (Fig. 3e–g).

IL-4 and Arginase-1 are two cytokines released by immune cells exhibiting anti-inflammatory response [43]. We observed significantly higher levels of Il-4 and Arg1 mRNA in keto D2 retina (Fig. 4a) and ON (Fig. 4d) compared to untreated D2 retina and ON. IL-4 protein levels were also significantly higher in keto D2 retina (Fig. 4b) and ON (Fig. 4c) compared to untreated D2. Immunohistochemistry analysis showed plentiful Arginase-1 labeling in keto retina (Fig. 4e, f) and ON (Fig. 4e, g), while barely detectable Arginase-1 labeling was observed in untreated D2 retina and ON (Fig. 4e–g). We quantified Arginase-1 protein levels in the retina and ON by western blot and capillary electrophoresis, respectively, detecting enhanced levels of Arginase-1 in keto D2 retina (Fig. 4h, i) and ON (Fig. 4j) compared to untreated D2 retina and ON. These results suggest that the ketogenic diet ameliorates neuroinflammation in D2 glaucoma mice by inhibiting pro-inflammatory while inducing anti-inflammatory response.

Ketogenic diet induces HCAR1 expression

The primary ketone body produced by the liver on a ketogenic diet is β-hydroxybutyrate (βHB). Apart from use as an alternative energy source during energy demand, βHB can act as a signaling molecule via binding to hydroxyl-carboxylic acid receptors (HCARs) [11, 44]. As a result, we investigated whether the ketogenic diet alters the expression of HCARs in D2 glaucoma mice. By qRT-PCR analysis, we detected significantly increased levels of Hcar1 mRNA in keto D2 retina compared to untreated D2 retina (Fig. 5a). We observed no change in Hcar2 mRNA levels in D2 retina after ketogenic diet

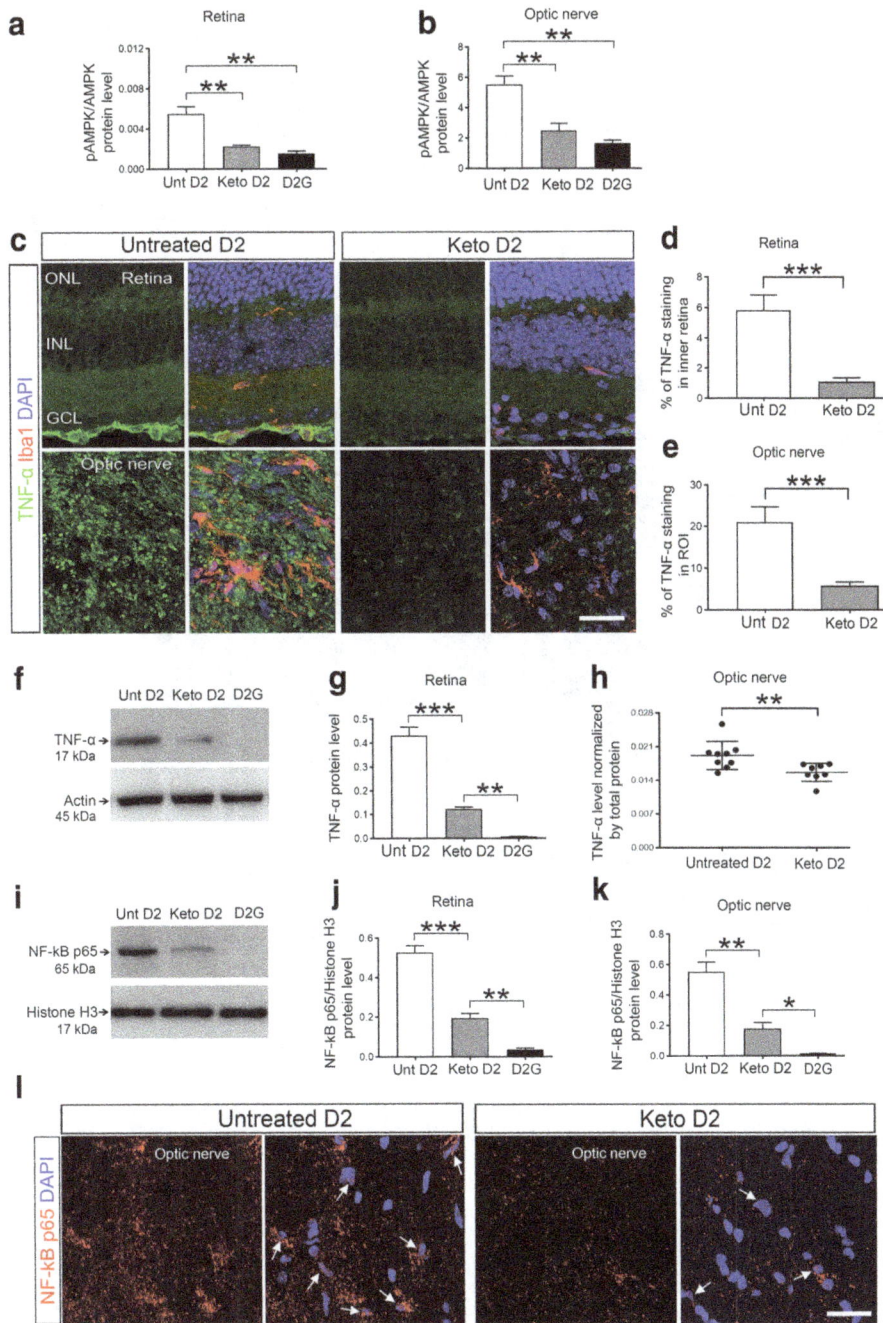

Fig. 2 Analysis of AMPK phosphorylation, TNF-α expression, and nuclear translocation of NF-κB p65 in D2 and D2G retina and ON. **a**, **b** The ratio of pAMPK to AMPK protein in the retina (**a**), **p = 0.0034, **p = 0.0016; n = 4 per group and ON (**b**), **p = 0.0018, **p = 0.0013, as analyzed by capillary electrophoresis; n = 6 Keto D2 and 3 D2G ON per group. **c** Immunohistochemical analysis of TNF-α (green) expression in untreated (Unt) and keto D2 retinas and ONs. Iba1 (red) labels microglia (**c**) and DAPI (blue) stains nuclei. **d**, **e** Percentage of mean fluorescence of TNF-α in the inner retina (**d**), ***p = 0.0001, and in the ROI of the proximal ON (**e**), ***p = 0.0001; n = 5 retinae per group, with five sections analyzed per retina. **f** Western blot analysis of TNF-α in untreated and keto D2 and D2G retinas. **g** Bar graph showing the quantification by densitometry of TNF-α protein levels normalized to actin levels in the retina, **p = 0.0035, ***p = 0.0001; n = 3 blots per group, each with independent samples. **h** TNF-α protein levels in ON analyzed by ELISA, **p = 0.0032; n = 8 per group. **i** Western blot analysis of NF-κB p65 levels in retinal nuclear protein fraction. **j** Quantification by densitometry of NF-κB p65 levels normalized to total histone H3 levels, **p = 0.0032, ***p = 0.0001; n = 3 blots per group, each with independent samples. **k** NF-κB p65 levels in nuclear fraction of the ON protein normalized to total histone H3 levels, as quantified with capillary electrophoresis, *p = 0.00593, **p = 0.0023; n = 3 ON per group. **l** NF-κB p65 (red) immunohistochemistry in the ON. Arrows indicate nuclear translocation of NF-κB. All bar graphs are presented as the mean ± SEM, n = 5–9 analyzed by two-tailed unpaired t test. **d**, **l** Scale bar, 20 µm

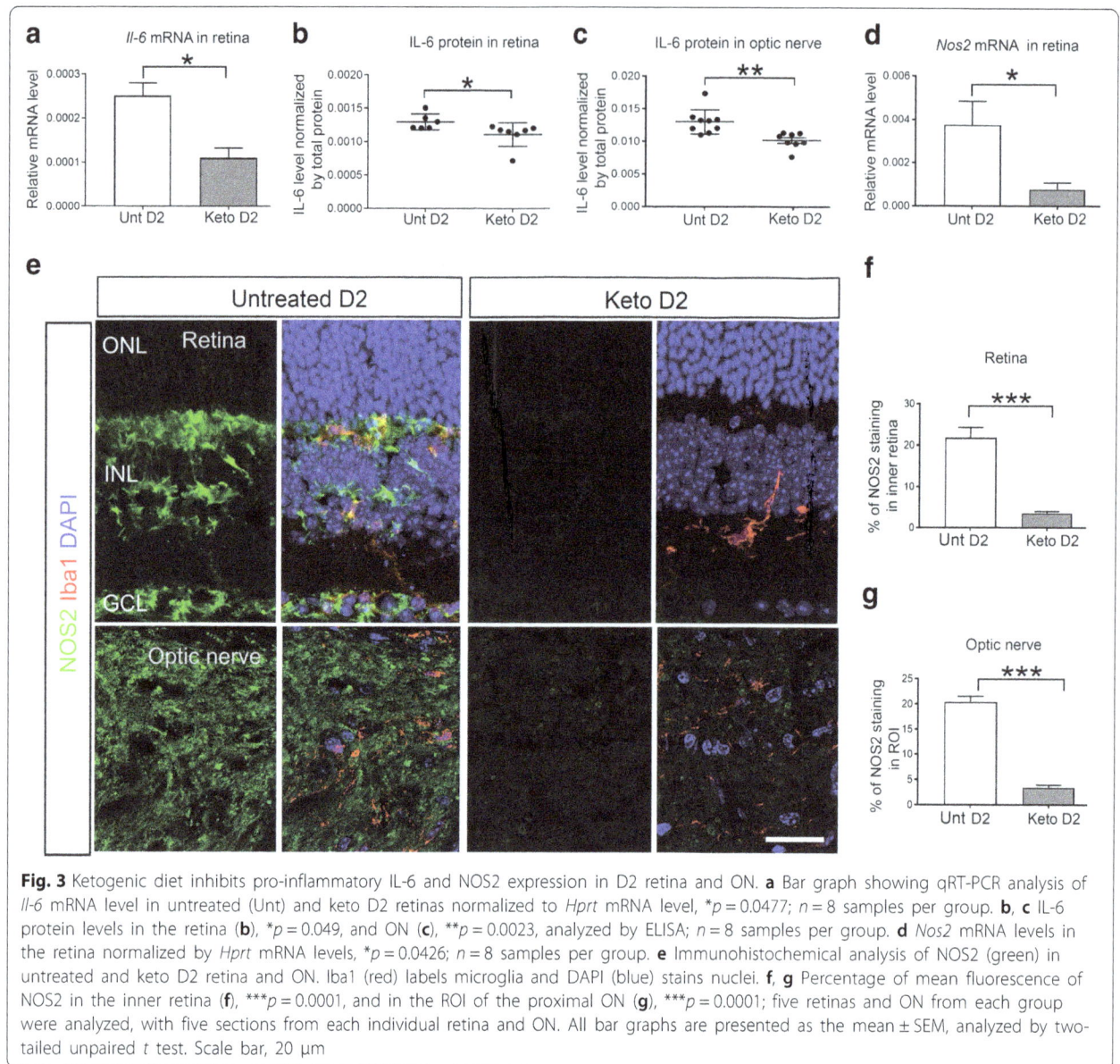

Fig. 3 Ketogenic diet inhibits pro-inflammatory IL-6 and NOS2 expression in D2 retina and ON. **a** Bar graph showing qRT-PCR analysis of *Il-6* mRNA level in untreated (Unt) and keto D2 retinas normalized to *Hprt* mRNA level, *$p = 0.0477$; $n = 8$ samples per group. **b, c** IL-6 protein levels in the retina (**b**), *$p = 0.049$, and ON (**c**), **$p = 0.0023$, analyzed by ELISA; $n = 8$ samples per group. **d** *Nos2* mRNA levels in the retina normalized by *Hprt* mRNA levels, *$p = 0.0426$; $n = 8$ samples per group. **e** Immunohistochemical analysis of NOS2 (green) in untreated and keto D2 retina and ON. Iba1 (red) labels microglia and DAPI (blue) stains nuclei. **f, g** Percentage of mean fluorescence of NOS2 in the inner retina (**f**), ***$p = 0.0001$, and in the ROI of the proximal ON (**g**), ***$p = 0.0001$; five retinas and ON from each group were analyzed, with five sections from each individual retina and ON. All bar graphs are presented as the mean ± SEM, analyzed by two-tailed unpaired *t* test. Scale bar, 20 μm

treatment (Fig. 5b). Immunohistochemistry analysis showed higher HCAR1 labeling in keto D2 retina (Fig. 5c, d) and ON (Fig. 5c, e) compared to untreated D2 retina and ON. HCAR1 colocalized with Iba1+ microglia and GFAP+ astrocyte somata (arrows), indicating the expression of HCAR1 in microglia and astrocytes. HCAR1 immunolabel was observed in many cell types in the retina, with high expression in the photoreceptor layer, the inner nuclear layer, and the ganglion cell layer. We quantified HCAR1 protein levels in retina and ON, detecting significantly higher levels of HCAR1 in both keto D2 retina (Fig. 5f, g) and ON (Fig. 5h) than in untreated D2 retina and ON. Thus, these data indicate that the ketogenic diet induces HCAR1 expression both in the retina and ON of D2 glaucoma mice.

Ketogenic diet inhibits inflammasome component NLRP3 and inflammatory cytokine IL-1β release via activation of HCAR1-ARRB2 signaling

Stimulation of HCAR by βHB ameliorates neuroinflammation via inhibition of inflammasome formation [31, 45]. To explore HCAR function in ketogenic diet-induced anti-inflammatory effects in D2 glaucoma mice, we analyzed inflammasome components NLRP3 and expression of IL-1β in keto D2 retina and ON. Consistent with inhibition of the NLRP3 inflammasome, we found significantly decreased levels of *Nlrp3* (Fig. 6a) and *Il-1β* (Fig. 6b) mRNA in keto D2 retina compared to untreated D2 retina. We measured NLRP3 and mature IL-1β protein levels by western blot, detecting significantly lower levels of NLRP3 ((Fig. 6c, d) and IL-1β (Fig. 6c, e) in keto D2 retina

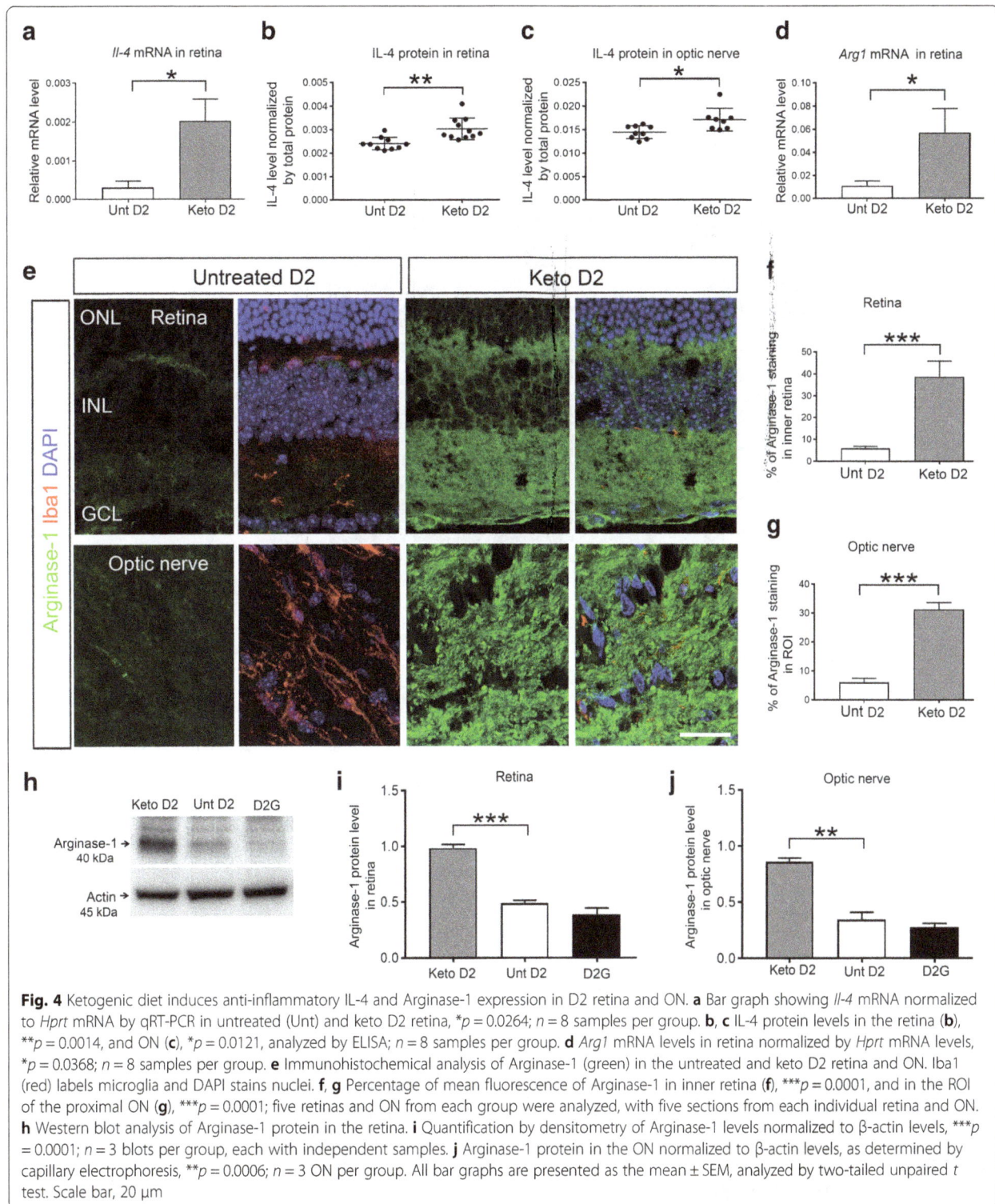

Fig. 4 Ketogenic diet induces anti-inflammatory IL-4 and Arginase-1 expression in D2 retina and ON. **a** Bar graph showing *Il-4* mRNA normalized to *Hprt* mRNA by qRT-PCR in untreated (Unt) and keto D2 retina, *$p = 0.0264$; $n = 8$ samples per group. **b, c** IL-4 protein levels in the retina (**b**), **$p = 0.0014$, and ON (**c**), *$p = 0.0121$, analyzed by ELISA; $n = 8$ samples per group. **d** *Arg1* mRNA levels in retina normalized by *Hprt* mRNA levels, *$p = 0.0368$; $n = 8$ samples per group. **e** Immunohistochemical analysis of Arginase-1 (green) in the untreated and keto D2 retina and ON. Iba1 (red) labels microglia and DAPI stains nuclei. **f, g** Percentage of mean fluorescence of Arginase-1 in inner retina (**f**), ***$p = 0.0001$, and in the ROI of the proximal ON (**g**), ***$p = 0.0001$; five retinas and ON from each group were analyzed, with five sections from each individual retina and ON. **h** Western blot analysis of Arginase-1 protein in the retina. **i** Quantification by densitometry of Arginase-1 levels normalized to β-actin levels, ***$p = 0.0001$; $n = 3$ blots per group, each with independent samples. **j** Arginase-1 protein in the ON normalized to β-actin levels, as determined by capillary electrophoresis, **$p = 0.0006$; $n = 3$ ON per group. All bar graphs are presented as the mean ± SEM, analyzed by two-tailed unpaired *t* test. Scale bar, 20 μm

compared to untreated D2 retina. We also measured IL-1β protein levels in ON by ELISA and detected significantly lower levels in keto D2 ON than untreated D2 ON (Fig. 6f). HCAR1-mediated anti-inflammatory effects are dependent on its adapter protein ARRB2 that acts on the NLRP3 inflammasome and ultimately reduces inflammation [32], so we examined whether ARRB2 expression is induced in keto D2 retina and ON. We detected significantly enhanced levels of ARRB2 protein in keto retina compared to untreated D2 retina

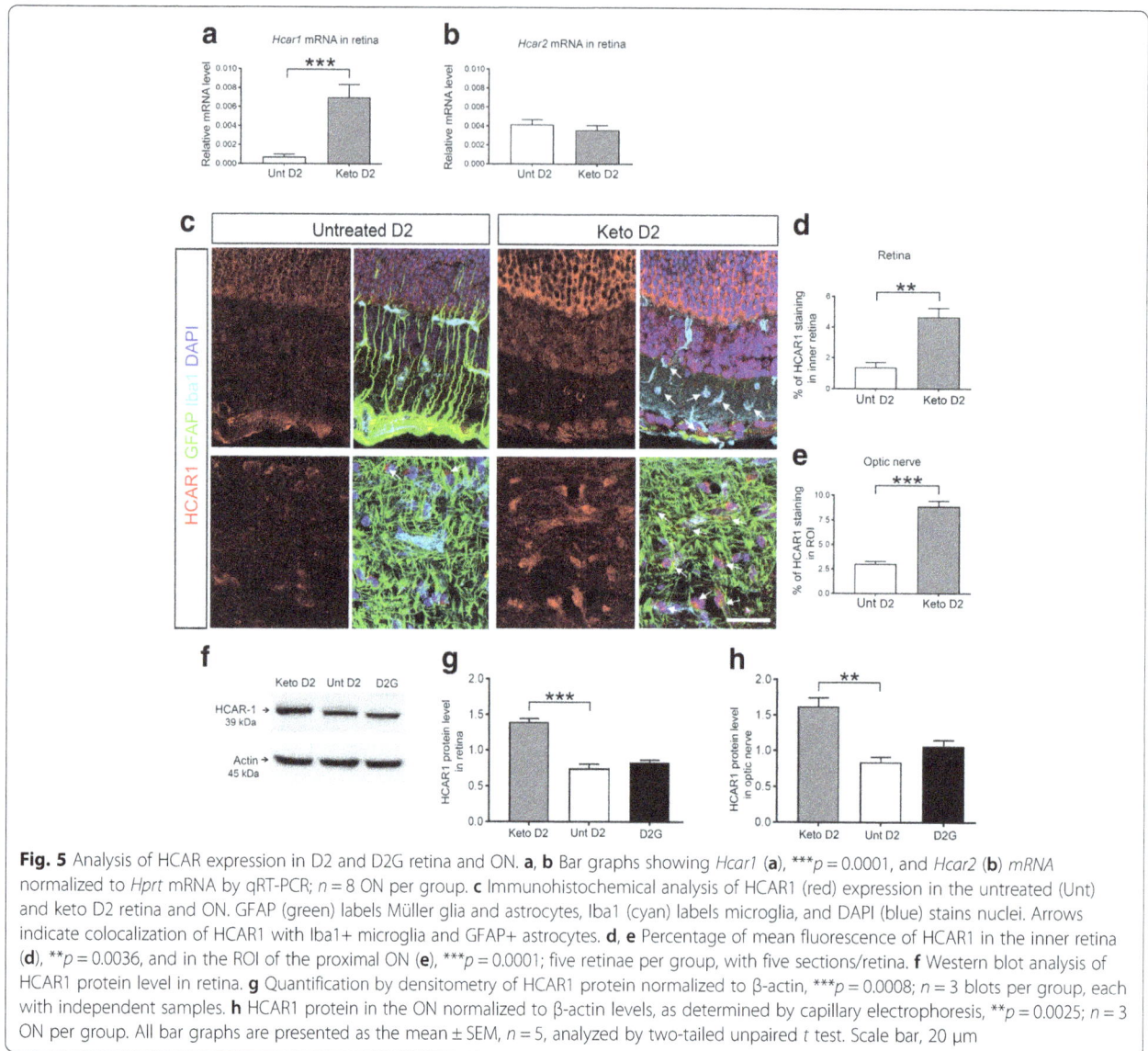

Fig. 5 Analysis of HCAR expression in D2 and D2G retina and ON. **a**, **b** Bar graphs showing *Hcar1* (**a**), ***p = 0.0001, and *Hcar2* (**b**) *mRNA* normalized to *Hprt* mRNA by qRT-PCR; n = 8 ON per group. **c** Immunohistochemical analysis of HCAR1 (red) expression in the untreated (Unt) and keto D2 retina and ON. GFAP (green) labels Müller glia and astrocytes, Iba1 (cyan) labels microglia, and DAPI (blue) stains nuclei. Arrows indicate colocalization of HCAR1 with Iba1+ microglia and GFAP+ astrocytes. **d**, **e** Percentage of mean fluorescence of HCAR1 in the inner retina (**d**), **p = 0.0036, and in the ROI of the proximal ON (**e**), ***p = 0.0001; five retinae per group, with five sections/retina. **f** Western blot analysis of HCAR1 protein level in retina. **g** Quantification by densitometry of HCAR1 protein normalized to β-actin, ***p = 0.0008; n = 3 blots per group, each with independent samples. **h** HCAR1 protein in the ON normalized to β-actin levels, as determined by capillary electrophoresis, **p = 0.0025; n = 3 ON per group. All bar graphs are presented as the mean ± SEM, n = 5, analyzed by two-tailed unpaired t test. Scale bar, 20 μm

(Fig. 6g, h). We analyzed ARRB2 protein level in ON by capillary electrophoresis and found significantly increased levels of ARRB2 protein in keto ON compared to untreated D2 ON (Fig. 6i). Hence, these results demonstrate that the ketogenic diet further promotes an anti-inflammatory response by inhibiting inflammasome formation in D2 glaucoma mice.

Discussion

Inflammation is a major pathophysiological process of secondary damage following CNS insult, including traumatic brain and spinal cord injury, Alzheimer's disease, and Parkinson's disease [46, 47]. Glaucoma is an age-related chronic degenerative disease with inflammatory response reminiscent of many other chronic neurodegenerative diseases. In this study, we investigated the contribution of metabolic vulnerability to the inflammation evident in D2

glaucoma mouse retina and optic nerve. Our data show that limited energy supply in the D2 ON and retina triggers the primary cellular energy sensor, AMPK, that activates NF-κB signaling and consequently induces the observed pro-inflammatory response. Treatment with ketogenic diet satisfies the energy demand, inhibits AMPK activation, and reduces inflammation. Lactate or ketones from the ketogenic diet also inhibit NLRP3 inflammasome-mediated inflammation through the HCAR1 receptor in D2 retina and ON.

Beneficial effects of the ketogenic diet have been reported in many neurodegenerative diseases including epilepsy, Alzheimer's disease, and Parkinson's disease [48]. Free fatty acids used in epilepsy treatment can reduce IL-1β levels, possibly through activation of PPARα [20], and the ketogenic diet metabolite βHB reduces inflammation [45]. Other than the impact of the diet on inflammation, our recent study showed the ketogenic diet directly

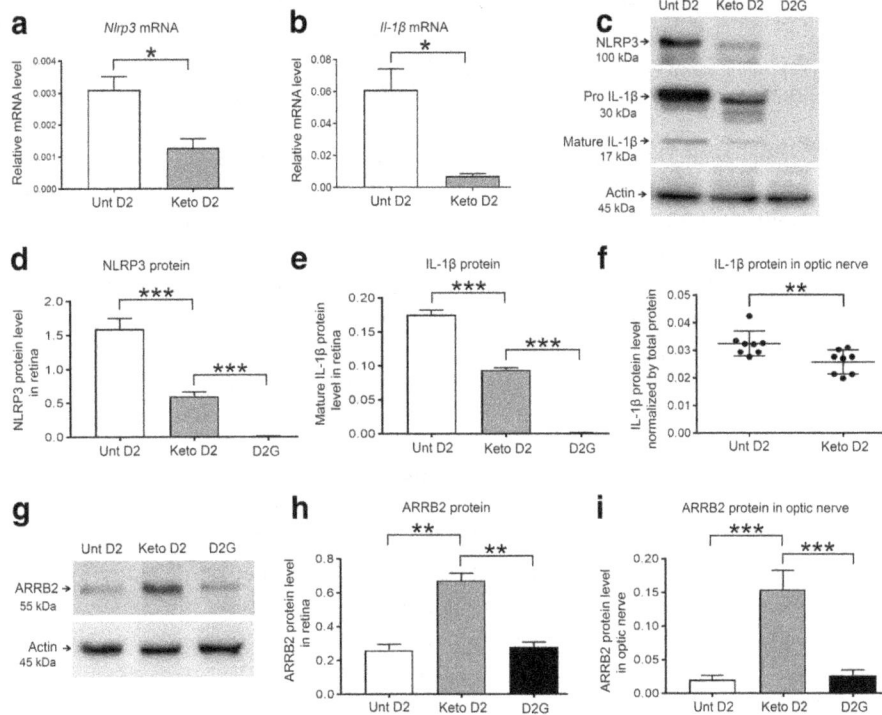

Fig. 6 Analysis of NLRP3, IL-1β, and ARRB2 expression in untreated (Unt) and Keto D2 and D2G retina and ON. **a**, **b** *Nlrp3* (**a**), *p = 0.0219, and *Il-1β* (**b**), *p = 0.0151 mRNA levels normalized to *Hprt* mRNA levels determined by qRT-PCR; *n* = 8 samples per group. **c** Western blot analysis of NLRP3 and IL-1β protein levels in the retina. **d**, **e** Quantification by densitometry of NLRP3 (**d**), ***p = 0.0001, ***p = 0.0001, and mature IL-1β (**e**), ***p = 0.0001, ***p = 0.0001 protein levels normalized to β-actin levels; *n* = 3 blots per group, each with independent samples. **f** IL-1β protein levels in the ON analyzed by ELISA, **p = 0.0092; *n* = 8 samples per group. **g** Western blot analysis of ARRB2 protein levels in the retina. **h** Quantification by densitometry of ARRB2 protein normalized to β-actin; *n* = 3 blots per group, each with independent samples. **i** Capillary tube electrophoresis of ARRB2 protein levels in the optic nerve normalized to β-actin ***p = 0.0001, ***p = 0.0001; *n* = 3 ON per group. All bar graphs are presented as the mean ± SEM, *n* = 5–9, analyzed by two-tailed unpaired *t* test

impacts energy management by inducing mitochondrial biogenesis, reversing monocarboxylate transporter decline, and inducing a robust antioxidant response. These alterations protect RGCs and their axons from degeneration, allowing them to maintain physiological signaling to the brain [8]. These data accord with evidence that βHB treatment protects cortical neurons through maintenance of neuronal respiratory capacity [49].

We first investigated microglial activation in energy-compromised D2 retina and ON. Studies have indicated that excessive and prolonged activation of microglia leads to degeneration of neurons, including RGCs [50, 51]. We detected activated microglia as shown by morphological change, including rounded shape, increased somal size, and ramified clusters in D2 retina and ON, which is consistent with previous studies showing microglia activation in glaucomatous retina and optic nerve head [50, 52]. Next, we examined how low energy in D2 retina and ON triggers inflammation. In low energy conditions, AMPKα1 is activated by phosphorylation of its Threonine 172 residue; it then works to switch cellular processes from an anabolic to a catabolic state, thereby improving energy balance by liberating ATP [53]. Our previous study showed AMPK activation early, at 6 months in the D2 ON, when glaucoma pathology is not obvious. AMPK was more highly activated at 10 month of age, indicating sustained AMPK activation in the D2 ON [8]. Activated AMPK contributes to mechanisms of inflammation [53]. Knockdown of AMPKα1 reduced LPS-induced NF-κB activation and IL-1β cytokine release [22, 23]. NF-κB is a master transcription factor for the production of cytokines; when activated, NF-κB translocates to the nucleus and induces the transcription of multiple inflammatory cytokines [54, 55]. We observed reduced NF-κB p65 activation and reduced release of pro-inflammatory cytokines TNFα, IL-6, IL-1β, and NOS2 after ketogenic diet treatment. Each of these cytokines has been associated with glaucoma pathogenesis in other studies; for example, TNFα is released by retinal glia and leads to RGC axon degeneration [56] through the upregulation of Ca^{++}-permeable AMPA receptors [57]. IL-6 is synthesized by RGCs following elevation of intraocular pressure [58]. IL-1β is upregulated prior to axon degeneration or RGC loss in the D2 model of glaucoma [52]. Moreover, we observed increased expression of the anti-inflammatory cytokines IL-4 and Arginase-1 in keto D2 retina and ON. Therefore, our data suggests that the ketogenic diet-induced anti-inflammatory response is due to inhibition of AMPK-mediated NF-κB signaling in D2 glaucoma mice. Our data are consistent with a recent study showing ketogenic diet-mediated inhibition of NF-κB signaling and attenuation of inflammation after spinal cord injury [18].

Inflammation has many feed-forward mechanisms for signal amplification, many of which involve cytokine binding to toll-like receptors (TLRs) [59] that promote NF-κB translocation and greater production of cytokines. High levels of TLR expression were reported in glaucomatous human retina as well as in the D2 retina and optic nerve head [60, 61]. Given this, we investigated a pathway downstream of TLR signaling and NF-κB, the NLRP3 inflammasome. An activating signal from a pattern recognition receptor (PRP) on the cell surface leads to the upregulation of NLRP3 as a priming reaction. This activating signal can originate from many different stimuli, including HCAR1 (see below). In fact, mechanical strain of astrocytes, as might occur in optic nerve head glial cells in glaucoma, can trigger the NLRP3 inflammasome [62]. Activated TLRs stimulate a protein cascade that results in NLRP3 inflammasome assembly, which activates caspase-1, the enzyme responsible for the maturation and release of pro-inflammatory cytokine IL-1β [32, 33]. The reduction in NF-κB signaling in our data indicates that pro-form IL-1β should be reduced, but any existing pools of IL-1β could become mature through NLRP3 inflammasome activity. Interestingly, in the context of type 2 diabetes, the NLRP3 inflammasome is a sensor of metabolic stress [63]. We observed downregulation of the NLRP3 inflammasome with the ketogenic diet. Our data also shows that NLRP3 inflammasome inhibition may occur through the activity of lactate and ketone bodies on HCAR1.

Lactate or ketone body binding to the HCARs on macrophages or monocytes can also reduce inflammation [32, 45]. We detected significantly increased mRNA and protein levels of HCAR1 but not HCAR2 in D2 retina and ON, indicating that ketogenic diet treatment induces HCAR1 expression in glaucoma mice. The HCAR1 expression was observed throughout the retina. Higher levels of HCAR1 have been detected at excitatory synapses than vascular endothelium and astrocytic end feet in the retina, suggesting that HCAR1 signaling is important for various cellular functions including metabolism, synaptic function, and blood flow in the retina [29]. Lactate or ketone body-induced anti-inflammatory effects through HCAR1 require the cytosolic signaling molecule ARRB2 [64]. We observed significantly increased ARRB2 protein levels in both the keto retina

and ON, demonstrating that ARRB2 expression is induced by the ketogenic diet. ARRB2 directly interacts with HCAR1 and exerts an anti-inflammatory effect by antagonizing NLRP3 inflammasome pathways [65]. A co-immunoprecipitation study suggested that ARRB2 interacts directly with NLRP3; accordingly, knockdown of ARRB2 markedly diminishes its ability to inhibit NLRP3 [66]. We observed reduced expression of NLRP3 after the ketogenic diet treatment in D2 retina and ON, which suggests lactate or ketone bodies trigger HCAR1-ARRB2 signaling to reduce the expression of the NLRP3 inflammasome. Our findings are consistent with the study showing HCAR1-mediated inhibition of the NLRP3 inflammasome in liver and pancreatic injury [31]. βHB-induced inhibition of NLRP3 inflammasome in macrophages was shown to be independent of HCAR2 signaling [45], but the study did not rule out the possibility that HCAR1 could be involved, as our data suggests. We detected significantly reduced levels of mature Il-1β after ketogenic diet treatment that corroborates HCAR1-mediated inhibition of NLRP3 inflammasome in D2 glaucoma mice. Knockdown of HCAR1 strongly induces hepatic IL-1β and NLRP3 expression and increases hepatocyte apoptosis, indicating a critical role for HCAR1 in endogenous dampening of inflammatory response [31]. Therefore, our data suggests that the ketogenic diet exerts its anti-inflammatory response in glaucoma not only through the inhibition of AMPK-NF-κB signaling but also via induction of HCAR1-mediated inhibition of NLRP3 inflammasome.

Conclusion

These data provide evidence that metabolic vulnerability observed in glaucoma contributes to an extended inflammatory response through chronic stimulation of AMPK that activates NF-κB signaling and subsequently induces pro-inflammatory response. Treatment with the ketogenic diet resolves energy demand and ameliorates the inflammation by inhibition of AMPK activation and by activating HCAR1 signaling that inhibits NLRP3 inflammasome-mediated inflammation. Hence, these findings reveal a neuroprotective mechanism of ketogenic diet in regulating inflammation in chronic glaucoma and provide potential therapeutic targets of glaucoma and other related inflammatory diseases.

Abbreviations
AMPK: AMP-activated protein kinase; ARRB2: Arrestin β-2; cAMP: Cyclic adenosine monophosphate; D2: DBA/2J mouse strain; D2G: DBA/2J-*Gpnmb* + mouse strain; ELISA: Enzyme-linked immunosorbent assay; GPR109A: G-protein-coupled receptor 109 A; GPR109B: G-protein-coupled receptor 109 B; GPR81: G-protein-coupled receptor 81; HCAR: Hydroxycarboxylic acid receptor; IL-1β: Interlekin-1 beta; IL-4: Interlukin-4; IL-6: Interlukin-6; IOP: Intraocular pressure; IκB: I kappa B; keto: Ketogenic diet; NF-κB: Nuclear factor-kappa B; NLRP3: NLR family, pyrin domain containing 3; NMNAT2: Nicotinamide mononucleotide adenylyltransferase 2; NOS2: Nitric oxide synthase 2; Nrf2: Nuclear factor (erythroid-derived 2)-like 2; ON: Optic

nerve; PPARα: Peroxisome proliferator-activated receptor alpha; qRT-PCR: Quantitative real-time polymerase chain reaction; RGC: Retinal ganglion cell; ROI: Region of interest; TLRs: Toll-like receptors; TNF-α: Tumor necrosis factor alpha; Unt: Untreated; βHB: β-Hydroxybutyrate

Acknowledgements

The authors thank Dr. Jason R. Richardson for sharing the primers and antibodies.

Funding

This work was supported by the National Institutes of Health Grant EY-026662 (DMI).

Authors' contributions

MHR conceptualized, designed, and conducted all the experiments and was involved in the analysis and interpretation of data as well as writing and revising the manuscript. DMI conceptualized and designed the studies, interpreted the data, and assisted in the critical revision of the manuscript. Both authors read and approved the final manuscript.

Competing interests

The authors declare that they have no competing interests.

References

1. Buckingham BP, Inman DM, Lambert W, Oglesby E, Calkins DJ, Steele MR, Vetter ML, Marsh-Armstrong N, Horner PJ. Progressive ganglion cell degeneration precedes neuronal loss in a mouse model of glaucoma. J Neurosci. 2008;28:2735–44.
2. Wojcik-Gryciuk A, Skup M, Waleszczyk WJ. Glaucoma - state of the art and perspectives on treatment. Restor Neurol Neurosci. 2015;34:107–23.
3. Quigley HA, Broman AT. The number of people with glaucoma worldwide in 2010 and 2020. Br J Ophthalmol. 2006;90:262–7.
4. Almasieh M, Wilson AM, Morquette B, Cueva Vargas JL, Di Polo A. The molecular basis of retinal ganglion cell death in glaucoma. Prog Retin Eye Res. 2012;31:152–81.
5. Quigley HA. Neuronal death in glaucoma. Prog Retin Eye Res. 1999;18:39–57.
6. Gerdts J, Summers DW, Milbrandt J, DiAntonio A. Axon self-destruction: new links among SARM1, MAPKs, and NAD+ metabolism. Neuron. 2016;89: 449–60.
7. Tsutsui S, Stys PK. Metabolic injury to axons and myelin. Exp Neurol. 2013; 246:26–34.
8. Harun-Or-Rashid M, Pappenhagen N, Palmer PG, Smith MA, Gevorgyan V, Wilson GN, Crish SD, Inman DM. Structural and functional rescue of chronic metabolically stressed optic nerves through respiration. J Neurosci. 2018;38: 5122–39.
9. Baltan S, Inman DM, Danilov CA, Morrison RS, Calkins DJ, Horner PJ. Metabolic vulnerability disposes retinal ganglion cell axons to dysfunction in a model of glaucomatous degeneration. J Neurosci. 2010;30:5644–52.
10. Coughlin L, Morrison RS, Horner PJ, Inman DM. Mitochondrial morphology differences and mitophagy deficit in murine glaucomatous optic nerve. Invest Ophthalmol Vis Sci. 2015;56:1437–46.
11. Newman JC, Verdin E. Ketone bodies as signaling metabolites. Trends Endocrinol Metab. 2014;25:42–52.
12. Henderson ST, Vogel JL, Barr LJ, Garvin F, Jones JJ, Costantini LC. Study of the ketogenic agent AC-1202 in mild to moderate Alzheimer's disease: a randomized, double-blind, placebo-controlled, multicenter trial. Nutr Metab (Lond). 2009;6:31.
13. Hertz L, Chen Y, Waagepetersen HS. Effects of ketone bodies in Alzheimer's disease in relation to neural hypometabolism, beta-amyloid toxicity, and astrocyte function. J Neurochem. 2015;134:7–20.
14. Paoli A, Rubini A, Volek JS, Grimaldi KA. Beyond weight loss: a review of the therapeutic uses of very-low-carbohydrate (ketogenic) diets. Eur J Clin Nutr. 2013;67:789–96.
15. Yang X, Cheng B. Neuroprotective and anti-inflammatory activities of ketogenic diet on MPTP-induced neurotoxicity. J Mol Neurosci. 2010;42:145–53.
16. Zhao Z, Lange DJ, Voustianiouk A, MacGrogan D, Ho L, Suh J, Humala N, Thiyagarajan M, Wang J, Pasinetti GM. A ketogenic diet as a potential novel therapeutic intervention in amyotrophic lateral sclerosis. BMC Neurosci. 2006;7:29.
17. Reger MA, Henderson ST, Hale C, Cholerton B, Baker LD, Watson GS, Hyde K, Chapman D, Craft S. Effects of beta-hydroxybutyrate on cognition in memory-impaired adults. Neurobiol Aging. 2004;25:311–4.
18. Lu Y, Yang YY, Zhou MW, Liu N, Xing HY, Liu XX, Li F. Ketogenic diet attenuates oxidative stress and inflammation after spinal cord injury by activating Nrf2 and suppressing the NF-kappaB signaling pathways. Neurosci Lett. 2018;683:13–8.
19. Shimazu T, Hirschey MD, Newman J, He W, Shirakawa K, Le Moan N, Grueter CA, Lim H, Saunders LR, Stevens RD, et al. Suppression of oxidative stress by beta-hydroxybutyrate, an endogenous histone deacetylase inhibitor. Science. 2013;339:211–4.
20. Rho JM. How does the ketogenic diet induce anti-seizure effects? Neurosci Lett. 2017;637:4–10.
21. Hallows KR, Fitch AC, Richardson CA, Reynolds PR, Clancy JP, Dagher PC, Witters LA, Kolls JK, Pilewski JM. Up-regulation of AMP-activated kinase by dysfunctional cystic fibrosis transmembrane conductance regulator in cystic fibrosis airway epithelial cells mitigates excessive inflammation. J Biol Chem. 2006;281:4231–41.
22. Wang W, Chen J, Li XG, Xu J. Anti-inflammatory activities of fenoterol through beta-arrestin-2 and inhibition of AMPK and NF-kappaB activation in AICAR-induced THP-1 cells. Biomed Pharmacother. 2016;84:185–90.
23. Wang W, Zhang Y, Xu M, Zhang YY, He B. Fenoterol inhibits LPS-induced AMPK activation and inflammatory cytokine production through beta-arrestin-2 in THP-1 cell line. Biochem Biophys Res Commun. 2015;462:119–23.
24. Nabel GJ, Verma IM. Proposed NF-kappa B/I kappa B family nomenclature. Genes Dev. 1993;7:2063.
25. Hatada EN, Nieters A, Wulczyn FG, Naumann M, Meyer R, Nucifora G, McKeithan TW, Scheidereit C. The ankyrin repeat domains of the NF-kappa B precursor p105 and the protooncogene bcl-3 act as specific inhibitors of NF-kappa B DNA binding. Proc Natl Acad Sci U S A. 1992;89:2489–93.
26. Siomek A. NF-kappaB signaling pathway and free radical impact. Acta Biochim Pol. 2012;59:323–31.
27. Offermanns S, Colletti SL, Lovenberg TW, Semple G, Wise A, AP IJ. International Union of Basic and Clinical Pharmacology. LXXXII: nomenclature and classification of hydroxy-carboxylic acid receptors (GPR81, GPR109A, and GPR109B). Pharmacol Rev. 2011;63:269–90.
28. Ahmed K, Tunaru S, Offermanns S. GPR109A, GPR109B and GPR81, a family of hydroxy-carboxylic acid receptors. Trends Pharmacol Sci. 2009;30:557–62.
29. Kolko M, Vosborg F, Henriksen UL, Hasan-Olive MM, Diget EH, Vohra R, Gurubaran IR, Gjedde A, Mariga ST, Skytt DM, et al. Lactate transport and receptor actions in retina: potential roles in retinal function and disease. Neurochem Res. 2016;41:1229–36.
30. Lauritzen KH, Morland C, Puchades M, Holm-Hansen S, Hagelin EM, Lauritzen F, Attramadal H, Storm-Mathisen J, Gjedde A, Bergersen LH. Lactate receptor sites link neurotransmission, neurovascular coupling, and brain energy metabolism. Cereb Cortex. 2014;24:2784–95.
31. Hoque R, Farooq A, Ghani A, Gorelick F, Mehal WZ. Lactate reduces liver and pancreatic injury in Toll-like receptor- and inflammasome-mediated inflammation via GPR81-mediated suppression of innate immunity. Gastroenterology. 2014;146:1763–74.
32. Rahman M, Muhammad S, Khan MA, Chen H, Ridder DA, Muller-Fielitz H, Pokorna B, Vollbrandt T, Stolting I, Nadrowitz R, et al. The beta-

hydroxybutyrate receptor HCA2 activates a neuroprotective subset of macrophages. Nat Commun. 2014;5:3944.

33. Lerch MM, Conwell DL, Mayerle J. The anti-inflammasome effect of lactate and the lactate GPR81-receptor in pancreatic and liver inflammation. Gastroenterology. 2014;146:1602–5.

34. Vohra R, Tsai JC, Kolko M. The role of inflammation in the pathogenesis of glaucoma. Surv Ophthalmol. 2013;58:311–20.

35. Anderson MG, Libby RT, Gould DB, Smith RS, John SW. High-dose radiation with bone marrow transfer prevents neurodegeneration in an inherited glaucoma. Proc Natl Acad Sci U S A. 2005;102:4566–71.

36. Ding C, Wang P, Tian N. Effect of general anesthetics on IOP in elevated IOP mouse model. Exp Eye Res. 2011;92:512–20.

37. Schindelin J, Arganda-Carreras I, Frise E, Kaynig V, Longair M, Pietzsch T, Preibisch S, Rueden C, Saalfeld S, Schmid B, et al. Fiji: an open-source platform for biological-image analysis. Nat Methods. 2012;9:676–82.

38. Neal ML, Boyle AM, Budge KM, Safadi FF, Richardson JR. The glycoprotein GPNMB attenuates astrocyte inflammatory responses through the CD44 receptor. J Neuroinflammation. 2018;15(1):73-86.

39. Saijo K, Glass CK. Microglial cell origin and phenotypes in health and disease. Nat Rev Immunol. 2011;11:775–87.

40. Imai Y, Ibata I, Ito D, Ohsawa K, Kohsaka S. A novel gene iba1 in the major histocompatibility complex class III region encoding an EF hand protein expressed in a monocytic lineage. Biochem Biophys Res Commun. 1996;224:855–62.

41. Garcia D, Shaw RJ. AMPK: mechanisms of cellular energy sensing and restoration of metabolic balance. Mol Cell. 2017;66:789–800.

42. Gutierrez H, Davies AM. Regulation of neural process growth, elaboration and structural plasticity by NF-kappaB. Trends Neurosci. 2011;34:316–25.

43. Orihuela R, McPherson CA, Harry GJ. Microglial M1/M2 polarization and metabolic states. Br J Pharmacol. 2016;173:649–65.

44. Cotter DG, Schugar RC, Crawford PA. Ketone body metabolism and cardiovascular disease. Am J Physiol Heart Circ Physiol. 2013;304:H1060–76.

45. Youm YH, Nguyen KY, Grant RW, Goldberg EL, Bodogai M, Kim D, D'Agostino D, Planavsky N, Lupfer C, Kanneganti TD, et al. The ketone metabolite beta-hydroxybutyrate blocks NLRP3 inflammasome-mediated inflammatory disease. Nat Med. 2015;21:263–9.

46. Faden AI, Loane DJ. Chronic neurodegeneration after traumatic brain injury: Alzheimer disease, chronic traumatic encephalopathy, or persistent neuroinflammation? Neurotherapeutics. 2015;12:143–50.

47. Wang YT, Lu XM, Chen KT, Shu YH, Qiu CH. Immunotherapy strategies for spinal cord injury. Curr Pharm Biotechnol. 2015;16:492–505.

48. Augustin K, Khabbush A, Williams S, Eaton S, Orford M, Cross JH, Heales SJR, Walker MC, Williams RSB. Mechanisms of action for the medium-chain triglyceride ketogenic diet in neurological and metabolic disorders. Lancet Neurol. 2018;17:84–93.

49. Laird MD, Clerc P, Polster BM, Fiskum G. Augmentation of normal and glutamate-impaired neuronal respiratory capacity by exogenous alternative biofuels. Transl Stroke Res. 2013;4:643–51.

50. Bosco A, Inman DM, Steele MR, Wu G, Soto I, Marsh-Armstrong N, Hubbard WC, Calkins DJ, Horner PJ, Vetter ML. Reduced retina microglial activation and improved optic nerve integrity with minocycline treatment in the DBA/2J mouse model of glaucoma. Invest Ophthalmol Vis Sci. 2008;49:1437–46.

51. Fischer AJ, Zelinka C, Milani-Nejad N. Reactive retinal microglia, neuronal survival, and the formation of retinal folds and detachments. Glia. 2015;63:313–27.

52. Wilson GN, Inman DM, Dengler Crish CM, Smith MA, Crish SD. Early pro-inflammatory cytokine elevations in the DBA/2J mouse model of glaucoma. J Neuroinflammation. 2015;12:176.

53. Hardie DG, Ashford ML. AMPK: regulating energy balance at the cellular and whole body levels. Physiology (Bethesda). 2014;29:99–107.

54. Kanarek N, Ben-Neriah Y. Regulation of NF-kappaB by ubiquitination and degradation of the IkappaBs. Immunol Rev. 2012;246:77–94.

55. Yang C, Ling H, Zhang M, Yang Z, Wang X, Zeng F, Wang C, Feng J. Oxidative stress mediates chemical hypoxia-induced injury and inflammation by activating NF-kappab-COX-2 pathway in HaCaT cells. Mol Cells. 2011;31:531–8.

56. Kitaoka Y, Kitaoka Y, Kwong JM, Ross-Cisneros FN, Wang J, Tsai RK, Sadun AA, Lam TT. TNF-alpha-induced optic nerve degeneration and nuclear factor-kappaB p65. Invest Ophthalmol Vis Sci. 2006;47:1448–57.

57. Cueva Vargas JL, Osswald IK, Unsain N, Aurousseau MR, Barker PA, Bowie D, Di Polo A. Soluble tumor necrosis factor alpha promotes retinal ganglion

cell death in glaucoma via calcium-permeable AMPA receptor activation. J Neurosci. 2015;35:12088–102.

58. Chidlow G, Wood JP, Ebneter A, Casson RJ. Interleukin-6 is an efficacious marker of axonal transport disruption during experimental glaucoma and stimulates neuritogenesis in cultured retinal ganglion cells. Neurobiol Dis. 2012;48:568–81.

59. Kawai T, Akira S. The role of pattern-recognition receptors in innate immunity: update on Toll-like receptors. Nat Immunol. 2010;11:373–84.

60. Howell GR, Macalinao DG, Sousa GL, Walden M, Soto I, Kneeland SC, Barbay JM, King BL, Marchant JK, Hibbs M, et al. Molecular clustering identifies complement and endothelin induction as early events in a mouse model of glaucoma. J Clin Invest. 2011;121:1429–44.

61. Howell GR, Walton DO, King BL, Libby RT, John SW. Datgan, a reusable software system for facile interrogation and visualization of complex transcription profiling data. BMC Genomics. 2011;12:429.

62. Albalawi F, Lu W, Beckel JM, Lim JC, McCaughey SA, Mitchell CH. The P2X7 receptor primes IL-1beta and the NLRP3 inflammasome in astrocytes exposed to mechanical strain. Front Cell Neurosci. 2017;11:227.

63. Schroder K, Zhou R, Tschopp J. The NLRP3 inflammasome: a sensor for metabolic danger? Science. 2010;327:296–300.

64. Ge H, Weiszmann J, Reagan JD, Gupte J, Baribault H, Gyuris T, Chen JL, Tian H, Li Y. Elucidation of signaling and functional activities of an orphan GPCR, GPR81. J Lipid Res. 2008;49:797–803.

65. Yan Y, Jiang W, Spinetti T, Tardivel A, Castillo R, Bourquin C, Guarda G, Tian Z, Tschopp J, Zhou R. Omega-3 fatty acids prevent inflammation and metabolic disorder through inhibition of NLRP3 inflammasome activation. Immunity. 2013;38:1154–63.

66. Lin C, Chao H, Li Z, Xu X, Liu Y, Bao Z, Hou L, Liu Y, Wang X, You Y, et al. Omega-3 fatty acids regulate NLRP3 inflammasome activation and prevent behavior deficits after traumatic brain injury. Exp Neurol. 2017;290:115–22.

16

New insights into meningitic *Escherichia coli* infection of brain microvascular endothelial cells from quantitative proteomics analysis

Wen-Tong Liu[1†], Yu-Jin Lv[1,2†], Rui-Cheng Yang[1], Ji-Yang Fu[1], Lu Liu[1], Huan Wang[1], Qi Cao[1], Chen Tan[1,3], Huan-Chun Chen[1,3] and Xiang-Ru Wang[1,3*] (iD)

Abstract

Background: Bacterial meningitis remains a big threat to the integrity of the central nervous system (CNS), despite the advancements in antimicrobial reagents. *Escherichia coli* is a bacterial pathogen that can disrupt the CNS function, especially in neonates. *E. coli* meningitis occurs after bacteria invade the brain microvascular endothelial cells (BMECs) that form a direct and essential barrier restricting the entry of circulating microbes and toxins to the brain. Previous studies have reported on several cellular proteins that function during meningitic *E. coli* infections; however, more comprehensive investigations to elucidate the potential targets involved in *E. coli* meningitis are essential to better understand this disease and discover new treatments for it.

Methods: The isobaric tags for relative and absolute quantification (iTRAQ) approach coupled with LC-MS/MS were applied to compare and characterize the different proteomic profiles of BMECs in response to meningitic or non-meningitic *E. coli* strains. KEGG and gene ontology annotations, ingenuity pathways analysis, and functional experiments were combined to identify the key host molecules involved in the meningitic *E. coli*-induced tight junction breakdown and neuroinflammatory responses.

Results: A total of 13 cellular proteins were found to be differentially expressed by meningitic *E. coli* strains PCN033 and RS218, including one that was also affected by HB101, a non-meningitic *E. coli* strain. Through bioinformatics analysis, we identified the macrophage migration inhibitory factor (MIF), granzyme A, NF-κB signaling, and mitogen-activated protein kinase (MAPK) pathways as being biologically involved in the meningitic *E. coli*-induced tight junction breakdown and neuroinflammation. Functionally, we showed that MIF facilitated meningitic *E. coli*-induced production of cytokines and chemokines and also helped to disrupt the blood-brain barrier by decreasing the expression of tight junction proteins like ZO-1, occludin. Moreover, we demonstrated the significant activation of NF-κB and MAPK signaling in BMECs in response to meningitic *E. coli* strains, which dominantly determined the generation of the proinflammatory cytokines including IL-6, IL-8, TNF-α, and IL-1β.

(Continued on next page)

* Correspondence: wangxr228@mail.hzau.edu.cn
†Wen-Tong Liu and Yu-Jin Lv contributed equally to this work.
[1]The Cooperative Innovation Center for Sustainable Pig Production, Huazhong Agricultural University, Wuhan 430070, Hubei, China
[3]State Key Laboratory of Agricultural Microbiology, College of Veterinary Medicine, Huazhong Agricultural University, Wuhan 430070, Hubei, China
Full list of author information is available at the end of the article

(Continued from previous page)

Conclusions: Our work identified 12 host cellular targets that are affected by meningitic *E. coli* strains and revealed MIF to be an important contributor to meningitic *E. coli*-induced cytokine production and tight junction disruption, and also the NF-κB and MAPK signaling pathways that are mainly involved in the infection-induced cytokines production. Characterization of these distinct proteins and pathways in BMECs will facilitate further elucidation of meningitis-causing mechanisms in humans and animals, thereby enabling the development of novel preventative and therapeutic strategies against infection with meningitic *E. coli*.

Keywords: iTRAQ, Proteomics, Blood-brain barrier, BMECs, Meningitic *E. coli*

Background

Bacterial meningitis is a severe, life-threatening infection of the central nervous system (CNS) with high morbidity and mortality. It is currently recognized as one of the top ten killers in infection-related deaths worldwide, with almost half of the survivors suffering from diverse neurological sequelae (e.g., mental retardation, hearing impairment and blindness), despite the advancements made in the field of antimicrobial treatment [1–3]. Most bacterial meningitis cases are initiated by hematogenous spread and develop when the circulating bacteria penetrate the blood-brain barrier (BBB), destroy brain parenchyma, and finally cause CNS disorders [1]. Among the meningitis-causing microbes, extraintestinal pathogenic *Escherichia coli* (ExPEC) has recently emerged as an important zoonotic bacterial pathogen with the potential to colonize multiple tissues outside the intestine and cause severe infections, with one typical outcome being meningitis. The evidence from recent in vivo and in vitro studies indicates that meningitic *E. coli* strains possess the ability to invade the brain, and the infection-induced BBB disruption that occurs is the hallmark event in the development of *E. coli* meningitis [4, 5].

The availability of in vitro and in vivo BBB infection models has made the study of meningitic *E. coli* penetration of the brain possible [6–9]. The in vitro BBB model uses brain microvascular endothelial cells (BMECs) that form distinctive tight junctions and exhibit high trans-endothelial electrical resistance, thereby mimicking the features of the natural in vivo barrier that protects the brain from circulating microorganisms and toxins [10–13]. The in vivo model is established by inducing experimental hematogenous meningitis in newborn rats and mice [9, 14, 15]. With these models, it is now well-established that successful traversal of the BBB by circulating *E. coli* strains requires the following prerequisites: a high bacteremia, binding to and invasion of BMECs, rearrangement of actin cytoskeleton, and crossing the BBB as live bacteria [1, 2]. These require a series of complicated interactions between meningitic *E. coli* and the host. So far, several host targets have been found to be associated with this invasion process, including certain intracellular signaling molecules like focal adhesion kinase, phosphatidylinositol 3-kinase (PI3K), Rho GTPases, cytosolic phospholipase A2, nuclear factor-κB (NF-κB), inducible nitric oxide synthase (NOS), and several cellular surface molecules/receptors such as caveolin-1, Toll-like receptors, the intercellular adhesion molecule (ICAM-1), and some actin-binding molecules like ERM family proteins (ezrin, radixin, and moesin), most likely through their influences on the aforementioned prerequisites [8, 16–19]. We have previously identified and characterized two essential cellular targets, S1P and EGFR, which are exploited by meningitic *E. coli* for successful invasion of the BBB [20]. In other work, we have also found that vascular endothelial growth factor A (VEGFA) and Snail-1, which are inducible by meningitic *E. coli*, can mediate the BBB disruption [5]. Despite these advances, the mechanisms involved in CNS infection by meningitic *E. coli* are still poorly understood, and a more comprehensive investigation to elucidate the cellular targets in infected BMECs is now required.

In the current study, we compared the different proteomic profiles of BMECs in response to meningitic and non-meningitic *E. coli* strains via the isobaric tags for relative and absolute quantification (iTRAQ) approach and investigated the potential host factors and mechanisms that were hijacked by meningitic *E. coli* to penetrate the BBB. Characterization of these potential host targets will expand our current knowledge on meningitic *E. coli*-induced CNS infections and provide new strategies to prevent this infection and develop novel therapeutic reagents against it.

Methods

Bacterial strains, cell culture, and infection

The *E. coli* K1 strain RS218 (O18:K1:H7) [GenBank: CP007149.1], whose genomic sequencing has been finalized and annotated, is a well-characterized cerebrospinal fluid (CSF) isolate from a neonatal meningitis case [21]. The porcine-originated ExPEC strain PCN033 (O11: K2) [GenBank: CP006632.1], which was isolated from swine CSF in China [22, 23], is evidenced to be highly virulent and capable of invading and disrupting the BBB, thereby causing CNS dysfunction [5, 24]. *E. coli* K12 strain HB101 is an avirulent and non-meningitic strain normally used as a negative control strain [25, 26]. All *E.*

coli strains were grown aerobically at 37 °C in Luria–Bertani medium unless otherwise specified.

The immortalized human BMECs (hereafter called hBMECs) were kindly provided by Prof. Kwang Sik Kim in Johns Hopkins University School of Medicine and routinely cultured in RPMI 1640 supplemented with 10% fetal bovine serum, 2 mM L-glutamine, 1 mM sodium pyruvate, essential amino acids, nonessential amino acids, vitamins, and penicillin and streptomycin (100 U/mL) in a 37 °C incubator under 5% CO_2 until monolayer confluence was reached [20, 27]. Confluent cells were washed with Hank's balanced salt solution (Corning Cellgro, Manassas, VA, USA) and starved in serum-free medium for 16–18 h before further treatment. For bacterial challenge, the cells were infected with *E. coli* PCN033, RS218, or HB101 strains each at a multiplicity of infection of 10 for 2 h. In some assays, the cells were pretreated with specific inhibitors prior to bacterial challenge.

Reagents, antibodies, and inhibitors

The p38 inhibitor SB202190, extracellular signal-regulated kinases 1 and 2 (ERK1/2) inhibitor U0126, c-Jun N-terminal kinase (JNK) inhibitor SP600125, NF-κB inhibitor BAY11-7082, and (S, R)-3-(4-hydroxyphenyl)-4, 5-dihydro-5-isoxazole acetic acid methyl ester (ISO-1), an inhibitor of macrophage migration inhibitory factor (MIF), were purchased from MedChem Express (Monmouth, NJ, USA). Recombinant MIF protein was purchased from Novoprotein (Summit, NJ, USA). The nucleic acid dye, 4′-6-diamidino-2-phenylindole (DAPI), was obtained from Solarbio (Beijing, China). Anti-ZO-1, anti-MIF, anti-TATA box-binding protein-like protein 1 (TBPL1), anti-legumain (LGMN), anti-ERK1/2, and anti-phospho-ERK1/2 antibodies (all rabbit) were purchased from ABclonal (Wuhan, Hubei, China). Anti-occludin, anti-dystrophin (DMD), anti-HISTIHIC, anti-JNK, and anti-p38 mitogen-activated protein kinase (MAPK) antibodies (all rabbit) were purchased from Proteintech (Chicago, IL, USA). Anti-phospho-JNK (rabbit) antibody was from R&D Systems (Minneapolis, MO, USA). Anti-phospho-p38, anti-p65, anti-phospho-p65, and anti-IκBα antibodies (all rabbit) were purchased from Cell Signaling Technology (Danvers, MA, USA). Cy3-labeled goat anti-rabbit antibody was purchased from Beyotime Institute of Biotechnology (Shanghai, China). Anti-GAPDH (mouse) antibody was purchased from Beijing Biodragon Immunotechnologies Co., Ltd. (Beijing, China).

Protein isolation, digestion, and labeling with iTRAQ reagents

Bacterial-infected and non-infected cells in 10 cm dishes were collected 2-h post-infection and gently washed with pre-chilled PBS buffer. The cells were lysed in 1 mL lysis buffer, and the soluble protein fraction was harvested by 5 min of ultrasonication treatment (pulse on 2 s, pulse off 3 s, power 180 W) followed by centrifugation at 20000×*g* for 30 min at 4 °C, and the protein concentration was determined via the Bradford protein assay method with BSA as the standard substance. The proteins were reduced with 10 mM iodoacetamide at room temperature for 45 min in the dark and then precipitated in acetone at – 20 °C for 3 h. After centrifugation at 20000×*g* for 20 min, the protein pellet was resuspended and ultrasonicated in pre-chilled 50% (*w/v*) tetraethyl-ammonium bromide (TEAB) buffer supplemented with 0.1% SDS. The proteins were obtained after centrifugation at 20000×*g* and their concentrations were measured by Bradford assays.

Subsequently, protein (100 μg) in TEAB buffer was incubated with 3.3 μL of trypsin (1 μg/μL) (Promega, Madison, WI, USA) at 37 °C for 24 h in a sealed tube. The tryptic peptides were lyophilized and dissolved in 50% TEAB buffer, and iTRAQ labeling was performed according to the manufacturer's instructions (AB Sciex, Foster City, CA, USA). Briefly, one unit of iTRAQ reagent was thawed and reconstituted in 24 μL isopropanol and the peptides were incubated at room temperature for 2 h. The peptides from the control, HB101, PCN033, and RS218 groups were designated 114, 115, 116, and 117, respectively. The labeled samples were then mixed and dried with a rotary vacuum concentrator. The labeling efficiency was examined by mass spectrometry (MS).

Strong cation exchange chromatography (SCX) fractionation and liquid chromatography (LC)–MS/MS analysis

The labeled samples were pooled and purified using an SCX column (Phenomenex, USA), and separated by LC using an LC-20AB HPLC pump system (Shimadzu, Japan). The peptides were then mixed with nine times their volume in buffer A (25% ACN, 10 mM KH_2PO_4, pH = 3) and loaded onto a 4.6 × 250 mm Ultremex SCX column containing 5-μm particles (Phenomenex). The peptides were eluted at a flow rate of 1 ml/min in a buffer B (25% ACN, 2 M KCL, 10 mM KH_2PO_4, pH = 3) gradient as follows: 0–5% buffer B for 30 min, 5–30% buffer B for 20 min, 30–50% buffer B for 5 min, 50% buffer B for 5 min, 50–100% buffer B for 5 min, and 100% buffer B for 1 min before equilibrating with buffer A for 10 min prior to the next injection. Next, the eluted peptides were desalted with a Strata X C18 column (100 mm × 75 mm, 5-um particles, 300A aperture) (Phenomenex, Torrance, CA, USA) and vacuum dried. The fractions were then dissolved in aqueous solution containing 0.1% formic acid (FA) and 2% ACN and centrifuged at 12000*g* for 10 min at 4 °C. Five micrograms supernatant was loaded on an LC-20AD nano HPLC (Shimadzu, Kyoto, Japan) by the autosampler onto a 2 cm C18 trap column (inner diameter 200 μm, Waters), and the peptides were eluted onto a resolving 10 cm analytical C18 column (inner diameter 75 μm, Waters). The mobile phases used were composed of solvent A (0.1% FA and 5% ACN) and solvent B (0.1% FA and 95% ACN). The gradient was run at 400 nL/min for 48 min at 5–80% solvent B, followed by running a linear gradient to 80% for 7 min, maintained at 80% B for 3 min, and finally returned to 5% in 7 min.

The peptides were subjected to nano-electrospray ionization followed by tandem mass spectrometry (MS/MS) in a Q EXACTIVE (Thermo Fisher Scientific, San Jose, CA, USA) coupled to the HPLC. Intact peptides were detected in the Orbitrap at a resolution of 70,000 and a mass range of 350–2000 m/z. Peptides were selected for MS/MS using high-energy collision dissociation (HCD), and ion fragments were detected in the Orbitrap at a resolution of 17,500. The electrospray voltage applied was 1.8 kV. MS/MS analysis was required for the 15 most abundant precursor ions, which were above a threshold ion count of 20,000 in the MS survey scan, including a following dynamic exclusion duration of 15 s.

iTRAQ data analysis

The raw data files acquired from the mass spectrometers were converted into MGF files using 5600 MS Converter. Protein identification and quantification were performed using the Mascot Server (http://www.matrixscience.com/search_form_select.html) against the Uniprot_2015_human database (Matrix Science, London, UK; version 2.3.0) and Proteome Discoverer 1.3 (Thermo Fisher Scientific Inc.). To reduce the probability of false peptide identification, only peptides with significance scores at the 95% confidence interval as determined by a Mascot probability analysis were included. The quantitative protein ratios were weighted and normalized by the median ratio in Mascot. Statistical significance analyses were evaluated using two-way ANOVA. The proteins were considered to be differentially expressed if the ratio of mean fold change > 1.2 (or < 0.83) with an Exp pr > 0.05 and a Group pr < 0.05 (Exp pr, three-experiment p value; Group pr, group p value; fold change = experiment + group + error).

The Gene Ontology (GO) annotation of the identified proteins was performed via the online GO program (http://geneontology.org/). The biological functions, networks, and signaling pathways of the differentially expressed proteins (DEPs) were analyzed with Ingenuity Pathways Analysis (IPA) software (version 7.5, http://www.ingenuity.com) (Additional files 8, 9 and 10).

RNA extraction and quantitative real-time PCR

Total RNA from the uninfected or infected cells was extracted with RNAiso Plus reagent according to the manufacturer's instructions (TakaRa, Japan). Any genomic DNA contamination was eliminated by DNase I treatment, and the RNA was reverse-transcribed into cDNA using the PrimeScript™ RT reagent kit with gDNA Eraser, following the manufacturer's instructions (Takara, Japan). Quantitative real-time PCR was performed in triplicate using the Power SYBR Green PCR Master Mix (Applied BioSystems, Foster City, CA, USA). The PCR primers for these experiments are listed in Table 1. The expression levels of the target genes were normalized to GAPDH by the $2^{-\Delta\Delta CT}$ method.

Western blotting

Uninfected and infected hBMECs were collected and lysed in RIPA buffer supplemented with a protease inhibitor cocktail (Sigma-Aldrich, St. Louis, MO, USA) and then sonicated and centrifuged at 10,000×g for 10 min at 4 °C. The soluble protein concentration in the supernatants was measured using the BCA protein assay kit (Beyotime, China). Aliquots from each sample were separated by 12% SDS-PAGE, and then transferred to polyvinylidene difluoride membranes (Bio-Rad, CA, USA). The blots were blocked with 5% BSA in Tris-buffered saline with Tween 20 at room temperature for 1 h and then incubated overnight at 4 °C with primary antibodies against GAPDH, DMD, MIF, HIST1H1C, TBPL1 or LGMN. The blots were subsequently washed and incubated with horseradish peroxidase-conjugated anti-rabbit or anti-mouse IgG at 37 °C for 1 h, and visualized with ECL reagents (Bio-Rad, USA). The blots were densitometrically quantified and analyzed with Image Lab software (Bio-Rad).

Immunofluorescence microscopy

Uninfected and infected hBMECs were fixed with 4% paraformaldehyde and permeabilized with 0.2% Triton X-100. After 2 h of blocking in PBS buffer with 5% BSA, the cells were incubated with the primary antibody (1:100) overnight at 4 °C, washed thrice with PBS, and then incubated with fluorescently labeled anti-mouse or anti-rabbit IgG (1500) for 1 h. Nuclei were stained with DAPI

Table 1 Primers used for real-time PCR in this study

Primers	Nucleotide sequence(5'-3')	Gene symbol(s)
P1	ACGAATCTCCGACCACT	IL-1β
P2	CCATGGCCACAACAACTGAC	
P3	CTCAGCCTCTTCTCCTTC	TNF-α
P4	GGGTTTGCTACAACATGG	
P5	CCACTCACCTCTTCAGAA	IL-6
P6	GGCAAGTCTCCTCATTGA	
P7	GACATACTCCAAACCTTTCC	IL-8
P8	ATTCTCAGCCCTCTTCAAA	
P9	TGCCTCCTGCACCACCAACT	GAPDH
P10	CGCCTGCTTCACCACCTTC	

(0.5 μg/mL) for 30 min. Finally, the cells were mounted and then visualized with fluorescence microscopy.

Electric cell substrate impedance sensing (ECIS)

To explore the influence of recombinant MIF on the permeability of the BBB, hBMECs were seeded at 7×10^4 cells on collagen-coated, gold-plated electrodes in 96-well chamber slides (96W1E+) linked to ECIS Zθ equipment (Applied BioPhysics, Troy, NY, USA) and continuously cultured until confluence, and the trans-endothelial electric resistance (TEER) was monitored to reflect the formation of the barrier [28]. After stable maximal TEER was reached, the recombinant human MIF protein was added into the cells at multiple dosages (10, 100, and 200 ng/mL), and the possible TEER alteration of the monolayer cells was automatically recorded by the ECIS system.

Statistical analysis

Data were expressed as the mean ± standard deviation (mean ± SD) from three replicates. Statistical significance of the differences between each group was analyzed by a one-way analysis of variance (ANOVA) or two-way ANOVA embedded in GraphPad Prism, version 6.0 (GraphPad Software Inc., La Jolla, CA, USA). $P < 0.05$ (*) was considered statistically significant, and $p < 0.01$ (**), as well as $p < 0.001$ (***) were all considered extremely significant.

Results

Differential protein profiling of hBMECs in response to E. coli infection

The protein extracts prepared from the hBMECs with or without meningitic E. coli challenge were subjected to the iTRAQ proteomics analysis. The whole work flow

was shown in Fig. 1. Approximately 3000 different proteins were identified and quantified by iTRAQ-coupled LC-MS/MS analysis of the hBMECs infected with E. coli HB101, PCN033, or RS218 strains (Additional file 1: Table S1, Additional file 2: Table S2, Additional file 3: Table S3). As shown in Fig. 2a–d, four proteins were identified as being significantly upregulated and two were significantly downregulated upon HB101 infection, six were significantly upregulated, and 72 were significantly downregulated upon PCN033 infection, while 16 significantly upregulated and 27 significantly downregulated proteins were identified in cells challenged with RS218. The details of these differentially expressed proteins (DEPs) are listed in Tables 2, 3, and 4. The meningitic E. coli PCN033 group displayed 65 unique proteins, while the RS218 group displayed 27 unique proteins. They both shared 13 DEPs with 12 of them being distinct proteins in the hBMECs in response to meningitic strains PCN033 and RS218 (Fig. 2e, Table 5). Only one protein, EXOSC4, was shared by the three groups, and it showed a 0.74-, 0.759-, and 0.8-fold decrease in HB101, PCN033 and RS218 groups, respectively (Fig. 2e, Table 5). In contrast, infection with the non-meningitic HB101 strain induced only two unique, differentially altered proteins. Four proteins were shared between HB101 and RS218 groups, and the three of them altered in response to HB101 and RS218 were specific host proteins in both of these human isolates (Fig. 2e).

Western blot verification of the DEPs

We next used western blotting to further test the DEPs identified by iTRAQ. We selected several proteins from the iTRAQ results from both PCN033 and

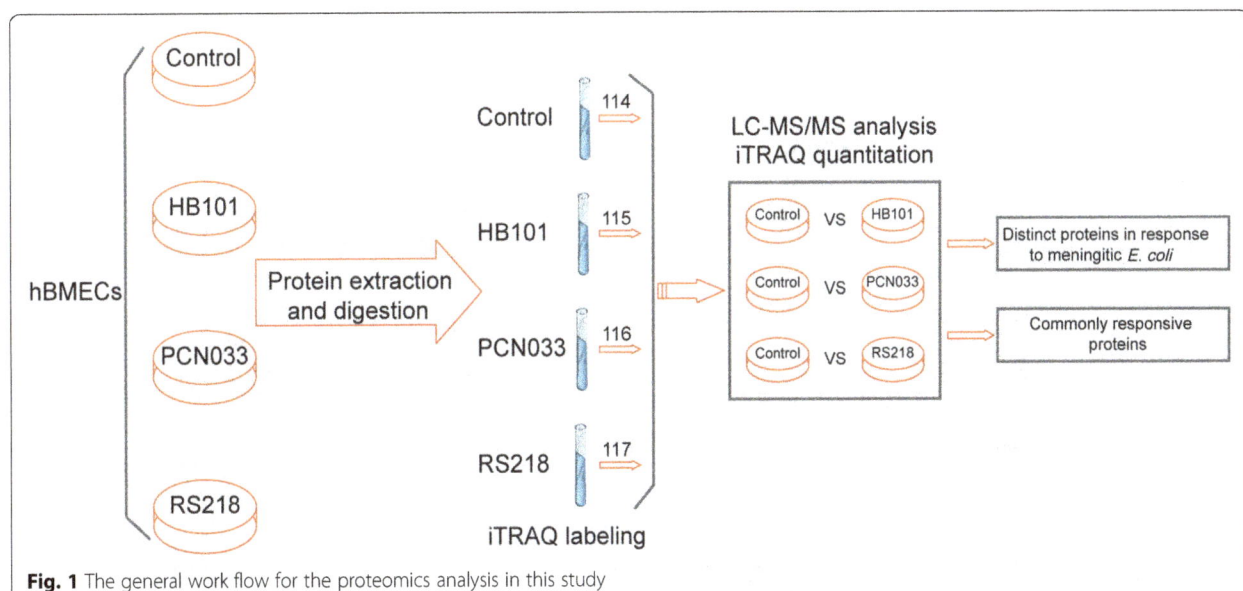

Fig. 1 The general work flow for the proteomics analysis in this study

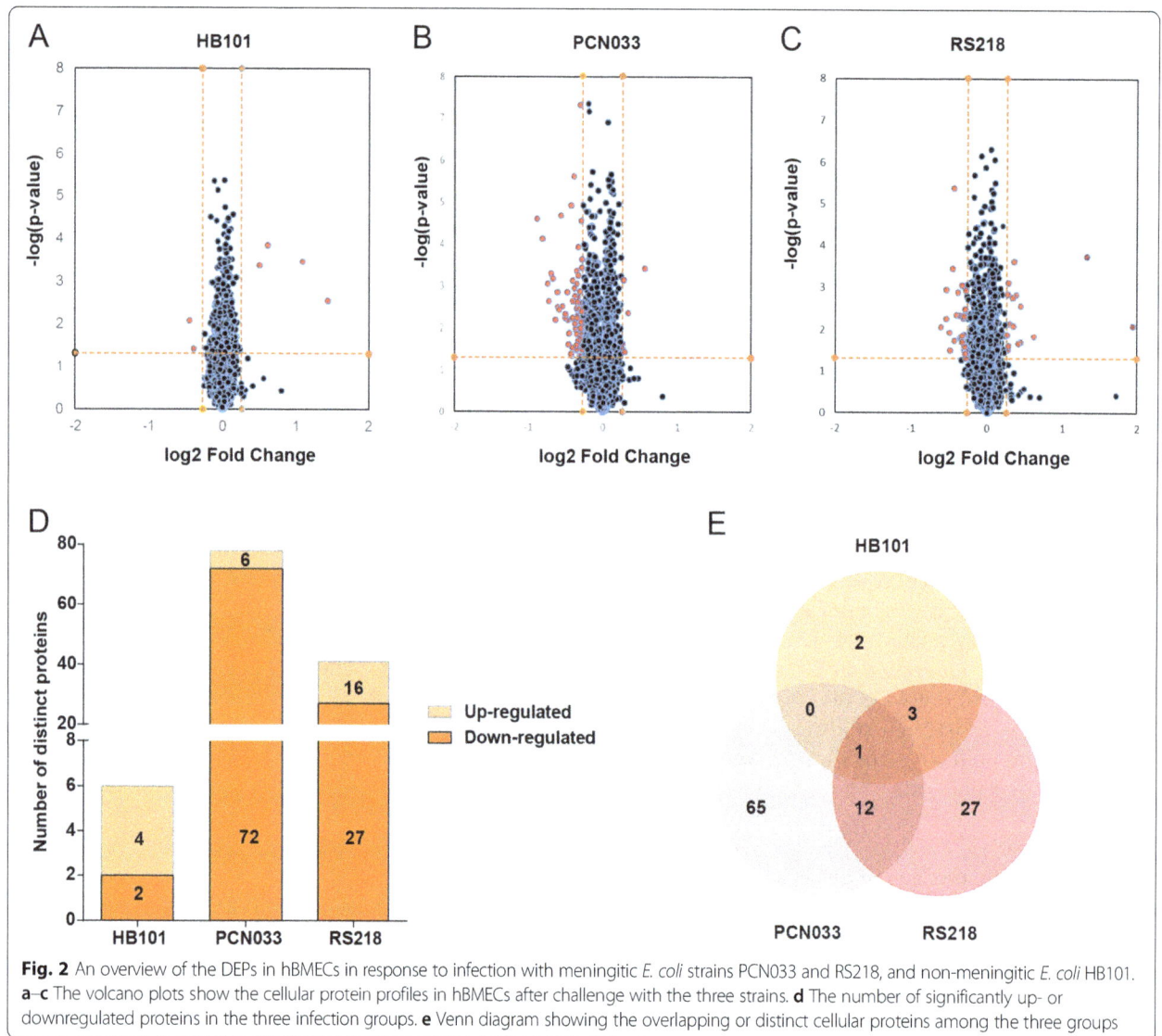

Fig. 2 An overview of the DEPs in hBMECs in response to infection with meningitic *E. coli* strains PCN033 and RS218, and non-meningitic *E. coli* HB101.
a–c The volcano plots show the cellular protein profiles in hBMECs after challenge with the three strains. **d** The number of significantly up- or downregulated proteins in the three infection groups. **e** Venn diagram showing the overlapping or distinct cellular proteins among the three groups

RS218 groups. The test proteins were HIST1H1C, TBPL1, and MIF for the PCN033 group (Fig. 3a), and DMD, LGMN, and HIST1H1C for the RS218 group (Fig. 3c). The western blot and densitometry analyses produced the similar expression alteration to those of the iTRAQ results following either PCN033 or RS218 infection (Fig. 3b, d).

Bioinformatic analysis of the DEPs in hBMECs

We next investigated and characterized the DEPs by searching the GO and UniProt databases. The DEPs were assigned to the categories of different "biological processes," "cellular components," and "molecular functions." Within the biological processes class, the DEPs from the three groups (RS218, PCN033, and HB101)

Table 2 Significantly changed proteins in HB101-infected hBMECs

Accession	Description	MW [kDa]	Fold change	P value[a]
P02656	Apolipoprotein C-III	10.8	1.544	0.000144***
Q07020	60S ribosomal protein L18	21.6	1.422	0.000429***
Q96HP4	Oxidoreductase NAD-binding domain-containing protein 1	34.8	2.715	0.002873**
Q9NPD3	Exosome complex component RRP41	26.4	0.737	0.008415**
Q9Y2Q5	Ragulator complex protein LAMTOR2	13.5	0.769	0.038574*
O14556	Glyceraldehyde-3-phosphate dehydrogenase, testis-specific	44.5	2.134	0.000347***

[a]$P < 0.05$ (*) was considered significant, and $P < 0.01$ (**), as well as < 0.001 (***) were all considered extremely significant

Table 3 Significantly changed proteins in PCN033-infected hBMECs

Accession	Description	MW [kDa]	Fold change	P value[a]
A6ZKI3	Protein FAM127A	13.2	0.756	0.028947*
O00625	Pirin	32.1	1.228	0.037445*
O43633	Charged multivesicular body protein 2a	25.1	0.758	0.002376**
O43752	Syntaxin-6	29.2	0.79	0.025619*
O60524	Nuclear export mediator factor NEMF	122.9	0.83	0.004194**
O75190	DnaJ homolog subfamily B member 6	36.1	0.799	0.020038*
O75251	NADH dehydrogenase [ubiquinone] iron-sulfur protein 7, mitochondrial	23.5	0.711	0.004822**
O75817	Ribonuclease P protein subunit p20	15.6	0.815	0.017814*
O95229	ZW10 interactor	31.3	0.668	0.003727**
P04004	Vitronectin	54.3	0.808	0.003548**
P07305	Histone H1.0	20.9	0.776	0.008176**
P11532	Dystrophin	426.5	0.691	0.003088**
P14174	Macrophage migration inhibitory factor	12.5	1.486	0.000377***
P16401	Histone H1.5	22.6	0.631	0.000673***
P16402	Histone H1.3	22.3	0.6	0.000896***
P16403	Histone H1.2	21.4	0.572	7.57E−05***
P35251	Replication factor C subunit 1	128.2	0.786	0.013936*
P35527	Keratin, type I cytoskeletal 9	62	0.72	0.001431**
P39060	Collagen alpha-1(XVIII) chain	178.1	0.792	0.031694*
P46013	Antigen KI-67	358.5	0.793	0.005934**
P48651	Phosphatidylserine synthase 1	55.5	0.83	0.000234***
P49585	Choline-phosphate cytidylyltransferase A	41.7	0.608	0.002306**
P50914	60S ribosomal protein L14	23.4	0.71	0.005946**
P52756	RNA-binding protein 5	92.1	0.758	0.005815**
P56377	AP-1 complex subunit sigma-2	18.6	0.765	2.4E−06***
P61966	AP-1 complex subunit sigma-1A	18.7	0.814	4.81E−08***
P62277	40S ribosomal protein S13	17.2	0.792	0.002441**
P62380	TATA box-binding protein-like protein 1	20.9	0.621	0.000503***
Q13625	Apoptosis-stimulating of p53 protein 2	125.5	0.724	0.006481**
Q14241	Transcription elongation factor B polypeptide 3	89.9	0.647	0.006556**
Q14686	Nuclear receptor coactivator 6	219	0.792	0.005234**
Q15388	Mitochondrial import receptor subunit TOM20 homolog	16.3	0.823	0.007395**
Q15629	Translocating chain-associated membrane protein 1	43	0.809	0.023084*
Q17RN3	Protein FAM98C	37.3	0.821	0.010317*
Q4V339	COBW domain-containing protein 6	43.9	0.747	1.2E−05***
Q567U6	Coiled-coil domain-containing protein 93	73.2	0.814	0.001351**
Q5SSJ5	Heterochromatin protein 1-binding protein 3	61.2	0.828	0.000364***
Q6N069	N-alpha-acetyltransferase 16, NatA auxiliary subunit	101.4	0.775	0.001734**
Q709C8	Vacuolar protein sorting-associated protein 13C	422.1	0.799	0.000576***
Q7Z422	SUZ domain-containing protein 1	17	0.808	0.002542**
Q8IXJ9	Putative Polycomb group protein ASXL1	165.3	0.807	0.007037**
Q8N2K0	Monoacylglycerol lipase ABHD12	45.1	0.786	0.0034**
Q8N884	Cyclic GMP-AMP synthase	58.8	0.82	0.013058*
Q8NC44	Protein FAM134A	57.8	0.78	0.010814*

Table 3 Significantly changed proteins in PCN033-infected hBMECs *(Continued)*

Accession	Description	MW [kDa]	Fold change	P value[a]
Q8NC60	Nitric oxide-associated protein 1	78.4	0.81	0.013637*
Q8NEY1	Neuron navigator 1	202.3	0.797	0.020924*
Q8TEM1	Nuclear pore membrane glycoprotein 210	205	0.833	0.032212*
Q8WUP2	Filamin-binding LIM protein 1	40.6	0.809	0.002633**
Q8WVV9	Heterogeneous nuclear ribonucleoprotein L-like	60	0.804	0.013638*
Q8WXA3	RUN and FYVE domain-containing protein 2	75	0.744	0.041934*
Q92604	Acyl-CoA:lysophosphatidylglycerol acyltransferase 1	43.1	0.789	0.033787 *
Q96A57	Transmembrane protein 230	13.2	0.786	0.000449***
Q96LB3	Intraflagellar transport protein 74 homolog	69.2	0.543	2.53E−05***
Q96RU3	Formin-binding protein 1	71.3	0.679	2.07E−05***
Q96T37	Putative RNA-binding protein 15	107.1	0.728	0.024086*
Q9GZP8	Immortalization upregulated protein	10.9	1.207	0.032624*
Q9H074	Polyadenylate-binding protein-interacting protein 1	53.5	1.266	0.004395**
Q9H5N1	Rab GTPase-binding effector protein 2	63.5	0.77	0.001156**
Q9H5X1	MIP18 family protein FAM96A	18.3	0.8	0.000118***
Q9HB40	Retinoid-inducible serine carboxypeptidase	50.8	1.215	0.000733***
Q9HC52	Chromobox protein homolog 8	43.4	1.201	0.023152*
Q9NPD3	Exosome complex component RRP41	26.4	0.759	0.000746***
Q9NRY4	Rho GTPase-activating protein 35	170.4	0.792	0.011172*
Q9NS87	Kinesin-like protein KIF15	160.1	0.785	0.010039*
Q9NSP4	Centromere protein M	19.7	0.802	0.021316*
Q9NTI5	Sister chromatid cohesion protein PDS5 homolog B	164.6	0.826	0.003399**
Q9NWU5	39S ribosomal protein L22, mitochondrial	23.6	0.812	0.016677*
Q9NZQ3	NCK-interacting protein with SH3 domain	78.9	0.661	0.00317**
Q9P0V3	SH3 domain-binding protein 4	107.4	0.797	0.001833**
Q9UBL6	Copine-7	70.2	0.823	2.73E−05***
Q9UJW0	Dynactin subunit 4	52.3	0.823	0.012604*
Q9UNP9	Peptidyl-prolyl cis-trans isomerase E	33.4	0.75	0.044207*
Q9Y2R0	Cytochrome c oxidase assembly protein 3 homolog, mitochondrial	11.7	0.792	0.003694**
Q9Y5Y2	Cytosolic Fe-S cluster assembly factor NUBP2	28.8	0.787	0.000891***
Q9Y6I9	Testis-expressed sequence 264 protein	34.2	0.814	0.047637*
Q9Y3Y2	Chromatin target of PRMT1 protein	26.4	0.828	0.008622**
Q9Y4R8	Telomere length regulation protein TEL2 homolog	91.7	0.735	0.013443*
P10412	Histone H1.4	21.9	0.655	0.001429**

[a]$P < 0.05$ (*) was considered significant, and $P < 0.01$ (**), as well as < 0.001 (***), were all considered extremely significant

were mainly divided into metabolic processes, localization, cellular process, and cellular component organization or biogenesis. The immune system process and developmental process classes were found in both RS218 and PCN033 infection groups, but not in the HB101 group. Within the cellular component class, the DEPs were mainly divided into organelle, macromolecular complex, and cell parts, and the membrane-associated ones were only identified in the meningitic strains RS218 and PCN033, not in HB101. As for molecular function, the DEPs were mainly associated with structural molecule activity, catalytic activity, and binding (Fig. 4a, Additional file 4: Table S4).

We next performed canonical pathway prediction through IPA on the DEPs. The top ranked canonical pathways in each group are shown in Fig. 4b. We found that protein kinase A signaling, eumelanin biosynthesis, EIF2 signaling, and granzyme A signaling were simultaneously enriched in both RS218 and PCN033 infection groups, but not in the HB101 group (Fig. 4b). Noticeably, granzyme A signaling was much more significantly

Table 4 Significantly changed proteins in RS218-infected hBMECs

Accession	Description	MW [kDa]	Fold change	P value[a]
O00592	Podocalyxin	58.6	1.214	0.001481**
O14556	Glyceraldehyde-3-phosphate dehydrogenase, testis-specific	44.5	2.514	0.000183***
O43598	2'-Deoxynucleoside 5'-phosphate N-hydrolase 1	19.1	0.8	0.020803*
O76024	Wolframin	100.2	0.732	0.000347***
O76095	Protein JTB	16.3	0.815	0.026287*
O95989	Diphosphoinositol polyphosphate phosphohydrolase 1	19.5	0.821	0.003332**
P05067	Amyloid beta A4 protein	86.9	0.813	0.004913**
P10412	Histone H1.4	21.9	1.271	0.001736**
P11532	Dystrophin	426.5	0.799	0.014535*
P14174	Macrophage migration inhibitory factor	12.5	1.276	0.008267**
P16401	Histone H1.5	22.6	1.221	0.025445*
P16402	Histone H1.3	22.3	1.306	0.001514**
P16403	Histone H1.2	21.4	1.332	0.021727*
P30154	Serine/threonine-protein phosphatase 2A 65 kDa regulatory subunit A beta isoform	66.2	0.809	0.005474**
P35527	Keratin, type I cytoskeletal 9	62	0.822	0.038701*
P42167	Lamina-associated polypeptide 2, isoforms beta/gamma	50.6	0.826	0.0494*
P46781	40S ribosomal protein S9	22.6	1.207	0.013518*
P50402	Emerin	29	0.8	0.000916***
P52756	RNA-binding protein 5	92.1	0.74	4.23E−06***
P55789	FAD-linked sulfhydryl oxidase ALR	23.4	1.537	0.014932*
P61313	60S ribosomal protein L15	24.1	1.286	0.000236***
P62380	TATA box-binding protein-like protein 1	20.9	0.66	0.008696**
Q07020	60S ribosomal protein L18	21.6	1.367	0.002799**
Q4V339	COBW domain-containing protein 6	43.9	0.756	0.00457**
Q8N4H5	Mitochondrial import receptor subunit TOM5 homolog	6	1.223	0.000783***
Q8ND56	Protein LSM14 homolog A	50.5	0.793	0.017061*
Q96BZ8	Leukocyte receptor cluster member 1	30.5	0.693	0.005542**
Q96HP4	Oxidoreductase NAD-binding domain-containing protein 1	34.8	3.845	0.008111**
Q96KR1	Zinc finger RNA-binding protein	116.9	0.811	0.01368*
Q96LB3	Intraflagellar transport protein 74 homolog	69.2	0.71	0.012006*
Q96P47	Arf-GAP with GTPase, ANK repeat and PH domain-containing protein 3	95	0.783	0.004713**
Q99538	Legumain	49.4	0.692	0.001173**
Q9BTA9	WW domain-containing adapter protein with coiled-coil	70.7	0.743	0.01886*
Q9BZF9	Uveal autoantigen with coiled-coil domains and ankyrin repeats	162.4	0.824	0.031539*
Q9H7B2	Ribosome production factor 2 homolog	35.6	1.367	0.020862*
Q9HCD5	Nuclear receptor coactivator 5	65.5	0.771	0.001324**
Q9NPD3	Exosome complex component RRP41	26.4	0.784	0.015931*
Q9NZR1	Tropomodulin-2	39.6	1.216	0.030742*
Q9UI10	Translation initiation factor eIF-2B subunit delta	57.5	0.828	0.001214**
Q9UIC8	Leucine carboxyl methyltransferase 1	38.4	0.811	0.0312*
Q9UK41	Vacuolar protein sorting-associated protein 28 homolog	25.4	0.715	0.032545*
Q9Y4R8	Telomere length regulation protein TEL2 homolog	91.7	0.807	0.019858*
Q9Y5V3	Melanoma-associated antigen D1	86.1	1.238	0.007536**

[a]P < 0.05 (*) was considered significant, and P < 0.01 (**), as well as < 0.001 (***), were all considered extremely significant

Table 5 The distinct differential proteins in hBMECs in response to meningitic *E. coli* strains PCN033 and RS218

ID	Name	Protein	Fold Change		
			RS218	PCN033	HB101
Q9NPD3	EXOSC4	Exosome complex component RRP41	0.8	0.759	0.74
Q96LB3	IFT74	Intraflagellar transport protein 74 homolog	0.7	0.543	/
P11532	DMD	Dystrophin	0.8	0.691	/
P52756	RBM5	RNA-binding protein 5	0.7	0.758	/
Q4V339	CBWD6	COBW domain-containing protein 6	0.8	0.747	/
Q9Y4R8	TELO2	Telomere length regulation protein TEL2 homolog	0.8	0.735	/
P35527	KRT9	Keratin, type I cytoskeletal 9	0.8	0.72	/
P62380	TBOL1	TATA box-binding protein-like protein 1	0.7	0.621	/
P16403	HIST1H1C	Histone H1.2	1.3	0.572	/
P16402	HIST1H1D	Histone H1.3	1.3	0.6	/
P10412	HIST1H1E	Histone H1.4	1.3	0.655	/
P16401	HIST1H1B	Histone H1.5	1.2	0.631	/
P14174	MIF	Macrophage migration inhibitory factor	1.3	1.486	/

enriched in the DEPs from both meningitic groups, suggesting a potential role for granzyme A in meningitic *E. coli* invasion of the BBB. Additionally, phosphatidylcholine biosynthesis I, choline biosynthesis III, and glioma invasiveness signaling were only enriched in the PCN033 group, while neuronal NOS signaling and regulation of eIF4 and p70S6K signaling were only identified in the RS218 group, which exhibited distinct signaling pathways that might have strain specificity (Fig. 4b).

The IPA tool was used to further analyze the potential networks based on the DEPs from the *E. coli* infections.

Two networks were drawn for these differential cellular proteins in response to HB101 infection (Fig. 5a, b, Additional file 5: Table S5). In addition, four networks were generated based on the DEPs from the PCN033 infection (Fig. 5c–f, Additional file 6: Table S6), while two networks were generated from the DEPs upon RS218 infection (Fig. 5g, h, Additional file 7: Table S7). It should be noted that the NF-κB complex, as well as ERK, were included in the networks of both PCN033 and RS218 groups, while they were not observed in the cells in response to the non-meningitic HB101 strain, suggesting that these two essential signaling molecules exert regulatory effects during meningitic *E. coli* penetration of the BBB.

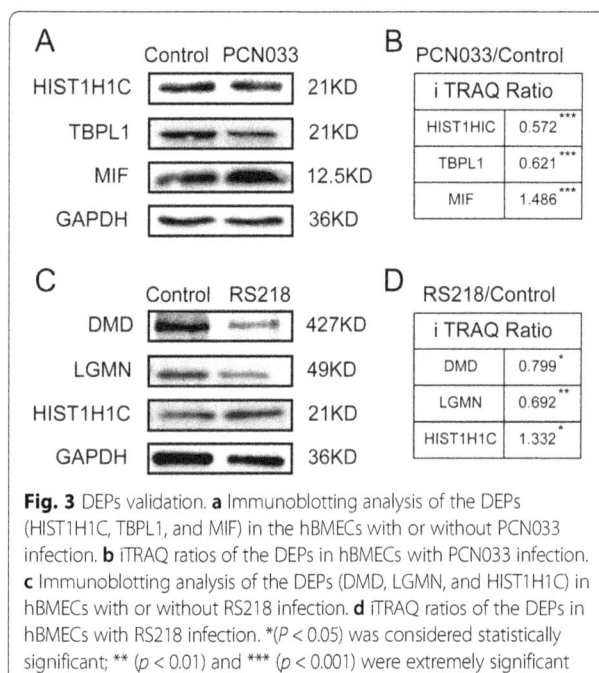

Fig. 3 DEPs validation. **a** Immunoblotting analysis of the DEPs (HIST1H1C, TBPL1, and MIF) in the hBMECs with or without PCN033 infection. **b** iTRAQ ratios of the DEPs in hBMECs with PCN033 infection. **c** Immunoblotting analysis of the DEPs (DMD, LGMN, and HIST1H1C) in hBMECs with or without RS218 infection. **d** iTRAQ ratios of the DEPs in hBMECs with RS218 infection. *(P < 0.05) was considered statistically significant; ** (p < 0.01) and *** (p < 0.001) were extremely significant

MIF contributes to meningitic *E. coli*-induced cytokine production and tight junction disruption

Based on the aforementioned network analysis, we noticed the presence of MIF in the meningitic PCN033 and RS218 strain groups, suggesting potential roles for it in meningitic *E. coli* invasion of the BBB. Here, by pretreating the hBMECs with 20 μM ISO-1 (a MIF inhibitor), we found that the multiple cytokines [e.g. interleukin (IL)-6, IL-8, tumor necrosis factor (TNF)-α, IL-1β] significantly induced by meningitic *E. coli* PCN033 or RS218 infection had decreased levels (Fig. 6a, b). Moreover, the ECIS system was applied to evaluate the potential effects of recombinant MIF protein on the barrier function of hBMECs. The results showed that recombinant MIF obviously decreased the resistance formed by the cells in a dose-dependent manner (Fig. 6c). We also observed that treatment with recombinant MIF (200 ng/ml) for 12 and 24 h led to decreased expression of tight junction proteins like ZO-1 and occludin (Fig. 6d); moreover, use of the

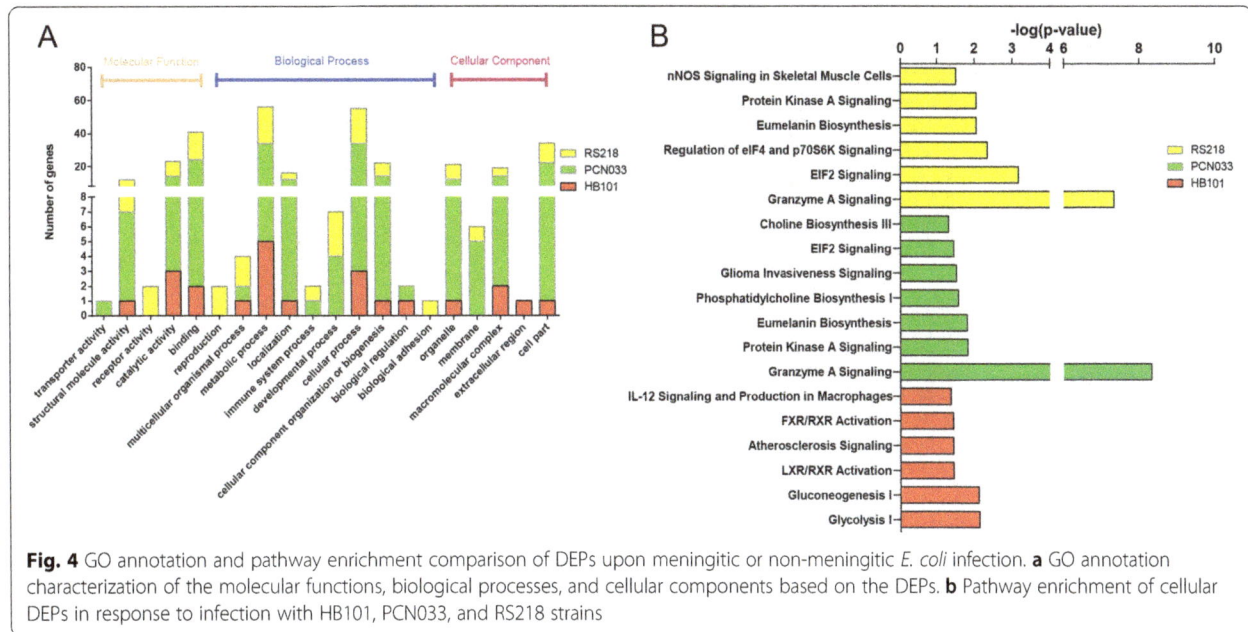

Fig. 4 GO annotation and pathway enrichment comparison of DEPs upon meningitic or non-meningitic *E. coli* infection. **a** GO annotation characterization of the molecular functions, biological processes, and cellular components based on the DEPs. **b** Pathway enrichment of cellular DEPs in response to infection with HB101, PCN033, and RS218 strains

MIF inhibitor ISO-1 could partially recover the PCN033 or RS218 infection-caused downregulation of tight junction proteins like ZO-1 and Occludin (Fig. 6e, f). Together, these observations support the conclusion that MIF contributes to the induction of proinflammatory cytokines and the decrease in tight junction proteins during meningitic *E. coli* invasion of the BBB.

Meningitic *E. coli* activation of NF-κB signaling mediates the production of cytokines

As mentioned above in the network analysis, involvement of the NF-κB complex was observed in cells following the challenge with meningitic *E. coli* strains PCN033 and RS218, but not with non-meningitic HB101. Therefore, we investigated NF-κB signaling activation in hBMECs in response to infection. Phosphorylation of the NF-κB p65 subunit increased significantly in response to PCN033 and RS218 infection, and this was much higher than that observed during the response to HB101 infection. Also, degradation of IκBα upon PCN033 or RS218 infection was much greater than that upon HB101 infection (Fig. 7a, b). Using immunofluorescence microscopy, we also observed p65 translocation to the nucleus upon PCN033 and RS218 infection (Fig. 7c), while this nuclear translocation was barely observed in response to HB101 infection (Fig. 7c). These results indicate that the NF-κB signaling pathway is activated during meningitic *E. coli* interaction with hBMECs. Moreover, by using the NF-κB inhibitor BAY11-7082, we observed that the meningitic *E. coli* PCN033- or RS218-induced cytokines production (including IL-6, IL-8, TNF-α, and IL-1β) was significantly decreased when compared with DMSO treatment (Fig. 7d, e). Together, these data firmly support our network analysis

that the NF-κB signaling pathway is involved in both PCN033 and RS218 infection of hBMECs, and their activation of NF-κB signaling in hBMECs mediates the induction of proinflammatory cytokines.

MAPK signaling pathways are involved in proinflammatory cytokine induction by meningitic *E. coli* strains

Because ERK was assumed to be involved in infections with PCN033 and RS218 based on our network prediction, we next investigated the activation of MAPK pathways in hBMECs in response to meningitic *E. coli*. The results showed that the phosphorylation of p38, JNK, and ERK1/2 significantly increased in response to meningitic strains PCN033 or RS218 (Fig. 8a, b), indicating the activation of all three MAPK pathways in hBMECs upon meningitic *E. coli* challenge. After demonstrating the significant induction of several proinflammatory cytokines above, we next investigated whether the MAPK pathways were involved in these cytokines production. Following pretreatment with U0126 (a specific ERK1/2 inhibitor), SB202190 (a selective inhibitor of p38), and SP600125 (a JNK-specific inhibitor), the proinflammatory cytokines (IL-6, IL-8, TNF-α, IL-1β) induced in hBMECs upon PCN033 or RS218 infection were significantly reduced (to different extents), compared with that in each DMSO control group (Fig. 8c). These results indicate that the MAPK signaling pathways, including MAPK-p38, MAPK-ERK1/2, and MAPK-JNK, were all activated and at least participated in meningitic *E. coli*-induced neuroinflammatory responses.

Discussion

The iTRAQ-based proteomics, a powerful approach for obtaining comprehensive and quantitative protein

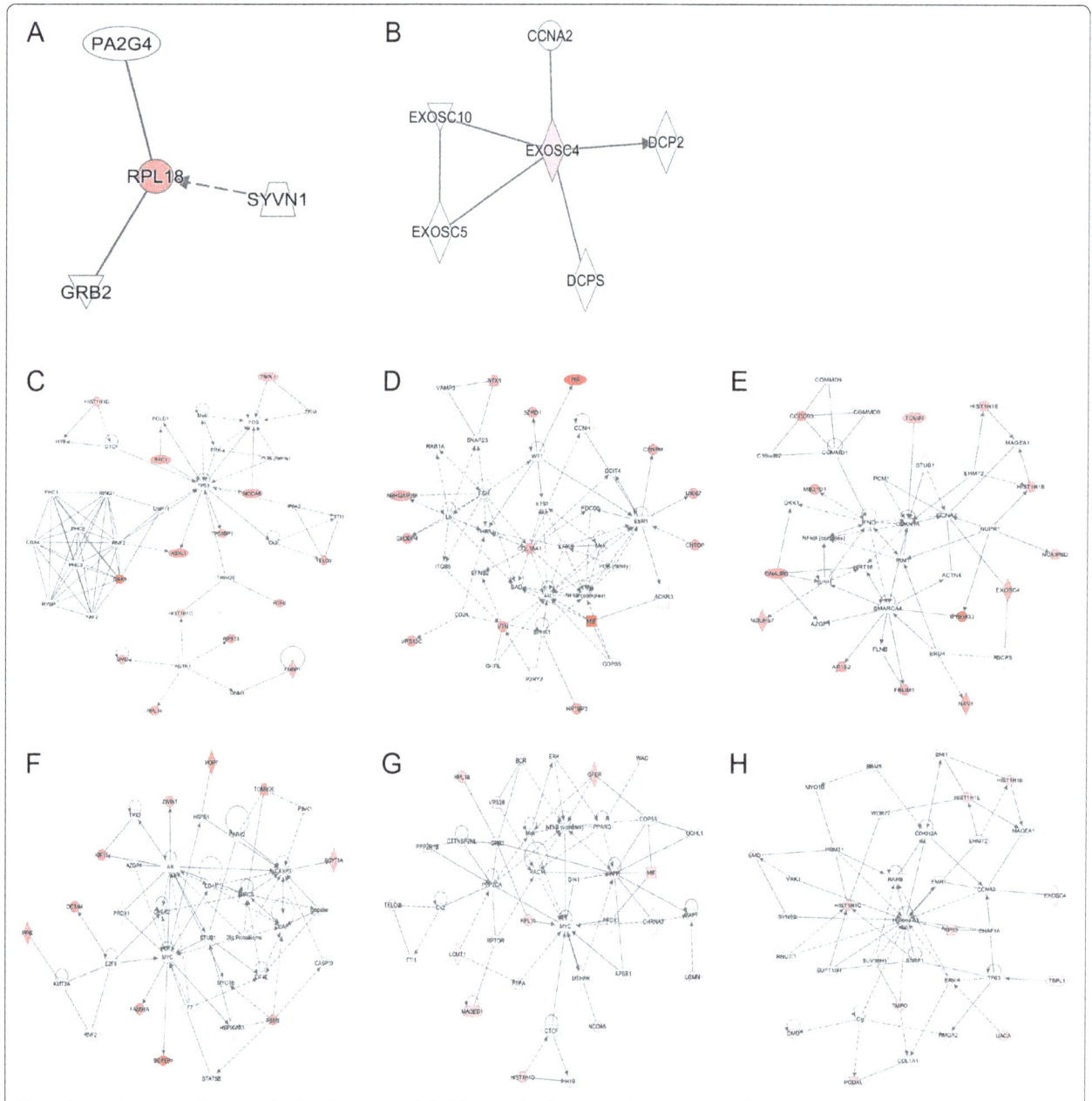

Fig. 5 Network analysis of significantly altered proteins in hBMECs upon *E. coli* infection. For the HB101 infection, two networks were constructed: **a** cellular assembly and organization, gastrointestinal disease, hepatic system disease; **b** RNA damage and repair, connective tissue disorders, developmental disorder. For the PCN033 infection, four networks were constructed: **c** lymphoid tissue structure and development, organ morphology, organismal development; **d** cellular movement, cancer, organismal injury and abnormalities; **e** inflammatory disease, inflammatory response, organismal injury and abnormalities; **f** cell death and survival, cellular development, cellular growth and proliferation. For the RS218 infection two networks were constructed: **g** neurological disease, organismal injury and abnormalities, cell cycle; **h** gene expression, cellular assembly and organization, DNA replication, recombination, and repair. The red nodes indicate significantly altered protein expression, and the white ones are those known to be involved in the networks, but not identified in this study. Arrows indicate the interrelationship between two molecules. Solid lines indicate direct interactions and dashed lines indicate indirect interactions

expression profiling data, has been used widely to identify and characterize potential cellular targets. In current study, we used iTRAQ to explore the proteomic differences in hBMECs in response to meningitic or non-meningitic *E. coli* infections. The *E. coli* strains PCN033 and RS218 were selected for this study because they are representative meningitis-causing strains capable of penetrating the BBB as well as inducing severe neuroinflammation [5, 20], while the *E. coli* strain HB101 is avirulent and non-meningitic and was therefore used as the negative control.

Based on our data, 13 significantly differentiated proteins in total were found to be shared by PCN033 and

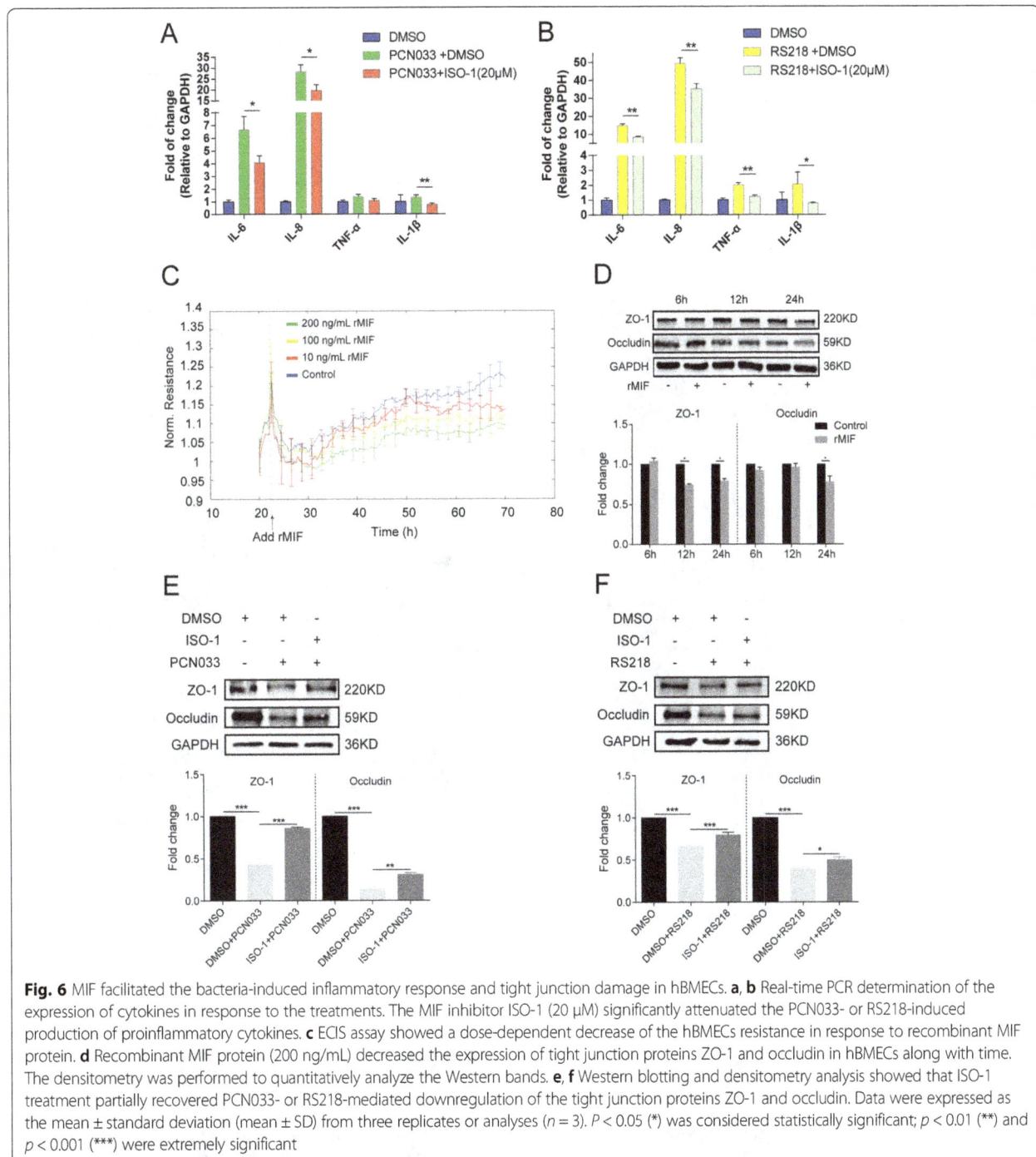

Fig. 6 MIF facilitated the bacteria-induced inflammatory response and tight junction damage in hBMECs. **a, b** Real-time PCR determination of the expression of cytokines in response to the treatments. The MIF inhibitor ISO-1 (20 μM) significantly attenuated the PCN033- or RS218-induced production of proinflammatory cytokines. **c** ECIS assay showed a dose-dependent decrease of the hBMECs resistance in response to recombinant MIF protein. **d** Recombinant MIF protein (200 ng/mL) decreased the expression of tight junction proteins ZO-1 and occludin in hBMECs along with time. The densitometry was performed to quantitatively analyze the Western bands. **e, f** Western blotting and densitometry analysis showed that ISO-1 treatment partially recovered PCN033- or RS218-mediated downregulation of the tight junction proteins ZO-1 and occludin. Data were expressed as the mean ± standard deviation (mean ± SD) from three replicates or analyses ($n = 3$). $P < 0.05$ (*) was considered statistically significant; $p < 0.01$ (**) and $p < 0.001$ (***) were extremely significant

RS218 (Fig. 1). They are TELO2, IFT74, CBWD6, EXOSC4, TBOL1, RBM5, KRT9, HIST1H1C, HIST1H1D, HIST1H1B, HIST1H1E, MIF, and DMD (Table 5). Among these, EXOSC4 was the only protein that was also significantly changed in response to non-meningitic *E. coli* HB101 (Fig. 2, Table 5). EXOSC4, a non-catalytic component of the RNA exosome machinery, has 3′-5′ exoribonuclease activity and participates in a multitude of cellular RNA processing

and degradation events [29]. It was reported that EXOSC4 was a potential factor involved in the maintenance of genome stability, by eliminating the RNA processing by-products and non-coding "pervasive" transcripts thereby limiting or excluding their export to the cytoplasm, or by preventing translation of aberrant mRNAs [30–32]. In lung adenocarcinoma, EXOSC4 has been reported to be extremely highly expressed and closely associated with cancer cell proliferation and

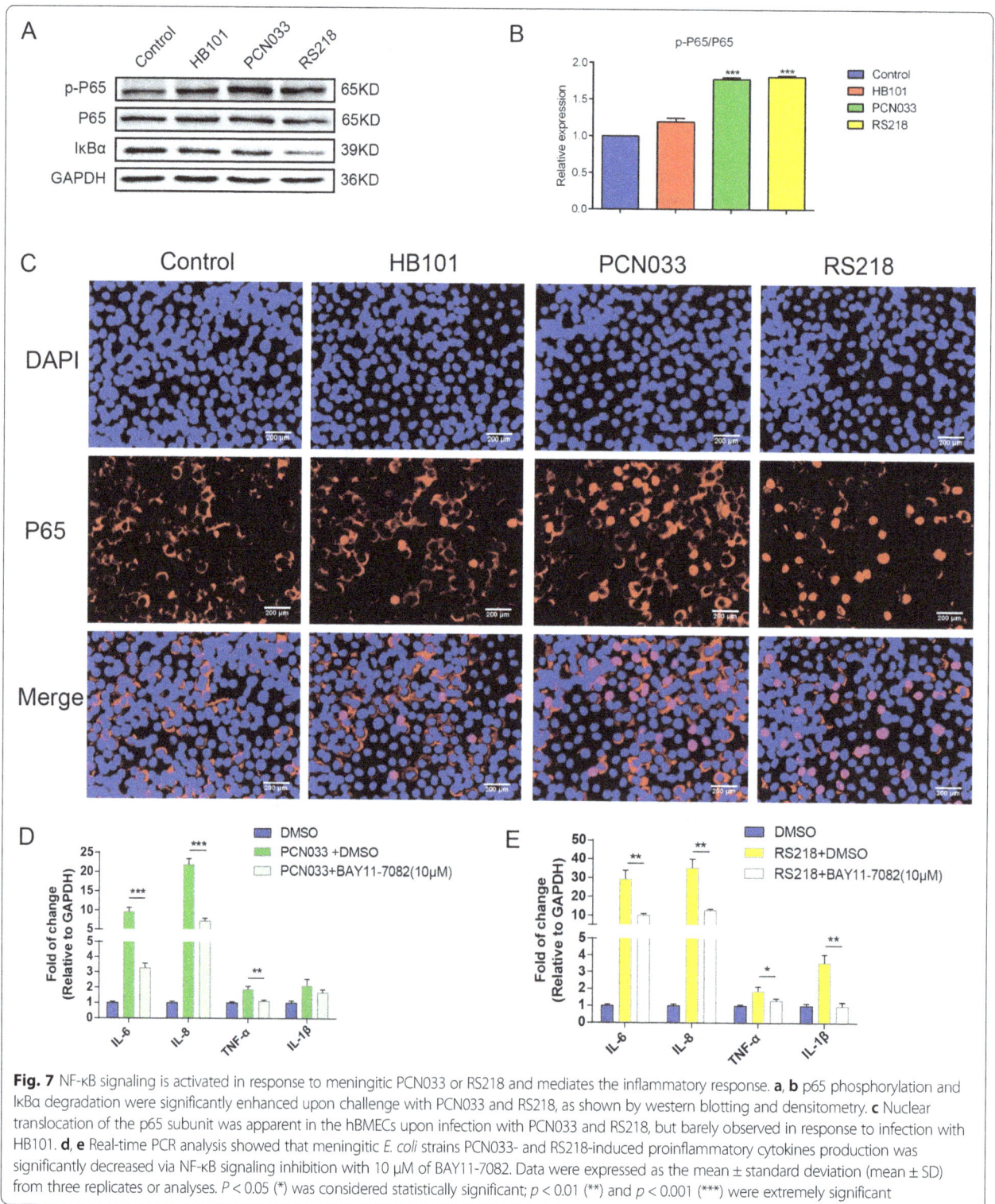

Fig. 7 NF-κB signaling is activated in response to meningitic PCN033 or RS218 and mediates the inflammatory response. **a, b** p65 phosphorylation and IκBα degradation were significantly enhanced upon challenge with PCN033 and RS218, as shown by western blotting and densitometry. **c** Nuclear translocation of the p65 subunit was apparent in the hBMECs upon infection with PCN033 and RS218, but barely observed in response to infection with HB101. **d, e** Real-time PCR analysis showed that meningitic *E. coli* strains PCN033- and RS218-induced proinflammatory cytokines production was significantly decreased via NF-κB signaling inhibition with 10 μM of BAY11-7082. Data were expressed as the mean ± standard deviation (mean ± SD) from three replicates or analyses. $P < 0.05$ (*) was considered statistically significant; $p < 0.01$ (**) and $p < 0.001$ (***) were extremely significant

was, therefore, recognized as a new prognostic marker [30]. Similarly, in patients with liver cancer, the EXOSC4 gene was found to be highly expressed, and its knock-down commonly inhibited cancer cell growth and invasion [33]. Here, we found that EXOSC4 was commonly targeted by the meningitic and the non-meningitic *E. coli* strains, indicating that this cellular protein is a non-specific infection-related protein. Other than EXOSC4, the remaining 12 proteins were shared by the meningitic strains (PCN033 and RS218)

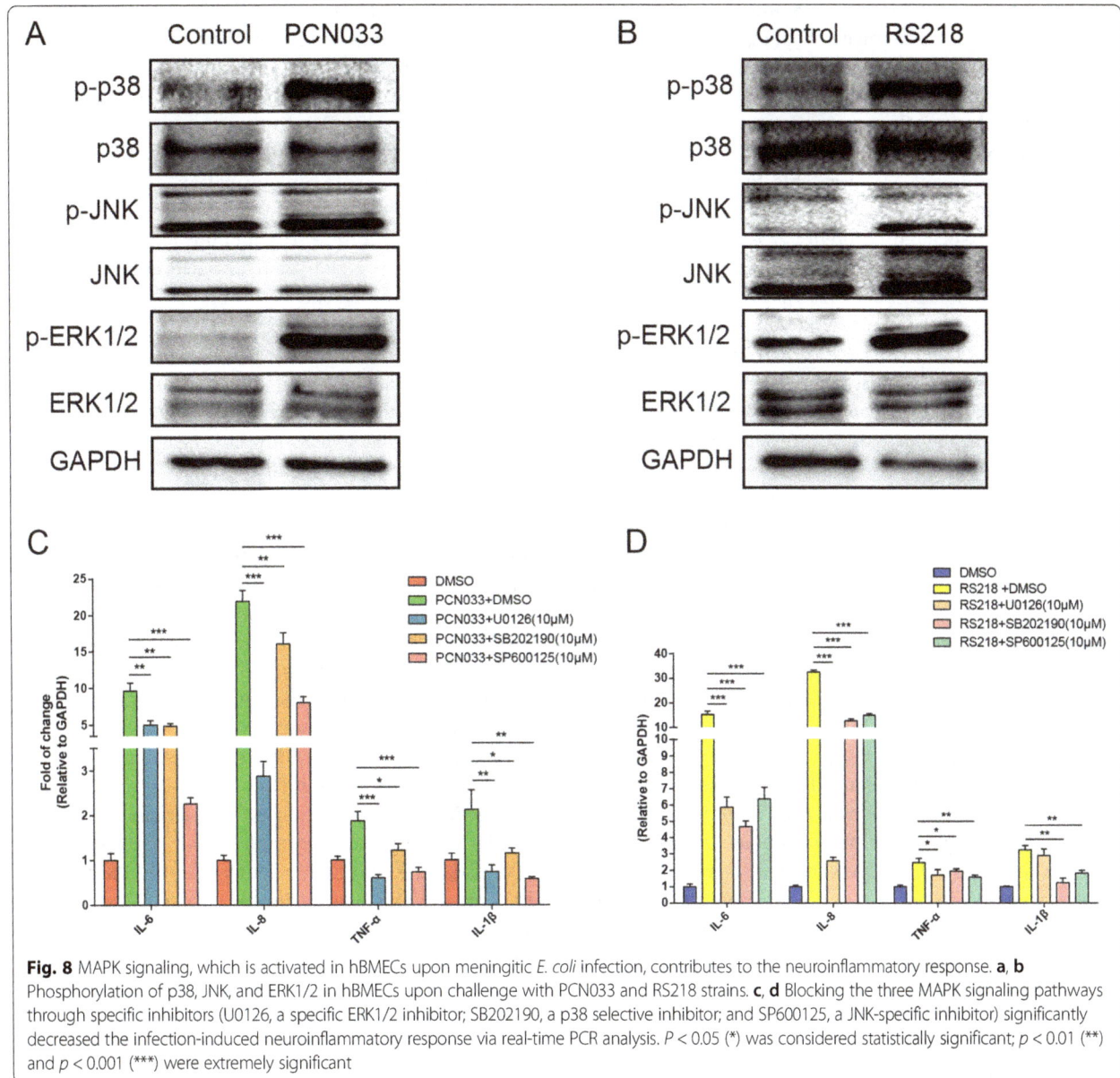

Fig. 8 MAPK signaling, which is activated in hBMECs upon meningitic *E. coli* infection, contributes to the neuroinflammatory response. **a, b** Phosphorylation of p38, JNK, and ERK1/2 in hBMECs upon challenge with PCN033 and RS218 strains. **c, d** Blocking the three MAPK signaling pathways through specific inhibitors (U0126, a specific ERK1/2 inhibitor; SB202190, a p38 selective inhibitor; and SP600125, a JNK-specific inhibitor) significantly decreased the infection-induced neuroinflammatory response via real-time PCR analysis. $P < 0.05$ (*) was considered statistically significant; $p < 0.01$ (**) and $p < 0.001$ (***) were extremely significant

alone, suggesting that these proteins might represent the potential targets hijacked by these meningitic *E. coli* strains.

Among these 12 meningitic *E. coli*-specific "cellular responders," we firstly focused on MIF, which was the only one to exhibit common upregulation in response to both meningitic *E. coli* PCN033 and RS218 (Table 5). MIF is a proinflammatory cytokine, which has been highlighted as a key player in infection and septic shock [34, 35]. It is reported to be involved in the cytokine storm, which facilitates the uncontrolled release of cytokines into the circulation during pathogen infection or sepsis [36]. As previously evidenced in *E. coli*-induced meningitis, cytokines and chemokines potentially contribute to BBB damage [5]. The burst of proinflammatory cytokines

during infection may lead directly to dysfunction of the endothelial barrier and an increase in vascular permeability in the brain, thus finally leading to severe CNS injury. Moreover, MIF may be secreted by a wide variety of cells upon stimulation, and once MIF binds to its receptors (e.g., CXCR2, CXCR4, and/or CD74 [37, 38]), several downstream signal molecules such as PI3K/Akt or MAPK/ERK become activated, thus mediating the inflammatory response [39, 40]. In the present study, the effects of MIF on meningitic *E. coli*-induced inflammation were also verified by the observation that the MIF inhibitor ISO-1 significantly decreased meningitic *E. coli* PCN033- or RS218-induced upregulation of IL-6, IL-8, IL-1β, and TNF-α (Fig. 5). Noticeably however, although the ISO-1 inhibitory effects were significant, there was still a significant induction of IL-6 and IL-8 in response to PCN033 and RS218 infection, suggesting that other "switches" for proinflammatory cytokine and chemokine generation commonly exist in response to infection. Except for its role in inflammation, we also observed the involvement of MIF in BBB damage, as evidenced by the fact that recombinant MIF was able to deconstruct the endothelial barrier by inducing a significant decrease in the junction-associated protein ZO-1 and occludin (Fig. 6). Furthermore, when MIF inhibitor ISO-1 was used, the PCN033- and/or RS218-induced downregulation of ZO-1 and occludin was largely restored (Fig. 6). Considering the potential roles of MIF in mediating the neuroinflammatory response as well as in inducing BBB disruption, it is possible that MIF may represent a novel and potential target for clinical prevention and therapy for *E. coli* meningitis.

Our IPA-based canonical pathways prediction suggested that protein kinase A signaling, eumelanin biosynthesis, EIF2 signaling, and granzyme A signaling were simultaneously enriched in hBMECs upon infection with RS218 and PCN033, but not with HB101. Among these processes, granzyme A signaling was much more significantly enriched. In the RS218 group, HIST1H1B, HIST1H1C, HIST1H1E, and HIST1H1D are included in granzyme A signaling, while in the PCN033 group, HIST1H1B, HIST1H1C, HIST1H1E, HIST1H1D, and H1F0 are involved (Additional file 6: Table S6). Granzyme A was identified as a cytotoxic T lymphocyte protease with multiple roles in infectious diseases. For example, several studies have shown that granzyme A is highly expressed in patients with tuberculosis and may represent a promising diagnostic marker distinct from IFN-γ to discriminate between patients with tuberculosis and other pulmonary diseases [41–43]. Granzyme A is also considered to participate in the host defense response in multiple ways, such as by generating superoxide and inactivating the oxidative defense enzymes that kill intracellular parasites [44], by unfavorably impairing host defenses during *Streptococcus pneumoniae* pneumonia [45], by performing as a proinflammatory protease that cleaves IL-1β intracellularly into bioactive IL-1β [46, 47], or by causing detachment of alveolar epithelial A549 cells accompanied by promotion of IL-8 release [48]. Here, in the present study, granzyme A signaling was significantly enriched by cellular differentiated proteins in response to both meningitic *E. coli* strains, but not in non-meningitic *E. coli* HB101. This result probably indicates that granzyme A could be a potential indicator of *E. coli* meningitis, but further supportive evidences are needed.

Based on the IPA functional network analysis, we also noticed that the NF-κB complex and MAPK/ERK signaling were involved in both PCN033 and RS218 infection

of hBMECs, but barely in the HB101 group. The NF-κB complex comprises a family of closely related transcription factors with important roles in regulating the gene expression involved in inflammation and the immune response [49]. The NF-κB activation process is induced by the phosphorylation of serine residues in IkB proteins, which are subjected to ubiquitination and proteasome degradation and, subsequently, phosphorylation and nuclear translocation of the p65 subunit. Early studies have shown that NF-κB is activated in bacteria-induced CNS infections [50], and NF-κB inhibitors have been found to reduce neuroinflammation [51] as well as protect rat brains from inflammatory injury following transient focal cerebral ischemia [52] and pneumococcal meningitis [53]. In *E. coli*, it has been evidenced that OmpA⁺*E. coli* can induce ICAM-1 expression in hBMECs by activating NF-κB signaling [54] and that the IbeA⁺*E. coli* K1 strain can also induce activation and nuclear translocation of NF-κB in hBMECs [55]. In the current study, by western blotting, we also showed that the NF-κB pathway was activated more in hBMECs infected by meningitic strains PCN033 and RS218 compared with that by HB101 infection, where the phosphorylation of p65 and degradation of IκBα were compared, as well as with the immunofluorescence experiments that showed the nuclear translocation of p65. Not unexpectedly, treating hBMECs with the NF-κB inhibitor BAY11-7082 significantly attenuated those cytokines induction during meningitic *E. coli* infection, suggesting that NF-κB signaling works potently in mediating the neuroinflammatory response.

Likewise, we found that the effects of MAPK signaling were similarly associated with both PCN033 and RS218 infection of hBMECs. MAPK signaling cascades actually involve three major pathways: JNK (which acts as mediator of extracellular stress responses), ERK1/2 (which mediates proliferative stimuli), and p38 (which is also involved in mediating extracellular stress responses, particularly by regulating cytokine expression) [56]. Our IPA network analysis indicated the involvement of ERK during infection with meningitic *E. coli* PCN033 and RS218, which is consistent with our previous finding that MAPK/ERK signaling is involved in infection and mediates the induction of VEGFA and Snail-1 by the meningitic strain PCN033 [5]; however, via western blotting we showed the activation of all these three signaling molecules in response to PCN033 and RS218 infection. Also, by using specific inhibitors against ERK1/2, p38, and JNK, we observed that inhibition of all three MAPK pathways significantly decreased the infection-induced upregulation of proinflammatory cytokines IL-6, IL-8, IL-Iβ, and TNF-α. Therefore, collectively these data largely support the viewpoint that all three major MAPK signaling pathways play potent roles in meningitic *E. coli* infection and induce neuroinflammatory responses.

Conclusions

In our study, using the iTRAQ proteomics approach, we compared and analyzed the DEPs in hBMECs infected with meningitic or non-meningitic *E. coli* strains. Twelve DEPs were identified as the commonly responding proteins in hBMECs upon infection with meningitic *E. coli* strains PCN033 and RS218, except for only one cellular protein shared by both meningitic and non-meningitic strains. Our data revealed MIF to be an important contributor to meningitic *E. coli*-induced cytokine production and tight junction disruption, while also showing that the NF-κB and MAPK signaling pathways are involved in the infection process. Comparing and profiling these differential cellular proteins in hBMECs in response to meningitic *E. coli* strains should open up further research on host responses against meningitic strains and help with the development of more targets for better prevention and therapeutic control of *E. coli* meningitis.

Additional files

Additional file 1: Table S1. Protein profile of HB101-infected hBMECs. (XLSX 287 kb)

Additional file 2: Table S2. Protein profile of PCN033-infected hBMECs. (XLSX 290 kb)

Additional file 3: Table S3. Protein profile of RS218-infected hBMECs. (XLSX 289 kb)

Additional file 4: Table S4. GO term annotation of DEPs. (DOCX 15 kb)

Additional file 5: Table S5. Ingenuity Canonical Pathways of HB101-infected group. (XLSX 71 kb)

Additional file 6: Table S6. Ingenuity Canonical Pathways of PCN033-infected group. (XLSX 70 kb)

Additional file 7: Table S7. Ingenuity Canonical Pathways of RS218-infected group. (XLSX 71 kb)

Additional file 8: Table S8. The potential networks in HB101-infected group. (XLSX 70 kb)

Additional file 9: Table S9. The potential networks in PCN033-infected group. (XLSX 72 kb)

Additional file 10: Table S10. The potential networks in RS218-infected group. (XLSX 71 kb)

Abbreviations

BBB: Blood-brain barrier; BMECs: Brain microvascular endothelial cells; CNS: Central nervous system; CSF: Cerebrospinal fluid; DEPs: Differentially expressed proteins; DMD: Dystrophin; *E. coli*: *Escherichia coli*; ECIS: Electric cell-substrate impedance sensing; EGFR: Epidermal growth factor receptor; ERK1/2: Extracellular signal-regulated kinases 1 and 2; ExPEC: Extraintestinal pathogenic *Escherichia coli*; GO: Gene Ontology; ICAM-1: Intercellular adhesion molecule-1; IL-1β: Interleukin 1 beta; IL-8: Interleukin-8; IPA: Ingenuity Pathways Analysis; ISO-1: (S, R)-3-(4-Hydroxyphenyl)-4, 5-dihydro-5-isoxazole acetic acid methyl ester DAPI4'-6-Diamidino-2-phenylindole; iTRAQ: Isobaric tags for relative and absolute quantification; JNK: c-Jun N-terminal kinase; KEGG: Kyoto encyclopedia of genes and genomes; LC-MS/MS: Liquid chromatography tandem mass spectrometry; LGMN: Legumain; MAPK: Mitogen-activated protein kinase; MIF: Macrophage migration inhibitory factor; NF-κB: Nuclear factor-κB; NOS: Nitric oxide synthase; PI3K: Phosphatidylinositol 3-kinase; S1P: Sphingosine-1-phosphate; SCX: Strong cation exchange chromatography; TBPL1: TATA box-binding protein-like protein 1; TEAB: Tetraethyl-ammonium bromide; TEER: Trans-endothelial electric resistance; TNF-α: Tumor necrosis factor-alpha; VEGFA: Vascular endothelial growth factor A; ZO-1: Zonula occludens-1, IL-6, interleukin-6

Acknowledgements

We would like to thank Prof. Kwang Sik Kim in Johns Hopkins University School of Medicine to kindly provide the hBMECs cells.

Funding

This work was supported by grants from the National Key R&D Program of China (2016YFD0500406), the National Natural Science Foundation of China (NSFC) (Nos. 31772736, 31502062), the Outstanding youth project of Natural Science Foundation in Hubei Province (2018CFA070), and the Fundamental Research Funds for the Central Universities (Program No. 2662018PY032).

Authors' contributions

WTL performed all experiments and analyzed the data. YJL drafted the manuscript. RCY, JYF, LL, HW, and QC participated in project planning, and all western blot experiments. XRW conceived of the project, coordinated and supervised the experiments, and revised the manuscript. XRW, CT, and HCC provide technical and administrative support. All authors read and approved the final manuscript.

Competing interests

The authors declare that they have no competing interests.

Author details

[1]The Cooperative Innovation Center for Sustainable Pig Production, Huazhong Agricultural University, Wuhan 430070, Hubei, China. [2]College of Veterinary Medicine, Henan University of Animal Husbandry and Economy, Zhengzhou 450046, Henan, China. [3]State Key Laboratory of Agricultural Microbiology, College of Veterinary Medicine, Huazhong Agricultural University, Wuhan 430070, Hubei, China.

References

1. Kim KS. Pathogenesis of bacterial meningitis: from bacteraemia to neuronal injury. Nat Rev Neurosci. 2003;4:376–85.
2. Kim KS. Mechanisms of microbial traversal of the blood-brain barrier. Nat Rev Microbiol. 2008;6:625–34.
3. Kim KS. Acute bacterial meningitis in infants and children. Lancet Infect Dis. 2010;10:32–42.
4. Candelario-Jalil E, Yang Y, Rosenberg GA. Diverse roles of matrix metalloproteinases and tissue inhibitors of metalloproteinases in neuroinflammation and cerebral ischemia. Neuroscience. 2009;158:983–94.
5. Yang RC, Liu WT, Miao L, Yang XP, Fu JY, Dou BB, Cai AL, Zong X, Tan C, Chen HC, Wang XR. Induction of VEGFA and Snail-1 by meningitic *Escherichia coli* mediates disruption of the blood-brain barrier. Oncotarget. 2016;7:63839–55.
6. Stins MF, Badger J, Sik Kim K. Bacterial invasion and transcytosis in transfected human brain microvascular endothelial cells. Microb Pathog. 2001;30:19–28.
7. Stins MF, Gilles F, Kim KS. Selective expression of adhesion molecules on human brain microvascular endothelial cells. J Neuroimmunol. 1997; 76:81–90.

8. Das A, Asatryan L, Reddy MA, Wass CA, Stins MF, Joshi S, Bonventre JV, Kim KS. Differential role of cytosolic phospholipase A2 in the invasion of brain microvascular endothelial cells by Escherichia coli and Listeria monocytogenes. J Infect Dis. 2001;184:732–7.

9. Kim KS, Itabashi H, Gemski P, Sadoff J, Warren RL, Cross AS. The K1 capsule is the critical determinant in the development of Escherichia coli meningitis in the rat. J Clin Invest. 1992;90:897–905.

10. Burkhart A, Thomsen LB, Thomsen MS, Lichota J, Fazakas C, Krizbai I, Moos T. Transfection of brain capillary endothelial cells in primary culture with defined blood-brain barrier properties. Fluids Barriers CNS. 2015;12:19.

11. Eigenmann DE, Xue G, Kim KS, Moses AV, Hamburger M, Oufir M. Comparative study of four immortalized human brain capillary endothelial cell lines, hCMEC/D3, hBMEC, TY10, and BB19, and optimization of culture conditions, for an in vitro blood-brain barrier model for drug permeability studies. Fluids Barriers CNS. 2013;10:33.

12. Abbott NJ. Blood-brain barrier structure and function and the challenges for CNS drug delivery. J Inherit Metab Dis. 2013;36:437–49.

13. Tajes M, Ramos-Fernandez E, Weng-Jiang X, Bosch-Morato M, Guivernau B, Eraso-Pichot A, Salvador B, Fernandez-Busquets X, Roquer J, Munoz FJ. The blood-brain barrier: structure, function and therapeutic approaches to cross it. Mol Membr Biol. 2014;31:152–67.

14. Hoffman JA, Badger JL, Zhang Y, Huang SH, Kim KS. Escherichia coli K1 aslA contributes to invasion of brain microvascular endothelial cells in vitro and in vivo. Infect Immun. 2000;68:5062–7.

15. Wang Y, Kim KS. Role of OmpA and IbeB in Escherichia coli K1 invasion of brain microvascular endothelial cells in vitro and in vivo. Pediatr Res. 2002; 51:559–63.

16. Reddy MA, Prasadarao NV, Wass CA, Kim KS. Phosphatidylinositol 3-kinase activation and interaction with focal adhesion kinase in Escherichia coli K1 invasion of human brain microvascular endothelial cells. J Biol Chem. 2000; 275:36769–74.

17. Khan NA, Wang Y, Kim KJ, Chung JW, Wass CA, Kim KS. Cytotoxic necrotizing factor-1 contributes to Escherichia coli K1 invasion of the central nervous system. J Biol Chem. 2002;277:15607–12.

18. Reddy MA, Wass CA, Kim KS, Schlaepfer DD, Prasadarao NV. Involvement of focal adhesion kinase in Escherichia coli invasion of human brain microvascular endothelial cells. Infect Immun. 2000;68:6423–30.

19. Chung JW, Hong SJ, Kim KJ, Goti D, Stins MF, Shin S, Dawson VL, Dawson TM, Kim KS. 37-kDa laminin receptor precursor modulates cytotoxic necrotizing factor 1-mediated RhoA activation and bacterial uptake. J Biol Chem. 2003;278:16857–62.

20. Wang X, Maruvada R, Morris AJ, Liu JO, Wolfgang MJ, Baek DJ, Bittman R, Kim KS. Sphingosine 1-phosphate activation of EGFR as a novel target for meningitic Escherichia coli penetration of the blood-brain barrier. PLoS Pathog. 2016;12:e1005926.

21. Wijetunge DS, Katani R, Kapur V, Kariyawasam S. Complete genome sequence of Escherichia coli strain RS218 (O18:H7:K1), associated with neonatal meningitis. Genome Announc. 2015;3:e00804-15.

22. Tan C, Xu Z, Zheng H, Liu W, Tang X, Shou J, Wu B, Wang S, Zhao GP, Chen H. Genome sequence of a porcine extraintestinal pathogenic Escherichia coli strain. J Bacteriol. 2011;193:5038.

23. Liu C, Zheng H, Yang M, Xu Z, Wang X, Wei L, Tang B, Liu F, Zhang Y, Ding Y, et al. Genome analysis and in vivo virulence of porcine extraintestinal pathogenic Escherichia coli strain PCN033. BMC Genomics. 2015;16:717.

24. Tan C, Tang X, Zhang X, Ding Y, Zhao Z, Wu B, Cai X, Liu Z, He Q, Chen H. Serotypes and virulence genes of extraintestinal pathogenic Escherichia coli isolates from diseased pigs in China. Vet J. 2012;192:483–8.

25. Zhu L, Maruvada R, Sapirstein A, Malik KU, Peters-Golden M, Kim KS. Arachidonic acid metabolism regulates Escherichia coli penetration of the blood-brain barrier. Infect Immun. 2010;78:4302–10.

26. Khan NA, Kim Y, Shin S, Kim KS. FimH-mediated Escherichia coli K1 invasion of human brain microvascular endothelial cells. Cell Microbiol. 2007;9:169–78.

27. Yang R, Huang F, Fu J, Dou B, Xu B, Miao L, Liu W, Yang X, Tan C, Chen H, Wang X. Differential transcription profiles of long non-coding RNAs in primary human brain microvascular endothelial cells in response to meningitic Escherichia coli. Sci Rep. 2016;6:38903.

28. Szulcek R, Bogaard HJ, Amerongen GPV. Electric cell-substrate impedance sensing for the quantification of endothelial proliferation, barrier function, and motility. J Vis Exp. 2014;85. https://doi.org/10.3791/51300.

29. Allmang C, Petfalski E, Podtelejnikov A, Mann M, Tollervey D, Mitchell P. The yeast exosome and human PM-Scl are related complexes of 3' --> 5' exonucleases. Genes Dev. 1999;13:2148–58.

30. O'Byrne K, Paquet N, Box JK, Adams M, Richard D. 17P examination of EXOSC4 as a new prognostic marker and a novel therapeutic avenue in lung adenocarcinoma. J Thorac Oncol. 2016;11:S63.

31. Basu U, Meng FL, Keim C, Grinstein V, Pefanis E, Eccleston J, Zhang T, Myers D, Wasserman CR, Wesemann DR, et al. The RNA exosome targets the AID cytidine deaminase to both strands of transcribed duplex DNA substrates. Cell. 2011;144:353–63.

32. Van Dijk EL, Schilders G, Pruijn GJ. Human cell growth requires a functional cytoplasmic exosome, which is involved in various mRNA decay pathways. RNA. 2007;13:1027–35.

33. Stefanska B, Cheishvili D, Suderman M, Arakelian A, Huang J, Hallett M, Han ZG, Al-Mahtab M, Akbar SM, Khan WA, et al. Genome-wide study of hypomethylated and induced genes in patients with liver cancer unravels novel anticancer targets. Clin Cancer Res. 2014;20:3118–32.

34. Rosado Jde D, Rodriguez-Sosa M. Macrophage migration inhibitory factor (MIF): a key player in protozoan infections. Int J Biol Sci. 2011;7:1239–56.

35. Delaloye J, De Bruin IJ, Darling KE, Reymond MK, Sweep FC, Roger T, Calandra T, Cavassini M. Increased macrophage migration inhibitory factor (MIF) plasma levels in acute HIV-1 infection. Cytokine. 2012;60:338–40.

36. Pang T, Cardosa MJ, Guzman MG. Of cascades and perfect storms: the immunopathogenesis of dengue haemorrhagic fever-dengue shock syndrome (DHF/DSS). Immunol Cell Biol. 2007;85:43–5.

37. Bernhagen J, Krohn R, Lue H, Gregory JL, Zernecke A, Koenen RR, Dewor M, Georgiev I, Schober A, Leng L, et al. MIF is a noncognate ligand of CXC chemokine receptors in inflammatory and atherogenic cell recruitment. Nat Med. 2007;13:587–96.

38. Schwartz V, Lue H, Kraemer S, Korbiel J, Krohn R, Ohl K, Bucala R, Weber C, Bernhagen J. A functional heteromeric MIF receptor formed by CD74 and CXCR4. FEBS Lett. 2009;583:2749–57.

39. Lue H, Kapurniotu A, Fingerle-Rowson G, Roger T, Leng L, Thiele M, Calandra T, Bucala R, Bernhagen J. Rapid and transient activation of the ERK MAPK signalling pathway by macrophage migration inhibitory factor (MIF) and dependence on JAB1/CSN5 and Src kinase activity. Cell Signal. 2006;18:688–703.

40. Lue H, Thiele M, Franz J, Dahl E, Speckgens S, Leng L, Fingerle-Rowson G, Bucala R, Luscher B, Bernhagen J. Macrophage migration inhibitory factor (MIF) promotes cell survival by activation of the Akt pathway and role for CSN5/JAB1 in the control of autocrine MIF activity. Oncogene. 2007;26:5046–59.

41. Garcia-Laorden MI, Blok DC, Kager LM, Hoogendijk AJ, van Mierlo GJ, Lede IO, Rahman W, Afroz R, Ghose A, Visser CE, et al. Increased intra- and extracellular granzyme expression in patients with tuberculosis. Tuberculosis (Edinb). 2015;95:575–80.

42. Guggino G, Orlando V, Cutrera S, La Manna MP, Di Liberto D, Vanini V, Petruccioli E, Dieli F, Goletti D, Caccamo N. Granzyme A as a potential biomarker of Mycobacterium tuberculosis infection and disease. Immunol Lett. 2015;166:87–91.

43. Laux da Costa L, Delcroix M, Dalla Costa ER, Prestes IV, Milano M, Francis SS, Unis G, Silva DR, Riley LW, Rossetti ML. A real-time PCR signature to discriminate between tuberculosis and other pulmonary diseases. Tuberculosis (Edinb). 2015;95:421–5.

44. Dotiwala F, Mulik S, Polidoro RB, Ansara JA, Burleigh BA, Walch M, Gazzinelli RT, Lieberman J. Killer lymphocytes use granulysin, perforin and granzymes to kill intracellular parasites. Nat Med. 2016;22:210–6.

45. Van den Boogaard FE, van Gisbergen KP, Vernooy JH, Medema JP, Roelofs JJ, van Zoelen MA, Endeman H, Biesma DH, Boon L, Van't Veer C, et al. Granzyme A impairs host defense during Streptococcus pneumoniae pneumonia. Am J Physiol Lung Cell Mol Physiol. 2016;311:L507–16.

46. Pardo J, Simon MM, Froelich CJ. Granzyme A is a proinflammatory protease. Blood. 2009;114:3968 author reply 3969-3970.

47. Hildebrand D, Bode KA, Riess D, Cerny D, Waldhuber A, Rommler F, Strack J, Korten S, Orth JH, Miethke T, et al. Granzyme A produces bioactive IL-1beta through a nonapoptotic inflammasome-independent pathway. Cell Rep. 2014;9:910–7.

48. Yoshikawa Y, Hirayasu H, Tsuzuki S, Fushiki T. Granzyme A causes detachment of alveolar epithelial A549 cells accompanied by promotion of interleukin-8 release. Biosci Biotechnol Biochem. 2008;72:2481–4.

49. Rothwarf DM, Karin M. The NF-kappa B activation pathway: a paradigm in information transfer from membrane to nucleus. Sci STKE. 1999;1999:RE1.

New insights into meningitic Escherichia coli infection of brain microvascular endothelial cells...

241

50. Ichiyama T, Isumi H, Yoshitomi T, Nishikawa M, Matsubara T, Furukawa S. NF-kappaB activation in cerebrospinal fluid cells from patients with meningitis. Neurol Res. 2002;24:709–12.

51. Yang XP, Fu JY, Yang RC, Liu WT, Zhang T, Yang B, Miao L, Dou BB, Tan C, Chen HC, Wang XR. EGFR transactivation contributes to neuroinflammation in *Streptococcus suis* meningitis. J Neuroinflammation. 2016;13:274.

52. Khan M, Elango C, Ansari MA, Singh I, Singh AK. Caffeic acid phenethyl ester reduces neurovascular inflammation and protects rat brain following transient focal cerebral ischemia. J Neurochem. 2007;102:365–77.

53. Koedel U, Bayerlein I, Paul R, Sporer B, Pfister HW. Pharmacologic interference with NF-kappaB activation attenuates central nervous system complications in experimental Pneumococcal meningitis. J Infect Dis. 2000;182:1437–45.

54. Selvaraj SK, Periandythevar P, Prasadarao NV. Outer membrane protein A of *Escherichia coli* K1 selectively enhances the expression of intercellular adhesion molecule-1 in brain microvascular endothelial cells. Microbes Infect. 2007;9:547–57.

55. Chi F, Bo T, Wu CH, Jong A, Huang SH. Vimentin and PSF act in concert to regulate IbeA+ *E. coli* K1 induced activation and nuclear translocation of NF-kappaB in human brain endothelial cells. PLoS One. 2012;7:e35862.

56. Ramsauer K, Sadzak I, Porras A, Pilz A, Nebreda AR, Decker T, Kovarik P. p38 MAPK enhances STAT1-dependent transcription independently of Ser-727 phosphorylation. Proc Natl Acad Sci U S A. 2002;99:12859–64.

Permissions

List of Contributors

Zhongyuan Tan, Jianhong Sun, Xianliang Ke, Caishang Zheng, Yuan Zhang, Penghui Li, Yan Liu, Hanzhong Wang and Zhenhua Zheng
CAS Key Laboratory of Special Pathogens and Biosafety, Center for Emerging Infectious Diseases, Wuhan Institute of Virology, Chinese Academy of Sciences, Wuhan 430071, China

Zhongyuan Tan and Penghui Li
University of Chinese Academy of Sciences, Beijing 100049, China

Wanpo Zhang and Wanpo Zhang
College of Veterinary Medicine, Huazhong Agricultural University, Wuhan 430070, China

Qinxue Hu
State Key Laboratory of Virology, Wuhan Institute of Virology, Chinese Academy of Sciences, Wuhan 430071, China

Sai Sampath Thammisetty, Jasna Kriz, Sai Sampath Thammisetty and Yuan Cheng Weng
CERVO Brain Research Centre, Université Laval, 2601 Chemin de la Canardière, Québec, QC G1J 2G3, Canada

Jordi Pedragosa and Anna Planas
IDIBAPS, Barcelona, Spain

Frédéric Calon
Research Centre of the CHUQ, Université Laval, Québec, QC G1J2G3, Canada

Sai Sampath Thammisetty and Frédéric Calon
Faculty of Pharmacy, Université Laval, Québec, QC G1J2G3, Canada

Jasna Kriz
Department of Psychiatry and Neuroscience, Faculty of Medicine, Université Laval, 2601 Chemin de la Canardière, Québec, QC G1J2G3, Canada

Stephanie M. Davis, Lisa A. Collier and Keith R. Pennypacker
Department of Neurology, University of Kentucky, 741 S. Limestone BBSRB B457, Lexington, KY 40536-0905, USA

Edric D. Winford
Department of Neuroscience, University of Kentucky, 800 Rose St. Lexington, Lexington, KY 40536, USA

Timothy J. Kopper and John C. Gensel
Department of Physiology, University of Kentucky, 800 Rose St. MS508, Lexington, KY 40536, USA
Spinal Cord and Brain Injury Repair Center, University of Kentucky, 741 S. Limestone BBSRB B463, Lexington, KY 40536, USA

Christopher C. Leonardo and Craig T. Ajmo Jr
Department of Molecular Pharmacology and Physiology, University of South Florida, 12901 Bruce B. Downs Blvd MDC 8, Tampa, FL 33612, USA

Elspeth A. Foran
Department of Molecular Medicine, University of South Florida, 12901 Bruce B. Downs Blvd MDC 7, Tampa, FL 33612, USA

Chin Wai Hui, Xuan Song, Fulin Ma, Xuting Shen and Karl Herrup
Division of Life Science and State Key Laboratory of Molecular Neurobiology, Hong Kong University of Science and Technology, Clear Water Bay, Kowloon, Hong Kong

Xuting Shen
School of Biomedical Sciences, The University of Hong Kong, Pokfulam, Hong Kong

Xiangrong Chen, Zhigang Pan, Zhongning Fang, Weibin Lin, Shukai Wu, Fuxing Yang, Yasong Li and Hongzhi Gao
Department of Neurosurgery, The Second Affiliated Hospital, Fujian Medical University, Quanzhou 362000, Fujian Province, China

Huangde Fu
Department of Neurosurgery, Affiliated Hospital of YouJiang Medical University for Nationalities, Baise 533000, Guangxi Province, China

Shun Li
Department of Neurosurgery, Affiliated Hospital of North Sichuan Medical College, Sichuan Province, Nanchong 637000, China

Taraneh Ebrahimi, Marcus Rust, Sarah Nele Kaiser, Jörg B. Schulz, Pardes Habib and Jan Philipp Bach
Department of Neurology, RWTH Aachen University, Aachen, Germany

Alexander Slowik and Cordian Beyer
Institute of Neuroanatomy, RWTH Aachen University, Aachen, Germany

Andreas Rembert Koczulla
Department of Internal Medicine, Pulmonary and Critical Care Medicine, University Medical Center Giessen and Marburg, Marburg, Germany

Jörg B. Schulz
JARA-Institute Molecular Neuroscience and Neuroimaging, Forschungszentrum Jülich GmbH and RWTH Aachen University, Aachen, Germany

Zhihua Yu, Lina Hou and Hongzhuan Chen
Department of Pharmacology and Chemical Biology, Shanghai Jiao Tong University School of Medicine, 280 South Chongqing Road, Shanghai 200025, China

Hongzhuan Chen
Shanghai University of Traditional Chinese Medicine, Shanghai 201203, China

Fangfang Dou
Basic Research Department, Shanghai Geriatric Institute of Chinese Medicine, Shanghai 200031, China

Yanxia Wang
Experimental Teaching Center of Basic Medicine, Shanghai Jiao Tong University School of Medicine, Shanghai 200025, China

Feng Zhou
Jiangsu Key Laboratory of Brain Disease Bioinformation, Research Center for Biochemistry and Molecular Biology, Xuzhou Medical University, Xuzhou 221004, Jiangsu, People's Republic of China.

Feng Zhou, Xiaomei Liu, Dongjiao Zuo, Lin Gao, Ying Yang, Jing Wang, Liping Niu, Qianwen Cao, Xiangyang Li, Hui Hua, Bo Zhang, Minmin Hu, Kuiyang Zheng and Renxian Tang
Jiangsu Key Laboratory of Immunity and Metabolism, Department of Pathogen Biology and Immunology and Laboratory of Infection and Immunity, Xuzhou Medical University, Xuzhou 221004, Jiangsu, People's Republic of China

Min Xue
Department of Physiology, Xuzhou Medical University, Xuzhou 221004, Jiangsu, People's Republic of China

Dianshuai Gao
Department of Neurobiology and Anatomy, Xuzhou Medical University, Xuzhou 221004, Jiangsu, People's Republic of China

Yoshihiro Izumiya
Department of Dermatology, University of California Davis (UC Davis) School of Medicine, Sacramento, CA, USA

Brian E. Dawes and Kendra Johnson
Department of Microbiology and Immunology, University of Texas Medical Branch, Galveston, USA

Junling Gao and Ping Wu
Department of Neuroscience, Cell Biology and Anatomy, University of Texas Medical Branch, Galveston, USA

Colm Atkins, Jacob T. Nelson and Alexander N. Freiberg
Department of Pathology, University of Texas Medical Branch, 301 University Boulevard, Galveston 77555-0609, USA

Alexander N. Freiberg
Center for Biodefense and Emerging Infectious Diseases, University of Texas Medical Branch, Galveston, USA
Sealy Institute for Vaccine Sciences, University of Texas Medical Branch, Galveston, USA

Brooke J. Wanrooy, Kathryn Prame Kumar, Shu Wen Wen and Connie H. Y. Wong
Centre for Inflammatory Diseases, Department of Medicine, School of Clinical Sciences at Monash Health, Monash Medical Centre, Monash University, Clayton, VIC 3168, Australia

Cheng Xue Qin and Rebecca H. Ritchie
Baker Heart and Diabetes Institute, Melbourne, Australia

Rebecca H. Ritchie
Department of Diabetes, Monash University, Melbourne, Australia

Pi-Ling Chiang, Hsiu-Ling Chen, Yueh-Sheng Chen, Meng-Hsiang Chen and Wei-Che Lin
Department of Diagnostic Radiology, Kaohsiung Chang Gung Memorial Hospital, Chang Gung University College of Medicine, 123 Ta-Pei Road, Niao-Sung, Kaohsiung 83305, Taiwan

Cheng-Hsien Lu and Nai-Wen Tsai
Department of Neurology, Kaohsiung Chang Gung Memorial Hospital, Chang Gung University College of Medicine, Kaohsiung, Taiwan

Kun-Hsien Chou
Brain Research Center, National Yang-Ming University, Taipei, Taiwan

Tun-Wei Hsu
Department of Radiology, Taipei Veterans General Hospital, Taipei, Taiwan

Shau-Hsuan Li
Department of Hematology and Oncology, Kaohsiung Chang Gung Memorial Hospital, Chang Gung University College of Medicine, Kaohsiung, Taiwan

Ting Zhang, Nan Zhang, Run Zhang, Weidong Zhao, Zilong Wang, Biao Xu, Mengna Zhang, Xuerui Shi, Qinqin Zhang, Yuanyuan Guo, Jian Xiao, Dan Chen and Quan Fang
Key Laboratory of Preclinical Study for New Drugs of Gansu Province, and Institute of Physiology, School of Basic Medical Sciences, Lanzhou University, 199 Donggang West Road, Lanzhou 730000, People's Republic of China

Yong Chen
Department of Neurology, School of Medicine, Duke University, Durham, North Carolina 27710, USA

Shinnosuke Yamada, Norimichi Itoh, Taku Nagai, Tsuyoshi Nakai and Kiyofumi Yamada
Department of Neuropsychopharmacology and Hospital Pharmacy, Nagoya University Graduate School of Medicine, 65 Turumai-cho, Showa-ku, Nagoya, Aichi 466-8560, Japan

Daisuke Ibi
Department of Chemical Pharmacology, Faculty of Pharmaceutical Science, Meijo University, 150 Yagotoyama, Tenpaku-ku, Nagoya, Japan

Akira Nakajima
Faculty of Agriculture and Life Science, Hirosaki University, 3 Bunkyo-cho, Hirosaki, Aomori 036-8561, Japan

Toshitaka Nabeshima
Advanced Diagnostic System Research Laboratory, Fujita Health University, Graduate School of Health Science and Aino University, 1-98 Dengakugakubo, Kutsukake-cho, Toyoake, Aichi 470-1192, Japan

Bhakta Prasad Gaire and Ji Woong Choi
College of Pharmacy and Gachon Institute of Pharmaceutical Sciences, Gachon University, Incheon 406-799, Republic of Korea

Mi-Ryoung Song
School of Life Sciences, Gwangju Institute of Science and Technology, Buk-gu, Gwangju 500-712, Republic of Korea

Mohammad Harun-Or-Rashid and Denise M. Inman
Department of Pharmaceutical Sciences, Northeast Ohio Medical University, 4209 State Route 44, Rootstown, OH 44272, USA

Wen-Tong Liu, Yu-Jin Lv, Rui-Cheng Yang, Ji-Yang Fu, Lu Liu, Huan Wang, Qi Cao, Chen Tan, Huan-Chun Chen and Xiang-Ru Wang
The Cooperative Innovation Center for Sustainable Pig Production, Huazhong Agricultural University, Wuhan 430070, Hubei, China

Yu-Jin Lv
College of Veterinary Medicine, Henan University of Animal Husbandry and Economy, Zhengzhou 450046, Henan, China

Chen Tan, Huan-Chun Chen and Xiang-Ru Wang
State Key Laboratory of Agricultural Microbiology, College of Veterinary Medicine, Huazhong Agricultural University, Wuhan 430070, Hubei, China

Index

www.ingramcontent.com/pod-product-compliance
Lightning Source LLC
Chambersburg PA
CBHW080508200326
41458CB00012B/4132

www.ingramcontent.com/pod-product-compliance
Lightning Source LLC
Chambersburg PA
CBHW080508200326
41458CB00012B/4132